CYTOLOGY

(CELL BIOLOGY AND MOLECULAR BIOLOGY)

CYTOLOGY

CELL BIOLOGY AND MOLECULAR BIOLOGY

For B.Sc., B.Sc. (Honours) and M.Sc. Students of all Indian Universities

Dr. P.S. VERMA
M.Sc. Ph.D., F.E.S.I., F.A.Z.
Reader (Retd.)

Dr. V.K. AGARWAL
M.Sc. (Ph.D.)
Reader and Head (Retd.)

Department of Zoology
Meerut College
Meerut

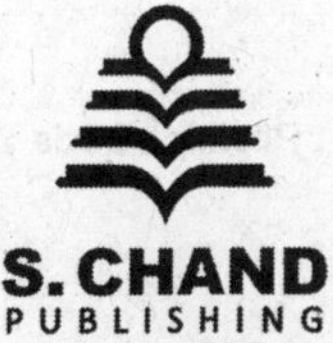

S Chand And Company Limited
(ISO 9001 Certified Company)

S Chand And Company Limited

(ISO 9001 Certified Company)

Head Office: Block B-1, House No. D-1, Ground Floor, Mohan Co-operative Industrial Estate, New Delhi – 110 044 | Phone: 011-66672000

Registered Office: A-27, 2nd Floor, Mohan Co-operative Industrial Estate, New Delhi – 110 044
Phone: 011-49731800

www.**schandpublishing.com**; e-mail: **info@schandpublishing.com**

Branches

Chennai	:	Ph: 23632120; chennai@schandpublishing.com
Guwahati	:	Ph: 2738811, 2735640; guwahati@schandpublishing.com
Hyderabad	:	Ph: 40186018; hyderabad@schandpublishing.com
Jalandhar	:	Ph: 4645630; jalandhar@schandpublishing.com
Kolkata	:	Ph: 23357458, 23353914; kolkata@schandpublishing.com
Lucknow	:	Ph: 4003633; lucknow@schandpublishing.com
Mumbai	:	Ph: 25000297; mumbai@schandpublishing.com
Patna	:	Ph: 2260011; patna@schandpublishing.com

First Edition 1978
Subsequent Editions and Reprints 1979, 80, 81, 83, 85, 86, 88, 91, 94, 95, 97, 98, 99, 2000, 2001, 2003, 2004, 2005, 2006, 2007, 2008, 2009, 2011, 2012
Revised and Enlarged Edition 2014; Reprints 2015, 2016, 2018, 2019, 2020, 2021

Reprint 2022 (Twice)

ISBN : 978-81-219-0814-6 **Product Code :** H6CYT68BIOL10ENZX14O

PRINTED IN INDIA

By Vikas Publishing House Private Limited, Plot 20/4, Site-IV, Industrial Area Sahibabad, Ghaziabad – 201 010 and Published by S Chand And Company Limited, A-27, 2nd Floor, Mohan Co-operative Industrial Estate, New Delhi – 110 044.

Affectionately Dedicated

to

My Departed Son

Sameer (Neetu)

Who left the family

in a mental Turmoil

Prem Singh

PREFACE TO THE REVISED EDITION

The release of this thoroughly revised and enlarged new edition of '**Cytology**' has provided twofold opportunities to the authors: firstly, to thank the readers for the overwhelming reception they accorded to the earlier editions of this book and secondly, to give a facelift to the old account. In fact cytology is one of the most exciting fields of biological science. The knowledge about the cell is increasing very year due to vast expansion of our understanding of the structure and function of various cellular organelles and macromolecules at biochemical and molecular biological levels. To cope with the current cytological understanding, the first three chapters of this edition have been thoroughly revised and revision questions have been added in each chapter. For explaining more adequately some of the recently understood cytological phenomena, several new diagrams have been added afresh.

In this revised edition, in the first three chapters, the subject matter has been altered as per new cytological advances and latest cytochemical techniques in this century. In chapter one, the feature of Nobel Prize Recipients has been updated. In chapter two, examples of optical microscopes have been covered in full detail. In chapter three, principles and types of chromatography have been expanded and covered adequately with diagrams. In chapter nine, the title has been altered to "Golgi Apparatus (Complex)" as per latest specification. New Glossary (with latest cytological terms) has been freshly incorporated.

Despite exhaustive efforts for the improvement of the book by the authors, they take refuge in a remark by **Max Delbruck** "*Any living cell carries with it the experiences of a billion years of experimentation by its ancestor. You cannot expect to explain so wise an old bird in a few simple words*".

The authors express their thanks to the generous readers and their friends for rendering the valuable suggestions for the improvement of the book. Suggestions for further improvement of the book will be thankfully acknowledged and incorporated in the future editions.

AUTHORS

PREFACE TO THE FIRST EDITION

It is trite but true that cell occupies the same central position in biology as the atom in the physical science. The cell is a vital unit of organisms and it can be considered as the anatomic and physiologic substrate of biologic phenomena. The biological studies of cell have provided enough convincing clues to most biological phenomena, such as growth, aging, metabolism, heredity, pathological disease and ecological interactions.

The cytology is comparatively a young biological science and it has made great advance during the past decade. In 1900, the rediscovery of Mendel's laws have aroused particular interest of biologists in the nucleus, more especially in the chromosomes which were thought as the carrier of hereditary factors. The rapid expansion of chromosomes studies led to a great development in cytology but primary workers remain especially concerned with the nucleus. After second world war, biologists made effective use of new techniques including electron microscopy, isotopic labelling, microsurgery, ultracentrifugation and great variety of other physical and chemical techniques in studying the cell and found cytoplasm equally fascinating for cytological studies. The rate of progress of cytology became steadily accelerated only after the recognition of central role of molecules in almost all cellular events. The discovery of molecular organization of both cytoplasmic and nuclear components and molecular interactions between different cellular organelles have opened new vistas in cytology. At present state of knowledge, most biological phenomena are explainable in terms of molecules.

Though there exist many test books of cytology or cell biology written by well reputed authors, but most of them have either too short or too detailed account that may become almost impossible for an Indian student to understand and appreciate the knowledge of them. By visualizing such difficulties of students, the present authors have attempted to provide a lucid, simple, detailed and well-illustrated account of cytology and molecular biology in this book. At every step, authors remained conscious about the genuine needs of students but even then the authors cannot claim about the perfectness of their attempt. Constructive suggestions from the readers will always he welcomed and entertained whole heartedly.

The authors express their thanks to their friends, colleagues and also students whose continuous inspiration have initiated them to bring out the book. The authors are also grateful to Shri Shyam Lal Gupta and Shri T.N. Goel, M.s S.Chand & Co., Ltd., New Delhi, for their whole hearted cooperation in the publication of this book.

Department of Zoology, *Dr. P.S. Verma*
Meerut College, Meerut *Dr. V.K. Agarwal*

CONTENTS

1 Chapter

INTRODUCTION

The **cytology** or **cell biology** is a biological science which deals with the study of cells from morphological, biochemical, physiological, developmental, genetical, pathological and evolutionary point of views. Recently, it has shown rapid progress and has become fundamental in the study of structure and function of living organism. The cell itself can be regarded as the vital unit of organisms and the anatomic and physiologic substrate of biologic phenomena. In its morphological aspect, modern cell biology has gone beyond simple description of structures visible to the light microscope ; by the application of new methods, an analysis has been started of sub-microscopic organization—the architectural arrangement of the molecules and micelles comprising living matter. In this functional aspect, it has transcended the stage of pure description of physiologic changes and seeks an explanation of them in the intimate physico-chemical and metabolic processes of protoplasm. Finally, we can say that the modern cytology or cell biology is attempting to interpret and explain the phenomena of metabolism, biosynthesis, heredity, sex, variation, mutation and evolution of living organisms in terms of molecules or macromolecules such as proteins, ribonucleic acids (RNAs) and deoxyribonucleic acid (DNA).

1.1 ADVENT OF CELL BIOLOGY: THREE HISTORICAL STRANDS

Modern cell biology involves the weaving togather of three distinctly different strands into a single cord (**Becker** *et al.*, 2006). Each of the strands had its own historical origins and most of the intertwining had occurred only within the last 75 years. Each strand should be appreciated in its own right, because each makes its own unique and significant contribution.

1. The first of these historical strands is **cytology** which is concerned primarily with cellular structure. The Greek prefix *cyto*—means "cell" as does the suffix—*cyte* + *logous* = to discourse. (Actually, the literal meaning of the Greek word *cytos* is "hollow vessel" which fits well with Hooke's initial impression of cells). As we will describe later on, cytology has its origin more than three centuries ago and depended heavily on the **light microscope** for its initial impetus. The advent of **electron microscopy** and several related optical techniques has led to considerable additional cytological activity and understanding.

2. The second strand represents the contributions of **biochemistry** to our understanding of cellular function. Most of the developments in this field have occurred within the last 80 years, though again the roots go back much further. Especially important has been the development of techniques such as **ultracentrifugation**, **chromatography** and **electrophoresis** for the separation of cellular components and molecules. The use of **radio-actively labeled compounds** in the study of enzyme-

catalyzed reactions and metabolic pathways is another very significant contribution of biochemistry to our understanding of how cells function.

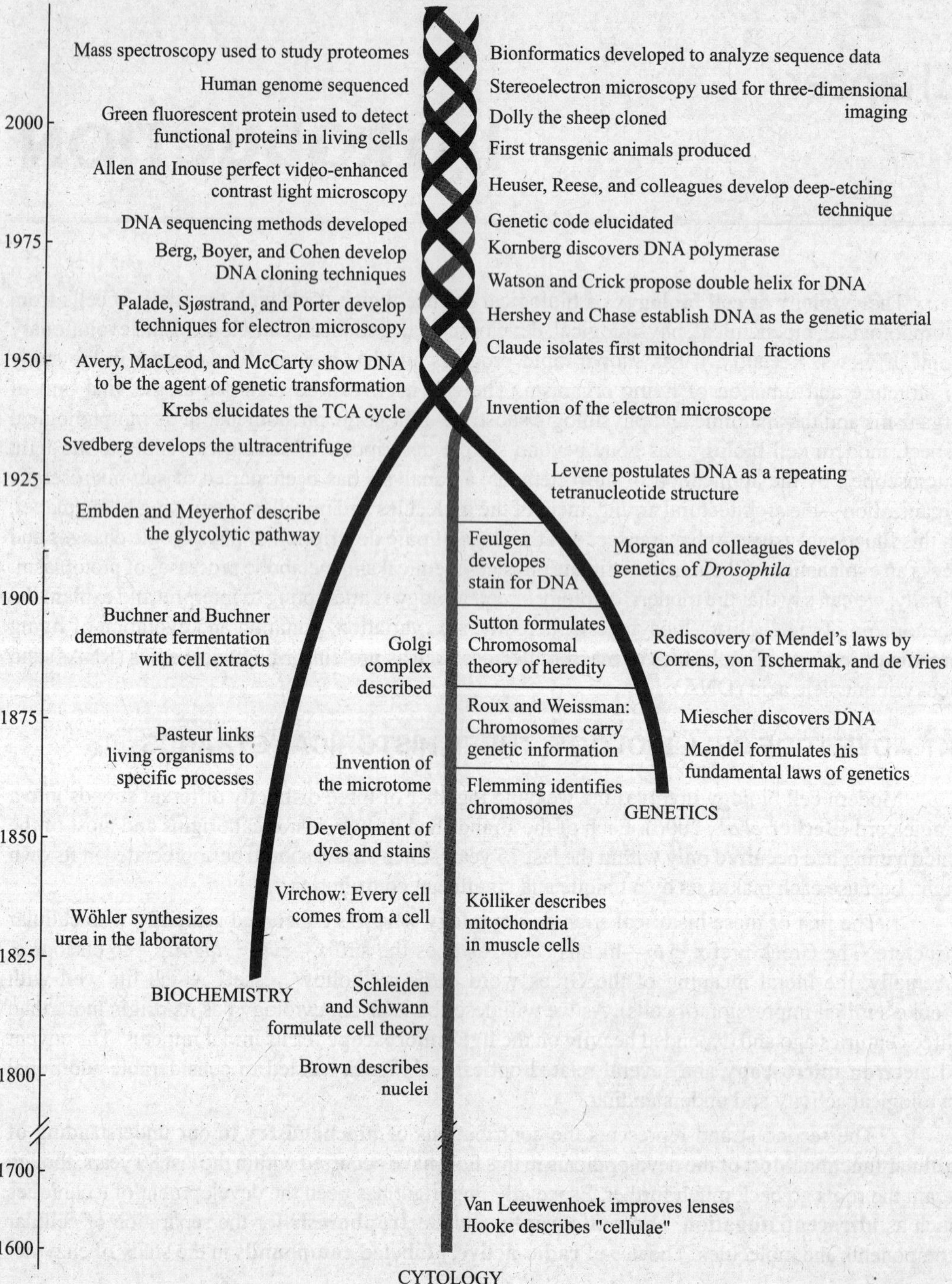

Fig. 1.1. A single cord of cell biology involves weaving together of three strands: Cytology, Biochemistry and Genetics during last 300 or more years.

3. The third strand is **genetics**. Here, the historical continuum stretches back more than 155 years to **Gregor Mendel**. Again, however, much of our present understanding has come within the last 80 years. An especially important landmark on the genetic strand came with the demonstration that DNA (deoxyribonucleic acid) is the bearer of genetic information in most life forms, specifying the order of subunits (= amino acids) and hence the properties, of the proteins that are responsible for most of the functional and structural features of the cells. Recent accomplishments on the genetic strand include the **sequencing** of the entire genomes (all of the DNA) of humans and other species and the **cloning** (production of genetically identical organisms) of mammals, including sheep, goat, cattle, camels and cats.

To understand present-day cell biology therefore means to appreciate its diverse roots and the important contributions that each of its component strands has made to our current understanding of what a cell is and what it can do.

1.2 HISTORICAL REVIEW

The cytology has taken its individual entity by the end of the nineteenth century. Its gradual development in the last centuries can be traced as follows:

Cytology before 19th Century

Ancient philosophers and naturalists, particularly **Aristotle** and **Paracelsus** concluded that "all animals and plants, however, complicated are constituted by few elements which are repeated in each one of them". They were referring to the macroscopic structures of an organism, such as roots, leaves and flowers common to different plants or segments and organs that are repeated in the animal kingdom. Many centuries later, owing to the invention of magnifying lenses, the world of microscopic dimensions was discovered.

The beginning of cytology can be visualized in the 15th century, when **da Vinci** in 1485 has stressed upon the use of lenses in viewing small objects. In the year 1658, **Jan Swammerdam** gave the first description of the cell in his account of the red blood cells of the frog. The cytology came in its actual existence with the discovery of cell in 1665, by an English botanist, **Robert Hooke** (1635–1703). While examining a thin slice of cork under his crude compound microscope, **Hooke** observed its honey-combed or porous structure. He found similar alveoli in other plant tissues and gave them the name "cells" (L., *cellula*—little room). What Hooke had seen of the cell was mainly its walls of thickened cellulose, and he ignored the existence of the substance occurring within the cell wall and thus, failed to grasp its true nature and significance.

In the year 1672, an Italian anatomist, **Marcello Malpighi** (1688–1694) and an English physician **Nehmian Grew**, without using the word cell mentioned that certain parts of plants were made up of minute elementary organisms—"utricles", "sacs", and "vesicles". **Malpighi** also studied a variety of animal tissues microscopically and therefore, he is generally considered as **the father of 'microscopic anatomy'**. During the 17th century, a Dutch microscopist, **A.V. Leeuwenhoek** (1632–1723) discovered the animalcules, infusoria (Protozoa), bacteria, etc., and made microscopical observations on Protozoa, ants, aphids, spermatozoa, red blood cells, muscles, nerves, skin, teeth and certain plants. Leeuwenhoek discovered the free living cells in pond water for the first time (1674) and in 1678 identified the sperm cells of humans, dogs, rabbits, frogs, fish and insects.

During the 18th century, little knowledge was added to cytology. However, some workers produced the accounts of plant cells and referred them by different names such as 'fibres' by **Haller** (1757) and **Bonnet**; 'cylinders' by **Fontana** (1781); 'otricles' by **Brisseau-Mirabel** and 'elementary vesicles' by **Oken**. In 1781, **F. Fontana** also described the nucleolus from the skin of an eel.

Cytology in 19th Century

The 19th century can be considered as the "classical era of cytology" because most important cytological investigations were made extensively in this century. By the beginning of the 19th century it was known that all the organs of animals were made up of tissues such as muscle, bone, cartilage and fat; and similarly that the stems, roots, leaves, and other organs of higher plants were also composed of distinct tissues. The cytological contributions of 19th century can be represented chronologically in the following Table 1.1:

Table 1.1. Chronological representation of certain significant cytological investigations of 19th century.

Year	Name of contributor	Cytological contribution
1808	**Mirabel**	Reported that plants consist of membranous cellular tissues.
1809	**J.B. Lamarck**	Stated that in the living organisms the cell has certain important functions.
1824	**R.J H. Dutrochet**	Showed that all animals and plants composed of cells and these cells remain united by simple adhesive forces.
1824	**[illegible] Prevost and J.B.A. Dumas**	Described cell division first of all by studying cleavage of the frog's egg.
1825	**F.V. Raspail**	Used iodine in the starch detection and developed the frozen-section technique; founder of cytochemistry.
1826	**Turpin**	Reported the occurrence of cell division.
1827	**Karl von Baer**	Discovered the mammalian ovum.
1828	**Wohler**	Synthesized urea and discredited the view that organic compounds could only be made by living things and thus paved the way for a systematic investigation of cellular reactions.
1828	**R. Brown**	Reported Brownian movement in cellular particles.
1830	**G.B. Amici**	Discovered fertilization in plants.
1830	**Meyen**	Suggested that each plant cell is an independent, isolated unit capable of receiving nourishment and building its own internal structures.
1831	**R. Brown**	Described the nucleus as a central feature in plant cells.
1835	**Felix Dujardin**	Described protoplasm ("sarcode") in Protozoa and considered it to be living matter.
1835	**H. von Mohl**	Described the cell division.
1838	**M.J. Schleiden**	Described the nucleoli and proposed "cell theory" along with T. Schwann.
1839	**T. Schwann**	Applied "cell theory" to animals.
1840	**J. E. Purkinje**	Named the cell contents as protoplasm.
1841	**Robert Remak**	Described amitotic cell division in the R.B.C. of the chick embryo.
1845	**A. Donne**	Studied spermatozoa and used photomicroscopy first time.
1845	**Kolliker**	Reported that the ova and spermatozoa are single cell products.
1846	**H. von Mohl**	Used the term protoplasm for the cytoplasm of modern time.
1846	**K. Nageli**	Reported that new plant cells arise from the pre-existing cells.
1849	**W. Hofmeister**	Studied nuclear divisions in stamens and fertilization. He drew figures of chromosomes of the nuclei of pollen mother cells of *Tradescantia.*
1855	**R. Virchow**	Stated that all cells arise from pre-existing cells.
1855	**Pringsheim**	Described the complete fertilization process in the alga.

Year	Name of contributor	Cytological contribution
1857	**Kolliker**	Discovered mitochondria in muscle.
1858	**R. Virchow**	Correctly asserted that as the functional units of life, cells are the primary site of disease.
1861	**Schultze**	Said that the cell is a living substance which possesses a nucleus and cell membranes. He used the term protoplasm for the living substances of cell and stated protoplasm as "physical basis of life".
1863	**Waldeyer**	Reported the utility of haematoxylin in staining the chromosomes of cell.
1865	**G. Mendel**	Discovered fundamental principles of genetics.
1866	**Haeckel**	Named plastids.
1867	**L. St. George**	Discovered what was later called the "Golgi-complex".
1870	**W. His**	Developed the microtome for cutting serial sections of tissue for cell study.
1871	**F. Miescher**	Discovered nucleoproteins and nucleic acid (Nuclein).
1873	**H. Fol**	Described the spindle and astral rays.
1875	**Strasburger**	Described chromosomes.
1876	**L. Pasteur**	Discovered anaerobic release of energy from cells (fermentation) in yeasts and moulds.
1876	**O. Hertwig**	Studied reproduction in sea urchin and concluded that fertilization involves the union of sperms and egg nuclei.
1877	**E. Abbe**	Discovered the oil-immersion objective.
1879	**H. Fol**	Observed the penetration of single sperm in the egg during fertilization.
1879	**W. Flemming**	Introduced the term chromatin and described splitting of chromosomes.
1881	**E.G. Balbiani**	Discovered the giant chromosomes of salivary glands of the larva of *Chironomus*.
1882	**W. Flemming**	Introduced the term mitosis, improved the techniques of fixation and staining and suggested relations of nucleic acid with the chromatin.
1882	**Strasburger**	Described mitosis in plant cells and introduced the terms cytoplasm and nucleoplasm.
1882	**W. Pfitzner**	Discovered chromomeres, the 'granules' on the chromosomes.
1883	**W. Roux**	Proposed that chromosomes contain hereditary units.
1883	**E. van Beneden**	Showed in *Ascaris* that gametes contain half of chromosomes than the body cells.
1883	**Schimper**	Introduced the term chloroplast.
1883	**Meyer**	Described details of chloroplast structure.
1883	**Metschnikoff**	Observed and named phagocytosis in cells.
1886	**R. Altmann**	Stained mitochondria and other granular components of cell and suggested their role in respiratory metabolism of the cell.
1886	**C. A. MacMunn**	Discovered cytochromes (originally "histohematins").
1887	**E. van Beneden**	Discovered centrioles.
1888	**T. Boveri**	Described the centrioles.
1888	**Waldeyer**	Introduced the term chromosome.
1888	**Kolliker**	Isolated mitochondria.

Year	Name of contributor	Cytological contribution
1890	**Boveri and Guignard**	Proved the re-establishment of a diploid chromosome number at fertilization, by joining of equal sets from the male and female gametes.
1892	**A. Weismann**	Proposed the germplasm theory and showed the chromosomes as the most important components of the nucleus.
1892	**T. Boveri**	Described spermatogenesis and oogenesis in *Ascaris*.
1897	**Granier**	Named and described the ergastoplasm.
1898	**C. Benda**	Named the mitochondrion.
1898	**C. Golgi**	Described the Golgi complex in nerve cells.

Cytology After 19th Century

In the 20th century various modern microtechniques have been employed in cytological (cell biological) investigations. For instance, new histochemical and cytochemical methods have been developed to detect various molecular components of the cell; various cellular components have been separated by ultracentrifugation; different biochemical events of the cell could be known in detail by autoradiography; and methods of tissue culturing have made possible the study of living cells. Moreover, micromanipulators, ultra-microtomes, chromatography, electrophoresis, electron microscopy, X-ray microscopy, phase contrast microscopy, spectrophotometry, X-ray structural analysis, etc., have provided new opportunities to cell biologists to investigate minute details of cell and its components.

Various important cytological investigations have been made in 20th century and many cytologists have received Nobel Prizes for their landmark cytological investigations. The cytological investigations of 20th century can be represented chronologically in the Table 1.2.

Table 1.2. Chronological tabulation of certain important cytological investigations of 20th century.

Year	Name of contributor	Cytological contribution
1900	**J. Loeb**	Discovered artificial parthenogenesis of eggs by chemical and mechanical methods.
1901	**T. H. Montgomery**	Showed that homologous chromosomes undergo pairing (synapsis) during reduction division.
1901	**Strasburger**	Introduced the term plasmodesmata.
1902	**C. E. McClung**	Identified the sex chromosomes in the Hemiptera.
1902	**W. S. Sutton**	Recognized the significance of reduction division and proposed the "chromosome theory" of heredity. He pointed out the parallels between genes and chromosome behaviour and suggested a chromosomal location for genes.
1903	**E. Buchner**	Discovered the enzyme and got Nobel Prize.
1904	**F. Meves**	Demonstrated the presence of mitochondria in plant cells.
1905	**J. B. Farmer**	Coined the term meiosis along with J. E. Moore.
1906	**M. Tswett**	Discovered chromatography.
1907	**R. G. Harrison**	Developed the technique for growing tissues in culture.
1909	**F. A. Janssens**	Stated chiasmata formed by the exchanges between two chromatids of non-homologous chromosomes.
1910	**A. Kossel**	Investigated the chemistry of the nucleus and got Nobel Prize.

Year	Name of contributor	Cytological contribution
1911	**T. H. Morgan**	Advanced his gene theory by proposing that genes are linearly arranged along chromosomes in a definite order.
1912	**Warburg**	Demonstrated that iron is essential to respiration.
1913	**Wilstatter and Stoll**	Isolated chlorophyll and later determined its structure.
1915	**R. M. Wilstatter**	Got Nobel Prize for the research on chlorophyll.
1923	**F. Pregl**	Got Nobel Prize for microanalysis of organic substances.
1923	**G. Hevesy**	Discovered the technique of isotopic tracing in which the fate of labelled isotope molecules can be traced through a metabolic pathway.
1923	**O. Warburg**	Discovered a method of measuring gaseous exchange in living tissue by manometry.
1924	**R. Feulgen and H. Rossenbeck**	Described a test for DNA.
1926	**T. Svedberg**	Got Nobel Prize for the discovery of ultracentrifuge.
1928	**F. Griffith**	Discovered genetic transduction in bacteria.
1929	**K. Lohmann**	Discovered ATP, the source of energy in biochemical reactions.
1931	**C. Stern, H. Creighton and B. McClintock**	Demonstrated cytologically the process of crossing over.
1931	**O. H. Warburg**	Got Nobel Prize for the discovery of respiratory enzymes and their actions.
1931	**Engelhardt**	Demonstrated that phosphorylation is coupled to oxygen consumption.
1931	**W. H. Lewis**	Discovered pinocytosis.
1932	**M. Knoll and E. Ruska**	Produced first electron microscope.
1933	**T. H. Morgan**	Received Nobel Prize for the discovery of function of chromosomes in transmission of heredity.
1933	**Keilin**	Partially reconstituted an electron transport chain.
1935	**W. M. Stanley**	Isolated tobacco mosaic virus in crystalline form.
1937	**Hans A.Krebs**	Formulated the critic acid cycle.
1937	**W. N. Haworth and P. Karrer**	Received Nobel Prize for the discovery of molecular structures of carbohydrates, vitamin C, and carotenoids, flavins, Vitamins A and B, respectively.
1938	**T. Caspersson**	Developed ultraviolet photomicrography for the study of nucleic acids.
1939–1941	**F. Lipmann**	Proposed a central metabolic role for ATP.
1943	**A. Claude**	Isolated cell components such as ribosomes, mitochondria and nuclei in relatively pure form by differential ultracentrifugation.
1944	**O. T. Avery, C. H. Mcleod and H. McCarty**	Showed the significance of DNA in hereditary transmission in bacteria.
1945	**K. R. Porter**	Discovered the endoplasmic reticulum.
1945	**F. Lipmann**	Discovered coenzyme A and got the Nobel Prize for this discovery in 1953.

Year	Name of contributor	Cytological contribution
1947–1950	**Lipmann and Kaplan**	Determined the structure of coenzyme A.
1948–1950	**Kennedy and Lehninger**	Showed that the citric acid cycle, oxidative phosphorylation and fatty acid oxidation take place in the mitochondria.
1948	**A. Boivin, R. Vendrely and C. Vendrely**	Demonstrated quantitative constancy of DNA material in various cells of same organism.
1952	**C. Du Duve**	Identified lysosomes.
1952	**G. E. Palade**	Analysed the fine structure of mitochondria and showed the presence of mitochondrial cristae.
1952	**M. Chase and A. D. Hershey**	Showed that the gene was DNA.
1953	**F. Zemike**	Received Nobel Prize for the discovery of phase contrast microscope.
1953	**H. A. Krebs**	Received Nobel Prize for the discovery of citric acid cycle.
1953	**J. D. Watson and F. H. C. Crick**	Proposed the double helix model for the DNA molecule and got Nobel Prize in 1962.
1954	**F. Sanger**	Gave the first complete structure of a protein molecule when he worked out the structure of the insulin molecule.
1956	**J. H. Tijo and A. Levan**	Gave the first correct human chromosome count (46 chromosomes in the diploid condition).
1957	**Seymour Benzer**	Gave the concept of the cistron (gene), the unit of function.
1957	**A. R. Todd**	Got Nobel Prize for the discovery of nucleotides and nucleotidic coenzymes.
1958	**F. Sanger**	Received Nobel Prize for the discovery of the structure of insulin.
1958	**G. W. Beadle and E. L. Tatum**	Received the Nobel Prize for the discovery that one gene regulates one definite chemical process.
1958	**F. H. C. Crick**	Proposed the central dogma of molccular biology that DNA determines the sequence of amino acids in polypeptide.
1959	**S. Ochoa**	Received the Nobel Prize for the synthesis of polyribonucleotide *in vitro*.
1959	**A. Kornberg**	Received the Nobel Prize for *in vitro* synthesis of polydeoxyribonucleotides.
1960	**Park and Pon**	Discovered quantosomes in the chloroplast.
1960	**J. Hurwitz, A. Stevens and S. Weiss**	Showed the role of the enzyme RNA polymerase in the synthesis of RNA from a DNA template.
1961	**F. H. C. Crick *et al.***	Produced direct evidence that the genetic code is a triplet one.
1961	**F. Jacob and J. Monod**	Discovered regulatory genes.
1961	**M. Calvin**	Received the Nobel Prize for the work on photosynthetic activity.
1964	**R. W. Holley**	Described the nucleotide sequence of alanine tRNA molecule of yeast.
1968	**M. W. Nirenberg and H. G. Khorana**	Received the Nobel Prize for the work on genetic code.
1968	**R. H. Holley**	Received the Nobel Prize for the discovery of base sequence of tRNA.

Year	Name of contributor	Cytological contribution
1969	**M. Delbrueck, A. D. Mershey and S. E. Luria**	Received the Nobel Prize for the discovery of reproductive patterns in viruses.
1970	**Knippers; Kornberg and Gefter; Moses and Richardson**	Isolated DNA-polymerase-II enzyme.
1972	**C. B. Anfinsen; S. Moore and W. H. Stein**	Got Nobel Prize (Chemistry) for the discovery of chemical structure and activity of the enzyme ribonuclease.
1974	**A. Claude, G. E. Palade and C. de Duve**	Were awarded Nobel Prize for their innovations that started the modern science of cell biology nearly 39 years ago, and for their major contributions to the understanding of the inner working of living cell.
1975	**R. Dulbecco, H. M.Temin and D. Baltimore**	Were awarded Nobel Prize for their discoveries concerning the interaction between tumour viruses and the genetic material of the cell.
1976	**D. C. Gajdusek**	Got Nobel Prize for his finding of the cause of a puzzling, fatal degenerative disease called Kuru. The agent responsible for Kuru was found to be a slow virus and this discovery has been considered a great achievement in medical genetics and neurobiology.
1977	**Rosalyn Talow, Roger Guillemin and Andrew Schally**	These three American endocrinologists got Nobel Prize in Physiology and Medicine for developing the techniques of radioimmunoassay for the estimation of hormones in blood and for isolating, characterising and synthesising three polypeptides involved in the control of the anterior pituitary gland from brain.
1978	**Daniel Nathans, Hamilton O. Smith and Werner Arber**	These three microbiologists were awarded Nobel Prize in Physiology and Medicine for their "discovery of restriction enzymes and their application to problem of molecular biology". The restriction enzymes provide the "chemical knives" that split chromosomes in their component genes.
1978	**Peter Dennis Mitchell**	Got Nobel Prize in Chemistry for his work in bioenergetics which concerns the chemical processes responsible for the energy supply in living cells.
1980	**Paul Berg, Frederick Sanger and Walter Gilbert**	Got Nobel Prize in Chemistry for their investigations in genetic engineering. Half of this year's Prize was shared by Sanger and Gilbert for developing tecbniques for decoding about 1000 alphabets of heredity from a DNA strand in one day. Another half of Prize was awarded to Berg for his invention of technique of gene-splicing which literally means joining together of the various pieces of gene or DNA.
1980	**George Snell, Jean Dausset and B. Benacerraf**	Got Nobel Prize in Physiology and Medicine for their research work in establishing links between genetics and immunology and to show ways to cure many human genetic diseases.

Discovery of Cell and its Organelles. Cells were discovered in 1665 by an English scientist, **Robert Hooke**. He saw cells for the first time in a thin slice of cork with his crude microscope. Hooke described the cork as made up of hundreds of little hexagonal boxes, giving a kind of honey-comb appearance. He called these little boxes **cells**. In 1833, a Scottish botanist, **Robert Brown** discovered and named the **nucleus** in a cell. **J.E. Purkinje** in 1839, used the term **protoplasm** for a living substance present inside the cell.

1.3 CELL THEORY

In 1838, a German botanist **Mathias Jacob Schleiden** (1804–1881) put forth the idea that cells were the units of structure in the plants. In 1839, his co-worker, a German zoologist, **Theodor Schwann** (1810–1882) applied Schleiden's thesis to the animals. Both of them, thus, postulated that the cell is the basic unit of structure and function in all life. This simple, basic and formal biological generalization is known as **cell theory** or **cell doctrine**. In fact, both **Schleiden** and **Schwann** are incorrectly credited for the formulation of the cell theory; they merely made the generalizations which were based on the works of their predecessors such as **Oken** (1805), **Mirabel** (1807), **Lamarck** (1809), **Dutrochet** (1824), **Turpin** (1826), etc. However, **Schleiden** was the first to describe the nucleoli and to appreciate the fact that each cell leads a double life—one independent, pertaining to its own development, and another, as integral part of a multicellular plant. **Schwann** studied both plant and animal tissues and his work with the connective tissues such as bone and cartilage led him to modify the evolving cell theory to include the idea that living things are composed of both cells and the products or secretions of the cells. **Schwann** also introduced the term **metabolism** to describe the activities of the cells.

In the coming years, the cell theory was to be extended and refined further. **K. Nageli** (1817–1891) showed in 1846 that plant cells arise from the division of pre-existing cells. In 1855, a German pathologist **Rudolf Virchow** (1821–1902) confirmed the Nageli's principle of the cellular basis of life's continuity. He stated in Latin that the cells arise only from the pre-existing cells (*viz.*, his actual aphorism was "*omnis cellula e cellula*"—every cell from a cell). **Virchow**, thus, established the significance of cell division in the reproduction of organisms. In 1858, **Virchow** published his classical textbook *Cellular Pathology* and in it he correctly asserted that as functional units of life, the cells were the primary sites of disease and cancer. Later, in 1865, **Louis Pasteur** (1822–1895) in France gave experimental evidence to support Virchow's extension of the cell theory.

The modern version of cell theory states that (1) All living organisms (animals, plants and microorganisms) are made up of one or more cells and cell products. (2) All metabolic reactions in unicellular and multicellular organisms take place in cells. (3) Cells originate only from other cells, *i.e.*, no cell can originate spontaneously or *de novo*, but comes into being only by division and duplication of already existing cells. (4) The smallest clearly defined unit of life is the cell.

The cell theory had its wide biological applications. With the progress of biochemistry, it was shown that there were fundamental similarities in the chemical composition and metabolic activities of all cells. **Kolliker** applied the cell theory to embryology—after it was demonstrated that the organisms developed from the fusion of two cells—the spermatozoon and the ovum. However, in the recent years, large number of sub-cellular structures such as ribosomes, lysosomes, mitochondria, chloroplasts, etc., have been discovered and studied in detail. Consequently, it may appear that cell is no longer a basic unit of life, because life may exist without cells also. Even then, the cell theory remains a useful concept.

Exceptions to cell theory. Cell theory does not have universal application, *i.e.*, there are certain living organisms which do not have true cells. All kinds of true cells share the following three basic characteristics: 1. **A set of genes** which constitute the blueprints for regulating cellular activities and making new cells. 2. A limiting **plasma membrane** that permits controlled exchange of matter and energy with the external world. 3. **A metabolic machinery** for sustaining life activities such as growth, reproduction and repair of parts. **Viruses** do not easily fit in these parameters of a true cell. Thus, they lack a plasma membrane and a metabolic machinery for energy production and for the synthesis of proteins. However, like any other cellular organism, viruses have (1) a definite genetically determined macromolecular organization; (2) a genetic or hereditary material in the form of either DNA or RNA; (3) a capacity of auto-reproduction; and (4) a capacity of mutation in their genetic substance. In consequence, viruses can only reproduce inside the host cells which may belong to animals, plants or bacteria (*i.e.*, microorganisms). They use their own genetic programme for reproduction but rely on the raw materials (*i.e.*, amino acids, nucleotides) and biosynthetic machinery of the host cells (*i.e.*, ribosomes, tRNA, enzymes) for their multiplication. Thus, a virus may be defined as an infectious, subcellular and ultramicroscopic particle representing an obligate cellular parasite and a potential pathogen whose reproduction (replication) in the host cell and transmission by infection cause characteristic reaction in the host cells. Outside the host cells, viruses are just like non-living inert particles and like the salt or sugar, they can be purified, crystallized and placed into jars on a shelf for years. Due to this fact, viruses have been variously described such as "*naked genes that had somehow acquired the ability to move from one cell to another*" or as "*cellular forms that have degenerated through parasitism*" or as "*primitive organisms that have not reached a cellular state*".

There are certain other organisms such as the protozoan *Paramecium*, the fungus *Rhizopus* and the alga *Vaucheria* (Fig. 1.2B) which do not fit into the purview of the cell theory. All of these organisms have bodies containing undivided mass of protoplasm which lacks cell-like organization and has more than one nucleus. They tend to raise the question that whether cell is a basic unit of structure in them.

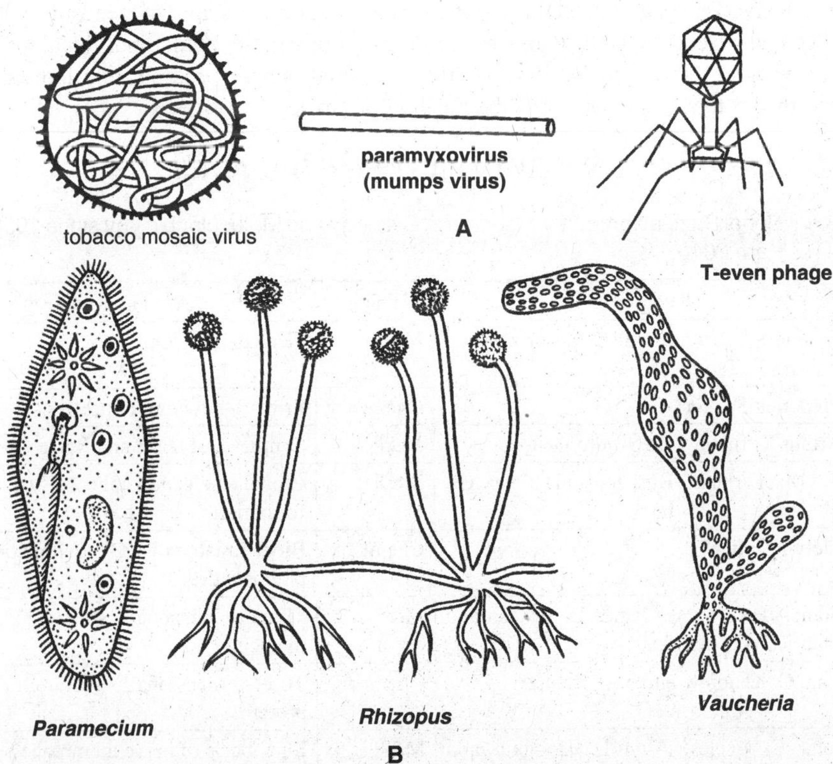

Fig. 1.2. Organisms forming exceptions to the cell theory: A—Three type of viruses; B—Three cases of cellular organization.

1.4 PROTOPLASM THEORY

Up to middle of the 19th century, greater emphasis was given to the cell wall and less to the cellular content. But soon cell biologists started to recognize the importance of "juicy" or "slimy" contents of the cells. In 1835, **Felix Dujardin** termed the jelly-like material within protozoans as sarcode. In 1835, **H.von Mohl** (1805–1875) described cell division. In 1839, the Czech biologist **J.E. Purkinje** (1787–1869) coined the term protoplasm to describe the contents of cells (animal embryos). **Von Mohl**, in 1846, applied the name protoplasm to the contents of embryonic cells of the plants. **Max Schultze**, in 1861, established similarity between sarcode and protoplasm of animal and plant cells and, thus, offering a theory which later on was improved and called protoplasm theory by **O. Hertwig** (1849–1922) in 1892.

Protoplasm theory holds that all living matter, out of which animals and plants are formed, is the protoplasm. The cell is an accumulation of living substance or protoplasm which is limited in space by outer membrane and possesses a nucleus. The protoplasm which is filled in the nucleus is called **nucleoplasm** and that exists between the nucleus and the plasma membrane is called **cytoplasm**.

1.5 ORGANISMAL THEORY

The organismal theory holds that the body of all multicellular organisms is a continuous mass of protoplasm which remains divided incompletely into small centres, the cells, for the various biological activities. Thus, a multicellular organism is a highly differentiated protoplasmic individual, differing with a unicellular Protozoa only in size and degree of differentiation of the protoplasm. The differentiation involves separation of the protoplasm into subordinate semi-independent compartments, the so-called cells. Even the embryological development of a multicellular individual includes only growth and progressive internal differentiation of a small single protoplasmic individual (egg). Organismal theory too fails to ascertain the position of viruses.

1.6 GROWTH OF CYTOLOGY IN LAST FIVE DECADES

Table 1.3. Nobel Prize awarded for research in Cytology and Molecular biology since 1958 (Source: Karp 2010).

Year	Recipient	Prize	Area of Research
1958	George W. Beadle, Joshua Lederberg and Edward L. Tatum	M&P	Gene expression
	Frederick Sanger	Chemistry	Primary structure of protein
1959	Arthur Kornberg and Severo Ochoa	M&P	Synthesis of DNA and RNA
1960	F. MacFarlane Burnet and Peter B. Medawar	M&P	Clonal selection theory of antibody formation
1961	Melvin Calvin	Chemistry	Biochemistry of CO_2 assimilation during photosynthesis
1962	Francis H.C. Crick, James D. Watson and Maurice H.F. Wilkins	M&P	Three-dimensional structure of DNA molecule
	John C. Kendrew and Max Perutz	Chemistry	Three-dimensional structure of globular proteins
1963	John C. Eccles, Alan L. Hodgkin and Andrew F. Huxley	M&P	Ionic basis of nerve membrane potential
1964	Dorothy C. Hodgkin	Chemistry	X-ray structure of complex biological molecules
1965	Francois Jacob, Andre M. Lwoff and Jacques L. Monod	M&P	Bacterial operons and messenger RNA
1966	Peyton Rous	M&P	Tumor viruses

Year	Recipient	Prize	Area of Research
1968	H. Gobind Khorana, Marshall W. Nirenberg and Robert W. Holley	M&P	Genetic code
1969	Max Delbruck, Alfred D. Hershey and Salvador E. Luria	M&P	Genetic structure of viruses
1970	Bernard Katz and Ulf von Euler	M&P	Nerve impulse propagation
	Leloir	Chemistry	Role of sugar in carbohydrate synthesis
1971	Earl W. Sutherland	M&P	Mechanism of hormone action and cyclic AMP
1972	Gerald Edelman and Rodney R. Porter	M&P	Immunoglobulin structure
	Christian B. Anfinsen	Chemistry	Relationship between primary and tertiary structure of proteins
1974	Albert Claude, Christian de Duve and George F. Palade	M&P	Structure and function of internal components of cells
1975	David Baltimore, Renato Dulbecco and Howard M. Temin	M&P	Reverse transcriptase and tumor virus activity
1976	D. Carleton Gajdusek	M&P	Prion-based diseases
1978	Werner Arber, Daniel Nathans and Hamilton O. Smith	M&P	Restriction endonuclease technology
	Peter Mitchell	Chemistry	Chemiosmotic mechanism of oxidative phosphorylation
1980	Paul Berg, Walter Gilbert and Frederick Sanger	Chemistry	Recombinant DNA technology and DNA sequencing technology
	Baruj Bennacerraf, Jean Dausset and George D. Snell	M&P	Major histocompatibility complex
1982	Aaron Klug	Chemistry	Structure of nucleic acid-protein complexes (TMV, Nucleosomes)
1983	Barbara McClintok	M&P	Mobile elements in the genome
1984	Georges Kohler, Cesar Milstein and Niels K. Jerne	M&P	Monoclonal antibodies
	Bruce Merrifield	Chemistry	Chemical synthesis of peptides
1985	Michael S. Brown and Joseph L. Goldstein	M&P	Regulation of cholesterol metabolism and endocytosis
1986	Rita Levi-Montalcini and Stanley Cohen	M&P	Factors that affect nerve outgrowth
1987	Susuma Tonegawa	M&P	DNA rearrangements responsible for antibody diversity
1988	Johann Deisenhofer, Robert Huber and Hartmut Michel	Chemistry	Bacterial photosynthetic reaction center
1989	J. Michael Bishop and Harold Varmus	M&P	Cellular genes capable of causing malignant transformation
	Thomas R.Cech and Sidney Altman	Chemistry	Ability of RNA to catalyze reactions
1991	Erwin Neher and Bert Sakmann	M&P	Measurement of ion flux by patch clamp recording (cell membrane function)
1992	Edmond Fischer and Edwin Krebs	M&P	Alteration of enzyme activity by phosphorylation/dephosphorylation
1993	Kary Mullis and Michael Smith	Chemistry	Polymerase chain reaction (PCR); Site directed mutagenesis (SDM)
	Richard J. Roberts and Phillip A. Sharp	M&P	Intervening sequences

Year	Recipient	Prize	Area of Research
1994	Alfred Gilman and Martin Rodbell	M&P	Structure and function of GTP-binding (G) proteins
1995	Edward B. Lewis, Christiane Nusslein-Volhard and Eric Wieschaus	M&P	Genetic control of embryonic development
1996	Rolf M. Zinkernagel, and Peter C. Doherty	M&P	Recognition of virus infected cells by the immune system
1997	Jens C. Skou, Paul Boyer, John Walker and Stanley B. Prusiner	Chemistry	Na^+/K^+-ATPase and mechanism of ATP synthesis
1998	Robert Furchgott Louis Ignarro and Ferid Murad	M&P	Nitric oxide (NO) as intercellular messenger
1999	Gunther Blobel	M&P	Protein trafficking
2000	Arvid Carlsson, Paul Greengard and Eric Kandel	M&P	Synaptic transmission and signal transduction
2001	Leland H. Hartwell, Tim Hunt and Paul Nurse	M&P	Control of cell cycle
2002	Sydney Brenner and John Sulston	M&P	Introduction of *Caenorhabditis elegans* as a model organism
	H. Robert Horvitz		Apoptosis in *C. elegans*
	John B. Fenn	Chemistry	Electrospray ionization in mass spectometry (MS)
	Koichi Tanaka		MALDI in MS (MALDI @ Matrix-assisted laser desorption ionization)
	Kurt Wuthrich		NMR analysis of proteins (NMR @ Nuclear magnetic resonance spectroscopy – a method for determination of three dimensional structure of small proteins)
2003	Peter Agre and Roderick Mackinnon	Chemistry	Structure of membrane channels
2004	Richard Axel and Linda B. Buck	M&P	Olfactory receptors
	Aaron Ciechanover and Avram Hershko	Chemistry	Ubiquitin and proteasome
2006	Andrew Z. Fire, Craig C. Mello and Roger D. Kornberg	M&P	RNA interference (RNAi)
2007	Mario R. Capecchi, Martin J. Evans and Oliver Smithies	M&P	Development techniques for knockout mice
2008	Francoise Barre-sinoussi, Luc Montagnier	M&P	Discovery of HIV
	Herald Zur Hausen		Role of HIV in cancer
	Martin Chalfie, Osamu Shimomura and Roger Tsien	Chemistry	Discovery and development of GFP (green fluorescent protein)
2010	Robert Edwards	M&P	IVF (*in vitro* fertilization) technique
*M&P, Medicine and Physiology			

In subsequent years *viz.*, 2011, 2012 and 2013, the Nobel Prize recipients are as follows:

Year	Recipient	Prize	Area of Research
2011	Dan Schectman	Chemistry	Discovery of quasi crystals

Year	Recipient	Prize	Area of Research
	Bruce A. Butler & Tules A. Hoffman	M&P	Discoveries concerning activation of innate immunity
	Ralph M. Steiman	M&P	Dendritic cells its role in adaptive immunity
2012	Robert J. Lefkowitz & Brian K. Kobilka	Chemistry	Studies of G. Proteins coupled receptors
	Sir John B. Govdon & Shinya Yamanaha	M&P	Discovery that mature cells can be reprogrammed to become pluripotent
2013	Matin Karpulus, Michael Levitt, Arieh Warshel	Chemistry	Development of multiscale models for complex systems
	James E. Rothman, Randy Schekman, Thomas C. Sudhof	M&P	Discoveries of machinery regulating vesicle traffic, a major transport system in cells.

1.7 RELATIONSHIP OF CYTOLOGY WITH OTHER BIOLOGICAL SCIENCES

The cytology has helped the biologists to understand various complicated life activities such as metabolism, growth, differentiation, heredity and evolution at the cellular and molecular levels. Due to its wide application in various branches of biological science, many new hybrid biological sciences have sprang up. Some of them are as follows:

1. Cytotaxonomy (Cytology and Taxonomy). Each plant and animal species has a definite number of chromosomes in its cells and the chromosomes of the individuals of a species resemble closely with one another in shape and size. These characteristics of the chromosomes are helpful to a taxonomist in determining the taxonomical position of a species. Further cytology furnishes strong support to the manner of origin of certain taxonomic units. Therefore, the cytotaxonomy can be defined as a cytological science which provides cytological support to the taxonomic position of any species.

2. Cytogenetics (Cytology and Genetics). Cytogenetics is that branch of cytology which is concerned with the cytological and molecular bases of heredity, variation, mutation, phylogeny, morphogenesis and evolution of organisms. The Weismann's germ plasm theory, Mendel's Laws of inheritance and the concept of gene could be well understood only after the application of cytological concept to the genetics.

3. Cell physiology (Cytology and Physiology). The cell physiology is the study of life activities, *viz.*, nutrition, metabolism, excitability, growth, reproduction or cell division and differentiation of the cells. The cell physiology has helped in understanding various complicated physiological activities at the cellular level.

4. Cytochemistry (Cytology and Biochemistry). The cytochemistry is that branch of cytology which deals with the chemical and physico-chemical analysis of living matter. For example, the cytochemical analysis has revealed the presence of carbohydrates, lipids, proteins, nucleic acids and other organic and inorganic chemical compounds in the cells.

5. Ultrastructure and Molecular Biology. These are the most modem branches of biology in which the merging of cytology with biochemistry, physiochemistry and especially macromolecular and colloidal chemistry becomes increasingly complex. Knowledge of the submicroscopic organisation or ultrastructure of the cell is of fundamental importance because practically all the functional and physiochemical transformations take place with the molecular architecture of the cell and at a molecular level. The recent discoveries in molecular biology such as the discovery of molecular model of **DNA** by **Watson** and **Crick** in 1953, molecular interpretation of protein synthetic mechanism, genetic code, etc., having an extraordinary impact on modern cytology and biology.

6. Cytopathology (Cytology and Pathology). The application of molecular biology to pathological sciences has helped in understanding various human diseases at molecular level. Because most diseases are caused due to disorder of genetic codes in DNA molecule which alter the synthetic process of enzymes and ultimately disturbs metabolic activities of the cell.

7. Cytoecology (Cytology and Ecology). The cytoecology is the science in which one studies the effects of ecological changes on the chromosome number of the cell. The cytological studies on plants and animals have revealed that the ecological habitat and geographical distribution have the correlation with chromosome numbers.

Now we can say that cytology or cell biology has given a great impetus to early and modern biologists to explore new vistas in biological sciences. The modern cytological studies are helpful in undersanding various life activities in terms of molecules, in the curing of various chronic human diseases and in improving the breeds of plants and animals.

1.8 APPLICATIONS OF MOLECULAR CELL BIOLOGY

Understanding the molecular biology of cells is an active area of research that is fundamental to all of the biological sciences. This is true not only from the standpoint of basic science, but also with respect to a growing number of applications in medicine, agriculture, biotechnolgy and biomedical engineering. Especially with the completion of the sequence of the human genome, progress in cell and molecular biology has opened new horizons in the practice of medicine. Striking examples include the development of new drugs specifically targeted to interfere with the growth of cancer cells and the potential use of stem cells to replace damage tissues and treat patients suffering conditions such as diabetes, Parkinson's disease, Alzheimer's disease, spinal cord injuries and heart disease (**Cooper** and **Hausman**, 2007).

REVISION QUESTIONS

1. Give detailed account of cell theory.
2. What are the landmark cytological discoveries of 19th and 20th centuries?
3. Write short notes on:
   (i) Cell Theory (ii) Protoplasm Theory
   (iii) Organismal Theory
4. What is cell biology? Who had discovered the cell?

2 Chapter

MICROSCOPY

A **microscope** is an optical instrument consisting of a single lens or a combination of lenses for magnifying objects too small to be seen or clearly observed by the naked eye. Thus, it is used to obtain magnified images of small objects such as cells of living organisms. Investigations or studies by means of the microscope is called **microscopy**. In cytology or cell biology, various types of microscopes are used to study the structure of cell; some important ones are the following:

1. Optical or light microscopes (simple, monocular, binocular and compound microscopes);
2. Electron microscope;
3. Phase contrast microscope;
4. X-ray diffraction microscope;
5. Interference microscope;
6. Polarized light microscope;
7. Ultra-violet microscope;
8. Ultra-microscope or Dark field microscope.

A **simple microscope** (also called dissecting microscope) has a single lens system. It is composed of a single convex lens. A **compound microscope** consists of two or more **lens systems** or **elements**. A **monocular microscope** contains one ocular or eyepiece while a **binocular microscope** has two oculars.

Here, only two types of microscopes, namely light microscope and electron microscope will be described.

2.1 RESOLVING POWER OF MICROSCOPE

In the search for information about the structure and composition of cells, the cell biologists immediately face two limitations: the exceedingly small dimensions of cells and their component parts and the transparent nature of cells. The diameters of the majority of cells fall within a range of 0.2 and 50 μm. The human eyes have limited distinguishing or resolving power. The ability of an observational instrument such as a human eye or a microscope to reveal details of structure is expressed in terms of **limit of resolution** (*l*) which is defined as *the smallest distance that may separate two points on an object and still permit their observation as distinct separate points*. The unaided human eye under optimal conditions in green light (to which it is most sensitive) cannot distinguish between points less than about 0.1 μm or 100 μm apart. Structural details smaller than this, *e.g.*, cell, is unresolved unless some instrument capable of higher resolution is used. **Magnification**, *the increase in size of optical image over the size of the object being viewed*, is of no use unless the observational system can resolve the various parts of the structure being examined. Increased magnification without improved resolution results only in a large blurred image. The human eye has no power of magnification, so magnifying glasses may be used to magnify images up to about 10 times. A light compound microscope in which many lenses are combined together has a useful magnification of about 1,500 times.

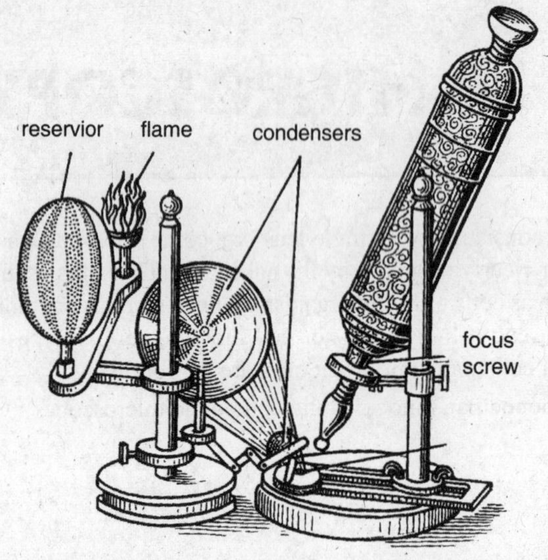

Fig. 2.1. Hooke's compound microscope.

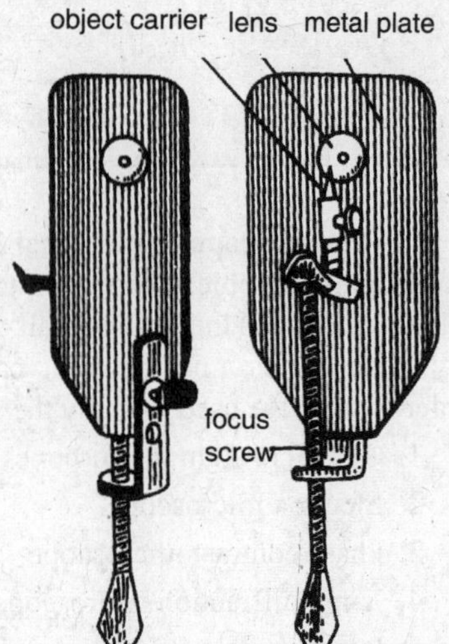

Fig. 2.2. Leeuwenhock's microscope.

The limit of resolution (*l*) of any optical instrument (*i.e.*, eye or microscope) is given approximately by the Abbe's relationships:

$$\text{Resolution } (l) = \frac{\text{wevelength } (\lambda)}{\text{numerical aperture } (n \sin \alpha)}$$

where λ (lambda) is the wavelength ("colour") of the illumination or radiation used to form the image, *n* is refractive index (a function of density) of the material (*i.e.*, mostly air or water) between the specimen and the first lens (or objective lens), and sin α is sine of the semi-angle of aperture of the first lens as viewed from the specimen. The quantity "*n* sin α" is often called the **numerical aperture (NA)**.

Abbe's relationships make it clear that high resolution in a microscope can only be achieved by manipulating a small number of variables: the wavelength of the illuminating radiation, the refractive index and the aperture. The **aperture** is limited to something less than 90° since that would have the lens and specimen in contact with one another. In fact, 85° is about the limit in good optical microscopes. Such angles require an excellent lens. In most cases, the aperture is less because the edges of the lens introduce distortions and so cannot be used. **Refractive index** is easy to alter, but only within narrow limits. It can be increased by using oils to fill the space between the specimen and the objective lens. Transparent immersion oils used in today's microscopes (*i.e.*, **oil immersion lens**) have *n* up to about 1.6. Still 1.6 is big improvement over air or water ($n = 1$). In a microscope, the smallest detectable detail is equal to about one-half the **wavelength** of light with which it is observed. The smaller the object, the shorter the wavelength of light required. Hence, the wavelength of light is the area which has great chances of improvement. One can, for example, use ultraviolet light instead of visible light, thus, improving resolution as much as two-fold. In order to do that however, special lenses (*e.g.*, of quartz) must be used since ordinary glass blocks much ultraviolet light. In such a microscope, called ultraviolet microscope, the eyes cannot be used to view the image directly, for they are insensitive to ultraviolet light. Lastly, a specimen cannot absorb light of wavelength below 0.3 μm.

Thus, a good light microscope, with a numerical aperture of 1.4 and using light of short wavelength (0.4 μm) will resolve two points at about 0.17 μm separations. By such a microscope though, one can see considerable details in most cells, there is also a great deal that cannot be seen. For instance, ribosomes and chromatin threads of nucleus are about 0.02 mm in diameter and quite invisible to the light microscope. For them electron microscope is used. In cell biological studies, the following two types of microscopes are most extensively used:

2.2 LIGHT MICROSCOPES (OPTICAL MICROSCOPES)

The compound light microscope (Fig. 2.3) is the simplest and most commonly used microscope. It consists of the following three lens system.

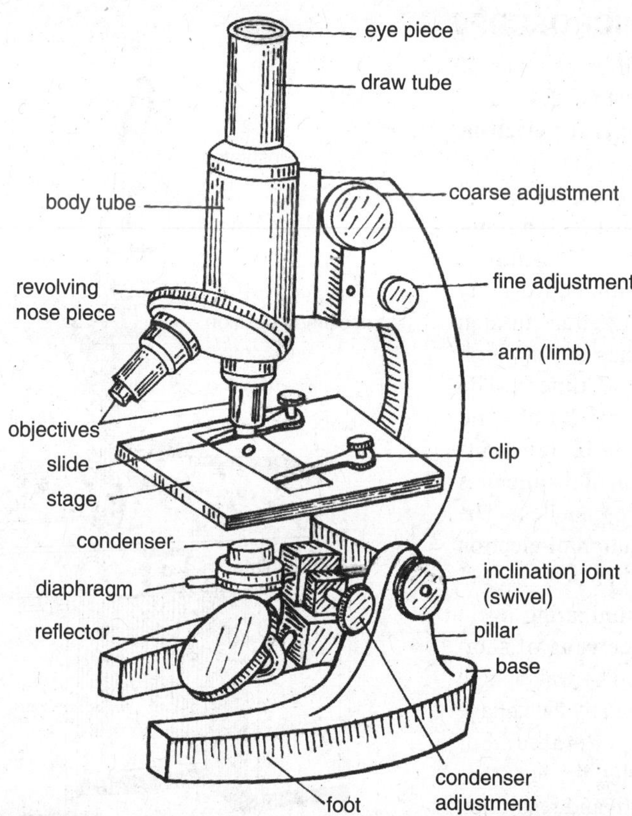

Fig. 2.3. Light or compound microscope.

(*i*) **Condenser lens system** occurs beneath the specimen and its function is the collection and focussing of the light rays on the object or specimen which is placed on the stage of the microscope.

(*ii*) **Objective lens system** remains near and above the specimen. It produces and magnifies the image of the specimen.

(*iii*) **Eye piece lens system** or ocular lens system remains near the eyes of the observer and it magnifies and forms the image (secondary) of the (primary) image previously produced by the objective.

Lenses. A simple lens can magnify an object only three times (3X). For getting a magnification of more than 3X, a combination of several lenses is used. Such a combination of several lenses (called **elements**) function as a single convex lens and a magnification of about 20X can be obtained. For example, an **eye piece lens** contains 2 to 3 lenses or elements. Likewise, the objective lens is made by placing 8 to 10 lenses or elements. Individual lenses are placed so close to each other that they act as a single lens. Only achromatic lenses are used in a microscope.

Working. Light rays from the light source (sunlight or bulb-light) are focussed on the object by the condenser lens. The objective lens produces the enlarged image, called **primary image**, of the object or material. The eye piece lens further magnifies the primary image into secondary image which is seen by our eye. Cellular organelles such as mitochondria and bacteria, both of which are 0.5 μm wide, are the smallest objects that can be clearly seen in the light microscope.

2.3 ELECTRON MICROSCOPE

Two basically different types of electron microscopes (Fig. 2.4) have been developed. **Transmission electron microscopes (TEMs)** form images from electrons that are transmitted through a specimen. Whereas **scanning electron microscopes (SEMs)** utilize electrons that have bounced off the surface of the specimen. A transmission electron microscope has a very high magnification (500,000 times). The TEM was designed by **Knoll** and **Ruska** of Germany in 1932. It permits direct study of biological ultrastructures (*e.g.*, structure of cell organelles). The practical limit of resolution of electron microscope is about 3 to 5 Å.

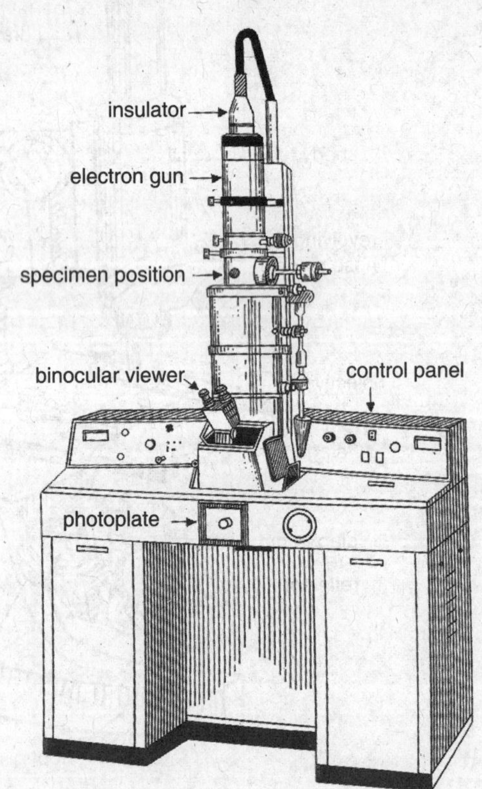

Fig. 2.4. An electron microscope.

In TEM, the illuminating agent is not light but the **electrons** of short wavelength (0.500 Å). The wavelength of electrons is determined by the voltage at which these are generated. For example, at 50,000 volts, the electrons have 0.50 Å wavelength and resolution power of electron microscope can be 0.50 Å/2 = 0.25 Å. Similarly, in an electron microscope with a voltage of 100,000 volts, the wavelength of an electron is 0.004 nm (or .04 Å). Theoretically the resolution of such a microscope should be 0.02 Å. But practical resolving power of most modern electron microscope is 0.5 μm or 5 Å. This is 400 times greater than that of a light microscope.

Structure

The transmission electron microscope comprises the following parts:

1. Electron gun and anode. In TEM, the source of illumination is electrons which are produced and concentrated into an electron beam by **electron gun**. Electron gun consists of an electrically heated **tungsten filament** or **cathode** that emits electrons. Outside the gun is an anode which attracts electrons. Thus, between the filament and anode the electrons attain a high velocity with wavelength of .005 to .003 nm.

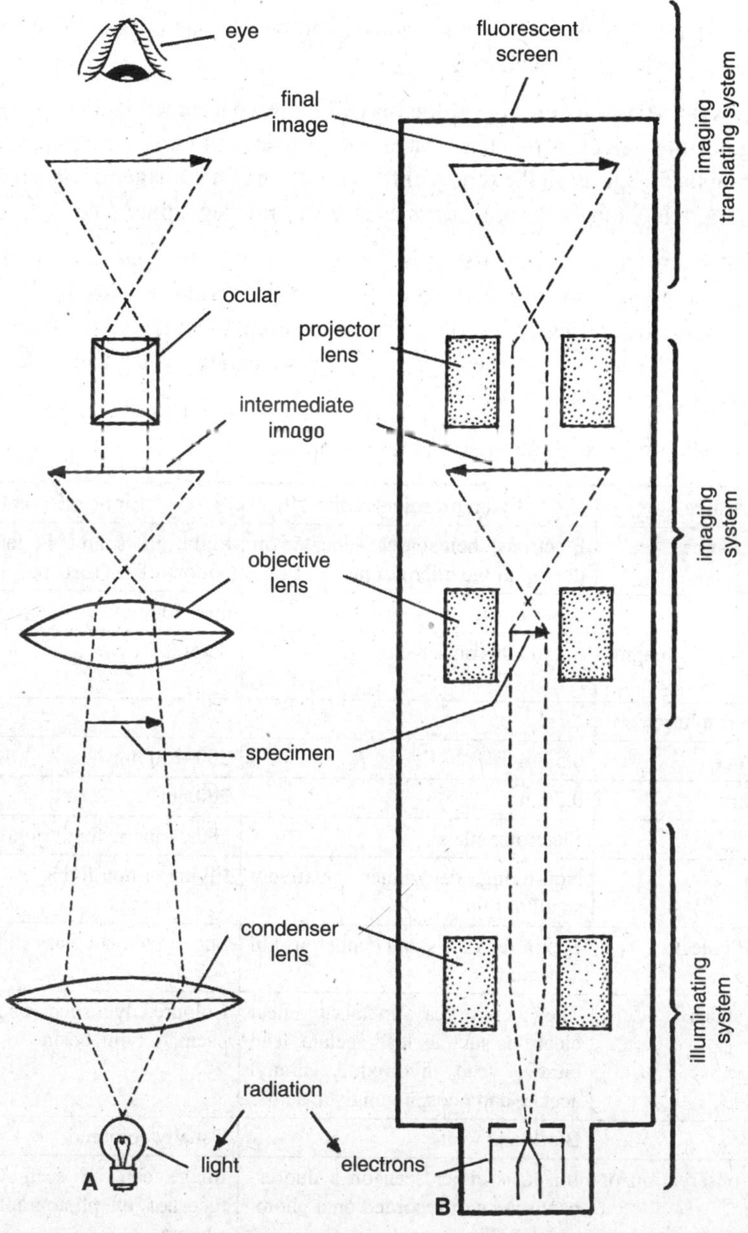

Fig. 2.5. A comparison of the lens systems of light (A) and electron microscope (B).

2. Microscope column. Electrons can travel in straight line in vacuum only, because in the air, these collide with oxygen or nitrogen atoms. The electron microscope, therefore, is enclosed in a evacuated metal tube.

3. Condenser lens. It is the **electromagnetic coil** which focusses or condenses the electron beam in the plane of object.

4. Objective lens. It is the **electromagnetic coil** which produces first magnified image of the object. It focusses the electrons which are reflected by the object and forms the first image.

5. Projector lens. It is also the electromagnetic coil which magnifies the first image formed by objective lens. It produces the final image.

6. Fluorescent screen or photographic plate. Fluorescent screen is used for observing the magnified image of the object. It remains coated with a chemical (*e.g.*, zinc sulphide) which on being excited form the image as on the screen of television. The final image can also be captured on photographic film; such photographs are known as **electron micrographs**.

In the light microscope, the focussing is done by moving the lens tube up and down. In TEM, focussing is done by changing the flow of current through the coils of the electromagnetic lenses. Further, in electron microscopy only dead and dried specimens are studied. With this microscope, living cells cannot be studied, since they possess water which causes large scattering of the electrons.

Table 2.1. Main differences in electron and light microscope.

	Feature	Electron microscope	Light microscope
1.	Radiation source	Electrons; their source is located on the top of the microscope	Light, its source is located at the bottom of microscope
2.	Wavelength	0.005 nm at 50 kV	400–700 nm
3.	Maximum useful magnification	× 250,000 (on screen)	× 1500
4.	Maximum resolution		
	(*i*) in practice	0.5 nm	200–250 nm
	(*ii*) in theory	0.2 nm	200 nm
5.	Lenses	Electromagnets	Glass (quartz for ultraviolet radiation)
6.	Specimen	Non-living, dehydrated, relatively small or thin.	Living or non-living
7.	Support of object	Supported on a small copper grid in a vacuum	Supported on a glass slide
8.	Common stains	They include heavy metals to reflect electrons such as lead acetate, lead citrate, lead hydroxide, uranyl acetate and phosphotungistic acid	Coloured dyes such as borax carmine, haematoxylin, eosin
9.	Image	Black and white	Usually coloured
10.	Mode of observation or recording	Image is either seen on a fluorescent screen or recorded on a photographic film	Image can be seen with eye or recorded on photographic film by camera

2.4 EXAMPLES OF OPTICAL MICROSCOPES

1. Phase Contrast Microscope

Phase contrast microscope was invented by **Frits Zernike** of Netherland in 1932. He got Nobel Prize for this invention in 1953.

Principle and working. Small, unstained specimens, such as a living cell, can be very difficult to see in a bright-field microscope. The phase contrast microscope has solved this problem by making highly transparent objects more visible. The ability to see different parts of an object depends on their capacity to affect light differently from one another. One basis upon which intracellular organelles differ is their refractive index. Cell organelles are made up of different proportions of various molecules: DNA, RNA, protein, lipid, carbohydrate, salts and water. Regions of different composition are likely to have different refractive indexes. Normally, however, such differences cannot be detected by our eyes. The phase contrast microscope converts differences in a refractive index into differences in intensity (relative brightness and darkness) which are then visible to the eye. The basis for this conversion centres on the ability to light waves to interact with one another, a property termed **interference**.

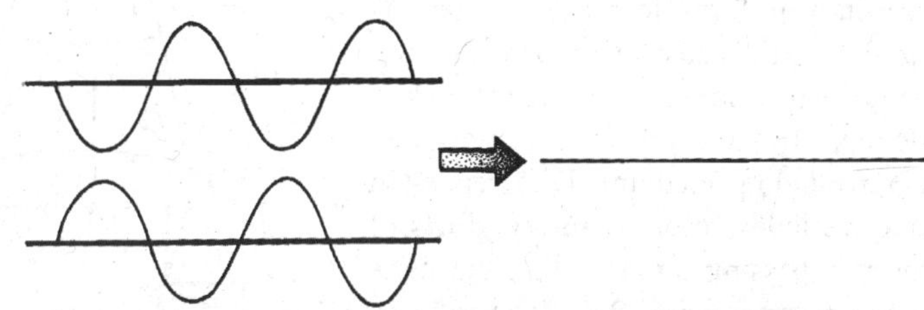

Fig. 2.6. Destructive interference. The two waves of light are one-half wavelength out of phase. When the waves meet, they combine to cancel each other out.

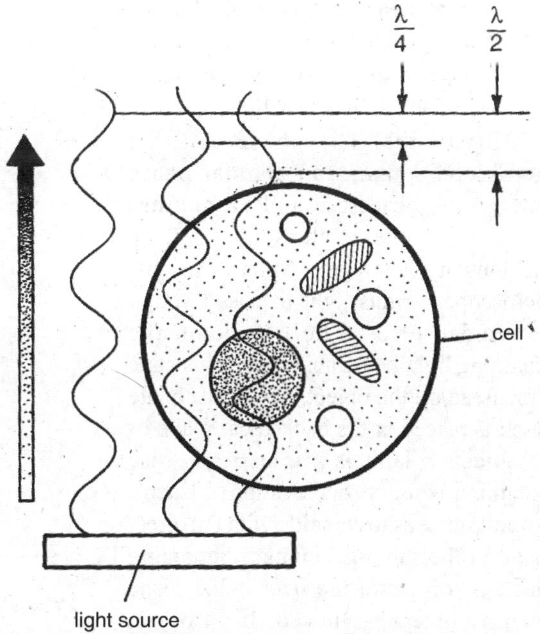

Fig. 2.7. Schematic diagram of retardation of light rays to varying degrees as they pass through different parts of a cell. Because the light rays that emerge from different parts of the cell are in *different phases* of their cycle, they interfere with the direct light to different degrees, producing different degrees of lightness and darkness in the final image.

In contrast to bright-field microscope, phase contrast microscope performs two functions:

1. It separates the direct light (the background light of the field) from the light diffracted by the object, and,
2. It causes these two types of waves to be approximately one-half wavelength out of phase with one another so that they can destructively interact and cause changes in intensity.

Suppose that all parts of the object being examined have exactly the same refractive index as the medium in which they are suspended. If this were the case, all the light from the object and the direct light would be one-half wave-length out of phase with one another, and **interference** would result in a uniform decrease in intensity (Fig. 2.6). Now consider an object whose various parts have different refractive indexes, all of which are greater than the surrounding medium. Differences in refractive index result in **phase shifts** of light rays passing through different parts of the specimen (Fig. 2.7). The relative brightness (**negative contrast**) or darkness (**positive contrast**) of each part of the image reflects the way in which the light from that part of the specimen interferes with the direct light. Since parts of the specimen have different refractive indexes, the various parts of the specimen appear in the image with varying intensity, thereby providing the necessary contrast to be visualized.

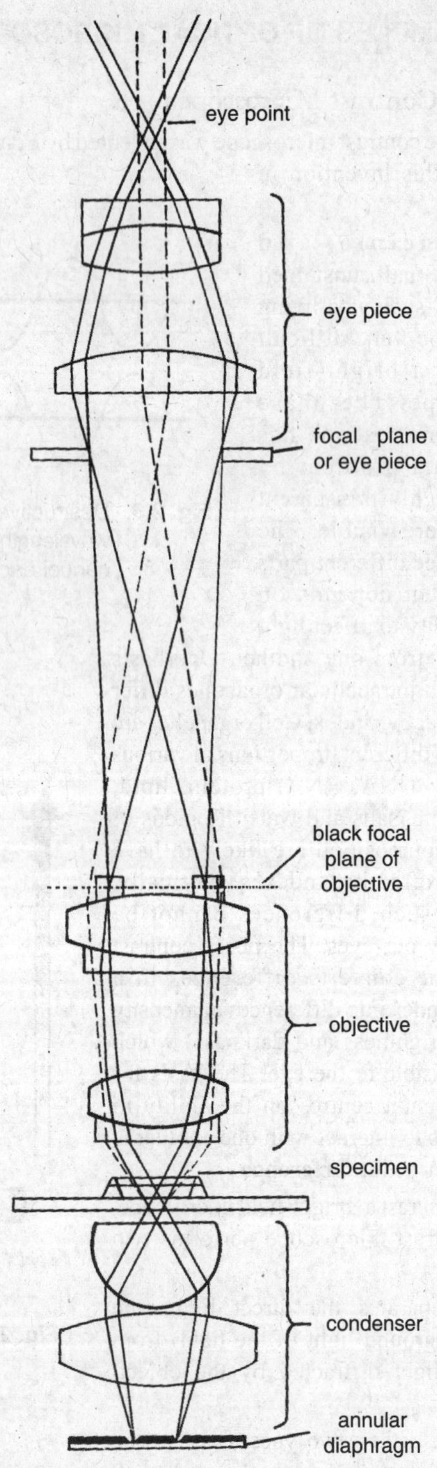

Fig. 2.8. Light path in phase contrast microscope.

Structure. The phase contrast microscope contains an annular phase plate in the objective and an annular diaphragm in the condenser (Fig. 2.8). The annular diaphragm of phase contrast microscope permits light to pass through the condenser as a hollow cone, the remaining light being absorbed. This cone is focussed on the object. The phase plate which is placed at the back focal plane of the objective lens, is a transparent disc containing a groove (or elevation) of such a size and shape as to coincide with the direct image of the substage annular diaphragm which is formed at the back focal plane when no object is viewed. If an object is placed between the condenser and the objective, in addition to direct image a number of overlapping diffracted images of the diaphragm then appear at the back focal plane of the objective. The depth of the groove (or the elevation) in the phase plate of the objective is so made that the two sets of rays forming the direct image and the diffracted image differ in optical path by a quarter wavelength of the illuminating beam of light. Under these conditions the phase difference, which is not seen by the eye, is converted to intensify difference which we see. In the bright contrast phase optical system the two sets of light rays are added to make a brighter image and in the dark contrast phase they partially cancel one another making a more contrasting darker image. The phase contrast microscope helps in the observation of behaviour of chromosomes of living cells during mitosis or meiosis and various other cellular components such as mitochondria and vacuoles. Observations of living cells on a television screen using a video camera provide especially dramatic portraits of the dynamic activities of a cell (Table 2.2).

Table 2.2. The differences between light microscope and phase contrast microscope.

	Light microscope		Phase contrast microscope
1.	The refracted light rays are delayed by about one-quarter wavelength (0.25 λ).	1.	The refracted light rays are delayed by one-half wavelength (0.50 λ).
2.	All points of the image look equally bright.	2.	The brightness of different points of image differs. It corresponds to differences in the refractive indexes of various cellular organelles.
3.	Difference in the wavelengths of refracted and unrefracted light rays is not changed.	3.	This increases the difference to produce maximum contrast (*i.e.*, interference) in the image.
4.	Both living and dead (stained) specimens may be seen by this instrument.	4.	Living (unstained) structures can be seen by this instrument.
5.	There is no phase plate.	5.	In this microscope, a glass phase plate is placed above the objective lens to increase the phase difference between the refracted and unrefracted light rays.

2. Dark Field Microscopy

Any ordinary light microscope in which light from the illuminating source is caused to converge on the specimen by the substage condenser, thereby forming a cone of bright light that can enter the objective lens, is called a **bright field microscope**. The cone of illuminating light is seen as a bright background against which the image of the specimen must be contrasted. Bright field microscopy is ideally suited only for specimens of high contrast, such as stained sections of tissues (Fig. 2.9).

The dark field microscope is an ordinary compound microscope which has a special condenser. In **dark field microscope**, an opaque disc is placed in the centre of the condenser. The light rays are thus removed from the centre and no direct light rays enter the objective. Due to opaque disc, light rays are directed from the sides and only scattered (oblique) rays tend to enter the objective lens. As a result,

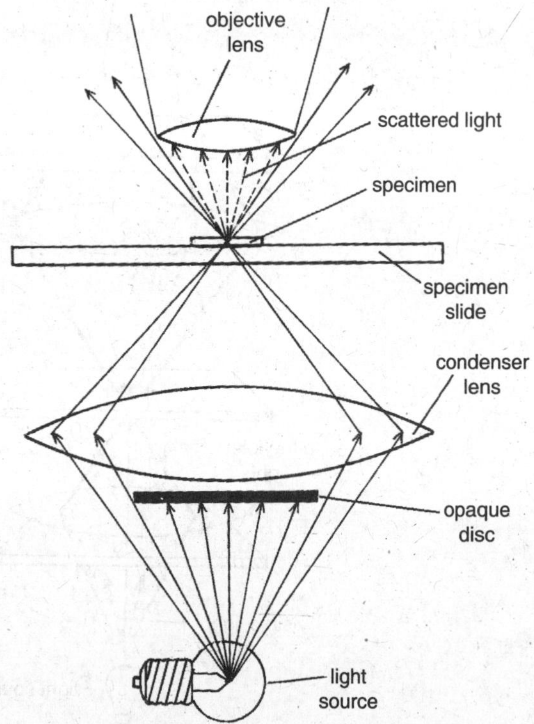

Fig. 2.9. Dark field microscope. Light path from the condenser to the objective lens.

the object appears illuminated (bright) against black background. Dark field microscopy improves visibility and resolution.

3. Fluorescence Microscopy

The fluorescence microscope is based on the phenomenon of fluorescence.

Fluorescence. It is found that when certain chemical compounds are illuminated by ultraviolet rays they become excited at molecular level and start to emit light of visible range. This phenomenon is known as **fluorescence**. The fluorescence may be of two kinds: **autofluorescence** and **secondary fluorescence**. Some substance, *e.g.*, chlorophyll become readily fluoresces or illuminates and produces red light, is an example of autofluorescence. When the fluorescence is induced in a substance by certain specific dyes or stains, the fluorescence is known as secondary fluorescence, *e.g.*, protein and carbohydrates, etc.

The source of illumination of fluorescence microscope (Fig. 2.10) is ultraviolet rays of higher wavelengths (3500 to 4000 Å). The different chemical compounds of the object to be seen when fluoresce by these ultraviolet rays, they emit rays of different wavelength. The rays of fluorescence can be detected and the chemical nature of the given object can be tested.

The ordinary compound microscope can be easily converted into the fluorescence microscope by placing a special filter in between the source of illumination and eye piece.

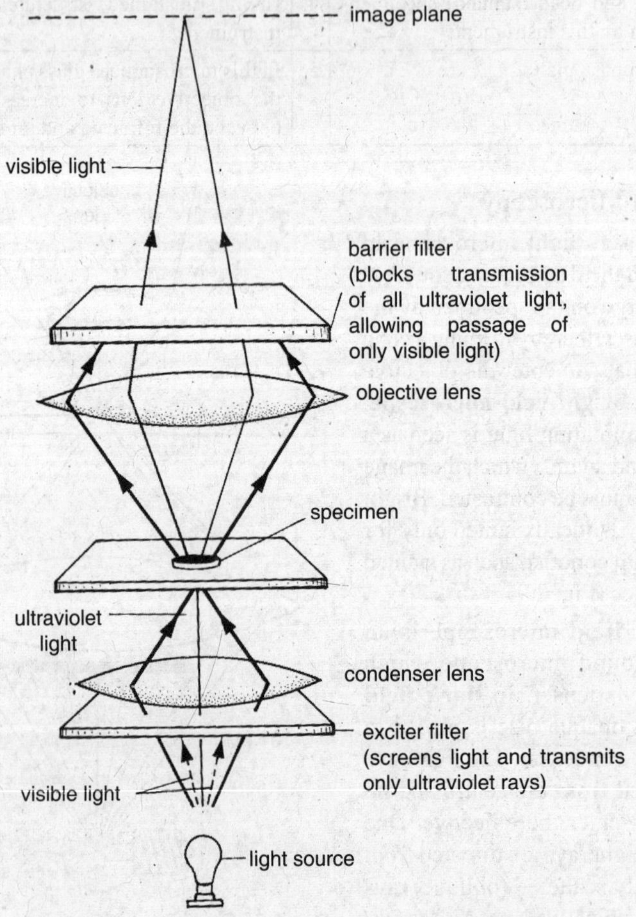

Fig. 2.10. Optics of the fluorescence microscope.

2.5 EXAMPLES OF ELECTRON MICROSCOPES

There are two types of electron microscopes:

1. Transmission electron microscope (TEM);
2. Scanning electron microscope (SEM).

The construction and operation of the TEM are very different from that of the SEM. The image formed by these two types of electron microscopes is also quite different.

1. Transmission Electron Microscope (TEM)

TEM (Fig. 2.11) is the most commonly used electron microscope. It is widely used to study the internal structure of the cell and has great resolving power. In TEM, an electric field propels electrons

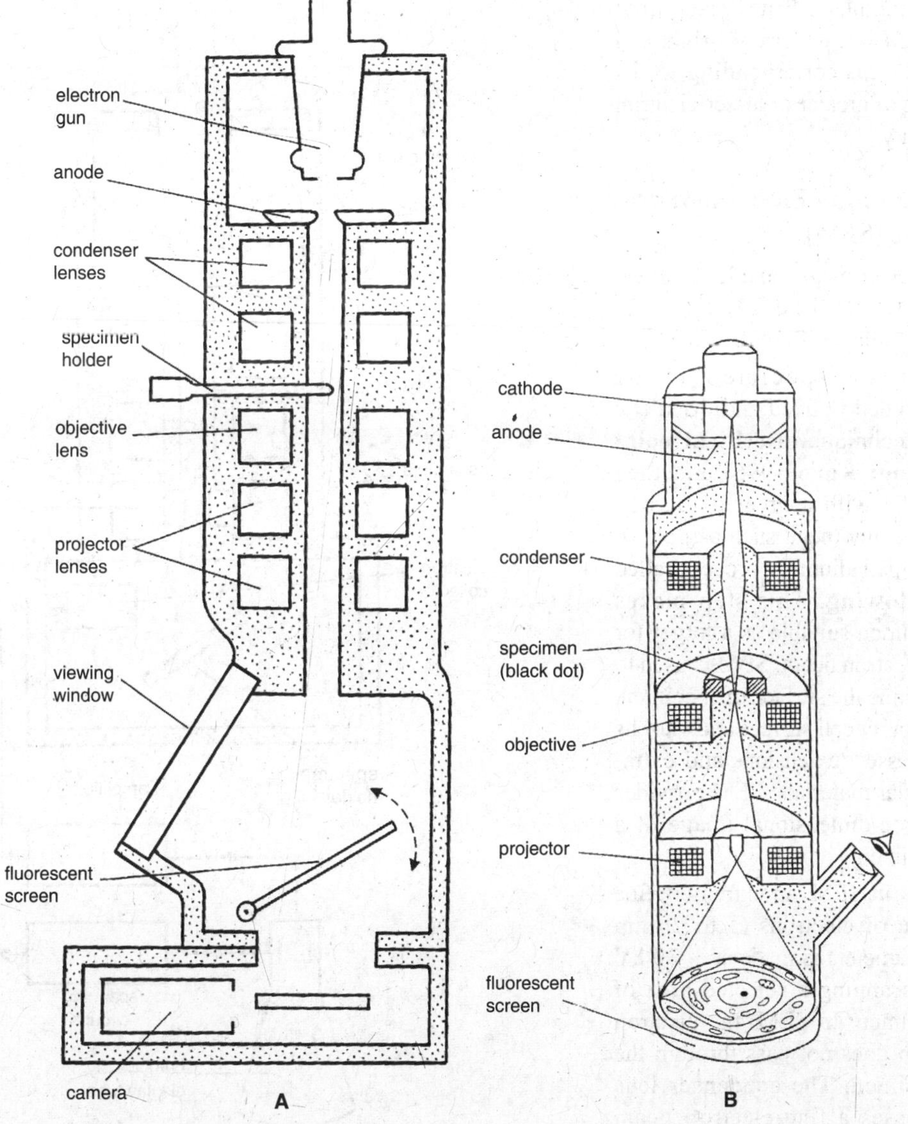

Fig. 2.11. Transmission electron microscope A–Diagrammatic view; B–Pathway of electron beam.

from a negatively charged electrode (**cathode** or electron gun). The electrons emitted from the gun are attracted towards the positively charged anode and then are focussed into beam by the electromagnetic **condenser**. This beam of electrons illuminates entire stained specimen. Many of these electrons pass right through the specimen and reach the electromagnetic objective. But some are absorbed or scattered by atoms of metallic stains that have combined with certain atoms of specimen. The **objective** magnifies the image of the specimen. This image is received by the third electromagnetic lens which works as **projection lens**. It further magnifies the image and projects it on a zinc sulphide or fluorescent screen at the bottom of TEM. This screen is similar to screen of a television tube. It is coated with a layer of crystals that respond to electrons by emitting visible light. The final image can also be captured on the photographic film.

Electrons that are not transmitted by the specimen leave correspondingly dark regions on the viewing plate. Thus, image from a TEM is a pattern of bright and dark areas corresponding to the areas of greater or lesser electron density.

2. Scanning Electron Microscope (SEM)

The electron gun and lens system of SEM is like TEM but its operation is different.

The specimen to be examined is fixed and dried (by the technique of **critical point drying; Karp** 1996) and then coated with a layer of carbon and heavy metal such as gold or gold-palladium—a process called **shadowing**. This step makes specimen suitable as a target for an electron beam. SEM is used to examine the surface of specimen, *i.e.*, outer cell surface and various processes, extensions and extra-cellular materials. SEM provides a three-dimensional image of a specimen.

In SEM, an extremely fine beam of electrons (5 to 20 nm in diameter) is made at 3–30 kV for scanning a selected area of specimen. In SEM, the electron beam does not pass through the specimen. The condenser lens focusses a fine electron beam on the surface of the specimen. The beam is moved rapidly back

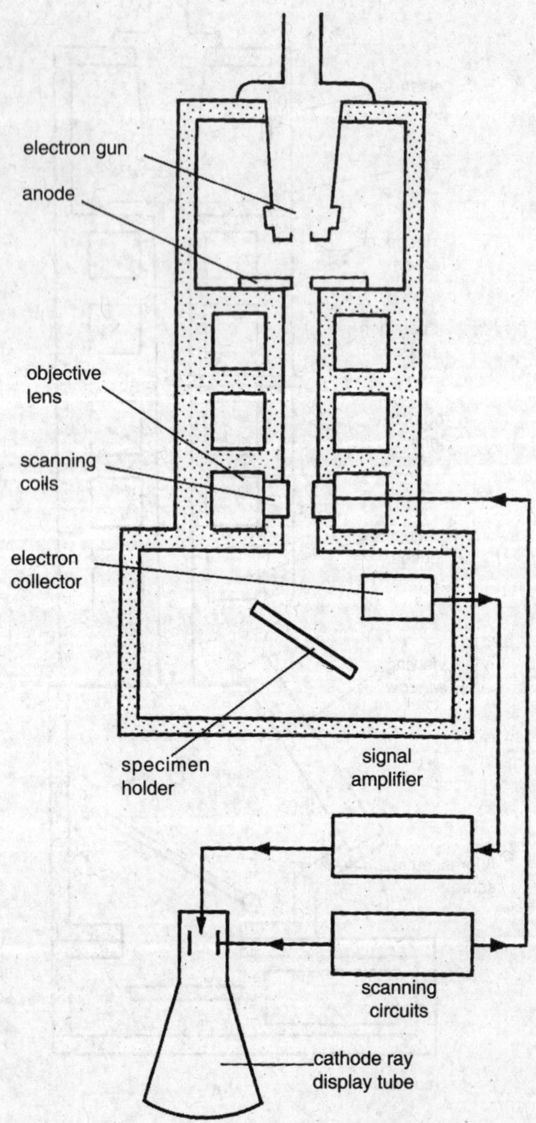

Fig. 2.12. A scanning electron microscope (SEM).

and forth by **beam deflectors** to scan the specimen surface. As the electron beam hits the surface of specimen it excites the specimen molecules to high energy levels. Due to the this, **secondary electrons** are emitted from the metallic surface. These secondary electrons are collected by the positively charged grid. The **collector** gives rise to a flash of light in a solid scintillator. The light output is amplified in a **photo-multiplier** or **video amplifier** (Fig. 2.12). The signal from the grid is transferred to a television tube which scans and forms the image on the screen. Thus image formation in the SEM is indirect compared to that in the TEM.

The amount of secondary electrons produced depends on the angle of specimen points with the scanning beam. Surface perpendicular to the beam produces maximum electrons while surfaces at greater angles release less electrons. Thus, the number of electrons produced depends on the three-dimensional shape of the specimen surface (or surface topology, *i.e.*, the crevices, hills and pits of the specimen). Accordingly the image contains bright (which correspond the elevations or ridges in specimen surface) and darker regions (which correspond to the valleys). These shadows give the image a three-dimensional appearance.

The resolving power of SEM is comparatively less than that of transmission electron microscope. It has an effective magnification upto 20,000 times.

REVISION QUESTIONS

1. Explain the principle, working and uses of phase contrast microscope.
2. How does an electron microscope differ from light microscope?
3. What is the resolving power of an optical system? State the working principle of phase contrast and dark field microscopy.
4. Write short notes on the following:
   (*i*) Electron microscopy
   (*ii*) Resolving power
   (*iii*) Compound microscope
   (*iv*) Fundamentals of TEM
   (*v*) Phase contrast microscope

3 Chapter CYTOLOGICAL AND CYTOCHEMICAL TECHNIQUES

3.1 CELL FRACTIONATION AND CENTRIFUGATION

Sometimes it becomes necessary to break up tissues and cells and to isolate various parts of the cell for structural or biochemical analysis. For this purpose, the technique of cell fractionation is employed. Cell fractionation method involves, essentially the homogenisation or destruction of cell boundaries by different mechanical or chemical procedures, followed by the separation of the subcellular fractions according to mass, surface and specific gravity by centrifuges.

The centrifuge is the most important tool available to cell biologists for the separation and analysis of subcellular organelles and their constituent macromolecules. Centrifugal force is generated by placing test tubes containing samples to be fractionated in a holder called a **rotor** and then spinning the rotor at high speeds by the help of a **motor** in a centrifuge. The ultra-centrifuge, developed by the Swedish chemist, **Theodor Svedberg** between 1920 to 1940, is a special high-speed instrument capable of spinning rotors at speeds of 100,000 revolutions per minute or more. The large forces generated by these high speeds make it possible to isolate not just organelles but macromolecules such as proteins and nucleic acids as well.

Stokes formula. The rate of movement of any particle subjected to a centrifugal force is given by **Stokes formula**:

$$\frac{dx}{dt} = \frac{2r^2(\rho_p - \rho_M)}{9^\eta} . g$$

where dx/dt is the velocity with which the particle moves towards the bottom of the tube, r is the particle radius, ρ_p and ρ_M are the respective densities of the particle and the suspending medium and g is the centrifugal force exerted on the particle. This formula tells us that when the density of a particle exceeds that of the medium, its velocity will be positive and the particle will migrate in the direction of the force field (towards the bottom of tube). If the particle is less dense than the medium, its velocity will be negative, meaning that it will move towards the top of the tube. Finally, if the density of particle is exactly equal to the density of the suspending medium, the particle will not move because the term, $\rho_p - \rho_M = 0$.

Types of Centrifugation

(*a*) **Velocity centrifugation** (It separates organelles and molecules based on differences in size);

(*i*) **Differential centrifugation;**

(*ii*) **Moving zone centrifugation**

(*b*) **Isodensity centrifugation** (It separates organelles and molecules on the basis of differences in density).

For these centrifugations, the following three centrifugation processes are employed:

1. **High speed centrifugation.** In high speed centrifugation rotor runs at a speed of about 20,000 rpm and generates a gravitational pull of about 50,000 g. At this speed most microorganisms, cell debris and cell organelles form sediments. It is used in **differential centrifugation**.
2. **Ultracentrifugation.** Ultracentrifuge (Fig. 3.1) of **Svedburg** operates at extremely high speed (about 75,000 rpm) and produces a gravitational pull of about 500,000 g. It is used for **differential centrifugation**, **zonal centrifugation**, **density gradient centrifugation** and **isopycnic centrifugation**.
3. **Analytical centrifugation.** This is the latest and most sophisticated instrument. Its sample container has a quartz window and the rotor has an optical system. It is possible to observe the material sedimenting and measure the sedimentation rate during the run.

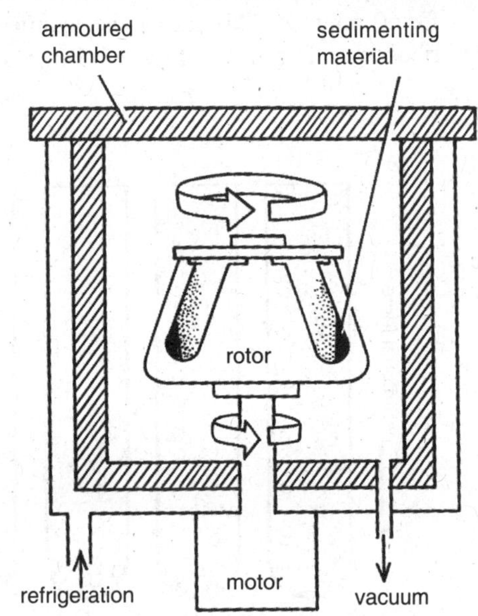

Fig. 3.1. The ultracentrifuge. The sample (*i.e.*, homogenate) is contained in tubes that are inserted into a ring of cylindrical holes in a metal rotor. Rapid rotation of the rotor generates immense centrifugal forces, which cause particles in sample to sediment. The vacuum tends to reduce friction, preventing heating of the rotor and allowing the refrigeration system to maintain the sample at 4°C.

Mechanism of Centrifugation (Cell Fractionation)

1. In the cell fractionation, the cells are gently broken by grinding a small piece of tissue in a homogeniser having a moving close-fitting glass or plastic pestle within a tube that contains a medium such as sucrose solution to preserve the cellular organelles (Fig. 3.3). The solution containing homogenised or disrupted cells, is called **homogenate**. In a homogenate the particles of different sizes are distributed homogeneously. The homogenate is subjected differential centrifugation of increasing velocity.
2. The tissue/liver homogenate is subjected first to low speed centrifugation at 700X g for 10 minutes. This sediments cell nuclei to the bottom of centrifuge tube. This **sediment-I** is called **nuclear fraction**. Nuclear fraction includes nucleus, intact cells, tissue debris and chloroplasts (in case of plant cells).
3. The overlying **supernatant-I** is transferred to another tube for second centrifugation at 10,000Xg for 20 minutes. The **sediment-II** is called **mitochondrial fraction**. It contains mitochondria and also lysosomes and peroxisomes.

4. Again the **supernatant-II** is removed and subjected to third centrifugation at (~ 100,000Xg) for 60 minutes. This causes the sedimentation of **microsomal fraction** which includes free ribosomes, fragments of smooth ER, rough ER, Golgi apparatus and plasma membrane.

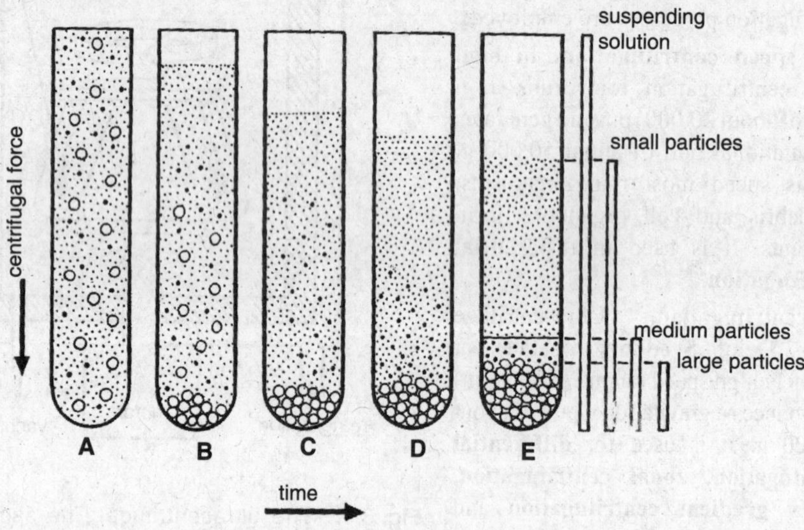

Fig. 3.2. Diagrammatic representation of the process of centrifugation and sedimentation of particles of different sizes.

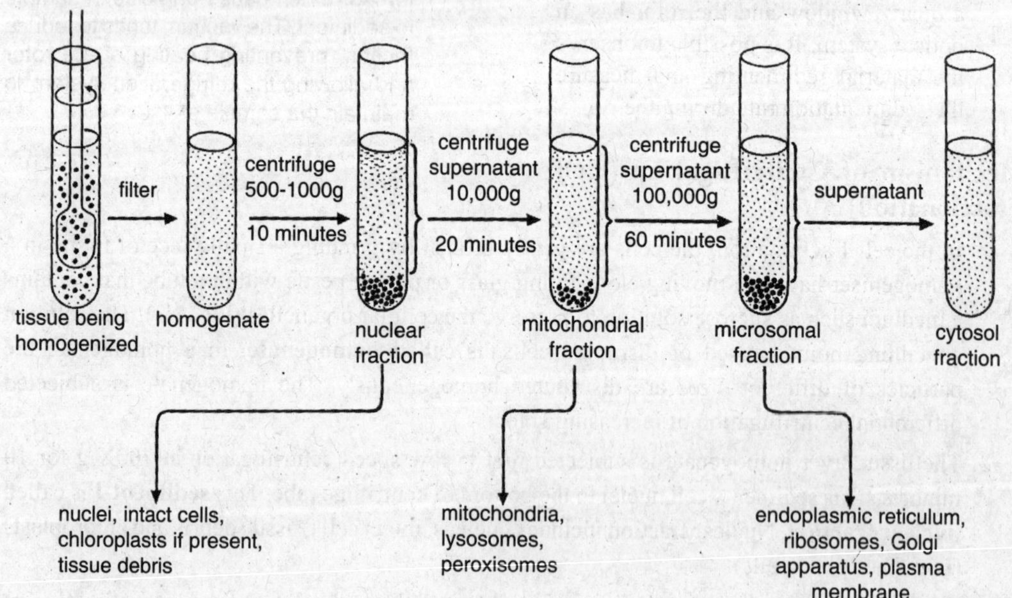

Fig. 3.3. Subcellular fractionation by differential centrifugation.

5. The **final supernatant** contains soluble molecules of cytoplasm and is called **cytosol fractions**. It contains proteins, soluble nucleic acids, soluble polysaccharides, lipid droplets and other particles. These are separated by **chromatography, dialysis** and **electrophoresis**.

The technique of cell fractionation has been improved through the use of **density gradient centrifugation**. In this method, centrifuge tube is loaded with layers of solution of varying densities of either sucrose, heavy water, cesium chloride or albumin, in a gradient from top to bottom. Once the gradient is formed, the homogenate is layered on the top and centrifuged until the particles reach equilibrium with the gradient. For this reason, this type of separation is called **equilibrium density** or **isopycnic centrifugation**.

3.2 AUTORADIOGRAPHY

Autoradiography is a technique which is used to locate radioactive isotopes in cells, tissues, organs and whole organisms. A specimen is exposed to a solution containing molecules that have been made radioactive by the incorporation of radioactive isotopes, such as tritium (^3H), carbon 14 (^{14}C), phosphorus (^{32}P) and sulphur (^{35}S). The tagged molecules are often precursor molecules used by the cell in the synthesis of other needed molecules. At intervals, samples are removed from the solution; in case of smaller tissues, the samples are sectioned and mounted on glass slides or grids. The sections are then coated with a photographic emulsion and stored in the dark for periods ranging up to several months.

When a radioactive atom emits a beta particle (*i.e.*, electron) the photographic emulsion is affected in a manner similar to the exposure of a photographic emulsion to light. Over a period of time sufficient radioactive emissions occur to affect the silver grains of the emulsion. Black spots will appear at those sites when the emulsion is developed. Such spots will mark sites in the tissues where the radioactive atoms have accumulated. These sites can be identified by examining the stained tissue sections under the light microscope.

In the technique of autoradiography, for the study of DNA metabolism of cell ^3H-thymidine is used; for RNA metabolism ^3H-uridine is used; for protein synthesis various tritiated (^3H-tagged) amino acids are used; and for polysaccharides and glycoproteins tritiated monosaccharides such as ^3H-mannose and ^3H-fucose are employed.

Pulse-labelling technique. This technique is used for those cases where biological molecules undergo considerable modifications after their synthesis (*e.g.*, ribosomal RNA). Here, actively growing cells are exposed to a radioactive precursor for a short period. The labelled precursor is then removed and replaced by 'cold' (unlabelled) precursor molecules. The unlabelled precursors are incorporated into the newly synthesized molecules and have the effect of 'chasing' the previously synthesized molecules containing the radioactive precursor through any maturation process. If the molecular species under investigation is sampled shortly after the start of the experiment, only the primary synthetic product will contain radioactivity. After longer time intervals, the original radioactive molecules will have been replaced with non-radioactive molecules. In this way the flow of radioactivity through a maturation process can be followed, together with any movement of molecular species within the cell.

3.3 CHROMATOGRAPHY

The separation of molecules from biological materials is an important part of biochemical work. Various methods are used for separating molecules. **Chromatography** is a method of separation which is utilised for separation and purification of both organic and inorganic molecules. The word 'chromatography' has its origin in Greek words '*chromo*' meaning colour and '*graphy*' meaning to measure. The Russian botatinst **Mikhail Tswett** is credited with the original development of this technique. In 1903, he reported the successful separation of a mixture of plant pigments using a column of calcium carbonate. The early methods of isolation and purification of compounds of mixtures were empirical, slow and laborious. But with the advancements in separation procedures over the years, chromatography has become a highly efficient technique for separation and purification of compounds.

Chromatography is based on the phenomenon of adsorption and differential migration of components of a mixture or a compound. This needs the following two basic things:

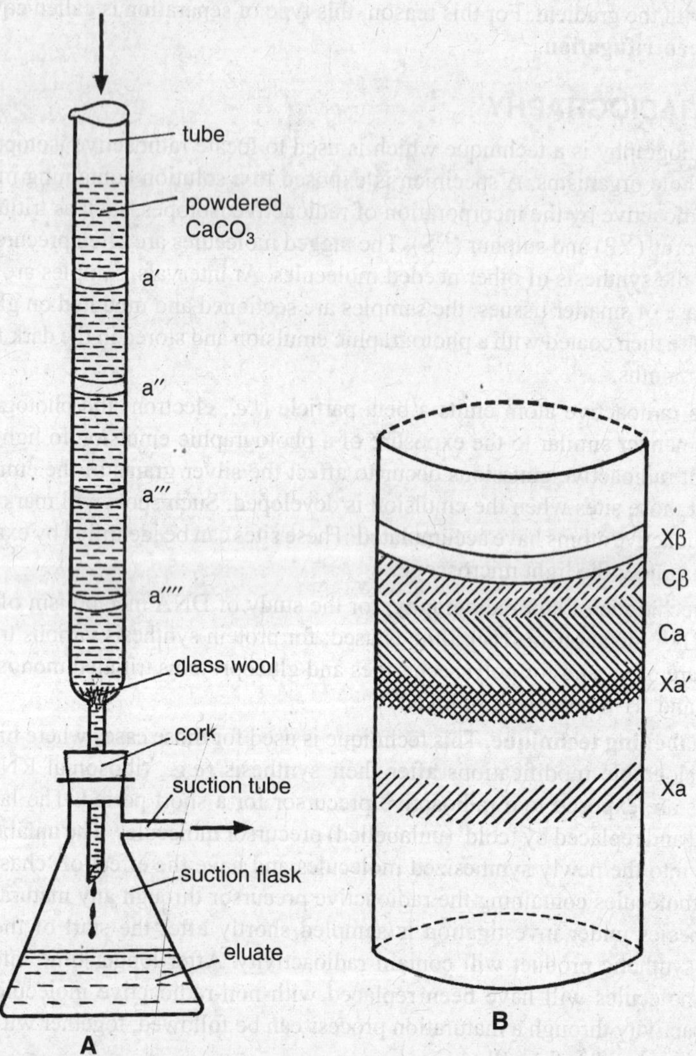

Fig. 3.4. A—An apparatus for column chromatography: B—Chromatogram of chlorophyll.

1. A force for propelling the molecules of any solution, mixture or cytosol. It is called **mobile phase** and it involves moving solvent.
2. A selective impedance causing differential movement of various molecules (*i.e.*, called **impeding medium** or **adsorbent**). It is called **immobile phase** and it involves the matrix (filter paper, $CaCO_3$, etc.) through which the solvent is moving.

During chromatography the mixture or solution is allowed to percolate in an insoluble medium or adsorbent or matrix which has different affinity for molecules of different substances. The molecules migrate through the medium (matrix) at different rates and are separated. For example, if a solution of leaf pigment, chlorophyll in petroleum ether is allowed to percolate through a column of powdered calcium carbonate, the pigments are initially absorbed by pure solvent (*i.e.*, petroleum ether), the individual pigments—carotene, chlorophyll and xanthophyll separate and appear as the coloured bands or zones on the calcium carbonate column like the light rays in spectrum. Such a preparation is called **chromatogram**.

The impeding medium (or immobile phase) is called **adsorbent**. The liquid that passes through adsorbent is **filterate** and the solution obtained after eluting adsorbed substances is **eluate**. The substances that are separated are **samples** or **solutes** and preparation having these solutes is called **chromatogram**.

Principle of Chromatography

Chromatography is based on **partition** or **distribution coefficient** (**Kd**). For two such immiscible (*i.e.*, liquids which are not able to be mixed together) phases A and B, the value for this coefficient is constant at a given temperature and is given as:

$$\text{Kd} = \frac{\text{Concentration in phase A}}{\text{Concentration in phase B}}$$

The term **effective distribution coefficient** is defined as the total amount of substance in one phase divided by the total amount present in the other phase.

$$\text{Effective distribution coefficient} = \frac{\text{Total amount in phase A}}{\text{Total amount in phase B}}$$

Basically all chromatographic systems consist of the **stationary phase** which may be a solid, gel, liquid or solid/liquid mixture that is immobilised, and the **mobile phase** which may be liquid or gas. The mobile phase flows over or through the stationary phase. The choice of stationary and mobile phase is made that the compounds to be separated have different distribution coefficient.

Types of Chromatography

Chromatography can be classified into various types depending upon the type of solid support, stationary phase and the mobile phase. Depending upon the physical state of the stationary phase, whether the stationary phase is solid or liquid, chromatography can be divided into two types:

1. **Adsorption chromatography.** The chromatography in which stationary phase is solid, *e.g.*, thin-layer chromatography and ion exchange chromatography are adsorption chromatography.

Table 3.1. Phase of various types of chromatographic techniques.

	Technique	Stationary phase	Mobile phase
1.	Adsorption chromatography	Solid	Liquid
	(*i*) Thin-layer chromatography	Solid	Liquid
	(*ii*) Ion-exchange chromatography	Solid	Liquid
	(*iii*) Affinity chromatography	Solid	Liquid
2.	Partition chromatography	Liquid	Liquid
	(*i*) Paper chromatography	Liquid (supported by cellulose fibers)	Liquid
	(*ii*) Gas-liquid chromatography	Liquid or solid	Gas

2. **Partition chromatography.** When the stationary phase is liquid, it is called partition chromatography, *e.g.*, paper chromatography.

In an alternative method, chromatography is divided into following two main types:

I. Column Chromatography

In column chromatography, the stationary phase is attached to a suitable matrix and it is packed into a glass or metal column (Fig. 3.4). The mobile phase is passed through the column either by gravity or by use of a pumping system. Adsorption, ion exchange, molecular exclusion, affinity and gas-liquid chromatographies are examples of column chromatography.

In column chromatography an insoluble medium is packed into a glass tube; the length and width of this tube influence the separation of the molecules. The molecules to be separated are applied to the top of the column and their migration is started by adding a solvent. The characteristic separation which results depends on the choice of solvent and carrier material. A positively charged carrier binds negatively charged molecules; other carriers contain pores which are penetrated by the smaller molecules, which are, therefore, slowed down. The solvent flows through the column, the *eluate* (the liquid emerging from the bottom of the column) is collected in many fractions (Fig. 3.5). The eluate fractions contain the separated classes of molecules. Column chromatography is important for the separations of mixtures of proteins, that is, for the isolation of enzymes such as cytochrome c or RNA polymerase.

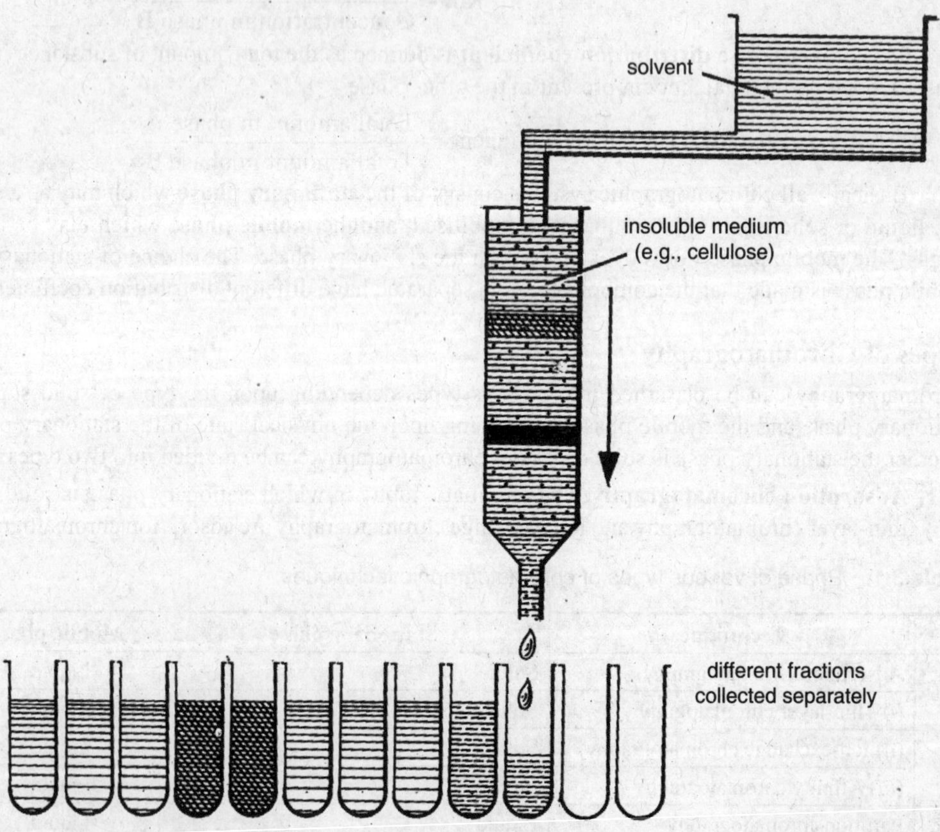

Fig. 3.5. Column chromatography.

Adsorbents and solvents. A few of the adsorbents used in column chromatography are carbonates of calcium, magnesium and sodium; various forms of charcoal activated in special ways;

Fuller's earth, bentonite, Lloyd's reagent, talcum, clays of different types; alumina, silica gel, cellulose, resin, starch, sucrose, inulin and benzoic acid, etc. The adsorbent column neither dissolves in the developing solvent nor reacts chemically with the solvent or the substance to be separated.

The **solvents** commonly used are water, aqueous solutions of various acids, alkalis and salts; alcohols, ketones and cyclohexanone, hydrocarbons such as benzene, chloroform and carbon tetrachloride, etc.

Table 3.2. Differences between column and partition chromatography.

	Column chromatography		Partition chromatography
1.	It was discovered by **Tswett**.	1.	It was discovered by **Martin Synge**.
2.	The adsorbent column may be of carbonates of calcium, magnesium or sodium; activated charcoal; Fuller's earth, resin, starch, etc.	2.	The adsorbent column may be of silica gel, cellulose or starch which are capable of holding water.
3.	Solvent used may be water, aqueous solution of inorganic acids or alkalies or salts, alcohol, ketones, hydrocarbons, benzene, chloroform or carbon tetrachloride.	3.	More than one solvents are used at a time. The substance to be separated are dissolved in alcohol and are then passed through the adsorbent column, already moistened with water.
4.	Column chromatography is based on the principle of differential rate of diffusion of the substances to be separated.	4.	Partition chromatography is based on the principle of differential solubility of substances to be separated in two or more immiscible solvents.
5.	This technique is used to separate any type of substances from any solvent.	5.	This technique is used to separate water soluble compounds from a mixture of two or more immiscible solvents.

II. Thin Layer Chromatography or Planer Chromatography

In this case, the stationary phase, attached to a suitable matrix is coated thinly on to a glass, plastic or metal foil plate. The mobile liquid phase passes across the thin-layer plate by capillary action.

Paper chromatography is a planer chromatography in which the stationary phase is supported by cellulose fibers of a paper sheet. The mobile phase passes over by capillary action over the stationary phase.

A. Adsorption chromatography. In includes the following five types of chromatographies:

1. Adsorption chromatography. This is most commonly used to separate non-ionic and water-insoluble compounds such as triglycerides, vitamins and some drugs.

In this technique, column is packed with an adsorbent. When the sample is passed through the column, the molecules with specific groups bind with adsorbent. The strength of binding of a particular anylate depends upon the functional groups present in its structure. Hydroxyl groups and aromatic groups tend to increase interaction depends upon the relative strength of the interaction of various molecules present in the eluent to the specific adsorption sites. As eluent is constantly passed down the column, differences in the binding strengths eventually lead to the separation of the analytes. The adsorption chromatography is influenced more by the presence of specific groups than by simple molecular size because only a specific group rather than the whole molecule can interact with the adsorption site.

2. Ion-exchange chromatography. In ion exchange chromatography molecules are separated by their difference in charge. The ion-exchange resin is used as chromatographic adsorbent which consists of porous polystyrene beads (polymers) to which ionizable groups are added chemically. Ion-exchange chromatography depends on the attraction between oppositely charged particles. The technique is used for the separation of many biological materials having ionizable groups such as amino acids and proteins.

Column is packed with an ion-exchanger which may be either cation or anion exchanger. **Cation exchangers** (*e.g.*, **DEAE-** or **diethylaminoethyl-cellulose**) possess negatively charged groups and attract positively charged anions. These are also known as **acidic ion-exchanger** as their negatively charges result from the ionization of acidic groups. **Anion-exchangers (*e.g.*, CM or carboxy methyl cellulose)** have positively charged groups that attract negative charged cations. These are also called **basic-ion exchange materials** since positively charges generally result from the association of protons with basic groups.

When a sample (a mixture of charged molecules such as proteins) is passed through the column carrying the ion-exchange material (*e.g.*, cation exchanger), the molecules with greater positive charges interact with the ion-exchange material and bind tighly to the molecules carrying lesser number of positive charges. Molecules with negative charge may just be washed out without any binding. Then, the bound molecules are eluted out one by one with an eluting buffer of a suitable pH. A number of ion-exchanger depends upon the stability of the sample components, their relative molecular mass and the specific requirements of the separation.

3. Molecular exclusion (permeation) chromatography. In molecular exclusion chromatography, the molecules are separated on the basis of their molecular size and shapes. A variety of porous materials act as molecular sieve, *e.g.*, glass granules and a number of the gels are used as molecular sieves. When the separation is carried out by using the gels as the molecular sieve, the technique is also called **gel filteration chromatography**. If porous glass granules are utilised as molecular sieve, the technique is called **controlled pore glass chromatography**. The term exclusion (permeation) chromatography describes all molecular separation processes using molecular sieves. When the mixture is poured over a column filled with gel particles or porous glass granules, large molecules in the mixture are completely excluded from the pores and pass through the interstitial spaces and appear in the eluate first. The smaller molecules are distributed between the mobile phase inside and outside the molecular sieve and then pass through the column at a slower rate, hence appear last in the eluate (Fig. 3.6).

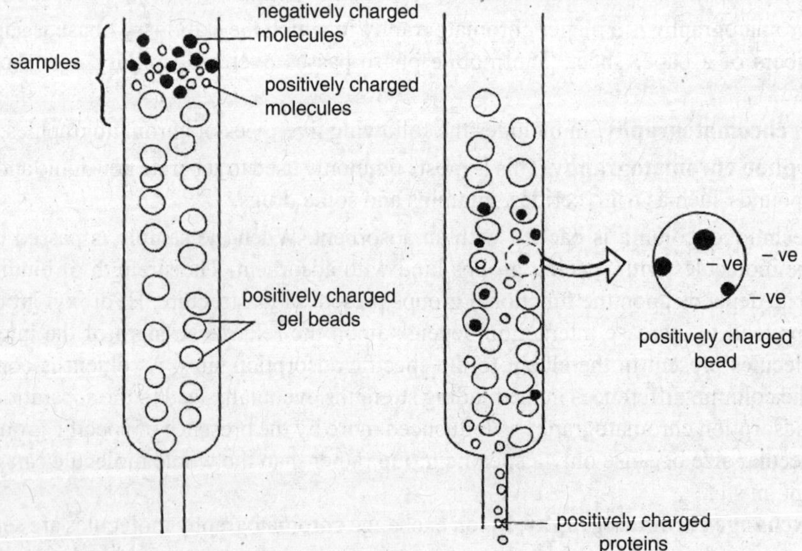

Fig. 3.6. Ion-exchange chromatography.

4. Affinity chromatography. Affinity chromatography is the method to separate all the molecules of a particular specificity from a mixture. It is basically a type of adsorption chromatography in which the molecules to be purified are specifically and reversibly adsorbed by a complimentary binding substance or ligand immobilised on insoluble support matrix. The technique is used for the separation of specific antibodies from the blood serum. For the purification of antibodies an immunoadsorbent is prepared which consists of a solid matrix to which antigen 'ag' has been coupled. The matrix used must be stable during binding of macromolecules and its subsequent elution. Agarose, sephadex and some derivatives of cellulose can be used as matrix. When the serum is passed over the immuno-adsorbent, the specific antibodies in the mixture (serum) will bind with the 'ag' and retained. Other antibodies and serum proteins will pass through unimpeded. Then a reagent is passed through the column to release the bound antibodies from the immunoadsorbent. The eluate is then dialyzed to remove the reagent used for elution (Fig. 3.7).

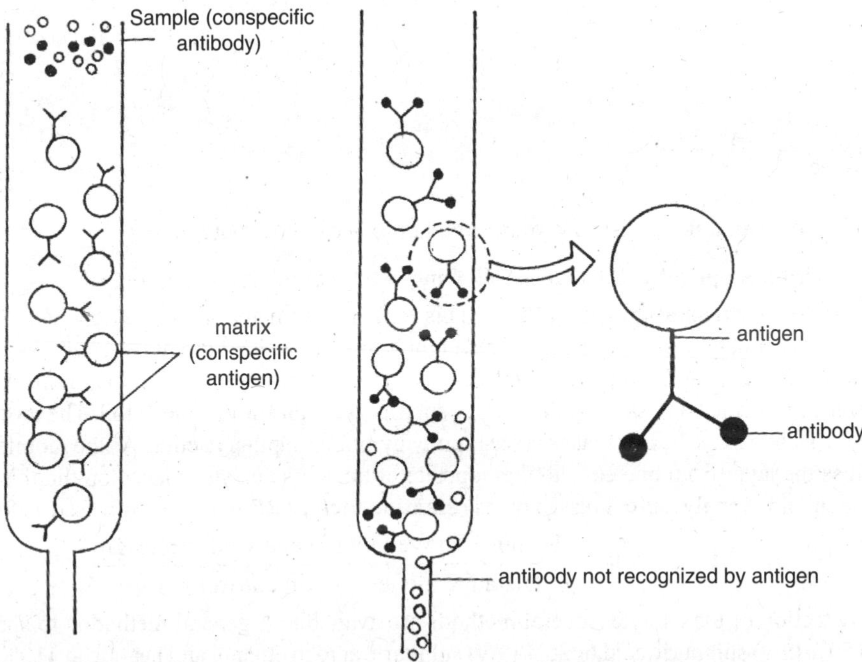

Fig. 3.7. Affinity chromatography.

5. Gas chromatography. This technique is used to separate volatile organic compounds. Gas chromatography is an efficient technique for identification of gases, pollutants, drugs, vitamins, alkaloids, etc. This technique was introduced by **Martin** and **Synge** (1952). This type of chromatography involves injecting the volatile materials into a column contaning a liquid or solid stationary phase. A gas chromatograph consists of a flowing mobile phase, an injection port, a separation column containing the stationary phase and a detector. The stationary phase may be either a liquid or solid. In gas-liquid chromatography (GLC), the mobile phase is a gas and the stationary phase is a thin layer of non-volatile liquid bound to a solid support. In gas-solid chromatography a solid adsorbent acts as the stationary phase and an adsorption process occurs. The organic compounds are separated due to differences in their partitioning behaviour between the mobile gas phase and stationary phase in the column.

In gas chromatography, the sample is injected into the injection port from where it is carried into the column. The eluate released from the column pass through a detector which is linked via an amplifier to a chart recorder which records a peak as a particular compound passes through a detector.

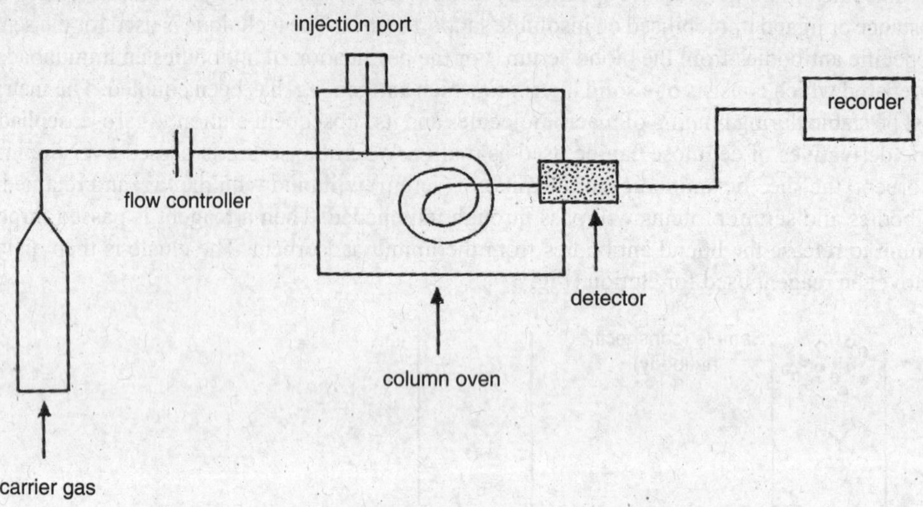

Fig. 3.8. Schematic representation of a gas chromatography.

B. Partition chromatography. It includes following two types of chromatographies:

1. Thin layer chromatography (TLC). This type of chromatography is extensively used in quantitative determination of high molecular weight compounds. Carbohydrates, dyes, pigments, vitamins, steroids, etc., can be separated and characterized by this method. In TLC, a thin layer of stationary phase is formed on a suitable flat surface such as glass, plastic or a metal foil. The movement of the mobile phase across the layer takes place rapidly by simple capillary action. As the mobile phase moves across the layer from one edge to the opposite, it transfers analytes placed on the thin layer. The movement of the analyte is expressed by its **retention factor (Rf)** which is expressed as follows:

$$Rf = \frac{\text{Distance moved by the analyte from origin}}{\text{Distance moved by solvent from origin}}$$

For detection of the analyte, several methods are available. A general method is to spray the plate with 50% (v/v) sulphuric acid or 25% (v/v) sulphuric acid in ethanol and heating at 110°C. This results in most of the compounds showing up as brown spots.

Table 3.3. Some differences between TLC and GLC.

	TLC or Thin-layer chromatography		GLC or Gas-liquid chromatography
1.	Adsorbent may be cellulose powder, alumina or cellulose.	1.	Adsorbent or the immobile phase is represented by liquid.
2.	The mobile phase is the solvent (liquid).	2.	The mobile phase is inert gas such as nitrogen, carbon dioxide, helium or argon.

2. Paper chromatography. Paper chromatography is a widely used technique in the separation of organic and biochemical products in laboratories. In this technique, stationary liquid phase is supported by cellulose fibres of a paper sheet. The mobile phase is developing solvent. The mobile phase passes over the stationary phase by capillary action. In paper chromatography the test solution is applied as a small spot on the chromatography paper (Whatman's No. 1 paper) and dried. The solvent is allowed to travel on the paper. As the solvent moves it carries the mixture components along with it. There are two types of paper chromatography: (*a*) **Ascending** (Fig. 3.9) and (*b*) **descending chroma-tography**. In ascending chromatography, the mobile phase (solvent) is at the bottom of the chromatographic chamber. The sample spot (loading spot) is kept in position just above the surface of the solvent. As the solvent moves vertically up on the paper, separation of the sample is achieved.

In descending chromatography, the mobile phase (solvent) is kept in the upper position of the chromatography chamber. The paper is inserted with the upper end with sample spot close to the mobile phase kept at the upper position of chromatographic chamber. Separation of the sample occurs as the solvent moves downwards due to capillary action and gravity.

A number of methods are available for the detection of eluate. Spraying with aqueous solution of 0.2% ninhydrin saturated with butyl alcohol is commonly employed for identification. The identification of a given compound is made on the basis of its Rf value.

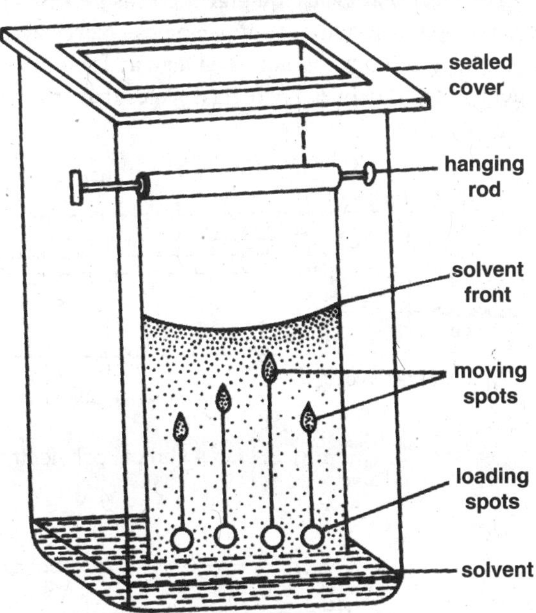

Fig. 3.9. Ascending paper chromatography.

3.4 ELECTROPHORESIS

Electrophoresis is a biochemical technique used to separate charged particles from a mixture (Fig. 3.10). The term 'electrophoresis' describes the migration of a charged particle under the influence of an electric field. This is a simple, rapid, sensitive and versatile analytical tool used to study and purify the charged molecules such as amino acids, peptides, proteins, nucleotides and nucleic acids. These molecules exist in solution as electrically charged species either as cations (–) and anions (+). Under the influence of an electric current these particles will migrate either to the cathode or anode, depending on the nature of their net charge.

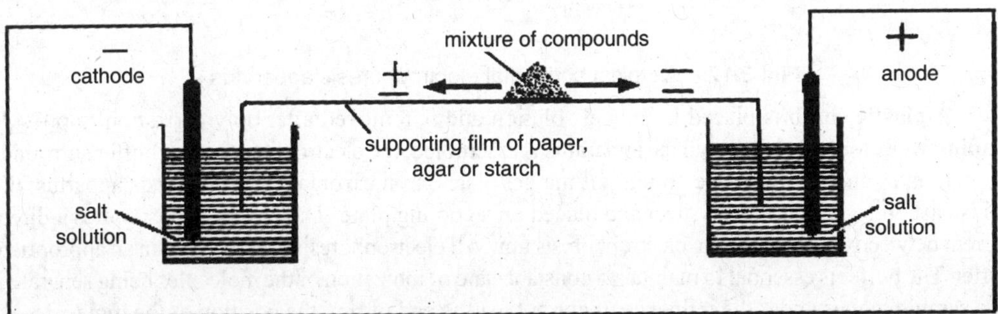

Fig. 3.10. Electrophoresis.

Electrophoresis is a technique, developed by **Tiselius** in 1937, for the analysis and separation of colloids and is based on the movement of charged colloidal particles in an electric field. **Arne Wilhelm Kaurin Tiselius** (1902–1971), Swedish Chemist awarded the 1948 Nobel Prize for Chemistry for his development in order to apply electrophoresis to the study of proteins, notably those of the blood.

The electrophoresis equipment consists of two units—a power pack and an electrophoresis unit. Electrophoresis units are of two types—**vertical** (Fig. 3.11) and **horizontal** (Fig. 3.12). Vertical slab gel units are commercially available and routinely used to separate proteins in acrylamide gel. The gel is formed between two glass plates that are clamped together.

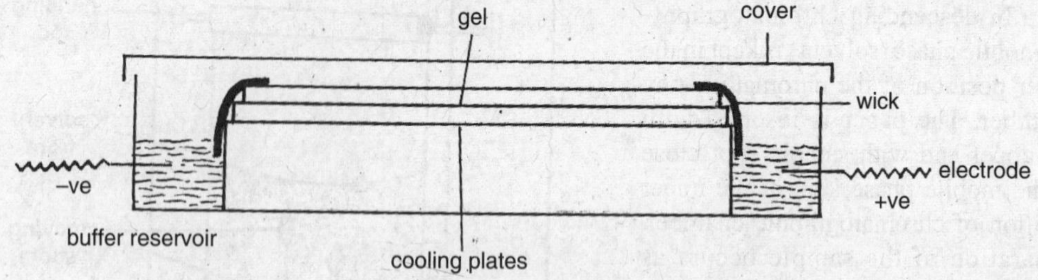

Fig. 3.11. A vertical gel electrophoresis apparatus.

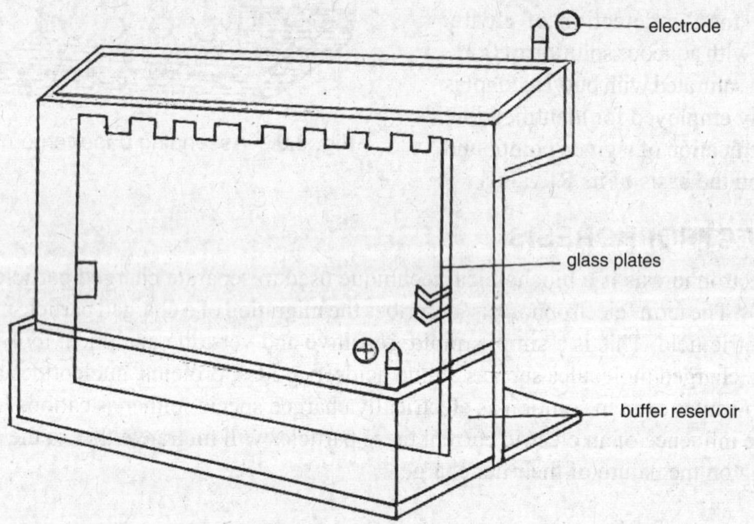

Fig. 3.12. A typical horizontal electrophoresis apparatus.

A **plastic comb** is placed in the gel solution and is removed after polymerization to provide **loading wells** for samples. When the apparatus is assembled, the electrophoresis tank buffer surrounds the gel plates and affords some cooling of the gel plates. In horizontal electrophoresis appartus, the gel is cast on a glass or plastic sheet and placed on a cooling plate. The power back supplies a direct current between the electrodes in electrophoresis unit. All electrophoresis is carried out in an appropriate buffer. The buffer is essential to maintain a constant state of ionization of the molecules being separated. The sample moves under the influence of current. At the end of run, the position of the molecules on the gel is fixed with a fixative to prevent simple diffusion. Then the separated components are stained to visualize them. The **bands** can be quantified (by elution or by scanning with densitometer) as the uptake of the dye is directly proportional to the concentration of the molecules in each band.

The rate of electrophoretic migration (or 'mobility') depends on the pH of the medium, strength of electric field, magnitude of the net charge on the molecule, and the size and shape of the molecule.

Types of Electrophoresis

1. Paper electrophoresis. It is most common type of electrophoresis which is run in clinical laboratories. This technique is used for separation of small molecules such as amino acids, peptides and carbohydrates.

2. Agarose gel electrophoresis. Starch, agarose or polysaccharide gels are used for electrophoretic techniques. Agarose is a linear polysaccharide made up of the basic repeat unit agarobiose. Agarose gel is formed by boiling dry agarose in aqueous buffer until a clean solution forms. This is allowed to cool at room temperature to form a rigid gel. The pore size in the gel depends upon the initial concentration of agarose. If the concentration is low large pore sizes are formed. Agarose is usually used at concentration between 1% and 3%. Agarose gels are used for electrophoresis of both proteins and nucleic acids. Agarose gel electrophoresis run by placing the gel under the level of buffer is most commonly employed in all the nucleic acid research applications such as DNA fingerprinting, sequencing and recombinant DNA technology. Agarose gel is also used in techniques such as immuno-electrophoresis (used for antigens and antibodies).

3. SDS-Page. SDS-polyacrylamide gel electrophoresis is a widely used technique for the qualitative analysis of protein mixtures. The relative molecular mass of proteins can also be determined by this method. Sodium dodecyl sulphate (SDS) is an anionic detergent. In this method the protein mixture (sample) is first boiled in a buffer containing β-merceptoethanol and SDS. This denatures the proteins and SDS binds with the proteins. The sample buffer also contains an ionizable tracking dye which allows the electrophoretic run to be monitored. It also contains sucrose and glycerol. These allow the sample to settle easily through the electrophoresis buffer to the bottom when injected into the loading wells. Once the samples are all loaded, a current is passed through the gel. Normally 15% polyacrylamide gel is used as the separating gel for separating proteins in the range of molecular mass of 100,000 to 10,000.

3.5 DIALYSIS

It is a sensitive method for separating lower molecular-weight component from macromolecules. A thin membrane in the form of a tube is filled with the solution containing the molecules to be separated. The pore size of the membrane allows the diffusion of small molecules such as salt or amino acids; larger molecules such as proteins or nucleic acids cannot pass through the pores and so remain inside the dialysis tube.

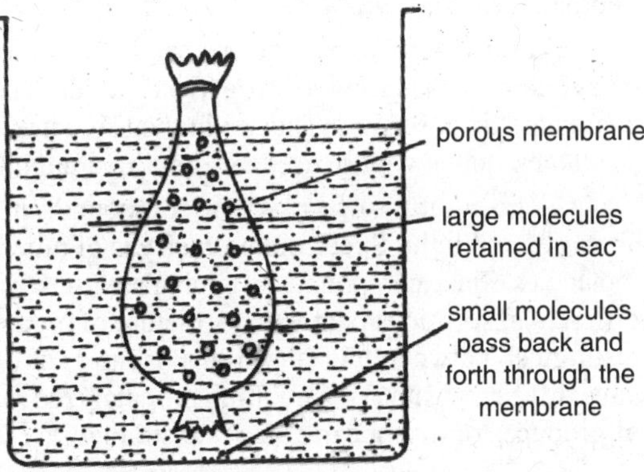

Fig. 3.13. Dialysis.

In dialysis, a protein solution is placed in a cylinder of cellophane tubing sealed at one end. The tubing is then sealed at the other end and suspended in a large volume of buffer. The cellophane membrane is semipermeable: high molecular weight proteins are too large to pass through the pores of the membrane so proteins remain inside the tubing while low molecular weight solutes including, in this case, ammonium and sulphate ions diffuse out and are replaced by solutes in the buffer.

3.6 SPECTROPHOTOMETRY

Spectrophotometry is the measurement of the intensity of different colours (wavelengths) present in a beam of light, normally using a prism or diffraction grating and a photoelectrical cell.

Spectrophotometer is an instrument for producing a spectrum and measuring the relation between absorption of electromagnetic radiation and frequency (or wavelength) of that radiation. It is a device used by researchers to determine how much radiation at various wavelengths a sample can absorb. The amount of absorption can be used to determine the concentration of particular molecules within a sample, because each type of molecule or macromolecule has its own characteristic wavelength(s) of absorption, called **absorption spectrum**. This instrument is used for colour comparison and in chemical analysis. Spectrophotometer is based on the principle of Beer–Lambert law.

A spectrophotometer typically has two light sources, which can emit ultraviolet or visible light. The light source is passed through a monochrometer, which emits light at a desired wavelength. This incident light then strikes a sample contained within a cuvette. Some of the incident light will be absorbed, and some will not. The unabsorbed light passes through the sample and is detected by the spectrophotometer. The amount of light which strikes the detector is substracted from the amount of incident light, yielding the measure of absorption. In this way, the spectrophotometer provides an absorption reading for the sample. This reading can be used to calculate the concentration of particular molecules or macromolecules in a sample.

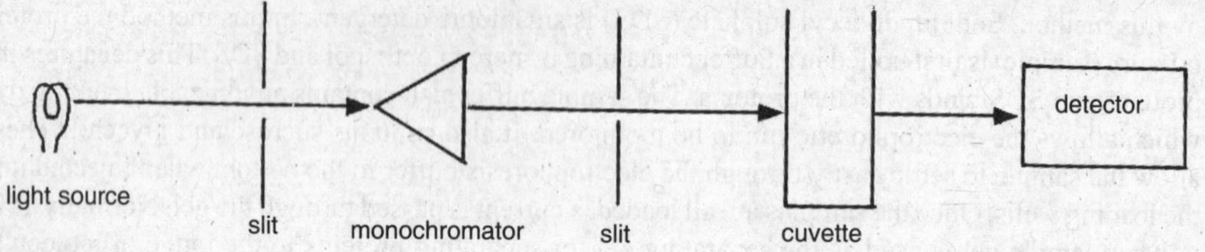

Fig. 3.14. Schematic representation of single beam spectrophotometer.

In detector, various types of photosensitive devices such as photovoltaic cells, phototubes or photoamultiplier tubes are used.

Applications of spectrometry. Spectrometry is one of most valuable analytical techniques of cytology. It has a wide variety of applications or uses. Compounds may be identified by their characteristic absorption spectra in the UV, visible or infrared regions of electromagnetic spectrum. The technique is widely used as a routine method of quantitative analysis of compounds.

Concentration of unknown compounds in a solution can be determined by measuring the absorption of light. Spectrophotometry is of much use in elucidating the structure of various organic molecules. Since compounds of similar structure have analogous absorption spectra, thus by comparing different absorption spectra, the structure of organic molecules can be elucidated. This technique can distinguish between 'cis' and 'trans' isomers of a complex. The geometrical isomers of compounds have different visible spectra. Enzyme catalyzed reactions can be studied by measuring the appearance of produces or disappearance of substrate with the help of spectrophotometry.

3.7 SAMPLE PREPARATION FOR MICROSCOPY

Cells are transparent and optically homogeneous: so either they are viewed as such by instruments such as phase contrast microscope or to produce necessary contrast, the cells are passed through various steps of slide preparation such as killing, fixation, dehydration, embedding, sectioning, staining and mounting.

Thus, superior specimens for microscopic examination can be obtained by **killing** the cells and coagulating or **fixing** the protoplasm by preservatives, called **fixatives** such as alcohols, formaldehyde, mercuric chloride, picric acid, acetic acid and mixture of these. The process of fixation involves the following events:

1. The proteins and other macromolecules are precipitated.
2. The intracellular hydrolytic enzymes are denatured, preventing autolysis.
3. Cross links are formed between macromolecules, making the preparation more stable and minimizing shrinkage upon drying.
4. Substances are introduced which prevent attack by microorganisms.
5. The tissues become stiffer, making their sectioning easier.
6. The affinity of the tissue for dyes (stains) is increased.

Fixation is generally followed by **dehydration** (*i.e.*, gradual removal of water vapours from the tissue) by the organic solvents such as ethanol. The dehydrated specimens are **embedded**, *i.e.*, they are infiltrated with molten paraffin which hardens upon cooling and provides enough support to allow thin sections to be cut with a **microtome**. By the microtome, serial sections, 5 to 10 μm thick can be cut and placed on slides in the order of cutting and permitting a sequence of specimens for observation. These sections are stained with a non-vital-stain to increase the contrast.

Stains are the chemicals that can selectively attach to particular molecules of specific cellular structures and make them stand out from other parts of the cell. The non-vital stains fall into two main classes: **acid stains** such as eosin, orange *G*, aniline blue and fast green, all of which combine with basic molecules such as proteins of the fixed cells; and **basic stains** such as methylene blue, crystal violet, haematoxylin, basic fuchsin, etc., all of which combine with nucleic acids and other acidic molecules of the fixed cells. The cellular structures that stain with acid stains are called **acidophilic** and those that stain with basic dyes are called **basophilic**.

Methods of Sample Preparation for Transmission Electron Microscopy

The standard procedure for the preparation of specimen for TEM entails fixation, dehydration, staining and sectioning similar to light microscopy (Table 3.4). However, the most significant difference being the need for ultra-thin sections. Following techniques of sample preparation are generally used for different types of methods of studying ultrastructure of the cell:

Table 3.4. Comparison between light and electron microscopy.

Steps	Electron microscopy	Light microscopy
Fixation	Osmium tetroxide, postassium permanganate, formalin, glutaraldehyde.	Bouin's solution; formalin; Zenker's fluid.
Dehydration	Increasing concentration of ethanol (or acetone) followed by propylene oxide.	Increasing concentration of ethanol followed by benzene.
Embedding	Araldite; Vestoplaw, Epan 812; Maraglas; Durcopan.	Paraffin.
Sectioning	Usually 10–100 nm thick sections cut with a glass or diamond knife on an ultramicrotome.	Usually 6 μm thick sections cut with a razor blade on a microtome.
Mounting	On a perforated metal disc (grid) usually covered with formvar or paralodian.	On a glass slide with an egg albumin adhesive. Deparaffinized in xylol for staining.
Staining	With salts of heavy metals such as lead acetate, lead citrate, lead hydroxide, urynyl acetate; phosphotungstic acid.	Selective chromatic stains (as haematoxylin and eosin), dehydrated in ethanol series, cleared in xylol and mounted for viewing in Canada balsam or Permount.
Viewing	Grid is placed between the condenser and objective lenses in vacuum and the image is viewed on phosphorescent screen.	Slide is placed between the condenser and objective lenses and the image viewed in the ocular lens.

1. Monolayer technique. Macromolecules such as DNA and RNA are studied by monolayer technique in which the macromolecules are extended on the air-water interface before being collected on a film.

2. Thin sectioning. This method uses a cutting device known as **ultramicrotome** to remove ultrathin (*i.e.*, 10 nm to 100 nm thick) sections from the specimen. To withstand the passage of ultrafine diamond or glass knife without tearing, the specimen is first embedded in a hard plastic such as, epoxy resin (Table 3.4). The resin is allowed to penetrate the sample before it is polymerized. Sections are floated from the knife of ultramicrotome onto the surface of water and picked up by touching them with a fine wire mesh or small circular copper grid (*i.e.*, small discs perforated with numerous openings). Prior to its use mesh or grid is coated with a thin monolayer film (7.5 to 15 nm thick) of plastic (such as formvar or collodion) or carbon to provide a support to the sections (or sample) (Fig. 3.15). The specimen is visualized through the holes of screen.

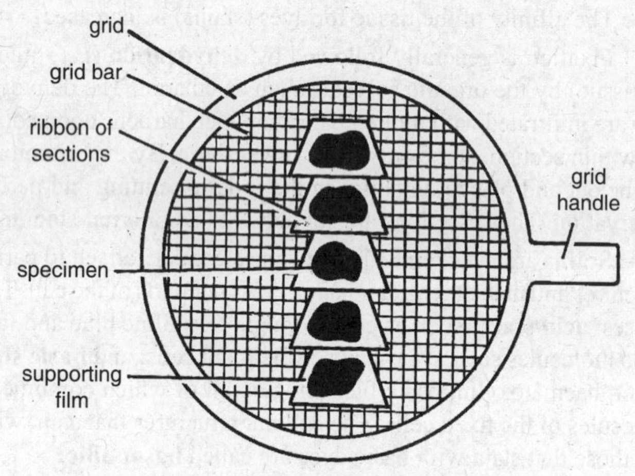

Fig. 3.15. Appearance of a ribbon of ultra-thin sections on the grid.

Sections to be examined with the electron microscope are generally not stained (since no colours are seen with the electron microscope). However, contrast may be improved by "post-staining" with **electron stains** or electron-dense materials such as urynyl acetate, urynyl citrate, lead citrate, osmium tetroxide, etc. The method of thin sectioning is used to study morphology of cell.

3. Negative staining. This technique is used to study small particles such as viruses or macromolecules. Here, the specimen is embedded in a droplet of electron dense material, such as, phosphotungstic acid ($H_3PW_{12}O_{40}$). The electron stain penetrates into all the empty spaces (*i.e.*, openings and crevices) between the macromolecules. The spaces appear well defined in negative contrast. The portions of sepecimen that exclude stain transmit electrons readily, so their images can be seen.

4. Shadow casting or heavy metal shadowing. This technique is used to study three-dimensional appearance of viruses and certain macromolecules such as DNA molecules and collagen fibres. It involves placing of specimen in an evacuated chamber and evaporating at an angle, a heavy metal such as chromium, palladium, platinum or uranium from a filament of incandescent tungsten. The vapour of heavy metal is deposited on one side of the surface of the elevated particles; on the other side a shadow forms, the length of which permits determination of the height of the particle. In such a specimen, during electron microscopy, the electrons pass readily through the area of light metal content, less readily through the plane on which the particle sits, and are scattered more severely by the side of the particle on which metal has accumulated. Thus, by shadow casting, shape and profile of a particle can be observed.

5. Tracers. Several biological processes such as pinocytosis, phagocytosis and transport of molecules across plasma membrane can be studied by the use of appropriate tracers (*e.g.*, gold, mercuric sulphide, iron oxide, etc.). These tracers are detected by their electron opacity. An ideal tracer should be non-toxic, physiologically inert, composed of small-sized particles of uniform and known size and preserved *in situ* during the processing of the tissue.

6. Freeze-fracture. This technique is used to study the molecular arrangement in the plasma membrane and other cellular membranes. It is carried out by rapidly cooling or freezing the sample (**cryofixation**) and then **fracturing** (cracking) it in the vacuum while it is still at –100°C. The knife does not cut cleanly under those conditions, but tends to **fracture** (crack) the specimen along the lines of natural weakness, such as the middle of a membrane that runs parallel to the cut (Fig. 3.16). After fracture, the sample is left in the vacuum long enough to allow some water to evaporate from the exposed surfaces, a process called **freeze etching**. The exposed face is then shadowed with electron-dense combination of carbon and metal such as platinum to provide the necessary contrast, after which organic material (*i.e.*, specimen itself) is removed by acids to leave a metal **replica** for examination in the electron microscope. Replica reveals a natural-looking representation of the surface of the freeze-etched object and is the only way of seeing membrane interior and certain other features of the cells.

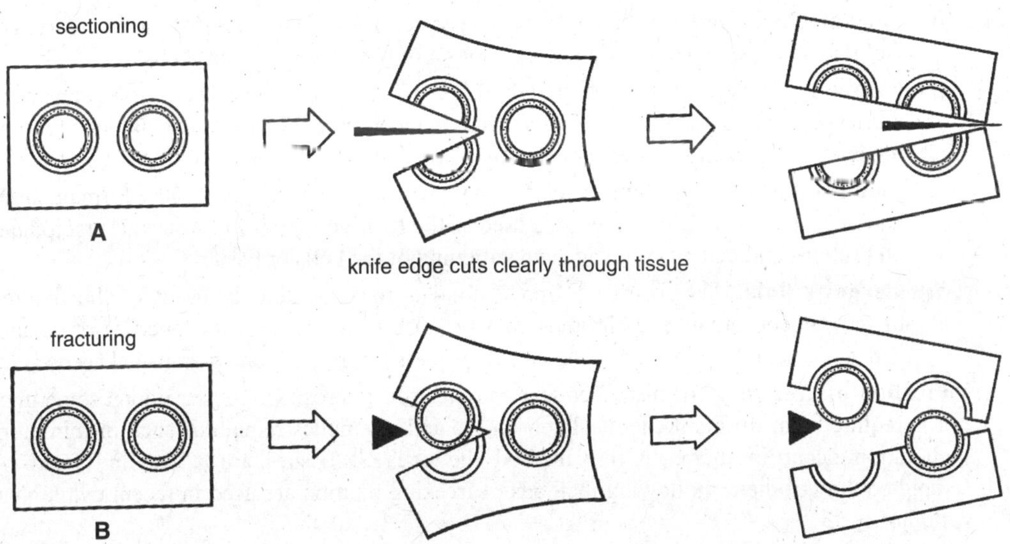

Fig. 3.16. A comparison of sectioning and fracturing tissues.

7. Whole mounts. They are often used to examine chromosomes and other relatively thick objects that can be isolated free of debris. In these methods, the specimen is neither sectioned nor stained. Thick areas will scatter electrons more strongly than thin areas, providing enough contrast to form an image.

Fixation

For microscopical study of dead cells, the process of killing and **fixation** brings about the sudden death of cells or tissues in such a manner that morphological organization and chemical composition of the cell remain unaltered up to greatest extent. The fixative or fixing solution performs following functions: it prevents bacterial decay and autolysis (self-digestion) of the cells; renders the components of the cell insoluble, reduces the cell distortion and shrinkage, increases the visibility of different cellular components and prepares the cells for the staining. The fixation of the cells can be achieved either by chemicals or cooling which is as follows:

(a) Chemical fixation. The choice of suitable fixative generally depends on the type of analysis and the chemical nature of different cells. For instance, for the study of the nucleus and chromosomes the **acid fixative** such as **Carnoy's solution** or **Bouin's fluid** is used. The commonly used fixatives are as follows:

(*i*) **Acetic acid**. The acetic acid is used from 0.3 to 50 per cent, alone or in mixtures. It does not fix cytoplasmic proteins, but precipitates nucleoproteins, destroys Golgi apparatus and mitochondria of the cells. Morever, the cells become swell up and soft. The acetic acid is used with basic dyes for the fixation of **nucleus** and **chromosomes**.

(*ii*) **Potassium dichromate**. Potassium dichromate is generally used in mixtures and in the percentage of 2–7. It renders proteins insoluble in water and fixes lipids. Potassium dichromate is used for the fixation of chromosomes and some cytoplasmic structures.

(*iii*) **Ethanol**. 70 to 100 per cent ethanol is used either alone or in mixture for the fixation of nucleus along with certain basic dyes. It does not precipitate proteins but dissolves lipids. Ethanol makes the cells to become hard but causes shrinkage.

(*iv*) **Formaldehyde**. The formaldehyde (4–10 per cent) is used in mixtures for the fixation of Golgi apparatus, mitochondria and enzymes along with some basic stains.

(*v*) **Osmium tetroxide**. Osmium tetroxide (0.5–2 per cent) fixes cytoplasm, Golgi apparatus, mitochondria and fats of the cell but causes blackening of cell due to its oxidation which renders difficulty in staining. This fixative is widely used for electron microscopy.

(*vi*) **Bouin's solution**. The Bouin's solution has 5 part picric acid, 5 parts 40% formaldehyde and one part glacial acetic acid. It is used as the fixative for chromosomes. It precipitates all proteins and causes shrinkage and softening of the cells or tissue.

(*vii*) **Carnoy's fluid**. The fixative Carnoy's fluid is most commonly used for the fixation of the nucleoproteins and chromosomes because it has combined properties of ethanol and acetic acid. Carnoy's fluid contains three parts ethanol and one part glacial acetic acid.

(b) Fixation by freezing. For histochemical and electron microscopic observations sometimes it is required that different chemical substances and organelles remain as such or minimum alteration occur in them. In this method the cells or tissues are killed and fixed by rapid cooling of them. Following methods of freezing fixation are used in recent cytological studies.

(*i*) **Fixation by freezing-drying method**. For the electron and X-ray microscopy, the tissues or cells are fixed by rapid freezing and are dehydrated in the vacuum at a low temperature. The rapid freezing of tissues is achieved by placing the living tissue in isopentane or propane cooled upto –160°C or –190°C by liquid nitrogen or helium. After freezing, the material is dried in vacuum at –30°C to –40°C.

By freezing-drying fixation method, the tissue does not shrink, homogeneous fixation of cell takes place, soluble substances are not extracted, the chemical composition of the cell is maintained without any alteration and the fixation takes place very quickly.

(*ii*) **Fixation by freezing-substitution method**. In the freezing-substitution fixation method, the living tissue is rapidly frozen and then kept frozen at a low temperature (–20 to –60°C) in a reagent that dissolves the ice-crystals. The reagent may be ethanol, methanol or acetone. This method of fixation is also used in electron microscopy and X-ray microscopy.

(*iii*) **Fixation by freezing-etching method**. In the freezing-etching method of fixation the specimen is placed in 20 per cent glycerol and is frozen at –100°C. It is mounted on a chilled holder and splintered with a knife along natural cleavage planes, usually along surfaces of membranes. Occasionally the structure is cross-fractured, giving cross sections of organelles. The splintered preparation is freeze-dried and covered with a platinum or carbon coating in the high vacuum of a freezing ultramicrotome. When the preparation is dried the vacuum is broken and the preparation is placed in water to float the replica off the carrier. The replica is then washed in basic solution to remove the cellular material and the replica is mounted on a grid and dried for elctron microscopy. Such replica gives the outlines of various cell structures and verify the structures seen in thin fixed and stained sections of various cellular organelles in various types of microscopy.

Staining

The process of colouring the cells, tissues of animal or plant bodies by certain inorganic or organic dyes is known as **staining**. The selection of dye or stain for a particular material usually depends on its chemical nature, the pH value of the fixative used and the chemical reactivity of stain to the material.

Stains. Most cytological stains are solutions of dyes of aromatic organic compounds which have two kinds of active chemical groups such as, **chromophoric** and **auxochromic** groups. The **chromophoric groups** gives the colour to the dye, *e.g.*, carboxyl (–COOH), azo (= N–), nitro ($-NO_2$), quinoid (O =⬡= O) and indamin (– N=) groups. The **auxochromic group** gives to the dye the ability to attach to the tissue or the material and to dissolve and dissociate, in the water, *e.g.*, *Hydroxy* (–OH) group.

The organic stains are classified into three groups:

1. Acidic stains;
2. Basic stains; and
3. Neutral stains.

1. Acidic stains. The acidic stains are usually used for the cytoplasm and proteins. These have great capacity for combining with the tissue at low pH than basic dyes. The most common cytological acidic stains are picric acid, acid fuchsin, Congo red, Janus green *B*, orange *G*, methyl blue, eosin, aniline blue, Bismark brown and fluorescein.

2. Basic stains. The basic stains are used to stain the nucleus, chromosomes and particularly the nucleic acids. The most common cytological basic stains are basic fuchsin, crystal violet, methyl green, safranine, acridine red, azures, methylene blue, thionine and haematoxylin.

3. Neutral stains. The neutral stains have both the properties of acidic and basic stains.

Acidiphilic and basiphilic tissues. The tissue, cell or cellular component taking acidic stains is known as **acidiphilic** tissue, cell or cellular component, *e.g.*, the cytoplasm. The nucleus, chromosomes and DNA have affinity for the basic stains and known as **basiphilic** organelles.

Metachromasia. Some basic dyes stain certain cell components with a different colour than their original colour. This property of stain is known as **metachromasia** and is very useful for **histochemical** and **physiochemical** tests. The property of metachromasia is displayed by the basic stains such as thionine, azure A and toluidine blue which react with mucopolysaccharides, nucleic acids and acidic lipids.

Mordant and lake. Certain dyes stain the proteins and cytoplasm in the presence of some metal or metallic compound which is known as **mordant**. Usually chemically a mordant is a double salt of potassium or ammonium or ferric sulphate. The mordant and the stain are collectively known as the **lake**. The most important mordant is ferric ammonium sulphate (iron alum), which is used along with the stain haematoxylin and carmine.

Staining for Light Microscopy

For light microscopy both acidic and basic stains are used for the staining of cells or tissue. The stains are specific for different types of cells and also for different organelles of cell. The cytoplasmic proteins and carbohydrates are stained by acidic stains, while the nucleus, chromosomes, etc., are stained by basic stains.

Staining for Electron Microscopy

Electron microscopy usually requires no stain because beside observing visually, the image is photographed and due to the contrast between cellular components a black and white photograph is received. But certain inorganic stains such as lead acetate, lead citrate, lead hydroxide, urynyl acetate, phosphotungstic acid, osmium tetroxide and potassium permanganate are used to increase contrast between cellular components. Sometimes certain organic stains as azure II, leucofuchsin, orcein, etc., are also used to increase the contrast.

Cytochemical Staining

In addition, there are certain specific stains, called **cytochemical** stains that bind selectively to some specific groups of cellular macromolecules such as proteins, nucleic acids, polysaccharides and lipids. For example, Millon reaction, diazonium reaction and Napthol Yellow 5 stain are used for the proteins; alkaline fast green is used for histone (basic protein); Feulgen reaction (using Schiff's reagent) is used for DNA; methyl green-pyronine stain (Unna-Pappenheim stain) is used in distinguishing between DNA and RNA and it stains DNA green and RNA red; acetocarmine and acetoorcein stains are used to stain chromosomes of dividing cells; periodic acid-Schiff (PAS) reaction is used for the demonstration of polysaccharide materials such as starch, cellulose, hemicellulose, and pectin in the plant cells and mucoproteins (glycoproteins), hyaluronic acid and chitin in animal cells; and fat soluble dyes such as Sudan Red and Sudan Black B are used for the lipids. The Sudan Black B is a specific stain for phospholipids and is used to stain Golgi apparatus.

Vital Staining

Vital stains selectively stain the intracellular structures of living cells without serious alteration of cellular metabolism and function. For example, Janus green B selectively stains mitochondria; neutral red stains plant vacuoles and methylene blue stains Golgi apparatus and also nuclear chromatin of dividing cells.

Immunostaining or usage of antibodies in Cell Biology. To use fluorescence microscopy for locating specific molecules or ions within cells, researchers must employ special indicator molecules called **fluorescent probe**. A fluorescent probe is a molecule capable of emitting fluorescent light that can be used to indicate the presence of a specific molecule or ion.

One of the most common application of fluorescent probes is **immunostaining**, a technique based on ability of **antibodies** to recognize and bind to specific molecules (the molecules to which antibodies bind are called **antigens**). Antibodies are proteins produced naturally by the immune system in response to invading microorganisms, but they can also be generated in the laboratory by injecting a foreign protein or macromolecule into an animal such as a rabbit or mouse. In this way, it is possible to produce antibodies that will bind selectively to virtually any protein that a scientist wishes to study. Antibodies are not directly visible using light microscopy, however, so they are linked to a fluorescent dye such as **fluorescein**, they emits a green fluorescence, or **rhodamine**, they emit a red fluorescence. More recently, antibodies have been linked to "**quantum dots**", which are tiny light-emitting crystals that are chemically more stable than traditional dyes. To identify the subcellular location of a specific protein, cell are simply stained with a fluorescent antibody directed against that protein and the location of fluorescence is then detected by viewing the cells with light of the appropriate wave-length.

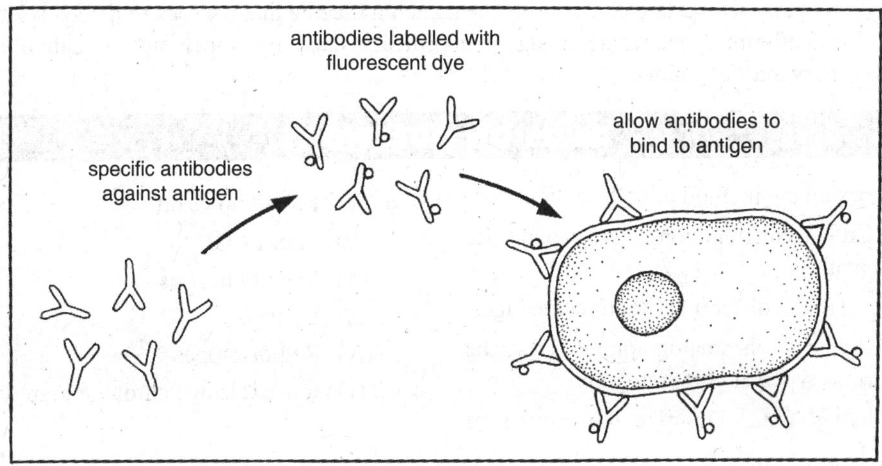

A. Immunofluorescence

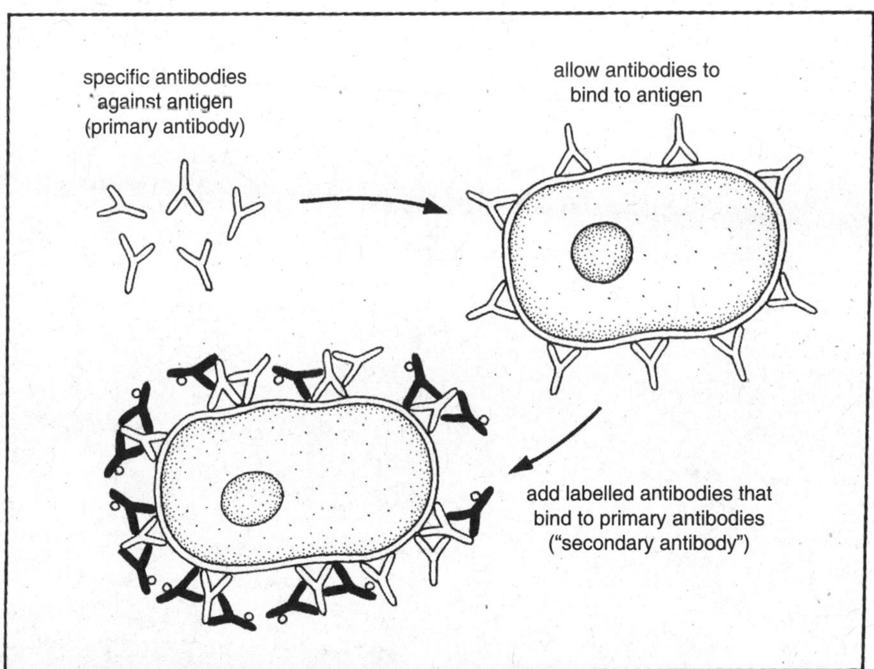

B. Indirect immunofluorescence

Fig. 3.17. Immunostaining using fluorescent antibodies (after Becker *et al.*, 2007).

Immunofluorescence microscopy can be performed using antibodies that are **directly labelled with fluorescent dye** (Fig. 3.17A). However, immunofluorescence microscopy is more commonly performed using **indirect immunofluorescence** (Fig. 3.17B). In indirect immunofluorescence, a tissue or cell is treated with an antibody that is not labelled with dye. This antibody is called **primary antibody** and it attaches to specific antigenic sites within the tissue or cell. A second type of antibody, called **secondary antibody**, is then added. The secondary antibody is labelled with a fluorescent dye, and it attaches to the primary antibody. Because more than one primary antibody molecule can attach to an antigen, and more than one secondary antibody molecules can attach to each primary antibody, more fluorescent molecules are concentrated near each molecule that we seek to detect. As a result, indirect immunofluorescence results in signal amplification, and it is much more sensitive than the use of a primary antibody alone.

REVISION QUESTIONS

1. Describe the method of cell fractionation.
2. What is Centrifugation? Describe in brief its method.
3. Write about different types of centrifuges.
4. What is chromatography? Describe various types of chromatography.
5. What is TLC? Describe the process of TLC.
6. Write short notes on:
   (*i*) SDS-PAGE
   (*ii*) Electrophoresis
   (*iii*) Dialysis
   (*iv*) Radioisotopes
   (*v*) Ion-Exchange chromatography

4
Chapter
CELL

The cell is the basic unit of organization or structure of all living matter. Within a selective and retentive semipermeable membrane, it contains a complete set of different kinds of units necessary to permit its own growth and reproduction from simple nutrients. **A.G. Loewy** and **P. Siekevitz** (1963) have defined a cell as "*a unit of biological activity delimited by a semipermeable membrane and capable of self-reproduccion in a medium free of other living systems*". This definition does not embrace the viruses, because they are the self-reproductive biological units which do not have a finite semipermeable membrane and are capable of self-reproduction only within the living cells. But because viruses are primitive and simpler units of life, therefore, demand priority in discussion.

4.1 VIRUSES

The viruses belong to the twilight zone between the living and non-living worlds. Depending upon one's definition of life, they can be considered living or non-living. They infect almost every kind of prokaryotic and eukaryotic cells and are obligate cellular parasites. In the extra-cellular or infectious state, the viruses are metabolically inert. They may even be crystallized much like molecules, although some kind of viruses can only be purified but not crystallized. When viruses gain entry to a host cell they may initiate the intra-cellular state of their existence and proceed to direct the replication of new virus particles.

The viruses (Latin, venum or poisonous fluid) are the simplest forms of life which instead of having cellular organization (*viz.*, plasma membrane, cytoplasm and nucleus), similar to the bacteria, blue green algae, protista (unicellular plants and animals), plants, fungi and animals, contain definite, genetically determined macromolecular organization, genetic material and characteristic mode of inheritance. Although viruses are not cells, their study has provided a great deal of information about the cells.

Historical

In 1798 an English physician, **Edward Jenner**, reported that infecting a young boy with a mild disease called cowpox made the child immune to small pox. The term "**vaccination**", from the Latin for cowpox (*Variolae vaccinae*, meaning small pocks of the cow), was coined to describe this procedure. In 1885, **Pasteur** perfected the second viral vaccine, that for rabies. In 1892, a Russian scientist, **D. Ivanovsky**, studied an infectious agent that causes a destructive mottling of the leaves of tobacco plants. He demonstrated that the agent, now called *tobacco mosaic virus* (*TMV*), is small enougth to pass filter of unglazed porcelain (a porcelain candle) that **Pasteur** and **C. Chamberlain** had earlier found capable of stopping all known forms of cellular life including bacteria. A few years later, **M.W. Beijerinck** confirmed Ivanovsky's observations, and in 1899 demonstrated that tobacco mosaic virus is not just a small cell, but something more fundamental: a subcellular form of life that can reproduce only as a parasite in living cells.

The concept of the virus as an obligate parasite was extended to the animal world through the experiments performed by **F. Loffler** and **P. Frosch**, who in 1898 showed that foot-and mouth disease in cattle is also caused by an agent that passes a porcelain filter—*i.e.*, the agent is a *filterable virus*. This word *virus*, meaning "poison", was first applied to all pathogens. Later, pathogens were divided into filterable and non-filterable viruses, using the porcelain filter as a test. Now filterable and non-cellular pathogens are considered as viruses.

In 1911, **Rous** found that a certain kind of cancer in chickens is transmitted by a filterable virus (the Rous sarcoma virus). In 1915, **F.W. Twort** reported a bacterial disease characterized by a "glassy transformation", of colonies growing on agar. In 1917, **Felix d'Herelle** independently found a lytic agent for dysentery bacterium and concluded that it was a bacterial virus or bateriophage. In 1935, **Wendell Stanley** crystallized TMV, permitting a careful chemical analysis of its composition. **Lwoff** proved in 1950, that lysogenic bacteria carry viral genes without carrying intact viruses. In 1952, **Hershey** and **Chase** demonstrated experimentally that phage DNA, not its protein, carried genetic information. **Fraenkel-Conrat** and **Williams** (1955) showed that TMV can be deassembled and reassembled in the laboratory. **Gierer** and **Schramm** (1956) demonstrated that the RNA from TMV is infective even without the protein.

Size

The viruses are submicroscopic entities and range in between 10 to 250 mμ or 100A° to 2500A° in size. Most viruses are smaller than bacteria, but, some viruses are larger than bacteria; for example, the psittacos is a virus measuring 0.75 μm in diameter, whereas a pleuropneumonia-like organism or PPLO bacterium measures only 0.25 μm in diameter.

Structure

The viruses possess a regular geometrical and macromolecular organization. Basically, all viruses consist of a core of only one type of nucleic acid (DNA or RNA) which remains wrapped in a coat of protein called **capsid**. The capsid is composed of numerous **capsomeres**. The capsomeres are of different shapes, such as hollow prism, hexagonal, pentagonal, lobular, or any other shape. The arrangement of capsomeres determine the shape of the virus particle or **virion**. Thus viruses have the following three different types of symmetry:

1. Spherical, cubical, polygonal or polyhedral symmetry. Crick and **Watson** have suggested that the polyhedral capsids can have three possible types of symmetry. *viz.*, **tetrahedral** (4-sided). **octahedral** (8-sided), and **icosahedral** (20-sided). **D.L.D. Caspar** and **A. Klug** (1962) showed that **icosahedron** is the most efficient shape for the packing and bonding of the subunits of a near spherical virus. Therefore, spherical, cubical or polygonal viruses are icosahedral rather than tetrahedral or octahedral in symmetry.

The icosahedron is related to the geodesic domes of **Buckminster Fuller**; it is a solid figure formed by 20 equilateral triangles giving 12 intersection points with five-fold symmetry. Each triangle consists of three equivalent structure units. The whole icosahedron consists of 60 structure units arranged in groups of 5 around the centres of symmetry on a surface. The smallest possible icosahedron consists of 12 pentameres of structure units. Larger icosahedron structures can be constructed by introducing specified numbers of additional triangles; the number of structure unit is always 60 T, where $T = H^2 + HK + K^2$, H and K being any integers.

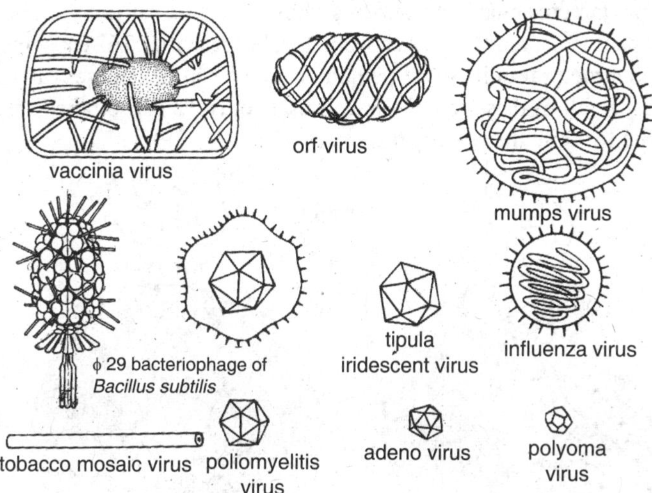

Fig. 4.1. Different kinds of viruses.

Studies of their physico-chemical properties, X-ray diffraction patterns and direct visualization of virus particles in the electron microscope have confirmed the geometry of such capsid or shell structures. Thus, a viral capsid consists of many capsomeres. Each capsomere is composed of a few **monomers** or **structural units**, each of which is made up of one or more polypeptide chains. A capsomere may have either 5 structural units (such a capsomere is called **pentamere**) or 6 structural units (such a capsomere is called **hexamere**). In each capsomere, the structural units are held together by strong bonds, each structural unit having bonds with two neighbouring structural units. The capsomeres are also held together by comparatively weaker bonds.

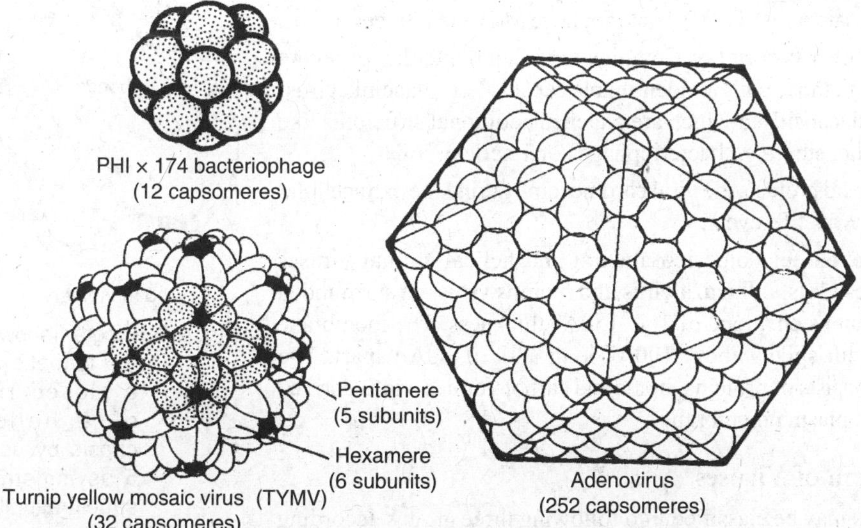

Fig. 4.2. Certain polyhedral (icosahedral) viruses.

According to the already mentioned rule of crystallography only certain numbers of capsomeres can be present in an icosahedral viral capsid. The minimum number of capsomeres can theoretically be 12, followed by its multiple like 32, 42, 72, 92, 162, 252, 362, 492, 642 and 812. The actual numbers of capsomeres found in different icosahedral viruses are: bacteriophage phi X 174, 12 capsomeres (60 structural units or 12 pentameres); turnip yellow mosaic virus (TYMV), 32 capsomeres (180 structural units or 12 pentameres plus 20 hexameres); poliovirus, 32 capsomeres; polyoma virus and papilloma virus, 72 capsomeres; reovirus, 92 capsomeres; herpes virus, 162 capsomeres; adenovirus, 252 capsomeres (1500 structural units or 12 pentameres and 240 hexameres) and tipula iridescent virus, 812 capsomeres. In all of these icosahedral viruses, only 12 capsomeres are pentameres and occupying the 12 corners, while the rest are hexameres.

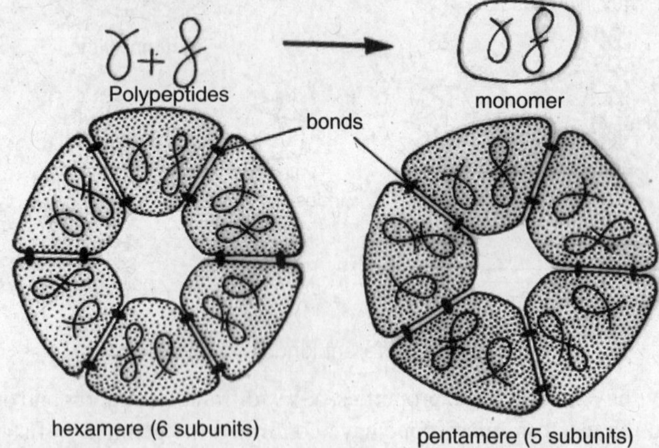

Fig. 4.3. Diagram showing the formation of a structural unit or monomer from two polypeptide chains and the mode of arrangement of monomers in the capsomeres.

2. Helical or cylindrical symmetry. The helical capsids consist of numerous identical structural units arranged into a helix because they are thicker at one end than the other (Fig. 4.4). The size and shape of the structural units determine the shape of the virus. Helical capsids occur in tobacco mosaic virus (TMV), bacteriophage M13 and influenza virus.

3. Complex symmetry. Complex viruses fall into the following two categories : those without identifiable capsids (*e.g.*, vaccinia virus) and those with capsids to which are attached additional structures like tail, basal plate, etc. (*e.g.*, bacteriophages of T series).

The capsid protects the viral chromosome during the extracellular phase of the virus life-cycle.

The envelope. Some icosahedral and helical animal viruses such as herpes virus, influenza virus and mumps virus are surrounded by a membranous envelope of 100–150A° thickness. The membrane is covered with spikes about 100A° long and 70–80A° apart. The membrane consists of proteins, lipids and carbohydrates and is derived from the host plasma membrane.

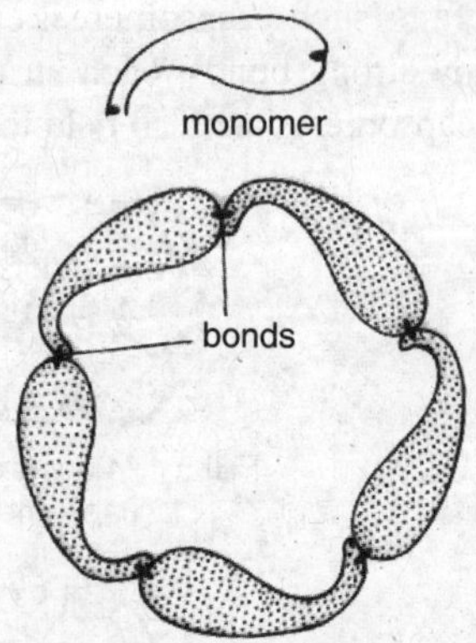

Fig. 4.4. Diagram showing the formation of a closed ring of a helical capsid by using 5 asymmetrical structural units.

Classification of Viruses

Viruses may be classified into following three groups according to the type of host:

A. The bacterial viruses or **bacteriophages**. Viruses that parasitize bacteria are called **bacteriophages** or **phages** (phage "to eat"). There are many varieties of bacteriophages, usually each kind of bateriophage will attack only one species, or even only one strain of bacteria. Their size and shape varies from species to species. Thus, some phages may be spherical or comma-shaped or may have a tail and resemble a tadpole.

The most widely studied bacteriophage is T_4 **bacteriophage** of T-even phages (T stands for "type") such as T_2, T_6 etc., that infects the colon bacillus, *Escherichia coli.* T_4 phage (or **coliphage**) is a highly organized structure and resembles with a landing module for the moon. It contains a polyhedral **head**, a short **neck** and **collar**, and a straight tail to which remain attached an end plate carrying tail **fibres**. T_4 phage is a complex virus: its head has icosahedral symmetry and its tail has helical symmetry. Thus, it has **binal symmetry**.

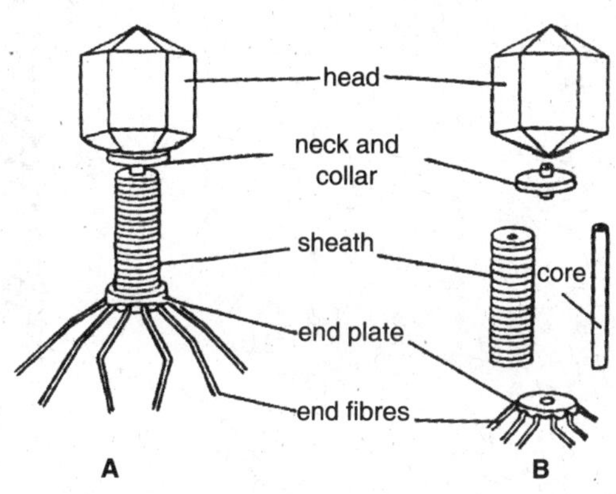

Fig. 4.5. The parts and structure of the T_4 bacteriophage.

The phage chromosome is a linear, double-stranded 53 μm long DNA molecule, containing more than 75 genes and remains highly coiled and tightly packed within protein envelope (capsid) of polyhedral head. The head has a length of 1250A° and width of 850A°. The capsid of head is made up of about 2000 similar subunits of capsomeres (proteins) and each protein subunit has molecular weight of about 80,000. A short neck containing collar connects the head with a tail. The tail consists of a central hollow core through which phage chromosome or DNA molecule passes on its way into the host cell. Around the core occurs a spring-like **contractile sheath** or **tube**. The contractile sheath is formed by 144 subunits, which are arranged in a hollow cylinder consisting 24 rings of six subunits each. Each subunit of contractile sheath has a molecular weight of about 50,000. The contractile sheath and core of the tail remain attached to a hexagonal end plate. Six slender fibres and six short **spikes** protrude from the end plate. Each of the tail-fibres and tail-spikes, is a bundle of polypeptide chains and of a molecular weight of about 100,000. Altogether, T_4 bacteriophage is a functioning, adaptive structure with functionally differentiated parts.

Mode of infection of T_4 bacteriophage. The mode of infection of T_4 bacteriophage is highly mechanised. At the time of infection, a T_4 bacteriophage becomes anchored to the bacterial wall by its tailfibres and tail-spikes so that the tail and head are perpendicular to the surface. Within a few minutes after attachment, the contractile sheath of the tail shortens, to less than half its original length, an enzyme of the core of the tail digests part of the bacterial cell wall so as, to produce a hole and finally, the phage DNA is injected into the bacterial cell. The capsid (protein coat of head and tail) of phage remains outside the bacterial cell.

The course of events within the bacterial cell is well known but will be summarized here. In brief, the bacterial DNA is disturbed, manufacture of bacterial protein stops and the viral genes take over: Among the first proteins to be made are the enzymes needed for viral DNA replication. This happens within the first 5 minutes after break through. Three minutes later another set of genes directs the synthesis of the structural proteins that will form the head components and tail components. The first completed virus particle appears 13 minutes after infection, and the process continues for another 12 minutes until about 200 such particles have been completed and the raw materials of the bacterial cell have been virtually exhausted. A viral enzyme, a lysozyme, then appears and attacks the cell wall, liberating the new viral particles.

B. Plant viruses. The plant viruses parasitize the plant cells and disturb their metabolism, which ultimately reflects into the disease of the plant. All plant viruses consist of ribomicleoproteins in their organization. The important plant viruses are tobacco rattle virus (TRV), tobacco mosaic virus (TMV), potato virus, beet yellow virus (BYV), southern bean mosaic virus (SBMV) and turnip yellow mosaic virus (TYMV).

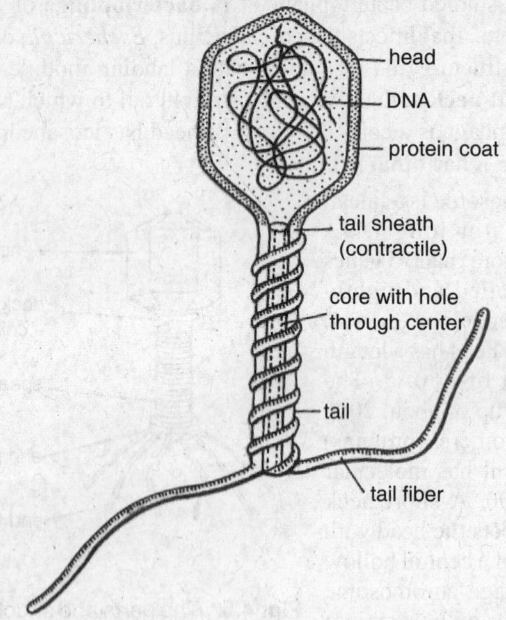

Fig. 4.6. Simplified structure of a T_4 bacteriophage.

TMV is the extensively studied plant virus. It is a helically symmetrical, rod-shaped virus that having the length of 3000A° and diameter of 180A°. X-ray diffraction studies have shown that TMV consists of a **protein tube** with a lumen of 20A° enclosing an elongated, single stranded, spirally or helically-coiled, chain-line polymer, the RNA which has 6500 nucleotides and carries all the genetic information of the virus. The tube is made up of 2,130 identical eleptical subunits (monomers) of proteins, which are arranged in a helix. Each protein subunit has a molecular weight of 18,000 and consists of a single polypeptide chain made up of 158 amino acids whose sequence has been worked out.

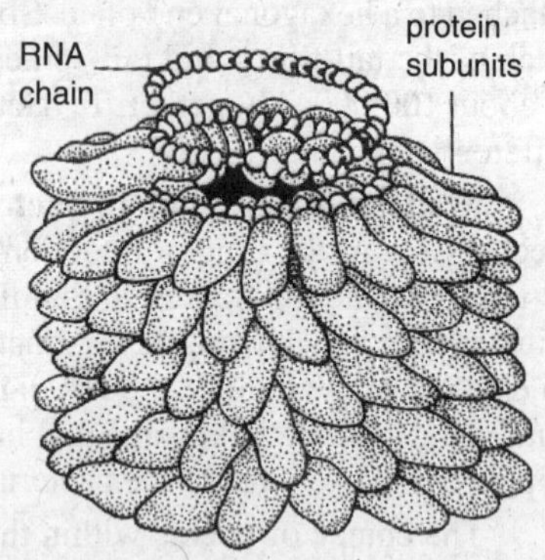

Fig. 4.7. The tobacco mosaic virus (TMV).

Another plant virus, the **turnip yellow mosaic virus** (**TYMV**) has a icosahedral symmetry. The capsid of TYMV contains ,180 structure units, each with a molecular weight of 20,100. These protein units are elongated and project out from the core of RNA in clusters of five or six units. There are 32 clusters, 12 with 5 units each (pentameres) and 20 with 6 units each (hexameres) (Fig. 4.2).

C. Animal viruses. The animal viruses infect the animal cells and cause different fatal diseases in animals including man. Generally, they have a polyhedron or spherical shape and genetic material in the form of DNA or RNA. The protein coat or capsid of animal viruses is also surrounded by an envelope. The important animal viruses are small pox virus, vaccinia virus, herpes virus, adeno virus, influenza virus, mumps, poliomyelitis, reo virus, etc.

Poliomyelitis is a most extensively studied animal virus. The polio virus has comparatively very simple organisation. It consists of a protein shell built up out of 60 structurally equivalent, asymmetric protein subunits of approximately 60A° in diameter, packed together in such a way that they form a spherical shell of about 300A° in diameter, enclosing the nucleic acid (RNA). Analysis shows that the shell contains about 49,600 amino acids and the nucleic acid about 5,200 nucleotides. The single-stranded RNA of poliovirus, thus, has triplet codes for 1,700 amino acids. During infection, to it alters cell metabolism drastically and leads to quick death of host cell.

Mode of infection of animal viruses. Animal viruses may enter cells by attaching to the surface; some are then engulfed by the cell through pinocytosis or phagocytosis. In such cases, uncoating of viral nucleic acid (chromosome) might occur within the cell. Inside the host cell they multiply and form numerous new viral particles. Usually, animal viruses release from the host cells by the rupturing and subsequent death of host cells (lysis). But sometimes, host cell destruction is less rapid, and the virus is released by inclusion in a bud pinched off at the cell surface. The bud remains around the virus. It is generally believed that in this way membrane-delimited viruses derive their membrane (or at least major lipid, polysaccharide, and protein components) from the host cell surface membrane and associated structures.

A Comparison of Cells and Viruses

Viruses are much simpler than cells and very different in both structure and life cycle. They range in size from about 10 nm to several hundred nm. The largest viruses, therefore, are at least as large as the smallest bacteria (mycoplasma, chlamydiae and rickettsiae) but there is a vast difference between them. In fact, even the tiniest cells may be parasitized by viruses.

Chlamydiae are similar to viruses in being able to reproduce only within living cells. However, chlamydiae are obligate cellular parasites becfause of their stringent nutritional requirements. Viruses are obligate cellular parasites because they are not cells, and only cells can be self-reproducing. Viruses have no metabolism and no cell membrane in the usual sense. In fact, the envelope that one finds around certain viruses has the same structure as a cell membrane, but it is not biologically active organ, only the remnant of one. In general, the molecular variety necessary to support an independent existence is simply not present in virus particles. There is no natural way in which their genes can be used to construct new virus particles without the help of a living cell (**Dyson**, 1978).

4.2 CLASSIFICATION OF CELLS OF CELLULAR ORGANISMS

The body of all living **organisms** (blue green algae, bacteria, plants and animals) except viruses and certain plants such as *Rhizopus*, *Vaucheria* etc., has cellular organization and may contain one or many cells. The organisms with only one cell in their body are called **Unicellular organisms** (*e.g.*, blue green algae, bacteria, some algae, Protozoa, etc.). The organisms having many cells in their body are called **multicellular organisms** (*e.g.*, most plants and animals).

The cells are found in an enormous variety of sizes and shapes representing their evolutionary adaptation to different environments or to different specialized functions within a multicellular organism. Cells range in size from the smallest bacteria, only a few tenths of μm in diameter, to certain marine algae and to various bird eggs with dimensions of centimeters. Besides all their apparent diversity, however, cells have many characteristics in common, the most basic of which is the potential for an independent existence. Thus, cells have the ability to continue living in the absence of any other cell; a capacity that requires first, a metabolic machinery capable of obtaining energy from the environment through capture of light or the degradation of chemical foodstuff; and second. the ability to use this energy to support essential life processes. These processes include the movement of components from one part of the cell to another, the selective transfer of molecules into and out of the cell, and the ability to transform molecules from one chemical configuration to another in order to replace parts as they wear out or to support growth and reproduction. In addition to this metabolic machinery, a cell must have a set of genes to act as blueprints for the synthesis of other components. And finally, a cell must have a physical delimiter, a boundary between it and rest of the world, called the **cell membrane** or **plasma membrane**.

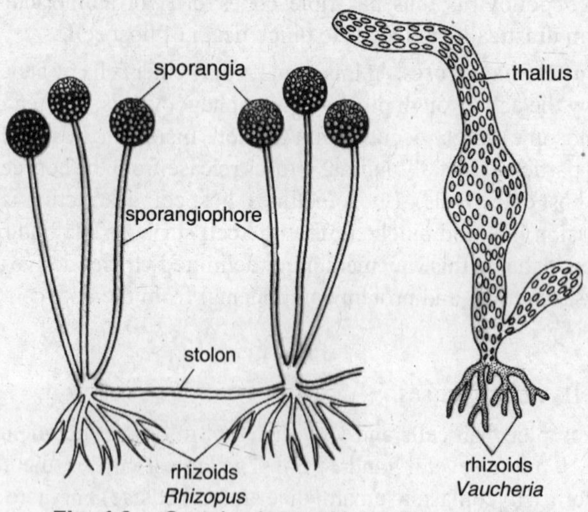

Fig. 4.8. Certain plants with acellular organization.

All cells are broadly divided into **prokaryotic cells** and **eukaryotic cells**, according to whether their genes are enclosed by a nuclear envelope. Eukaryotic cells have such an envelope where as prokaryotic cells do not. The term prokaryotic (*pro-* before; *karyon*-nucleus) and eukaryotic (*eu-* true) were suggested by **Hans Ris** in the early 1960's. Any cellular organism may have only one kind of cell from these two types of cells.

4.3 PROKARYOTIC CELLS

The *prokaryotic* (Gr., *pro* = primitive or before; *karyon* = nucleus) or pro-caryote cells—namely, bacteria, blue green algae, etc., are the most primitive cells from morphological point of view. They are essentially **one-envelope systems** organized in depth. They consist of central nuclear components (*viz.*, DNA molecule, RNA molecules and nuclear proteins) surrounded by cytoplasmic ground substance, with the whole enveloped by a plasma membrane. Neither the nuclear apparatus nor the respiratory enzyme systems are separately enclosed by membranes, although the inner surface of the plasma membrane itself may serve for enzyme attachment. The cytoplasm of a prokaryotic cell, lack in well defined cytoplasmic organelles such as endoplasmic reticulum, Golgi complex, mitochondria, centrioles, etc. The prokaryotic cells are so small that simple organic molecules could traverse the cell 100 or 200 times a second, and diffusion alone suffices to take care of metabolic transport needs. Few important prokaryotic cells are following:

(i) PPLO (The Pleuropneumonia-like Organisms)

The pleuropneumonia-like organisms or PPLO are the bacteria-like organisms which differ with the latter only in lacking the cell wall and mesosomes and in having very simple organization, small size and a deformable cytoplasmic or plasma membrane around their prokaryotic cells. **W.V. Iterson** (1969) has placed PPLO in the group Mycoplasmataceae of bacteria (Schizomycetes), but, **Novikoff** and **Holtzman** (1970) have considered them as simplest known cells and have excluded them from the bacteria. The diameters of the smallest PPLO are 0.1–0.3 μm, and of the largest on the order of a micron. Thus, in size, the PPLO's overlap with the largest viruses and with the smallest bacteria. The most widely studied genus of PPLO is *Mycoplasma*.

The Mycoplasmas are the smallest organisms that have been cultivated on cell-free media. Two types of Mycoplasmas exist in the nature. The first with *Mycoplasma laidlawii* (0.1 μm diameter) as the type species, is saprophytic. It is found in sewage, compost, earth, etc. The second type with *Mycoplasma gallisepticum* (0.25 μm diameter) as the type species, is parasite of the cells and cell exudates of respiratory organs of warm-blooded animals. It causes various chronic respiratory diseases in them.

Structure. The prokaryotic cells of PPLO remain bounded by a 75A° thick plasma membrane. The DNA molecule is contained in a nuclear region. DNA molecule may be in the form of either fibrils or a single circular double helix and it is not enveloped by any nuclear membrane. The nuclear region is surrounded by numerous ribosomes and other components involved in protein synthesis. The cytoplasm has some granules and vacuoles of uncertain significance. The vacuoles are said to be formed due to deep infoldings of the plasma membrane. At one side of the cell occurs bleb of ill understood function.

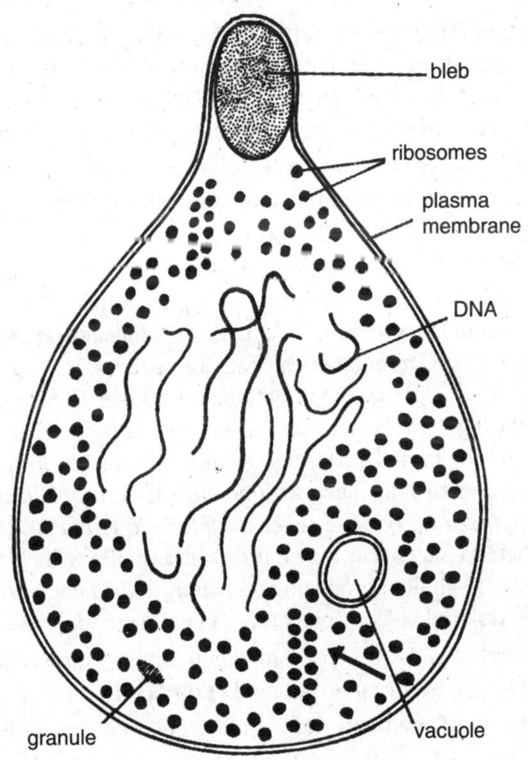

Fig. 4.9. Diagram of a typical prokaryotic cell of PPLO.

The PPLO cells have many enzymes which may be required for DNA replication, the transcription, and translation involved in protein synthesis, and the generation of adenosine triphosphate (ATP) by anaerobic breakdown of sugar. Unlike viruses, they are free living; they do not require host cells for duplication. PPLO reproduce by binary fission, budding, formation of small spore-like bodies and growth of large branched filament that ultimately fragment.

PPLO is probably far more complex than the primitive self-duplicating systems from which life arose. Yet, it may be close to the minimum size and complexity required for independent cellular life and reproduction under present-day conditions (**Morowitz**, 1966).

(*ii*) Chlamydiae and Rickettsiae

Chlamydiae and Rickettsiae are small bacteria that are parasites of cells in vertebrates. Like other bacteria, they have both DNA and RNA, a cell membrane surrounded by a cell wall and other typical cell organelles. They reproduce like true bacteria by cell division and are also sensitive to anti-bacterial chemicals, antibiotics.

Chlamydia or **Bedsonia** which are psittacosis-lymphogranuloma-trachoma (PLT) group of bacteria, are obligate intracellular parasites like the viruses. They cause the disease **psittacosis**, "parrot fever", transferred from birds to humans.

Rickettsiae cause several important diseases, including typhus fever, Rocky Mountain spotted fever, Q fever, and scrub typhus (tsutsugamushi fever). They are spread by blood-sucking arthropods (lice, fleas, ticks and mites).

(*iii*) Bacteria

The bacteria are microscopic, unicellular, achlorophyllous, asexually reproducing prokaryotes which occur in fresh and salt water, in soil and in plants and animals. They lead either a saprophytic or parasitic mode of existence. The saprophytic species of bacteria are of great economic significance for man. Some parasitic species of bacteria are pathogenic (disease-producing) to plants, animals and man.

Size of bacteria. Bacterial cells are very small, on an average the bacterial cell measures 1.25 µm in diameter. The smallest bacterium is *Dialister pneumosintes* (0.15 to 0.3 µm in length). The largest bacterium is *Spirillum volutans* (13 to 15 µm in length).

Form of bacteria. There are three basic shapes of bacteria—the spheroidal (**coccus**), rod-shaped or cylindrical (**bacillus**) and spiral (**spirillum** and **spirochetes**). The spheroidal forms occur either singly (called **micrococcus**); in groups of two (called **diplococcus**) *e.g.*, pneumonia causing bacteria, *Diplococcus pneumoniae*, and gonorrhea causing gonococcus; in long chains (called **streptococcus**, *e.g.*, *Streptococcus phyegens*, cause sore throat); or in irregular clumps, resembling bunches of grapes (called, **staphylococci**, *e.g.*, *Staphylococcus aureus*, causes boils). The rod-shaped bacteria or bacilli may occur as single rods or, as in the bacillus causing anthrax, as long chains of rods joined together. Certain notorious diseases of man, such as tuberculosis (*Mycobacterium tuberculosis*), diphtheria (*Corynebacterium diptheriae*), typhoid fever (*Salmonella typhosa*), etc., are all caused by bacilli. The spiral-shaped bacteria may occur in two forms: the **sprilla**, which are less coiled and sometimes resembled a comma (*e.g.*, cholera producing spirillum, *Vibrio comma*); and the **spirochetes**, which are highly coiled and resemble a corkscrew (*e.g.*, syphilis causing bacteria).

Structure of bacteria. All bacteria fundamentally contain prokaryotic cells in their body. A typical bacterial cell has an **outer covering**, and **cytoplasm**.

A. Outer covering of the bacterial cell. The outer covering of bacterial cells is made up of three layers:

1. Plasma membrane. The cytoplasm is delimited by a thin membrane of lipid and protein molecules, called **plasma membrane**. The plasma membrane of bacteria contains oxidative or respiratory chain enzymes and multienzyme complexes and performs the functions which are usually done by the mitochondria of eukaryotic cells. The bacterial plasma membrane may become differentiated to from other structures. For example, the plasma membrane of bacterium *Thiovulvum majus* sinks deep into the cytoplasm to form multilayered structures called the **desmosomes**. In some bacteria (*e.g.*, *Bacillus subtilis*) the plasma membrane giving out certain invaginations or infoldings of complex whorls of convoluted membranes called **mesosomes**, in the cytoplasm. The mesosomell have various functions, *viz.*, respiratory (respiratory enzymes remain in mesosomes), secretory (synthesize material for extracellular transport and for the formation of cell wall) and they receive the transforming DNA molecule from other bacterial cells during conjugation. Further, mesosomes always remain associated with the nuclear regions and are the sites of the DNA-replication enzymes. They also function in chromosome duplication and in distributing daughter chromosomes (DNA molecules) to each daugther cell.

2. Cell wall. The plasma membrane is followed and is coveted by a strong, rigid **cell wall**. The bacterial cell wall besides containing carbohydrates, lipids, proteins, phosphorus and certain inorganic salts, contains an amino acid, **diaminopimelic acid** (found only in bacteria and blue green algae) and a derivative of glucose called **muramic acid**. Electron micrographs reveal that cell walls of bacteria may be constructed of units 50 to 140 mμ (nm) in diameter that are arranged in a regular hexagonal or rectangular pattern.

The Gram reaction. Bacteriologists generally use a stain called **Gram stain** (a stain developed by a Danish scientist **C. Gram** in 1884) to distinguish two different major bacterial classes by light microscopy. Many bacteria (*e.g.*, *Diplococcus pneumoniae*, etc.,) are stainable by the Gram stain (crystal violet and iodine), so, usually are referred as **Gram-positive bacteria**, other bacteria (*e.g.*, *Eschericnia coli*, etc.) are not stained by Gram stain, therefore, are called **Gram-negative bacteria**. The cell walls of Gram-positive bacteria contain polysaccharides and mucopeptides. They also contain teichoic acid and traces of ribonucleic acid (RNA). The macromolecule of polysaccharides and mucopeptides remain extensively linked to one another, producing a complex multi molecular network that provides considerable strength to the wall. The cell walls of Gram-negative bacteria contain a similar network but have in addition an outer layer of lipids, complexed with protein and polysaccharides. They lack RNA and teichoic acid. The cell walls of Gram-negative bacteria are so thin that they appear like unit membrane in the electron microscope. Some of the outer layer components in Gram-negative cell walls are toxic to animals an may account for certain effects of bacterial infection.

3. Capsule. Outside to the cell wall of most bacteria occurs a slimy capsule which composed largely of polysaccharides. Capsule serves as additional protective layer to the bacterial cell.

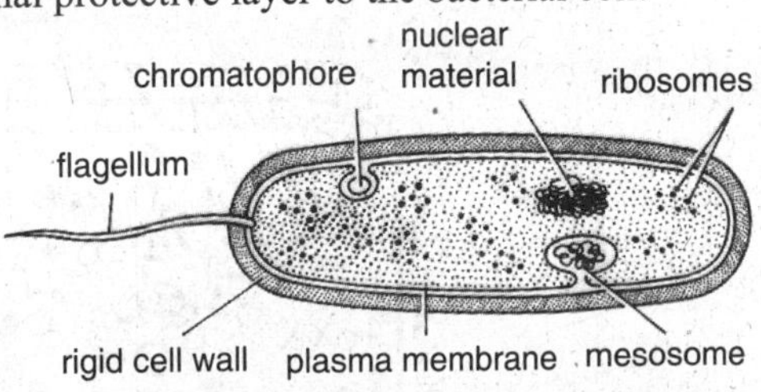

Fig. 4.10. A typical bacterial cell.

B. Cytoplasm. The cytoplasm of bacterial cells is dense, colloidal and contains granules of glycogen, proteins and fats. It also contains poly-β-hydroxy-butyric acid, granulose (a polymer of glucose), volutin (metaphosphate granules) and elemental sulphur as the stored food materials. It lacks most of the important membrane-delimited cellular organelles of eukaryotic cells, such as endoplasmic reticulum, Golgi complex, mitochondria, lysosomes, centrioles, etc. However, the bacterial cells have ribosomes which occur freely in the cytoplasm and do not remain bounded to membranes. Bacterial ribosomes are slightly smaller than the ribosomes of eukaryotes (they sediment at 70S as opposed to 80S) and contain slightly more RNA (60 per cent) than protein (eukaryotic ribosomes contain 40–50 per cent RNA). During protein synthesis many ribosomes reads the codes of mRNA and form the polyribosomes or poly somes.

The genetic informations of each bacterial cell is carried by DNA molecules which is often called **bacterial chromosomes** or **genophores**. The DNA is present in a distinct nuclear region, often called **nucleoid**. The nucleoid lacks any delimiting membrane. Cocci usually have one nucleoid per cell ; rod-like bacilli usually have two or more nucleoids per cell.

Certain photosynthetic bacteria have chromatophores which have **bacteriochlorophyll** and other photosynthetic pigments differ somewhat from the comparable pigments of eukaryotes. (Some bacteria utilize hydrogen sulphide in photosynthesis and do not evolve oxygen, the H_2S is oxidized to produce sulphur as higher plants oxidize H_2O to produce oxygen). The photosynthetic pigments and enzymes are associated with internal membranes that are arranged as lamellae, tubules or vesicles in different species to form the so called chromatophores.

Many bacteria are able to swim about by beating of whip-like; cellular outgrowths called **flagella**. Bacterial flagella consist of a single fibril 100–200A° thick and several microns long, protruding from an intracellular "basal granule" through the plasma membrane and cell-wall. The fibril is made largely of the protein **flagellin**. Most rod-and spiral-shaped bacteria have flagella; most spherical ones do not.

The cells of some bacteria contain certain hair-like extracellular outgrowths called **pili** ("hair", sing., **pilus**) or **fimbriae** ("fringe"), with diameters of 0.01 μm or less and lengths up to a μm or two. Most pili seem to have a construction somewhat similar to that of flagella, including a basal body anchor within the cytoplasm. However, male bacteria of certain strains carry one or two special hollow **sex pilí** that form a bridge (*i.e.*, conjugation canal) with the female cell during mating. In a few pathogenic strains of bacteria pili are responsible for recognizing and attaching to the host. In most bacteria pili are used for the attachment of bacterial cells to solid surface. Pili composed of helically arranged subunits of "**pilin**" protein.

Escherichia coli. *E. coli* is a gram-negative bacillus which is non-pathogenic and found in the mammalian digestive tract. It is a favourite experimental organism for cell biologists, geneticists, biochemists and molecular biologists. An *E. coli* cell is about 2 μm long and 0.8 to 1 μm thick. It has an outer cell wall of 100A° thickness. The cell wall composed of molecules of polysaccharides, lipids and proteins and also of certain mineral salts. The cell wall is followed by a true plasma membrane which contains the molecules of lipids and proteins like the 'unit membranes' of eukaryotic cells. Due to the absence of mitochondria, the respiratory mechanism of bacterial cell is performed by the plasma membrane. To the plasma membrane, therefore, many respiratory enzymes such as cytochromes, enzymes of Krebs cycle, NADH, acid phosphatase, etc., remain attached.

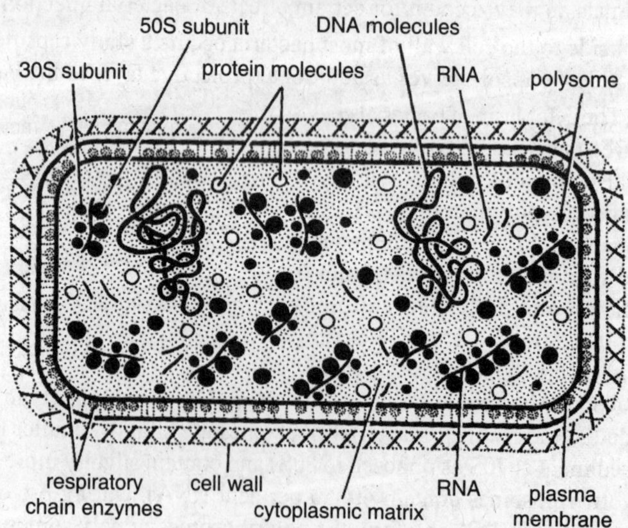

Fig. 4.11. A prokaryotic cell of *Escherichia coli.*

The cytoplasm of *E. coli* is colloidal containing roughly 5000 distinguishable components, ranging from water to DNA and other macromolecules (such as RNA, enzymatic proteins, glycogen, etc.). It has no endoplasmic reticulum, Golgi complex, mitochondria, centriole, lysosome, flagella and pili, but has about 20,000 to 30,000 particles of 200A° diameter, known as **ribosomes**. The ribosomes contain ribosomal RNA and proteins and are the sites for synthesis of proteins. During protein synthesis many ribosomes read the coded informations of messenger RNA (mRNA) simultaneo usly and they aggregate to form polyribosomes or polysomes.

All the genetic informations of an *E. coli* cell are carried by a single, double-stranded, circular and 1000–1500 μm long molecule of DNA. DNA molecule of *E. coli* does not remain wrapped in histone proteins like the DNA of eukaryotes, but, certain **polyamines** may be bound to some of its phosphate groups. It forms the bacterial chromosome or **genophore** and remains confined to the clear central region of cytoplasm which lacks nuclear membrane and is called **nucleoid**. Under certain artificial growth conditions of culture, a cell of *E. coli* may contain two or more nucleoids, each containing identical copies of one DNA molecule.

(*iv*) Blue Green Algae

The blue green algae is another group of prokaryotes which includes in it about 2000 species resembling bacteria in many regards. A few blue green algae are unicenular and grow as single separate cells, but, most species are multicellular and forming multicellular colonies of prokaryotic cells.

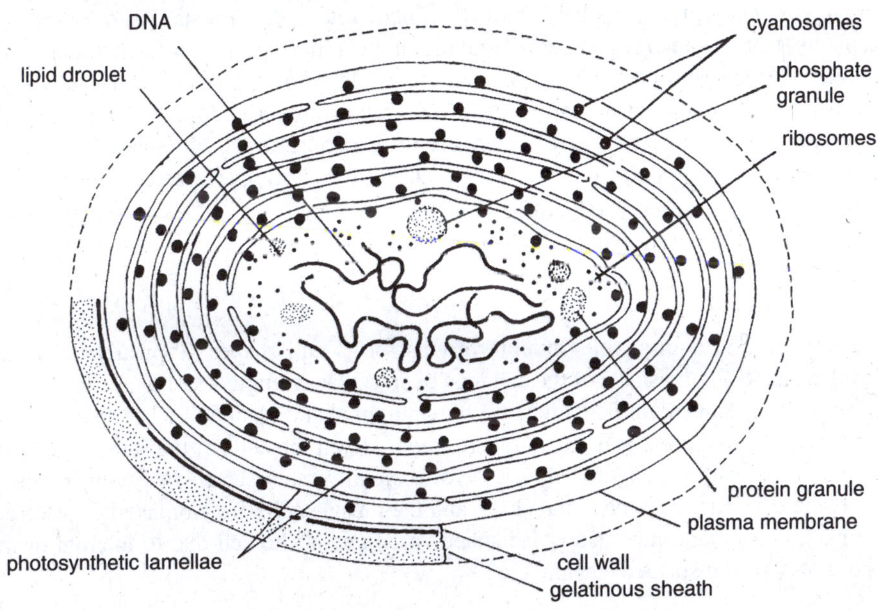

Fig. 4.12. Diagram of a blue-green algae cell.

A typical cell of a blue green alga is basically composed of outer cellular coverings and cytoplasm. The outer coverings of cell include an outermost **gelatinous** or **slimy layer**, a middle **cell wall** and an innermost lipoproteinous **plasma membrane**. The cell wall of blue green algae resembles to the cell wall of bacteria and contains molecules of lipoproteins, lipopolysaccharides and mucoproteins.

The cytoplasm of the blue gree algae lacks endoplasmic reticulum, Golgi complex, mitochondria, and lysosomes. It contains numerous 70S ribosomes which remain free and form polysomes during protein synthesis.

Because the metabolism of blue green algae is based on photosynthesis, therefore, the cells of blue green algae contain the photosynthetic, pigments such as **chlorophyll** and **carotenoid**. In addition to these pigments, these algae contain certain unique pigments, collectively called **phycobilin**; one of these pigments (**phycocyanin**) is blue and another (**phycoerythrin**) is red. The photosynthetic pigments (chlorophyll ahd carotenoids) are present in flattened sacs called **lamellae** which are arranged in parallel array. In between the lamellae occur certain granules of 400A° diameter. These granules contain phycobilin pigments and are called **cyanosomes** or **phycobilisomes**. Each phycobilisome contains about 10 subunits, each about 130A° in diameter and remains attached to outer lamellar membrane surface. Thus, the photosynthetic apparatus of blue green alga is not segregated into membrane-delimited, chloroplastids like the eukaryotes.

As in all prokaryotes the DNA is double-stranded helix and is not segregated into a nucleus separated from the cytoplasm by a nuclear envelope. The cells of blue green algae though lack cilia or flagella, but have the capacity to do movement by gliding and rotator motions.

4.4 EUKARYOTIC CELL

The eukaryotic cells (Gr., *eu* = good, *karyotic* = nucleus) are essentially two envelope systems and they are very much larger than prokaryotic cells. Secondary membranes envelop the nucleus and other internal organelles and to a great extent they pervade the cytoplasm as the endoplasmic reticulum. The eukaryotic cells are the true cells which occur in the Protista (Protozoa and Protophyta), fungi, plants (from algae to angiosperms) and the animals (from poriferans to mammals). Though the eukaryotic cells have different shape, size, and physiology; all the cells are typically composed of plasma membrane, cytoplasm and its organelles, *viz.*, mitochondria, endoplasmic reticulum, ribosomes, Golgi apparatus, etc., and a true nucleus. Here the nuclear contents *viz.*, chromatin fibres, nucleoplasm, nucleolus, etc., remain separated from the cytoplasm by the thin, perforated nuclear membranes.

Before going into the details of cell and its components, it will be advisable to consider the general features of different types of cells which are as follows:

Shape

The plant and animal cells exhibit various forms and shapes. Typically the animal cell is spherical in shape but the shape of the cell may be irregular, triangular, tubular, cuboidal, polygonal, cylindrical, oval, rounded or elongated in different animal and plant cells. The shape of the cell may vary from animal to animal and from organ to organ. Even the cells of the same organ may display variations in the shape. Generally the shape of the cell remains correlated with its functions. For example, the epithelial cells have flat shape and the muscle cells are elongated. Moreover, external or internal environment may also cause shape variations in the cell due to internal or mechanical stress or pressure and surface tension, etc.

Size

The eukaryotic cells are typically larger (mostly ranging between 10 to 100 μm) than the prokaryotic cells (mostly ranging between 1 to 10 μm).

The size of the cells of multicellular organisms ranges between 20 to 30 μm. Among animals, the smallest cells have a diameter of 4 μm (*e.g.*, polocytes); human erythrocytes being 7 to 8 μm in diameter. Largest animal cell is the egg of ostrich, having a diameter of 18 cm (its yolk or deutoplasm is about 5 cm in diameter); though, some nerve cells of human beings have a meter long "tails" or axons.

Number

The number of cells present in an organism varies from a single cell in a **unicellular organism** (Protists such as Protozoa and Protophyta) to many cells in multicellular organisms (most plants, fungi and animals). The number of cells in the multicellular organisms usually remains correlated with size of the organisms and, therefore, small-sized organisms have less number of cells in comparison to large-sized organisms. For example, a human being weighing about 80 kg may contain about 60 thousand billion cells in his body. This number would be more in certain other multicellular organisms.

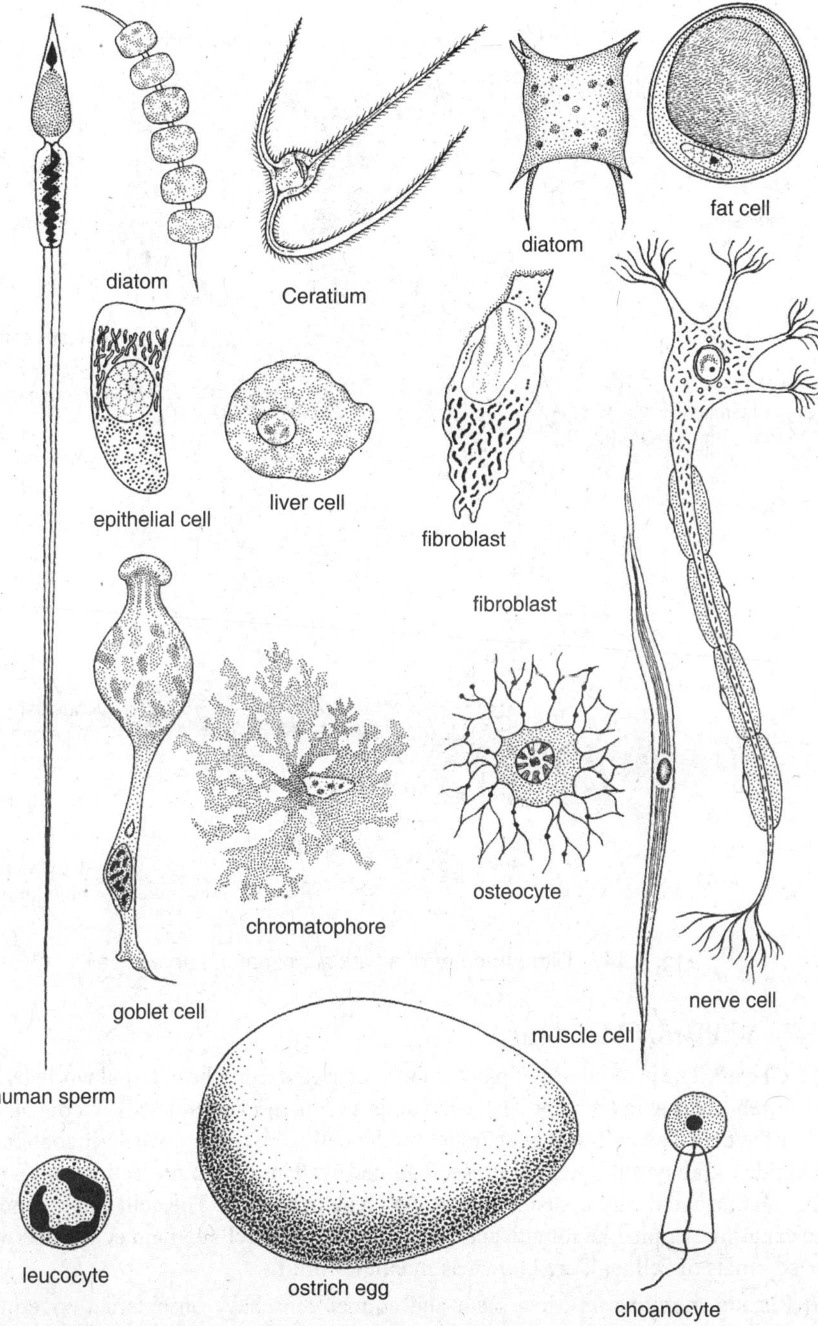

Fig. 4.13. Various types of eukaryotic cells showing different shapes.

Structure

An eukaryotic cell consists of the following components:

A. Cell wall and plasma membrane, B. Cytoplasm, and C. Nucleus.

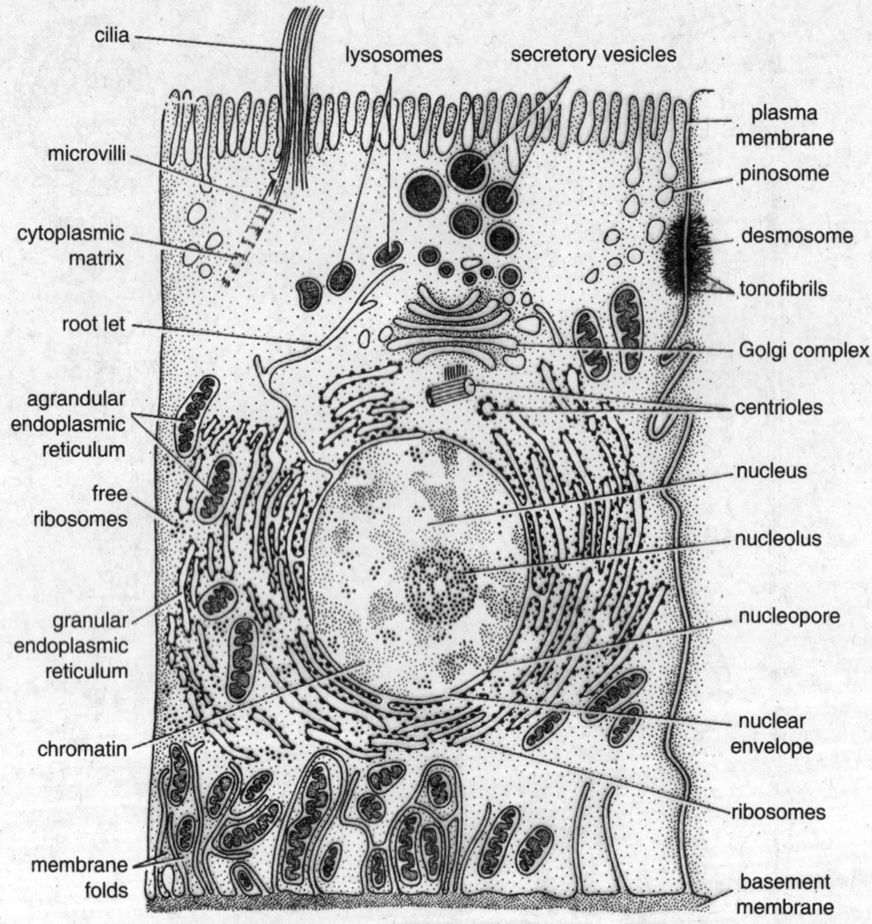

Fig. 4.14. Ultrastructure of a typical animal eukaryotic cell.

Cell Wall and Plasma Membrane

***(i)* Cell wall.** The protoplasm of plant cells is separated from the external world by the cell wall which is entirely lacking in animals. The cell wall is a semi-rigid, laminated, external and non-living covering of the cell. The cell wall is secreted by the cell itself and primarily it contains a complex polysaccharide carbohydrate, the cellulose. The cell wall provides protection and support to the plasma membrane and the cytoplasm, both of which lie beneath it. The cell wall of some plant cells has some canal-like or pit-like minute apertures by which the cells remain connected with adjacent cells. These canals of cell wall are known as **plasmodesmata**.

***(ii)* Plasma membrane.** Most plant and animal cells have an external covering known as plasmalemma, cell membrane, or plasma membrane. The plasma membrane is a living, ultra-thin, elastic, porous, semipermeable membranous covering of cell. Primarily the plasma membrane provides mechanical support and external form to the protoplasm (cytoplasm + nucleus) and it also delimits the protoplasm from the the exterior, checks the entry or exit of undesirable substances and due to its semipermeability it transmits necessary materials to and from the cell. It consists of an outer and inner layers of proteins and a middle layer of lipids. It is found to contain many pores through which exchange of molecules may occur.

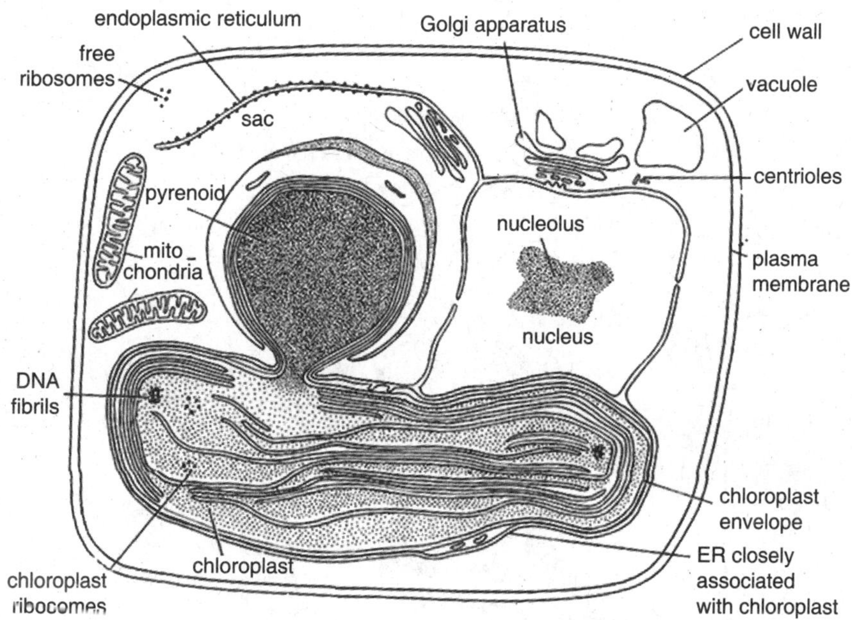

Fig. 4.15. Relationship among organelles in hypothetical brown algae. Note that the flat sacs within the plastid are arranged in extended parallel arrays other than separated into grana and stroma systems as in higher plants.

Cytoplasm

The plasma membrane is followed by distinguished into following structures.

A. Cytoplasmic matrix. The space between the plasma membrane and the nucleus is filled by an amorphous, transluscent, homogeneous colloidal liquid known as **hyaloplasm** or **cytoplasmic matrix**. The cytoplasmic matrix consists of various inorganic molecules such as water, salts of Na, K and other metals and various organic compounds, *viz.*, carbohydrates, lipids, proteins, nucleoproteins, nucleic acids (RNA and DNA) and a variety of enzymes. The peripheral layer of cytoplasmic matrix is relatively non-granular, viscous, clear and rigid and is known as the **plasmagel**, **cortex** or **cortical layer** or **ectoplasm** (Gr., *ecto*-outside, *plasm*-form). The inner portion of the cytoplasmic matrix is granular, less viscous and known as **endoplasm** (Gr., *endo*-inside, *plasm*-form).

B. Cytoplasmic structures. In the cytoplasmic matrix certain , non-living and living structures remain suspended. The non-living structures are called **paraplasm**, **deutoplasm** or **inclusions**, while the living structures are membrane bounded and are called **organoids** or **organelles**. Both kinds of cytoplasmic structures can be studied under the following headings:

(*a*) Cytoplasmic inclusions. The stored, food and secretory substances of the cell remain suspended in the cytoplasmic matrix in the form of refractile granules and forming the cytoplasmic inclusions. Cytoplasmic inclusions are not usually metabolically active in themselves but represent the storage sites for end products of metabolism. The cytoplasmic inclusions include oil drops, yolk granules, pigments, secretory granules, starch granules in plants and glycoge granules in animal cells. Inclusions are not membrane-bounded .

(*b*) Cytoplasmic organoid or organelles. The organoids or organelles are living structures of the cytoplasm. They perform various important biosynthetic and metabolic activities such as respiration biosynthesis, transportation, support, storage and reproduction. The most important cytoplasmic organelles are microtubules, centrosome, basal granules, cilia and flagella, endoplasmic reticulum, Golgi apparatus, lysosomes, cytoplasmic vacuoles, ribosomes, microbodies, mitochondria and plastids.

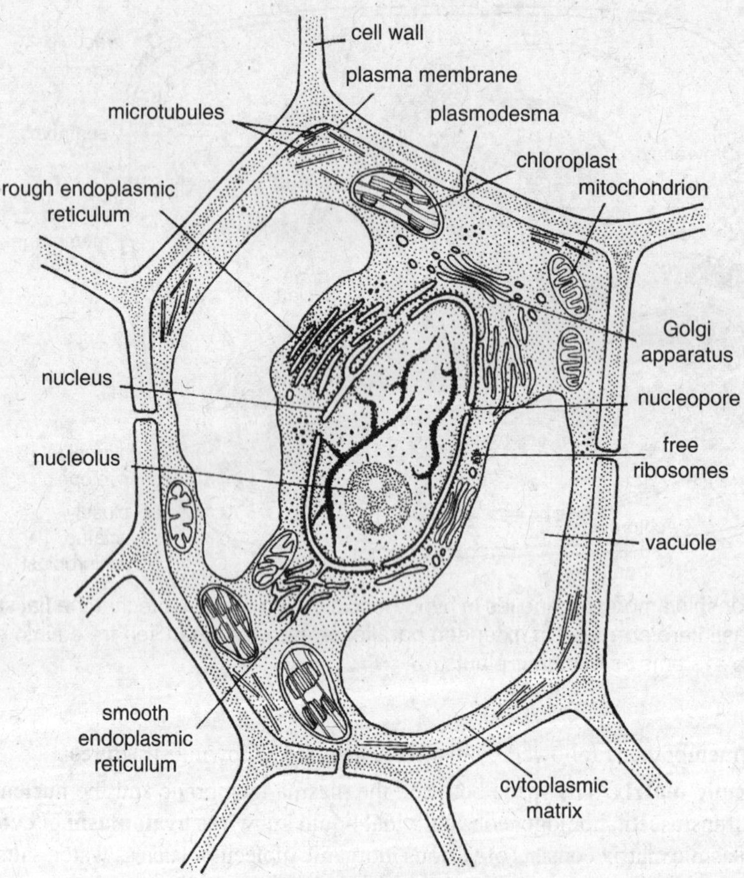

Fig. 4.16. Ultrastructure of a typical cell of a higher plant.

1. Microtubules. The cytoplasm of plant and animal cells is traversed by numerous ultrafine tubules of **tubulin** protein, called **microtubules**. Microtubules are complex sturctures generally comprised of 13 individual **protofilaments** arranged to form a hollow cylinder. The function of microtubules is the transportation of water ions or small molecules, cytoplasmic streaming (cylcosis) and the formation of fibres or asters of the mitotic or meiotic spindle during cell division. Moreover, they form the structural units of the centrioles, basal granules, cilia and flagella.

2. Cytoplasmic filaments. The cytoplasm is laced with ultrafine, proteinous and solid filaments of various sizes. There are three classes of cytoplasmic filaments. The smallest are the **microfilaments**, some 40–60 A° in diameter. They occur next to plasma membrane where they form a web in ectoplasm. The second class, the **myosin filaments** was found first in muscle cells, but the protein of which they are composed has recently been identified in numerous other cell types. The contraction of muscle is achieved by sliding filaments of **myosin** past filaments of **actin**. Actin filaments are very similar to universal microfilaments. This fact has proved that microfilaments are involved in many kinds of cell movements, including division, the amoeba-like crawling common to so many cells and various extensions of the cell surface, such as microvilli.

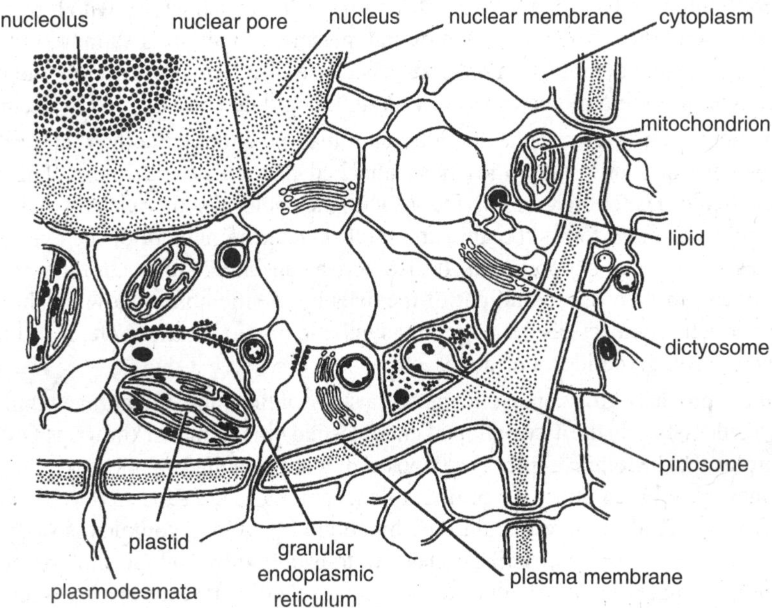

Fig. 4.17. Ultrastructure of plant cell (showing small portion of cell).

In addition to microfilaments and myosin filaments, a third class of filaments called simply **100A° (10 nm) filaments**. These filaments are found to be involved in movement, both of the cell itself and of materials within the cell.

3. Centrosome. The centrosome contains dense cytoplasm and is located near the nucleus of animal cells. During the cell division the centrosome is found to contain two rod-shaped granules known as **centrioles**. The centrioles consist of nine fibrillar units and each fibrillar unit is found to contain three microtubules. At the time of cell division the centrioles form the spindle of microtubules which help in the separation and movement of chromosomes during concluding stages of cell divisions.

4. Basal granules or kinetosomes. The animal or plant cells which are having locomotory organelles such as the cilia or flagella, contain spherical bodies known as **basal granules** or kinetosomes, at the base of the cilia or flagella. The kinetosomes remain embedded in the ectoplasm and are composed of nine fibrils. Each fibril consists of three microtubules, out of which two enter in the cilia or flagella. The basal granules may contain both DNA and RNA. The evidence is questionable.

5. Cilia and flagella. The cells of many unicellular organisms and ciliated epithelium of multicellular organisms consists of some hair-like cytoplasmic projections outside the surface of the cell. These are known as **cilia** or **flagella**. Cilia are typically 2–10 μm long by about 0.5 μm in diameter, and are numerous on those cells that have any at all. Flagella are longer (100–200 μm) and have the same diameter and the same structure, but usually there are no more, than one or two per cell. Both structures are composed of microtubular framework enclosed by an extension of the plasma membrane. The tubules are generally found in nine pairs arranged around the circumference, with two single tubules running down the centre. This is so called "9 + 2" construction, distinct from "9 + 0" construction of the basal body or centriole. The cilia and flagella are originated from the basal granules and chemically consist of tubulin and dynein proteins and adenosine triphosphate (ATP).

Cilia and flagella are motile appendages. Movement is achieved by sliding microtubules past one another. The cells lining the air passages in the lungs, for example, have cilia that beat in a synchronized, wave-like motion to sweep particles out of the lungs. Flagella are more often used to propel the cell itself, *e.g.*, sperm.

6. Endoplasmic reticulum. The cytoplasmic matrix is traversed by a vast reticulum or network of inter-connecting tubules and vesicles which is known as **endoplasmic reticulum** or ER. The endoplasmic reticulum is having a single vast and inter-connected cavity which remains bounded by a single unit membrane. The membrane of endoplasmic reticulum is supposed to be originated by inpushings of plasma membrane in the matrix because like the plasma membrane it has an outer and an inner layer of protein molecules sandwiching the middle layer of lipid molecules.

The membranes of the endoplasmic reticulum may be either smooth when they do not have attached ribosomes or rough when they have attached ribosomes with them. The membrane of endoplasmic reticulum is found to be continuous with the nuclear membrane and plasma membrane. The endoplasmic reticulum forms the ultrastructural skeletal framework of the cytoplasmic matrix and it provides mechanical support to it. It also acts as an intracellular circulatory system and it circulates various substances into and out of the cells by the membrane flow mechanism. Further, the endoplasmic reticulum acts as a storage and synthetic organ. For example, it synthesizes lipids, glycogen, cholesterol, glycerides, hormones, etc.

7. Golgi apparatus. In cytoplasmic matrix, a stack of flattened, membrane bounded, parallely arranged organelles occur in the association of endoplasmic reticulum and known as **Golgi apparatus** or **Golgi complex**. Each Golgi complex is composed of many lamellae, tubules, vesicles and vacuoles. The membranes of Golgi complex are of lipoproteins and these are supposed to be originated from the membranes of endoplasmic reticulum. The function of the Golgi complex is storage of proteins and enzymes which are secreted by ribosomes and transported by endoplasmic reticulum to them. Further the Golgi complex has most important secretory function. It secretes many secretory granules and lysosomes. In plant cells the Golgi complex is known as **dictyosome** and secretes necessary materials for cell wall formation during cell division.

8. Lysosomes. The cytoplasm of animal cells contains many tiny spheroid or irregular-shaped, membrane bounded vesicles known as **lysosomes**. The lysosomes are originated by Golgi complex and contain many digestive enzymes. Their function is the digestion of food material which comes in the cell by pinocytosis and phagocytosis. The lysosomes of plant cells are membrane-bounded storage granules containing hydrolytic digestive enzymes and are comprised of **spherosomes**, **aleurone grain** and **vacuoles**.

9. Cytoplasmic vacuoles. The cytoplasm of many plant and some animal cells (*i.e.*, ciliate protozoans) contains numerous small or large-sized, hollow, liquid-filled structures, the **vacuoles**. These vacuoles are supposed to be greatly expanded endoplasmic reticulum or Golgi complex. The **vacuoles** of animal cells are bounded by a lipoproteinous membrane and their function is the storage, transmission of the materials and the maintenance of internal pressure of the cell.

The vacuoles of the plant cells are bounded by a single, semipermeable membrane known as tonoplast. These vacuoles contain water, phenol, flavonols, anthocyanins (blue and red pigment), alkaloids and storage products, such as sugars and proteins.

10. Microbodies. The cytoplasmic matrix of many kinds of cells, *viz.*, Yeast, Protozoa, cells of higher plants, hepatocytes (liver cells) and kidney cells, contains certain roughly spherical, membrane bounded particles (0.3–1.5 μm diameter). These particles have a central granular or crystalloid core containing some enzymes, occur in intimate relation with endoplasmic reticulum, mitochondria and chloroplasts and are called **microbodies**. The microbodies use molecular oxygen like mitochondria, but instead of having cytochromes and capacity of ATP synthesis like mitochondria, they contain enzymes for hydrogen peroxide metabolism, purine metabolism, gluconeogensis (conversion of fat into carbohydrate) and photorespiration.

11. Ribosomes. Many minute, spherical structures knows as ribosomes are remain attached with the membrane of endoplasmic reticulum and form granular or rough type of ER. The ribosomes are originated in the nucleolus and consist of mainly the ribonucleic acids (RNA) and proteins. Each ribosome is composed of two structural units, a smaller subunit known as **40S subunit** and a larger subunit known as **60S subunit**. The ribosomes remain attached with the membranes of endoplasmic reticulum by the 60S subunits. The 40S subunits occur on the larger unit and form a cap-like structure. The ribosomes consist of 3 types of RNA's known as **ribosomal** RNA's or rRNA, *viz.*, 5S, 18S and 28S rRNA's. The 28S and 5S rRNA's occur in large (60S) subunit, while 18S rRNA occurs in the smaller ribosomal subunit. The ribosomes also occur freely in the cytoplasm. They are the sites of protein synthesis.

12. Mitochondria. In the cytoplasm of most cells occur many large-sized, rounded or rod-like structures known as **mitochondria**. The mitochondria occur singly or in groups and their shape and size vary from cell to cell. The mitochondria are bounded by two membranes of lipoproteins. The outer membrane forms a bag-like structure around the inner membrane which gives out many finger-like folds in the lumen of the mitochondria. The folds of inner mitochondrial membrane are known as **cristae**. The space between outer and inner mitochondrial membrane as well as the central space is filled up by a viscous **mitochondrial matrix**. The matrix, outer and inner membranes are found to contain many oxidative enzymes and coenzymes. The functions of mitochondria are respiration, oxidation of food, and metabolism of energy. Mitochondria are the only major site of oxygen consumption in the cell; hence, eukaryotic cells that do not have mitochondria (*e.g.*, mature mammalian red blood cells) cannot use oxygen. The mitochondria also contain a circular DNA molecule and ribosomes and are capable of synthesis of certain proteins.

13. Plastids. The plastids occur commonly in plant cells and their diameter varies from 4 μm to 6 μm. They may be colourless or coloured. The colour less plastids are known as **leucoplastids** or **leucoplasts** and coloured plastids as **chromoplastids** or **chromoplasts**. The leucoplasts usually have storage function and store starch and lipids and may be called **amyloplasts** and **lipoplasts**, respectively. The chromoplasts may have many forms and pigments, but those having the chlorophyll are most important. These are known as **chloroplasts**. The chloroplasts have complicated organization. They contain DNA, ribosomes and complete protein synthetic machinery. The chloroplasts help in the biosynthesis of food stuffs by the process of photosynthesis.

Nucleus

The nucleus is a centrally located and spherical cellular, component which controls all the vital activities of the cytoplasm and carries the hereditary material the DNA in it. The nucleus consists of three structures: (*i*) nuclear membranes, (*ii*) nucleoplasm and chromosomes, and (*iii*) the nucleolus.

(*i*) Nuclear membranes. The nucleus is bounded by two membranes of lipoprotein which are known as **nuclear membranes**. The nuclear membranes form a kind of envelope around the nucleus and this envelope is known as **nuclear envelope**. The nuclear envelope contains many pore-like octagonal perforations through which to and for movement of chemical substances takes place. The outer nuclear membrane of nuclear envelope remains continuous with the membranes of endoplasmic reticulum and plasma membrane.

(*ii*) Nucleoplasm and Chromosomes. The space between the nuclear membrane and nucleolus is filled by a watery substance known as **nucleoplasm** or **karyolymph**. The nucleoplasm contains dissolved phosphorus, ribose sugars, proteins, nucleotides and nucleic acids. The nucleoplasm contains certain thread-like elongated structures known as **chromosomes**. The chromosomes appear only during cell division otherwise they occur in the form of **chromatin granules**. The chromatin granules or chromosomes fundamentally consist of large molecules of deoxyrbonucleic acid (DNA) and many nucleoproteins.

(*iii*) Nucleolus. The nucleoplasm contains a conspicuous, darkly stained spherical body known as the **nucleolus**. Chemically nucleolus is composed of large amount of ribosomal proteins and ribosomal RNA. The nucleolus stores the rRNA molecules which are synthesized by nucleolar organizer region of DNA (called **rDNA**) and provides the raw materials such as different kinds of rRNA's and ribosomal proteins for the biogenesis of ribosomes.

Table 4.1. Functions of cellular organelles (of an eukaryotic cell).

Cell organelle	Functions
Plasma membrane	It is differentially permeable membrane through which extracellular substances may be selectively sampled and cell products may be liberated.
Cell wall (plant cells)	It forms a thick cellulose wall around the plasma membrane giving strength and rigidity to the cell.
Cytoplasm	It contains machinery for carrying out the instructions sent from the nucleus.
Hyaloplasm or matrix	It contains enzymes for glycolysis and structural materials such as sugars, fatty acids, amino acids, water, vitamins, nucleotides, etc.
Microtubules	They transport water, ions and small molecules of various substances, form structural unit of centrioles, basal granules, cilia, flagella and mitotic spindle and play active role in the cyclosis (amoeboid movement) of cytoplasm and in movement of chromosomes during the cell divisions.
Microfilaments	They maintain the structure of cell and form contractile components of muscle cell and cells performing amoeboid movement.
Centrioles	They form the spindle and have significant role in the movement of chromosomes during cell divisions.
Basal granules	They originate the cilia or flagella and have their importance in ciliary or flagellar movement.
Cilia and flagella	These are microtubule-containing extracellular projections of the cell which provide movement to the cells and serve various other roles of cells.
Endoplasmic reticulum	It provides greatly expanded surface area for biochemical reactions which normally occur at or across membrane surfaces and provide skeletal support to the colloidal complex of hyaloplasm. It also has transporting business of extracellular and intracellular chemical molecules.
Ribosomes	These are the sites for synthesis of protein molecules.
Golgi apparatus	It stores and modifies the synthetic proteins and enzymes of cells and forms secretory vesicles and lysosomes.
Lysosomes (animals only)	They contain intracellular digestive enzymes which aid in disposal of bacteria and other foreign bodies.
Peroxisomes (Microbodies)	They contain enzymes for hydrogen peroxide metabolism, purine metabolism, gluconeogenesis and photorespiration.
Sphaerosomes	They store fats.
Vacuoles	They are storage depots for excess water, waste products, soluble pigments, etc.
Mitochondria	They are the organelles for the oxidation of food by Krebs cycle, production of energy by electron transport chain and beta-oxidation of fatty acids.
Plastids (Plants only)	They are the structures for storage of starch, pigments, and other cellular products. Photosynthesis occurs in chloroplasts.
Nucleus	It regulates growth and reproduction of cell.
Nuclear membrane	It provides selective continuity between nuclear and cytoplasmic materials.
Nucleoplasm	It contains materials for building DNA and messenger molecules (different kinds of RNA molecules, *viz.*, rRNA, mRNA and tRNA) which act as intermediates between nucleus and cytoplasm.
Chromosomes	They are the bearers of hereditary instructions and regulations of cellular processes.
Nucleolus	It disappears during cellular replication and synthesizes the ribosomes.

Differences between Prokaryotic and Eukaryotic cells

Main differences between prokaryotic cells (of archaea, bacteria, blue green algae and mycoplasma) and eukaryotic cells (of protozoa, fungi, plants and animals) have been tabulated in Table 4.2.

Table 4.2. Some major differences between prokaryotic and eukaryotic cells.

		Feature	Prokaryotic cell	Eukaryotic cell
1.	Size		Mostly 1–10 μm	Mostly 10–100 μm
2.	Multicellular forms		Rare	Common, with extensive tissue formation
3.	Cell wall		Present in most but not in all cells	Present in plant and fungal cell only
4.	Plasma membrane		Present	Present
5.	Nucleus		Absent	Present
6.	Nuclear membranes		Absent	Present
7.	Chromatin with histone		Absent	Present
8.	Genetic material		Circular or linear, double-stranded DNA: genes are not interrupted by intron* (notable exception is archaea)	Linear double-stranded DNA: genes frequently interrupted by intron sequences, especially in higher eukaryotes (such genes are called **split genes**)
9.	Nucleoli and mitotic apparatus		Absent	Present
10.	Plasmids		Commonly present	Rare
11.	Cellular organelles:			
	(i)	Mitochondria	Absent	Present
	(ii)	Endoplasmic reticulum	Absent	Present
	(iii)	Vacuoles	Absent	Present
	(iv)	Lysosomes	Absent	Present
	(v)	Chloroplasts	Absent	Present (only in plants)
	(vi)	Centrioles	Absent	Present (absent in higher plants)
	(vii)	Ribosomes	Present (70S)	Present (80S)
	(viii)	Microtubules	Absent	Present
	(ix)	Flagellae	Simple structure composed of the protein flagellin	Complex 9 + 2 structure of tubulin and other proteins
12.	Respiration		Many strict anaerobes (oxygen fatal)	All aerobic, but some facultative anaerobes by secondary modifications
13.	Metabolic patterns		Great variations	All share cytochrome electron transport chains, Krebs cycle oxidation, Embden-Meyerhof glucose metabolism or glycolysis
14.	Photosynthetic enzymes		Bound to plasma membrane as composite chromatophores	Enzymes packaged in plastids bound by membrane

	Feature	Prokaryotic cell	Eukaryotic cell
15.	Sexual system	Rare: if present one way (and usually partial); transfer of DNA from donor to recipient cell occurs	Both sexes involved in sexual participation and entire genomes transferred; alternation of haploid and diploid generations is also evident

*Intron is an intervening sequence of nucleotides in DNA, located within a gene that is not included in the mature mRNA.

Differences between Plant and Animal Cells

Differences between typical animal and plant cells have been tabulated in Table 4.3.

Table 4.3. Differences between animal and plant cells.

	Animal cell		Plant cell
1.	Animal cells are generally small in size.	1.	Plant cells are larger than animal cells.
2.	Cell wall is absent.	2.	The plasma membrane of plant cells is surrounded by a rigid cell wall of cellulose.
3.	Except the protozoan *Euglena* no animal cell possesses plastids.	3.	Plastids are present.
4.	Vacuoles in animal cells are many and small.	4.	Most mature plant cells have a large central sap vacuole.
5.	Animal cells have a single highly complex and prominent Golgi apparatus.	5.	Plant cells have many simpler units of Golgi apparatus, called dictyosomes.
6.	Animal cells have centrosome and centrioles.	6.	Plant cells lack centrosome and centrioles.

REVISION QUESTIONS

1. Define the cell. How will you differentiate between the prokaryotic and eukaryotic cells?
2. What is a virus? Is it alive? How do viruses compare with cells in size and structure? What is a typical life cycle of a virus? What is meant by lysogeny? A provirus?
3. Which of the eukaryotic organelles are also found in prokaryotes? Are their structures the same in the two types of cells?
4. What structures are typically found in plant cells that are lacking in animal cells?
5. What cytoplasmic organelles are found in eukaryotic cells and what are the general functions of each?
6. Even today one can read in some books that a particular organism is "*Somewhere between a virus and a bacterium*". If it is upto you to decide into which category it falls, how would you go about it?

5 Chapter

CYTOPLASM

The part of the cell which occurs between the plasma membrane and nuclear envelope is known as cytoplasm (Gr., *kytos*-hollow, *plasma*-form). The cytoplasm forms the most essential part of the cell because it is the seat of all biosynthetic and bioenergetic functions. It is composed of two distinct types of structures, the matrix (L., *matrix*-womb) and the **organelles** (Gr., *organon*-instrument).

5.1 MATRIX

After the removal of all the organelles from the cytoplasm, there remains a transparent, homogeneous and colloidal substance called **matrix**. **Purkinje** (1840) has described the matrix by the name of **protoplasm**. The matrix is also known by various other names such as the ground cytoplasm, fundamental cytoplasm, hyaloplasm and kinoplasm, etc.

Physical Nature of Matrix

In past, there has been a lot of controversy about the physical nature of the matrix. Different workers advanced different theories about the physical characteristics of the matrix. Their theories can be represented as follows:

1. **Reticular theory** suggests that the matrix is composed of reticulum of fibres or particles in the ground substances (Fig. 5.1A).
2. **Alveolar theory** was proposed by **Butschili** in 1892 and according to it, the matrix consists of many suspended droplets or alveoli or minute bubbles resembling the foams of emulsion (Fig. 5.1B).
3. **Granular theory** was propounded by **Altmann** in 1893. This theory supports the view that the matrix contains many granules of smaller and larger size arranged differently. These granules were known as bioplasts (Fig. 5.1C).
4. **Fibrillar theory** was proposed by **Fleming** and it holds that the matrix is fibrillar in nature (Fig. 5.1D).
5. **Colloidal theory** has been forwarded very recently after the electron microscopical observations of the matrix. According to this recent concept, the matrix is partly a true **solution**, partly a **colloidal system**.

A solution is a mixture of liquid called **solvent** and any chemical substance in solid or liquid state, called **solute**. In a solution the particles of solute should be less than 1/10,000 millimetre in diameter. The solution part of the matrix consists of water as solvent in which various solutes of biological importance such as glucose, amino acids, fatty acids, electrolytes, minerals, vitamins, hormones and enzymes remain dissolved.

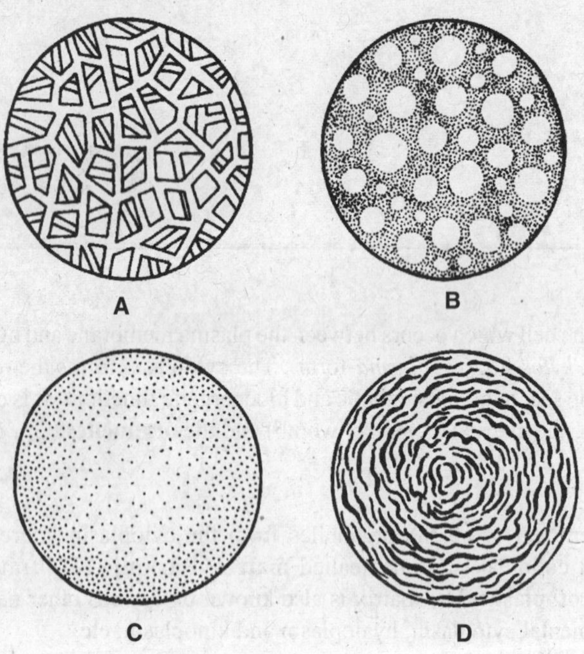

Fig. 5.1. Physical appearance of protoplasm. A—Reticular, B—Alveolar, C—Granular, and D—Fibrillar.

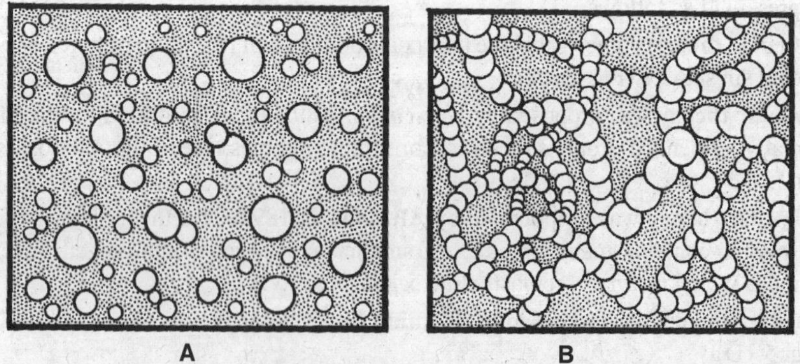

Fig. 5.2. Cytoplasm in sol (A) and gel (B) state.

A colloidal system can be defined as a system which contains a liquid medium in which the particles ranging from about 1/10,000,000 to 1/10,000 millimetre in diameter, remain dispersed. In other words, a colloidal system composed of two phases namely **liquid phase** and **dispersed phase**. The colloidal part of the matrix is polyphasic and consists of a liquid phase in the form of water and dispersed phase in the form of macromolecular solids such as proteins and nucleic acids and liquids such as oily fats (lipids).

Phase reversal. The colloidal system ot the matrix may occur fither in a semisolid or liquid state. The semisolid state is known as **gel phase** or **gel state**, while the liquid state is known as **sol phase** or **sol state**. In gel state the molecules of colloidal substances remain held, together by various types of chemical bonds or bond between H—H, C—H or C—N. The stability of gel depends on the nature and strength of chemical bonds.

Both the states of colloidal matrix are interchangeable according to the various physiological, mechanical and biochemical activities of the cell. Thus, a gel can change into sol by **solation** and a sol can change into gel by **gelation**. This property of colloidal matrix is called **phase reversal**.

Chemical Organization of Matrix

Chemically, the cytoplasmic matrix is composed of many chemical elements in the form of atoms, ions and molecules.

Chemical elements. According to **John Dalton** (1766–1844), a chemical element is a fundamental substance which cannot be broken down into two or more simpler substances. Uptil now, about 104 elements have been discovered in the universe. Out of these 104 elements, only 90 different elements [*viz.*, from hydrogen (1) to thorium (90)] occurring naturally on earth, and other 14 different elements *e.g.*, protactinium (91), Lawrencium (103), etc.] have been man made in the cyclotron, on nuclear reactor of laboratories of nuclear physics. From these 104 elements of universe, the cytoplasmic matrix consists of about 36 elements. The 36 elements occur in different percentage in the matrix and perform various important biological and chemical activities for the cell. Generally, they are grouped in the following three categories according to their percentage in the matrix and in molecules.

***(i)* Major constituents.** The elements which occur predominantly in the matrix are called **major constituents**. The major constituents of the matrix are oxygen, (O, 62%), carbon (C, 20%), hydrogen (H, 10%) and nitrogen (N, 3%). These elements occur in the wide array of chemical molecules (inorganic and organic) of great biological importance.

***(ii)* Trace elements.** The elements which occur in low percentage in the matrix are called **trace elements**. The trace elements of the matrix are: calcium (Ca, 2.5%), phosphorus (P, 1.14%), chlorine (Cl, 0.16), sulphur (S, 0.14%), potassium (K, 0.11%), sodium .(Na, 0.10%), magnesium (Mg, 0.07%), iodine (I, 0.014%) and iron (Fe, 0.10%). These elements occur in significant ratio in various biologically important molecules, for example, phosphorus is one of the main component of adenosine triphosphate (ATP) and deoxyribonucleic acid (DNA) and ribonucleic acid (RNA). Further, many trace elements required by the cell for its various physical and biochemical activities such as osmosis, diffusion, impulse conduction and other various physico-chemical activities.

***(iii)* Ultrastructure elements.** The rest 23 elements such as copper (Cu), cobalt (Co), manganese (Mn), zinc (Zn), molybdenum (Mo), boron (B), silicon (Si), etc., occur in the matrix in 0.756%. Most of them required by the cell as cofactors for various chemical reactions.

Atom and its structure. Each of the 104 elements known to man is composed of a characteristic kind of identical atoms. The atoms of an element are perfectly alike in shape, weight, and physicochemical properties. An atom can be defined as the smallest part of an element that can enter into combinations with other elements. Once the atoms were believed to be the ultimate, smallest units of matter, but now, it has become clear that atoms are divisible and are complex assemblage of tinier elementary particles or **subatomic particles**. Uptill now about twelve kinds of subatomic particles namely—**photon, neutrino, electron, muon, pion, kaon, proton, neutron, lambda, sigma, chi** and **omega**, have been found to occur in different kinds of atoms (for details see **C. Mande** and **A. Pimpale**, 1973). For our purpose, we need consideration of only three types of subatomic particles—**electrons** (e±) which have a negative electric charge and an extremely small mass or weight (0.511 Mev) : **protons** (P±) which have a positive electric charge and are 1836 times heavier than the electron and have mass 938.2 Mev; and **neutrons** (n), which have no electrical charge, but have essentially the same mass as protons (936.5 Mev). (1 Mev = 1.783×10^{-27} gm).

The centre of the atom, corresponding in position to the sun in our solar system, is the **nucleus**, containing protons and neutrons (both of which are also called **nucleons**); it comprises almost the total mass of the atom. Just as the solar system is mostly empty space, so is the atom, with electrons revolving around the nucleus in definite **paths**, **shells**, **energy levels** or **orbits**. The various types of atoms have different numbers of electrons circling in orbits and different numbers of protons and neutrons in their nuclei. In all atoms, the number of protons in the nucleus equals the number of electrons circling around it, so that a state of electric neutrality is maintained. Further, the number of protons present in the atomic nucleus of an atom of an element forms the atomic number, of that atom, For example, the simplest atom, **hydrogen** (H) has atomic number one and consists of a single proton in the nucleus and a single electron revolving around the nucleus in a spherical orbit; the atom of **helium** (He) consists of atomic number 2 and two protons and two neutrons in the nucleus and two electrons around the nucleus; and the atomic number of **carbon** (C) is 6, it has 6 protons, 6 neutrons and 6 electrons in two orbits, the inner orbit has only two electrons, while outer orbit has four electrons.

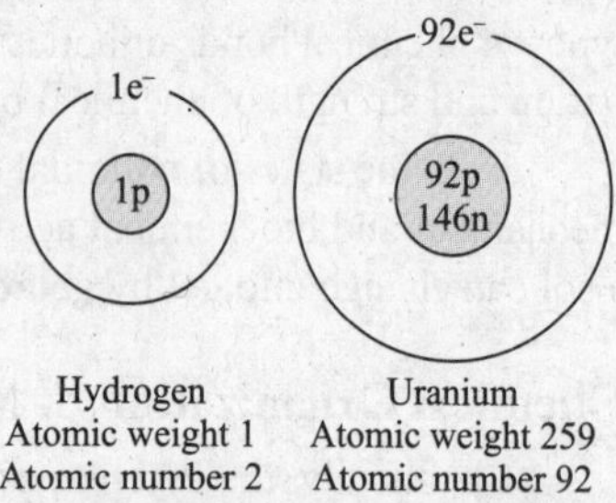

Fig. 5.3. Atomic structure of hydrogen and uranium.

Further, there are limits to the number of electrons that can be present at any single energy level or orbit. At the innermost energy level only two electrons can be present. The next level can hold a maximum of eight electrons. These are arranged in four pairs. The maximum number of electrons which can exist at any given level (n) can be computed from the expression—maximum number = $2n^2$. The arrangement of electrons in the atom plays a crucial role in its chemistry. Atoms are most stable when their outer shell contains its full quota of electrons. The so called inert gases (*e.g.*, neon and argon) have eight electrons in their outer shell.

Other atoms tend to gain or lose electrons until their outer shell also has the stable arrangement of the inert gases. Such unstable atoms are called charged atoms or **ions**. For example, atoms with one, two or three electrons in the outer shell usually lose these so that the next inner shell with a more stable set of electrons left exposed. These atoms are called **electro-positive atoms** or **cations**. The elements with atoms of this kind are the metals, such as sodium, magnesium, potassium and calcium. Atoms with four, five, six or seven electrons in their outer shell tend to add the necessary number of electrons to complete this shell. These atoms are **electronegative** or **anions**. The elements with this kind of atoms are the non-metals, such as carbon, nitrogen, oxygen, phosphorus, sulphur, and chlorine.

The cytoplasmic matrix consists of various kinds of ions. The ions are important in maintaining osmotic pressure and acid-base balance in the cells. Retention of ions in the matrix produces an increase in osmotic pressure and thus, the entrance of water in the cell. The concentration of various ions in the intracellular fluid (matrix) differs from that in the interstitial fluid. For example, in the cell K^+ and Mg^{++} can be high, and Na^+ and Cl^- high outside the cell. In muscle and nerve cells a high order of difference exists between intracellular K^+ and extracellular Na^+. Free calcium ions (Ca^{++}) may occur in cells or circulating blood. Silicon ions occur in the epithelium cells of grasses. The free ions of phosphate (primary, $H_2PO_4^-$ and secondary, HPO_4^-) occur in the matrix and blood. These ions act as a buffering system and tend to stabilize pH of blood and cellular fluids. The ions of different cells also include sulphate (SO_4^-), carbonate (CO_3^-), bicarbonate (HCO_3^-), magnesium (Mg^{++}) and amino acids.

Atomic weight. The weight of a quantity of the element in question relative to the weight of an equal quantity of carbon, which is taken as 12.01, is called the **atomic weight** of that element.

Thus, the atomic weights of some biologically important elements are following—nitrogen (14.01), oxygen (16.00), sodium (23.00), chlorine (35.46), potassium (39.01) and iron (55.85).

Compounds and molecules. Under specific conditions most atoms can become attached to certain other atoms. Such combinations of two or more atoms are called **compounds**. In a compound, the atoms are held together by specific bonding forces or chemical bonds. The fundamental or smallest unit of a compound is a molecule. A molecule is not a mere mixture of atoms of same or different types of elements, but in a molecule the atoms of different or same elements are bound in different proportions and by different kinds of chemical bonds. A molecule has a definite shape and properties. There are following two possible ways by which atoms of different elements may join each other to form a molecule of a compound:

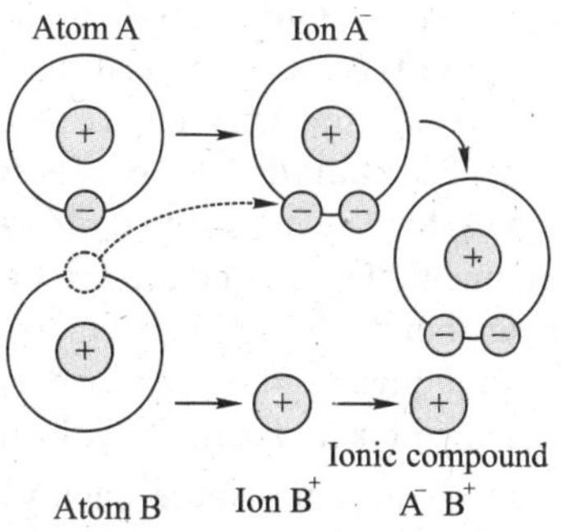

Fig. 5.4. Electron transfer and formation of ionic compound.

***(i)* Formation of an ionic compound.** When in a group of atoms of different types of elements, due to ionization some atoms become anions (electronegative) and other atoms become cations (electropositive), both electronegative and electropositive atoms start to attract each other. Subsequently, both atoms become united by a chemical bond, called **ionic** or **electrovalent bond** or **electrostatic bond** and form a compound. Such compounds which are formed by a transfer of electrons between atoms and a mutual attraction of the resulting ions are called **ionic compounds**.

The number of the ionic bonds in an ionic compound depends on the number of transferring electrons between two ionized atoms and that varies compound to compound. For example, NaCl is ionic compound. Its single molecule contains a cation (Na^+) and a anion (Cl^-) both of which remain united by a single ionic bond. In such electron transfers, atom that tend to lose electrons and thereby becomes positively charged ions are otherwise called **metals**, and atoms that gain electrons and become negatively charged ions arc **non-metals**. Sodium is metal and chlorine is non-metal.

***(ii)* Formation of molecular compounds.** In the previous paragraph, we have observed that the ionic compounds are typically formed when in a group of atoms, some (non-metal) attract electrons very strongly whereas others (metals) attract electrons quite weakly. But, when two or more atoms attract electrons with more or less equal force, another type of situation comes in existence. For example, when two atoms of oxygen (A and B) occur in close proximity, then the nucleus of oxygen atom A will attract some of the electrons of atom B, but the nucleus of oxygen atom B now also attracts some of electrons of atom A with equal force and thus, an electronic "tug of the war" will, therefore, take place and neither atom can "win". This mutual tugging will continue indefinitely and as a result the electrons of both atoms will remain linked together. In this case, thus, no transfer of electrons occurs and also no ion is formed. Instead, as each atom pulls on electrons of tbe other, some electrons of both atoms are shared in common.

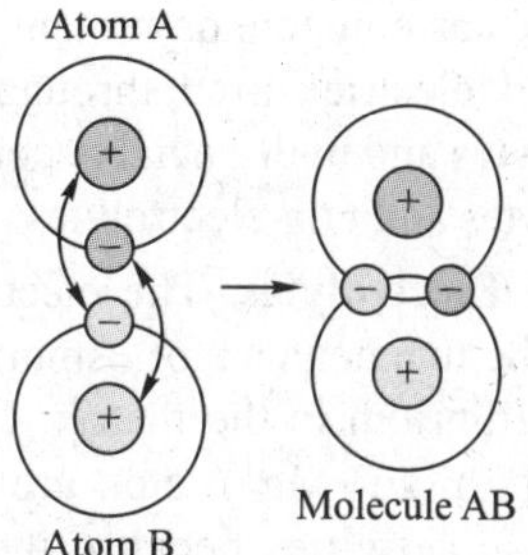

Fig. 5.5. Electron sharing and formation of molecular compounds.

Electron sharing represents a second major way in which compounds are formed. Compounds of this type are called **molecular compounds** or **simple molecules**. The chemical bonds within molecules are called **covalent bonds**. Covalent bonds are strong chemical links between atoms and contain a relatively large amount of chemical energy. The number of covalent bonds in a molecular compound is related directly to the number of electrons shared.

Chemical bonds. Covalent and electrostatic bonds are called **primary bonds** of molecules. They are the types of chemical linkages that hold atoms together in molecules. Many biological molecules such as water, proteins, nucleic acids, etc., are capable of forming weaker types of chemical bonds, called **secondary bonds**. These bonds are responsible for holding molecules together in larger aggregates, for causing one part of large molecules to bend or fold and become attached to other parts of the same molecule, and are responsible for the nature of liquid water's structure and properties. Secondary bonds are weaker chemical linkages, but they have great influence over molecular structure because although each secondary bond may be weak, there can be dozens or hundreds of such bonds associated with a molecule or with an aggregation of molecules such as is found in water.

One of the important secondary bonds is the **hydrogen bond** and this type of bond is responsible for many of the structural features of macromolecules, such as proteins or nucleic acids.

Dissociation. All chemical compounds of biological importance occur in the water medium of the matrix. When ionic compounds are dissolved in water, they generally exist as free ions physically separate from one another, water molecules become interposed between the ions of the compound. The process by which the atoms of a compound become separated as cations or anions is called **dissociation**. Similarly, when the molecular compounds are dissolved in water, one of two events may occur. Some types of molecular compounds simply continue to exist as whole, intact molecules with water interposed between individual ones. Ordinary sugar is a good example of such molecular compounds. By contrast, other types of molecular compounds do not remain intact in water, instead become dissociated mto ions like an ionic compound, such as follows:

$$\underset{\text{Sodium hydroxide}}{NaOH} \xrightarrow{H_2O} \underset{\text{Sodium ion}}{Na^+} + \underset{\text{Hydroxyl ion}}{OH^-}$$

$$\underset{\text{Acetic acid}}{CH_3COOH} \xrightarrow{H_2O} \underset{\text{Acetate}}{CH_3COO^-} + \underset{\text{Hydrogen ion}}{H^+}$$

Electrolytes and non-electrolytes. In as much as dissociation produces equal amounts of positive and negative electric charges (or cations and anions), solutions containing dissociated ionic or molecular compounds remain electrically neutral. However, the presence of free ions permits passage of electric current through such solutions. Dissociable compounds are, therefore, also called **electrolytes** and undissociable compounds are called **non-electrolytes**. The matrix consists of both electrolytes and non-electrolytes.

(*i*) Electrolytes. The electrolytes play a vital role in the maintenance of osmotic pressure and acid base equilibrium in the matrix. Certain ions such as the magnesium (Mg^+), etc., are essential for many enzymatic activities because these act as cofactor. The phosphate (PO_4) ion is the important constituent of adenosine triphosphate (ATP) which is the chief supplier of energy for most of the life processes.

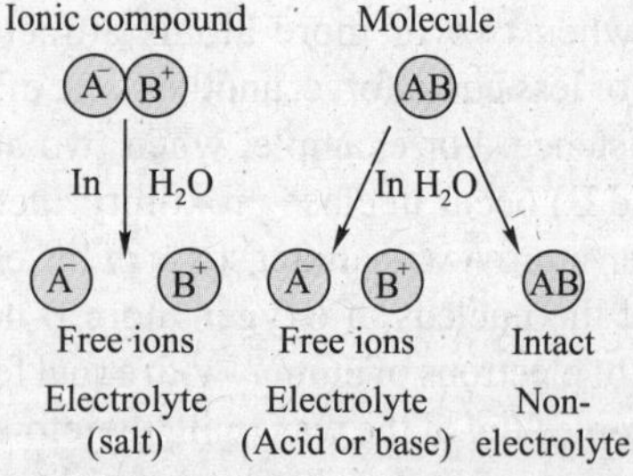

Fig. 5.6. Electrolytes and non-electrolytes.

(*ii*) Non-electrolytes. Some of minerals occur in matrix in non-ionzing state. The non-electrolytes of the matrix are Na, K, Ca, Mg, Cu, I, Fe, Mn, Fl, Mo, Cl, Zn, Co, Ni, etc. The iron (Fe) occurs in the haemoglobin, ferritin cytochromes and some enzymes as catalase and cytochrome oxidase. The calcium (Ca) occurs in the blood, matrix and the bones. The copper (Cu), manganese (Mn), molybdenum (Mo) and zinc (Zn) are useful as cofactors for enzymatic actions. The iodine and fluorine are essential for the thyroid and the enamel metabolism, respectively.

Acids, bases, and salts. The ionic and molecular compounds of the matrix generally belong to one of the three general classes: acids, bases or salts. An **acid** is a compound containing hydrogen which is replaceable by a metal or in other words an acid is a compound which in solution yields hydrogen ions.

$$\underset{\text{Hydrochloric acid}}{HCl} \rightarrow \underset{\text{Hydrogen ion}}{H^+} - \underset{\text{Chloride ion}}{Cl^-}$$

$$\underset{\text{Sulphuric acid}}{H_2SO_4} \rightarrow \underset{\text{Hydrogen ion}}{2H^+} + \underset{\text{Sulphate ion}}{SO_4^-}$$

A base is a compound in which a metal is combined with a hyd roxyl radical (OH^-) or in other words a base is a compound in which solution yields hydroxyl ions:

$$\underset{\text{Potassium hydroxide}}{KOH} \rightarrow \underset{\text{Potassium ion}}{K^+} + \underset{\text{Hydroxyl ion}}{OH^-}$$

The **salts** are composed of metals and non-metals combined in ways which do not qualify them as either acid or bases; that is, in solution salts yield neither hydrogen ions nor hydroxyl ions:

$$\underset{\text{Sodium chloride}}{NaCl} \rightarrow \underset{\text{Sodium ion}}{Na^+} + \underset{\text{Chloride ion}}{Cl^-}$$

5.2 TYPES OF COMPOUNDS OF MATRIX

The matrix contains both ionic and molecular compounds and these compounds are superficially classified into two main categories such as follows:

5.3 INORGANIC COMPOUNDS

The inorganic compounds are those compounds which normally found in the bulk of the physical, non-living universe, such as elements, metals, non-metals, and their compounds such as water, salts and a variety of electrolytes and non-electrolytes. In the previous section, we have discussed a lot about the inorganic substances except the water which will be discussed in the following; paragraph.

Water

The most abundant inorganic component of the matrix is the water. Water constitutes about 65 to 80 per cent of the matrix.

In the matrix the water occurs in two forms, *viz*., **free water** and **bound water**. The 95 per cent of the total cellular water is used by the matrix as the solvent for various inorganic substances and organic compounds and is known as **free water**. The remaining 5 per cent of the total cellular water remains loosely linked with protein molecules by hydrogen bonds or other forces and known as **bound water**.

The water contents of the cellular matrix of an organism depend directly on the age, habitat and metabolic activities. For instance, the cells of the embryo have 90 to 95 per cent water which decreases progressively in the cells of the adult organism. The cells of lower aquatic animals contain comparatively high percentage of the water than the cells of higher terrestrial animals, Further the percentage of the water in the matrix also varies from cell to cell according to the rate of the metabolism. It is believed that life originated in water and life is impossible without water. Water is essential to living systems, but its direct role in cellular processes is usually not known. The exact structure of liquid water is also, not known. However, its many unique properties which seem essential for living systems can be well understood by studying its molecular structure and bonding pattern.

Molecular structure of water. Water is formed by the combination of hydrogen and oxygen through the formation of covalent bonds, in which atoms, by sharing pairs of electrons, become linked together. Each oxygen atom has two electrons which it may share with two hydrogen bonds.

If the two bonds in the water molecule were completely covalent, that is, if there were an equal sharing of electrons between the oxygen and hydrogen atoms, theory states that the bond angle between the oxygen and hydrogens should be 90°. But the bond angle actually is 104.5° in water molecule. The main reason for this greater-than-expected bond angle is that the oxygen atom is more **electronegative** than the hydrogen atom. This simply means that the oxygen atom has a stronger attraction for the negatively charged electrons than does the hydrogen atom, and therefore the rapidly moving electrons tend to spend more time in the neighbourhood of the oxygen atom than of the hydrogen atom.

This unequal spatial distribution of electrons tends to give the oxygen atom of the water molecule a negative charge, and the absence of the electrons in the vicinity of the hydrogen atoms of the water molecule tends to give them a positive charge; they act almost as hydrogen ions (H^+). The water molecule is a charged molecule—a **dipole**—containing two charged groups. There is a negative charge in the region of the oxygen atom, and a positive charge in the region of the hydrogens. This unequal distribution of electrons between atoms of the water molecule tends to make the bonds of the water molecule somewhat electrostatic. The dipole nature of water molecule is responsible for many of the unique properties of water because the charges present on the molecules permit them to form weak chemical linkages with each other and with other molecules.

Further, whenever a covalent bond is formed between hydrogen and an electronegative atom, such as oxygen (O), the hydrogen becomes almost a bare proton (H^+), because it tends to lose its one electron to the electronegative atom. Such a hydrogen atom within a molecule with its positive charge can form a weak electrostatic bond with any other negatively charged chemical group.

The oxygen atom of a given water molecule is covalently bonded to its two hydrogen atoms and is also hydrogen-bonded to a hydrogen atom of each of two other water molecules. Thus water molecules form a three dimensional crystalline network structure in ice. When ice melts to form liquid water, about 15 per cent of the hydrogen bonds between water molecules are broken and water still retains a somewhat ice-like structure. But now there are free water molecules with more movement available to them. Liquid water is even more labile (changeable) than this, and it is thought that water molecules are constantly breaking and making hydrogen bonds between them. One model to show this type of labile structuring is the **flickering cluster model**, in which it is assumed that collections of water molecules are momentarily joined together by hydrogen bonds, forming small clumps of structured water, somewhat like miniature icebergs. These events which are taking place at the molecular level are extremely rapid; for example, such "icebergs" are thought to have an existence of only 10^{-11} second before they break apart. This type of structuring of water molecules has given unique properties to water molecules, such as follows:

Unique Properties of Water and its Uses

1. Water is one of the best solvents known, and this is useful to biological systems with a variety of different molecular types that exist in solution for normal cellular activities. The polar nature of water molecules makes it possible for them to attract other charged molecules or ions; and this attraction of such charged particles tends to separate them and allow them to become surrounded by water molecules. This is, in fact, exact what solution is : the surrounding of solute molecules by liquid medium (solvent), which prevents solute molecules from aggregating together and precipitating out of the solution. The more polar the solvent (*i.e.*, the more charged it is), the more molecules can be dissolved in it. Water is a very polar liquid, and therefore can act as a solvent for a wide variety of charged particles.

2. The water forms the good dispersion medium for the colloidal system of the matrix.

3. Water is also a stabilizer of the temperature of the atmosphere, the oceans and the bodies and cells of organisms. Water has a very high **heat capacity**. Heat capacity in terms of **specific heat**, is

a measure of the amount of heat that a substance can absorb to produce a given rise in temperature; it is the quantity of heat in calories or joules required to raise the temperature of 1 gram of substance 1 degree Celsius. One calorie is the amount of heat required to raise the temperature of 1 gram of water from 14.5 to 15.5°C. One calorie is equivalent to 4.185 Joules, the latter being the more accepted measure of heat today .

The higher the specific heat of a substance, the smaller is its rise in temperature upon the absorption of a given amount of heat. When substances absorb heat, the heat energy is transformed into the kinetic energy of the molecules (this is the energy of molecular motion). Under these conditions random molecular movement is increased, and this is what we measure and call **temperature**. When water is heated, the heat energy is first used to break the hydrogen bonds that are holding the water molecules together. Only after all the hydrogen bonds are broken can heat be absorbed by the water molecules themselves, with an increase in the motion of the now-freed water molecules and a corresponding rise in temperature. Here, again, the basic dipole nature of the water molecule and the resulting ability of hydrogen bonds to form between water molecules play a significant role in producing a liquid whose thermal properties are necessary to maintain a stable life environment.

The high specific heat of water is useful in aiding in the maintenance of the proper body temperatures of organisms. All cells are constantly producing heat as a result of chemical reactions that take place in the cell. As this heat is produced by body cells, much of it can be absorbed by body water with little rise in temperature, until such time as the organism can lose any excess heat. Cells generally can withstand only relatively small changes in temperature, so in them water acts to avoid drastic temperature changes and maintains a relatively constant thermal environment, inside cell.

4. Water also has a high **heat of vaporization**—the amount of heat energy required to convert 1 gram of liquid to its gaseous state. This is used to advantage by some organisms as a cooling mechanism in warmer environments or during strenuous exercise, when large amounts of heat is produced. By evaporating water from body surfaces or from respiratory passages, excess body heat is removed, with the use of only a relatively small amount of water. The reason of high heat of vaporization of water is that heat energy is used first to break the hydrogen bonds holding water molecules together. Only after the molecules are freed from these attachments can the heat be used to increase molecular motion and allow water molecules to separate far enough away from each other to form a gas. About 600 calories of heat are needed to convert 1 gram of water from the liquid to the gaseous state.

5. Other unique properties of water arise from its hydrogen-bonded nature. Water molecules show great coherence; that is, they hold together strongly. In fact, only mercury shows a greater coherence. Such a strong coherence means that water has a large surface tension.

A somewhat similar phenomenon is that of **capillary action**, in which; water is seen to move up a fine-bore tubing or through a piece of paper toweling, or through minute soil channels that allow water to reach plant roots. This movement of water is due to its **adhesion**, the ability of water to be attracted to and join with molecules of other substances.

6. The water has greater importance for the various metabolic functions because most of them require exclusively the aqueous media.

7. The water is used by the cell as a transporting media for the food, nitrogen wastes and other necessary substances.

8. The water is immiscible with the non-polar liquids as the lipids, so its molecules remain stable and unmixed with the lipid contents of the plasma membrane and other intracellular membranes.

9. The water is transparent to light, enabling the specialized photosynthetic organelles, the chloroplast, inside the plant cell to absorb the sunlight for the process of photosynthesis.

Organic Compounds (Micromolecules and Macromolecules)

The chemical substances which contain carbon (C) in combination with one or more other elements as hydrogen (H), nitrogen (N), sulphur (S), etc., are called **organic compounds.** The organic compounds usually contain large molecules which are formed by the similar or dissimilar unit structure known as the **monomers.** A monomer (Gr., *mono* = one, *meros* = part) is the simplest unit of the organic molecule which can exist freely. Some organic compounds such as carbohydrates occur in the matrix as the monomers. The monomers usually link with other monomers to form **oligomers** (Gr., *oligo* = few or little, *meros* = part) and **polymers** (Gr., *poly* = many, *meros* = part). The oligomers contain small number of monomers, while the polymers contain large number of monomers. The oligomers and polymers contain large-sized molecules or macromolecules. When a polymer contains similar kinds of monomers in its macromolecule it is known as **homopolymer** and when the polymer is composed of different kinds of monomers it is known as the **heteropolymer**.

Carbohydrates

The carbohydrates (L., *carbo*-carbon or coal, Gr., *hydro*-water) are the compounds of the carbon, hydrogen and oxygen. They generally conform to the empirical formula $(CH_2O)_n$—hence the name "hydrate of carbon" or carbohydrate. The most common carbohydrates are the sugars or **saccharides**. They form the main source of the energy for all living beings. Only green parts of plants and certain microbes have the power of synthesizing the carbohydrates from the water and CO_2 in the presence of sunlight and chlorophyll by the process of photosynthesis. All the animals, non-green parts of the plants (*viz.*, stem, root, etc.), non-green plants (*e.g.*, fungi), bacteria and viruses depend on green parts of plants for the supply of carbohydrates.

Chemically the carbohydrates are defined as polybydroxy aldehydes or ketones. This means that they contain many **hydroxy**, —OH groups and also carbon-oxygen (**carbonyl**) groups, —C=O, either at the end of a chain of carbon atoms (an **aldehyde**) or somewhere in the middle of a carbon chain (a **ketone**). There are following three general classes of carbohydrates:

A. Monosaccharides (Monomers),
B. Oligosaccharides (Oligomers), and
C. Polysaccharides (Polymers).

A. Monosaccharides. The monosaccharides are tbe simple sugars with the empirical formula $C_n(H_2O)_n$. They are classified and named according to the number of carbon atoms in their molecules as follows:

(*i*) **Trioses** contain three carbon atoms in their molecules, *e.g.*, glyceraldehyde and dihydroxy acetone.

(*ii*) **Tetrose** contain four carbon atoms in their molecules, *e.g.*, erythrose.

(*iii*) **Pentoses** contain five carbon atoms in their molecules, *e.g.*, ribose, deoxyribose, arabinose and xylulose.

(*iv*) **Hexoses** contain six carbon atoms in their molecules, *e.g.*, glucose, fructose and galactose.

(*v*) **Heptoses** contain seven carbon atoms in their molecules, *e.g.*, sedoheptulose.

The monosaccharides are named by specifying the position of the carbonyl, then the number of carbons and finally the ending "—ose". Thus, an "aldohexose" is a six-carbon sugar with the carbonyl at the end of the carbon chain, while a "2-ketopentose" has its carbonyl at the second of five carbons. Some aldoses of greatest biological importance are trioses, pentoses and hexoses. The most common ketoses are the ketotrioses and the pentuloses, hexuloses and heptuloses (Note the inserted "ul", indicating the ketose family).

The monosaccharides usually exist as isomers. For example, three hexose sugars—glucose, fructose, and galactose, contain the same number of carbon, hydrogen and oxygen atoms (*i.e.*, $C_6H_{12}O_6$), but they are different sugars because of different arrangements of the atoms within the molecules. Glucose and galactose are **optical isomers** or **stereoisomers**. If a carbon atom is present in a molecule which has four different chemical groups bonded to it, the groups can be arranged in two distinct spatial arrangements about the carbon atom (such a carbon atom is often called **asymmetric carbon atom**). These two different arrangements are known as the **mirror-images** and a convenient example of such mirror-image structures are the two human hands which are identically structured but which cannot be superimposed on each other. The two isomers are designated as '**D**' or '**L**' by analogy to D— and L— glyceraldehyde, which are aldotrioses.

Most of the monosaccharides are optically active, meaning that their asymmetric carbon(s) cause the rotation of plane of polarised light. Molecules that rotate the plane of polarization to the right, as one faces the light source, are called **dextrorotatory** and are designated d or (+), while the opposite case is **levorotation**, designated l or (–). It is important to remember that the small capitals D and L refer to structure, whereas the lower case *d* and *l* refer to optical activity, established before the structure could be determined (see **Dyson**, 1978). Thus, one sees references to D (+)-glucose, also called dextrose, and D (–)-fructose, also called levulose.

The optical isomers or stereoisomers exhibit different physical properties and have vastly different biochemical properties. Often one mirror-image compound is completely ineffectual in maintaining biological structure or function. For example, all naturally occurring sugars are D-sugars. Thus, even though it is possible to manufacture L-sugars, they cannot be utilized by organisms.

Further, for the sake of simplicity, sugars can be represented in a linear straight chain form. In fact, however, the more important configuration is the cyclic one; it is an isomer having an oxygen bridge between two of the carbons. Ring formation introduces a new assymetric carbon at position one, so the nomenclature must reflect the additional pair of isomers. If the hydroxyl (–OH) at position one is below the plane of the molecule, it is the α **anomer**; otherwise we have the β **anomer**. Thus, one can have α-D-glucose or β-D-glucose as well as the two anomers of L-glucose.

The ring forms of the saccharides are referred to as **furanoses** or **pyranoses** by analogy to furan and pyran, which are five and six-membered rings, respectively. Thus one may refer to α-D-glucose and β-D-fructose as, respectively, α-D-glucopyranose and β-D-fructofuranose.

(Aldone)	(Ketose)	(Ribulose)	(Ribose)	(D. Glucose)
HC = O	H_2C—OH	CH_2OH	HC = O	O=C—H
HC—OH	C = O	C = O	HC = OH	H—C—OH
H_2C—OH	H_2C—OH	H—C—OH	HC = OH	H—C—OH
		H—C—OH	HC—OH	HO—C—OH
		CH_2OH	H_2C—OH	H—C—OH
				CH_2OH
(Triose)		(Pentose)		(Hexose)

Fig. 5.7. Structure of some monosaccharides.

The monosaccharides are the monomers and cannot split further or hydrolysed into the simpler compounds. The pentoses and hexoses are the most abundantly occurring monosaccharides of the matrix.

The pentose sugar, **ribose** is the important constituent molecule of the ribonucleic acid (RNA) and certain coenzymes as nicotinamide adenine dinucleotide (NAD), NAD phosphate (NADP), adenosine triphosphate (ATP) and coenzyme A (CoA). Another pentose sugar tile **deoxyribose** is the important constituent of the deoxyribonucleic acid (DNA). The **ribulose** is a pentose sugar which is necessary for photosynthetic mechanism.

The **glucose**, a hexose sugar is the primary source of the energy for the cell. The other important hexose sugars of the matrix are the fructose and galactose.

B. Oligosaccharides. The oligosaccharides consist of 2 to 10 monosaccharides (monomers) in their molecules. The monomers remain linked with each other by the glycosidic linkages. Certain important oligosaccharides are as follows:

(*i*) **Disaccharides** contain two monomers, *e.g.*, sucrose, maltose, lactose, etc.

(*ii*) **Trisaccharides** contain three monomers, *e.g.*, raffinose, mannotriose, rabinose, rhaminose, gentianose and melezitose.

(*iii*) **Tetrasaccharides** contain four monomers, *e.g.*, stachyose and scordose.

(*iv*) **Pentasaccharides** contain five monomers, *e.g.*, verbascose.

The most abundant oligosaccbarides of the animal and plant cells are disaccharides such as sucrose, maltose and lactose. The sucrose and maltose occur mainly in the matrix of plant cells, while the lactose occurs exclusively in the matrix of animal cells. The molecules of sucrose are composed of D-glucose and D-fructose. The molecules of maltose consist of D-glucose. The molecules of lactose are composed of two - monomers, *viz.*, D-glucose and D-galactose.

Fig. 5.8. Chemical formula of Lactose.

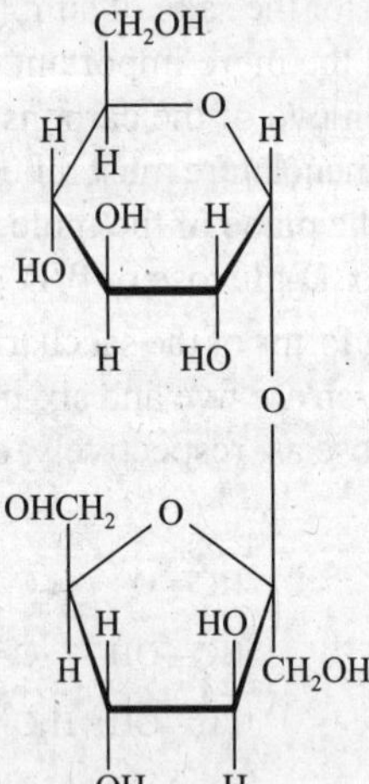

Fig. 5.9. Chemical formula of Maltose.

Fig. 5.10. Chemical formula of Sucrose.

C. Polysaccharides. The polysaccharides are composed of ten to many thousands monosaccharides as the monomers in their macromolecules. Their empirical formula is $(C_6H_{10}O_6)_n$. The molecules of the polysaccharides are of colloidal size having high molecular weights. The polysaccharides can be hydrolysed into simple sugars.

The matrix contains two kinds of polysaccharides, *viz.*, homo-polysaccharides and heteropolysaccharides.

Homopolysaccharides. The homopolysaccharides contain similar kinds of monosaccharides in their molecules. The most important homopolysaccharides of the matrix are the starch, glycogen and cellulose.

(*a*) Starch. The starch is the important storage food material of the plant cells. The true starches occur in two forms, amylose and amylopectin, found together in granules. **Amylose** is an unbranched α-1, 4 polymer of glucose (The disaccharide of the α-1, 4 polymers is maltose). The remainder of the starch granule is **amylopectin**, a branched polymer of glucose like glycogen. Its each branch is 24–30 units in length.

(*b*) Glycogen. The glycogen is a branched polymer of glucose molecules. It consists of α-D-glucose units, mostly linked 1–4, but highly branched via frequent 1–6 linkages, each of which starts other α-1, 4 chains of some 8–12 glucose units. A complete molecule of glycogen consists of several thousand glucose monomers that, because of branching, form a much more compact structure than cellulose. Being important storage food of animal cells, glycogen is also known as "animal starch". The glycogen though occurs in most animal cells in smaller amount but the cells of molluscs, liver and muscles are rich in glycogen contents.

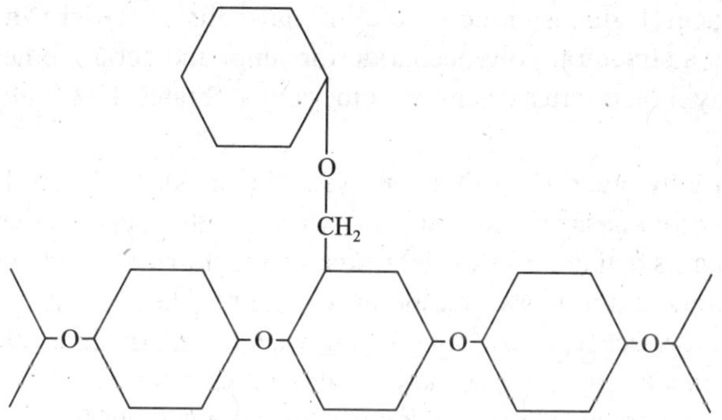

Fig. 5.11. Chemical formula of Glycogen.

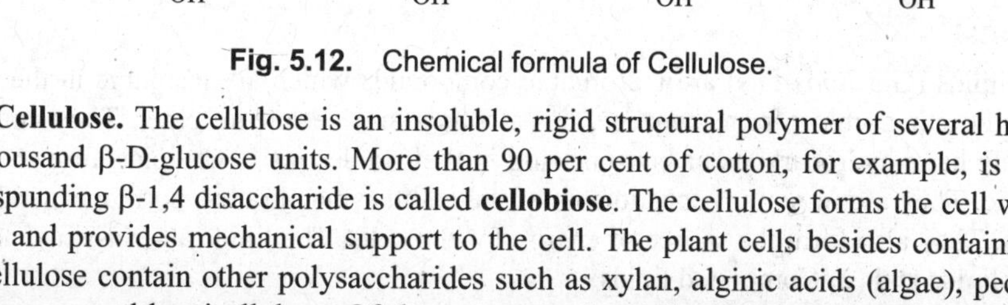

Fig. 5.12. Chemical formula of Cellulose.

(*c*) Cellulose. The cellulose is an insoluble, rigid structural polymer of several hundred to several thousand β-D-glucose units. More than 90 per cent of cotton, for example, is cellulose. The correspunding β-1,4 disaccharide is called **cellobiose**. The cellulose forms the cell wall of the plant cells and provides mechanical support to the cell. The plant cells besides containing starch and the cellulose contain other polysaccharides such as xylan, alginic acids (algae), pectic acids, inulin, agar-agar and hemicellulose. Of these, some polysaccharides provide mechanical support to the cell, while otners are used as stored food material. Glycogen and starches serve as depots for glucose. They give the cell a way of storing this important food molecule in a form that is compact, yet accessible to specialized enzymes. Cellulose on the other hand, is a structural component that is relatively rigid and insoluble.

Further, α-1, 4 polymers of starches, plant or animal, are **helical**, so they provide open spaces for solvent penetration. As a result, glycogen and starches are more flexible and more soluble, as human enzymes can hydrolyze the α-1, 4 glucoside bonds. However, β-1, 4 polymers of cellulose are

linear, hence cellulose is found in fibres of 100–200 parallel chains with few of hydroxyls exposed to the surrounding solvent. This configuration accounts for both its rigidity and its insolubility.

Except certain micro-organisms, no heterotroph (animals including man) has enzyme that can hydrolyze the β-1, 4 glucoside bond of cellulose, therefore, men like other carnivores derive no food value from cellulose. However, grazing animals utilize micro-organisms to break down the cellulose in their diet and then live by digesting the micro-organisms and their metabolic by-products.

Heteropolysaccharides. The polysaccharides which are composed of different kinds of the monosaccharides and amino-nitrogen or sulphuric or phosphoric acids in their molecules are known as heteropolysaccharides. The most important heteropolysaccharides are as follows:

(*a*) Neutral heteropolysaccharides. The neutral heteropolysaccharides contain monosaccharides and the acetylated amino nitrogen in their molecules and are known as **acetyl glucosamines**. The most important acetyl glucosamine of the animal cells is the **chitin** which is similar to cellulose and serves as a structural polysaccharide for fungi and certain other lower plants and as the exoskeleton of many insects, crustaceans and other invertebrates. It provides mechanical support to the cells.

(*b*) Acidic heteropolysaccharides (Mucopolysaccharides). The acidic heteropolysaccharides contain different kinds of monosaccharides and sulphuric or other acids in their molecules. Most of them contain amino sugars and are also called **mucopolysacharides** or **glycosaminoglycans**. The term **amino sugars** refers to a monosaccharide in which one—OH group is replaced by an—NR_2 or its derivative. The polysaccharide coat found on most cells and the intercellular material of most animal tissue contains much Mucopolysaccharides. Examples include, hyaluronic acid, chondroitin and chondroitin sulphate, dermatan sulphate, keratan sulphate and heparin.

The **hyaluronic** acid forms the cementing material of the connective tissues. It occurs in the skin, connective tissues and synovial fluid of the joints. The **chondroitin sulphate** occurs in the cells of the cartilage, skin, cornea, umbilical cord and it serves as a matrix for the bone formation. The **heparin** is a blood anticoagulant and found in the liver, lung, thymus, spleen and blood.

(*c*) Mucoproteins and Glycoproteins. When the acetyl glucosamines, monosaccharides and proteins unite together they form **mucoproteins** and **glycoproteins**. These include the blood group polysaccharides and occur in the red blood corpuscle, saliva, gastric mucin, ovomucoids, serum and albumins, etc.

Lipids (Fats)

The lipids (Gr., *lipos*-fats) are the organic compounds which are insoluble in the water but soluble in the ether, chloroform, benzene, hot alcohols and petroleum ether. They contain long chains of aliphatic hydrocarbons or benzene ring in their molecules. The lipids are non polar and hydrophobic. They are important constituents of the cellular membranes, hormones, and vitamins of the cells. They also form the source of energy for the cells. The lipids are classified as follows: (1) Simple lipids and (2) Compound lipids.

1. Simple lipids. Simple lipids are the esters of the alcohols or the triglycerides containing fatty acids and alcohols.

$$\text{Triglyceride} \xrightarrow[H_2O]{\text{Lipase}} \text{Glycerol} + 3 \text{ Fatty acids.}$$

The constituent fatty acids may be saturated, *e.g.*, palmatic, stearic acids, or unsaturated, *e.g.*, oleic, linoleic, linolenic, arachedonic and clupanadonic acids (Table 5.1). The lipids of the matrix of animal cells contain fatty acids, *viz.*, palmatic, stearic, palmitoleic, oleic, linoleic and linolenic acids. The simple lipids of the matrix are as follows:

Table 5.1. Some common fatty acids.

Formula	Common name	Formal name	Structure
1. $C_{16}H_{32}O_2$	Palmitic	n-hexadecanoic	$CH_3(CH_2)_{14}COOH$
2. $C_{18}H_{36}O_2$	Stearic	n-octadecanoic	$CH_3(CH_2)_{16}COOH$
3. $C_{16}H_{30}O_2$	Palmitoleic	9-hexadecenoic	$CH_3(CH_2)_5CH{=}CH(CH_2)_7COOH$
4. $C_{18}H_{34}O_2$	Oleic	Cis-9-octadecenoic	$CH_3(CH_2)_7CH{=}CH(CH_2)_7COOH$
5. $C_{18}H_{32}O_2$	Linoleic	Cis, cis-9-12-octadecadienoic	$CH_3(CH_2)_4(CH{=}CHCH_2)_2(CH_2)_6COOH$
6. $C_{18}H_{30}O_2$	Linolenic	9,12,15-octadecatrienoic	$CH_3CH_2(CH{=}CHCH_2)_3(CH_2)_6COOH$

***(i)* Natural fats.** The natural fats are the naturally occurring fats which occur in animal and plant cells as stored food substances.

***(ii)* Wax.** The waxes are the simple lipids and are the esters of fatty acids of high molecular weight with the alcohol except the glycerol. The most important constituent alcohol of the molecules of waxes is the cholesterol, *e.g.*, bees wax.

2. Compound lipids. The compound lipids contain fatty acids, alcohols and other compounds as phosphorus, amino-nitrogen carbohydrates, etc., in their molecules. The most important compound lipids of the matrix of animal and plant cells are as follows:

***(i)* Steroids.** These lipids contain a common cyclic nucleus of cyclopentano perhydrophenanthrene. The common steroids of the matrix of animal cells are the sex hormones (male androgens and female estrogens), adreno-cortical hormones, vitamin D, and bile acids.

The steroids which possess—OH groups in their molecules are known as **sterols**. The sterol alcohol **cholesterol** occurs in the bile, brain, adrernal gland, blood and other animal cells. The plant cells usually contain no cholesterol in their cellular matrix.

***(ii)* Phospholipids (Phospboglycerides).** The phospholipids or phosphotids contain in their molecules, the glycerol, fatty acids and phosphoric acids. The phospholipids are the main components of the lipids of the unit membranes of the cells. In animal cells the phospholipids occur along with the choline, ethanolamine or serine. For instance, the phosphotidylcholines or lecithins occur in most animal cells and are important for the metabolism of fats in the liver cells. The phosphotidyl ethanolamine and phosphotidyl serine are commonly called as **cephalios**. The other important phospholipids of the matrix are the phosphoinositides (occur mostly in the cells of liver, brain, muscle and soyabean), plasmologens and isositides.

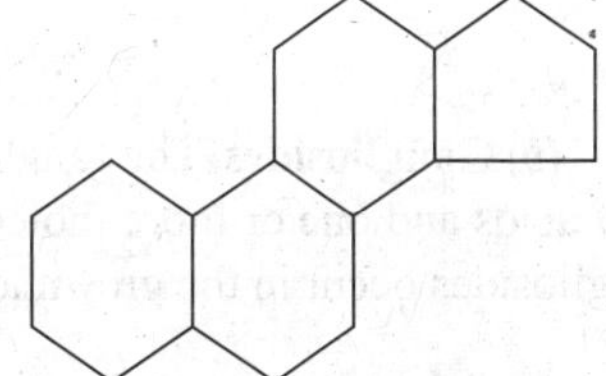

Fig. 5.13. Cyclopentano-perhydrophenanthrene nucleus of the steroids.

Fig. 5.14. Chemical formula of Cholesterol.

***(iii)* Sphingolipids.** The sphingolipids occur mostly in the cells of the brain. Instead of the glycerol, they contain in their molecules amine alcohol (sphingol or sphingosine). For instance, the myelin sheaths of the nerve fibres contain a lipid known as **sphingomyelin** which contains sphingosine and phospholipids in its molecules.

$$\begin{array}{l} CH_3 \\ | \\ (CH_2)_3 \\ | \\ CH \\ \| \\ CH \\ | \\ CH{-}OH \\ | \quad\quad\quad\;\; O \\ | \quad\quad\quad\;\; \| \\ CH{-}NH{-}C{-}R \\ | \quad\quad\quad\;\; O \\ | \quad\quad\quad\;\; \| \\ CH_2{-}O{-}P{-}O{-}CH_2CH_2{-}\overset{+}{N}(CH_3)_3 \\ \quad\quad\quad\;\; | \\ \quad\quad\quad\;\; O^- \end{array}$$

Fig. 5.15. General chemical formula of Sphingomyelin.

***(iv)* Glycolipids.** The glycolipids contain in their molecule the carbohydrates and the lipids. The matrix of the animal cells contain two kinds of glycolipids, *viz.*, cerebrosides and gangliosides.

(*a*) Cerebrosides. The cerebrosides contain in their molecules sphingosine, fatty acids and galactose or glucose. The cerebrosides are the important lipids of the white matter of the cells of brain and the myelin sheath of the nerve. The important cerebrosides are the kerasin, cerebron, nervon and oxynervons.

$$CH_3(CH_2)_{12}{-}CH{=}CH{-}\underset{OH}{CH}{-}\underset{NH_2}{CH}{-}\underset{OH}{CH_2}$$

Fig. 5.16. Chemical formula of Sphingosine.

(*b*) Gangliosides. The gangliosides have complex molecules which are composed of sphingosine, fatty acids and one or more molecules of glucose, lactose, galactosamine and neuraminic acid. The gangliosides occur in the grey matter of the brain, membrane of erythrocytes and cells of the spleen.

$$\begin{array}{l} \quad\quad\quad\quad\quad\quad\quad\quad CH_2 \\ \quad\quad\quad\quad\quad\quad\quad\quad \| \\ \quad\quad\quad\quad\quad CH_3 \quad\;\; CH \\ \quad\quad\quad\; HC{-} \quad\quad\quad\quad\quad {=}CH \\ \quad\quad\quad\quad\quad\quad\quad N \\ CH_2{=}CH{-} \quad\quad\quad\quad\quad\quad\quad\quad\quad {-}CH_3 \\ \quad\quad\quad\quad\quad N{-}Fe{-}N \\ CH_3{-} \quad\quad\quad\quad\quad\quad\quad\quad\quad\quad\quad {-}CH_2 \\ \quad\quad\quad\quad\quad\quad\quad N \quad\quad\quad\quad\quad\quad\; CH_2 \\ \quad\quad\quad\; HC{-} \quad\quad\quad\quad\quad {=}CH \quad\quad\; COOH \\ \quad\quad\quad\quad\quad CH_3 \quad\;\; CH_2CH_2COOH \end{array}$$

Fig. 5.17. Chemical formula of heme portion of haemoglobin.

(*v*) Lipoproteins. The lipoproteins contain lipids and proteins in their molecules and occur in blood of mammals in association with plasma proteins. In lipoproteins, cholesterol and, α and β globulins are found.

(*vi*) Carotenoids. The carotenoids are the compound lipids and they form the pigments of the animal and plant cells. There are about 70 carotenoids occurring in both type of cells. The important carotenoids of cells arc the α, β and γ carotenes, rctineve, xanthophylls, lactoflavin in milk, riboflavin (vitamin B_2), xanthocyanins, coenzyme Q, anthocyanins, flavones. flavonols and flavonones, etc., Chemically carotenoids are porphyrins. The porphyrin (Gr., *porphyra*-purple) are the cyclic compounds formed by four pyrole $(CH)_4NH$ rings linked by methylene bridges. The porphyrins linked with metals and proteins and forming the important pigments of animal and plant cells such as the chlorophyll and haemoglobin. The chlorophyll is a porphyrin which contains magnesium in its molecule. Many pigments of animal cells such as haemoglobin, myoglobin and cytochromes contain porphyrin in their molecules.

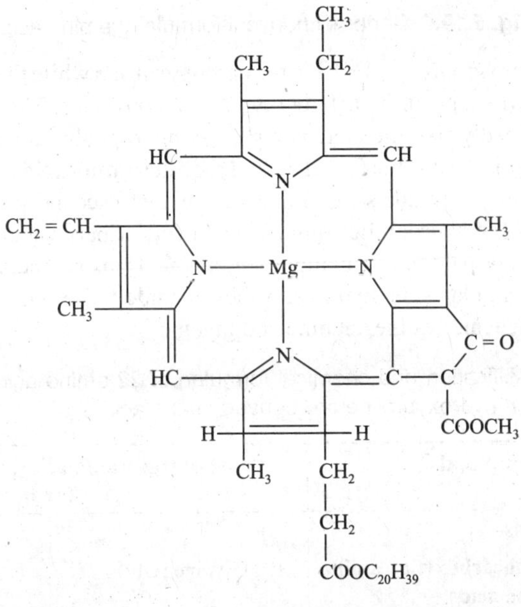

Fig. 5.18. Chemical formula of Chlorophyll.

Proteins

The proteins (Gr., *proteno*-occupy first place) are the important constituents of the matrix. The proteins are of primary importance to the continuous functioning of the cell. They provide many of the structural elements of a cell, and help to bind cells together into tissues. Proteins also catalyze most of the chemical reactions that occur in the cell. Some proteins act as contractile elements, to make movement possible; others control the activity of genes, transport needed material across membranes, and carry certain substances from one part of animal to another. Proteins in the form of **antibodies**, protect animals from disease and, in the form of **interferon**, mount an intracellular attack against viruses that have escaped destruction by the antibodies and other defences. And finally, some hormones are proteins.

Thus, the performance of so many different tasks requires many kinds of proteins, varying markedly in size and shape as well as in function. This diversity is possible because proteins are polymers of 20 or more different kinds of building blocks called **amino acids**—the short name for "α-amino carboxylic acid".

Amino acids. An organic compound containing one or more amino groups ($-NH_2$) and one or more carboxyl groups (–COOH) is known as amino acid. The amino acids occur freely in the cytoplasmic matrix and constitute the so called **amino acid pool**. The amino acids are derived from the organic acids in which the hydrogen in alpha position is replaced by the amino groups. For example, the amino acid **glycine** is formed by the acetic acid and **alanine** derived from propionic acid, is shown by following reactions:

$$\text{Acetic acids} + \text{Amino group} \rightarrow \text{Glycine}$$

$$\text{Propionic acids} + \text{Amino group} \rightarrow \text{Alanine}$$

The general molecular formula of amino acids is as follows:

```
       COOH
        |
H2N —  C — H
        |
        R
```

Fig. 5.19. General chemical formula of amino acids.

where the NH_2 is the amino group, —COOH is the carboxyl group while the 'R' represents variety of chemical combinations which occur in different types of amino acids. The matrix contains about 22 amino acids which are broadly classified into two groups: hydrophobic and hydrophilic, according to the nature of their side chains (see Table 5.2). The **hydrophilic amino acids**—those whose side chains interact strongly with water—include several that have either a second free amine or a second free carboxyl group. Examples of hydrophilic amino acids include aspartic acid, glutamic acid, cysteine, lysine, arginine, histidine, asparagine, glutamine, threonine, tyrosine and serine. The **hydrophobic amino acids** contain non-polar side chains and they include tryptophan, phenylalanine, proline, methionine, leucine, isoleucine, valine, alanine and glycine.

Table 5.2. Name, classification and chemical formulae of 22 amino acids of cytoplasmic matrix. (Cystine and hydroxyproline are derived amino acids).

Group of amino acids	Name of the amino acids, symbols and chemical formulae
A. Aliphatic amino acids.	
I. Monoamino-monocarboxylic amino acids or simple amino acids.	1. Glycine (Gly) H—CH(—NH_2)—COOH
	2. Alanine (Ala) CH_3—CH(—NH_2)—COOH
	3. Valine (Val) (CH_3)(CH_3)>CH—CH(—NH_2)—COOH
	4. Leucine (Leu) (CH_3)(CH_3)>CH—CH_2—CH(—NH_2)—COOH

Group of amino acids	Name of the amino acids, symbols and chemical formulae
	5. Isoleucine (Ilu) $CH_3—CH_2—CH—CH—COOH$ CH_3 NH_2
II. Mono-amino-dicarboxylic or acidic amino acids.	6. Aspartic acid (Asp) $HOOC—CH_2—CH—COOH$ NH_2 7. Glutamic acid (Glu) $HOOC—CH_2—CH_2—CH—COOH$ NH_2
III. Diamino-mono-carboxylic or basic amino acids.	8. Lysine (Lys) $H_2N—CH_2—CH_2—CH_2—CH_2—CH—COOH$ NH_2 9. Arginine (Arg) NH $\Vert$ $H_2N—C—NH—CH_2—CH_2—CH_2—CH—COOH$ NH_2 10. Histidine (His) $—CH_2—CH—COOH$ N NH NH_2
IV. Hydroxyl containing amino acids	11. Serine (Ser) $HO—CH_2—CH—COOH$ NH_2 12. Threonine (Thr) $CH_3—CH—CH—COOH$ OH NH_2
V. Sulphur containing amino acids.	13. Cysteine (Cys) $HS—CH_2—CH—COOH$ NH_2 14. Cystine (a dimer of cysteine) $S—CH_2—CH—COOH$ NH_2 $S—CH_2—CH—COOH$ NH_2

Group of amino acids	Name of the amino acids, symbols and chemical formulae
	15. Methionine (Met) $CH_3—S—CH_2—CH_2—CH(NH_2)—COOH$
B. Aromatic amino acids.	16. Phenylalanine (Phe) $C_6H_5—CH_2—CH(NH_2)—COOH$
	17. Tyrosine (Tyr) $HO—C_6H_4—CH_2—CH(NH_2)—COOH$
	18. Tryptophan (Try) (indole ring, N—H)$—CH_2—CH(NH_2)—COOH$
C. Secondary amino acids.	19. Proline (Pro) $H_2C—CH_2$; H_2C, $CH—COOH$; N; H
	20. Hydroxyproline (Hpro) $HO—CH—CH_2$; CH_2, $CH—COOH$; N; H
D. Amino acid amides.	21. Asparagine (Asn) $O=C(NH_2)—CH_2—CH(NH_2)—COOH$
	22. Glutamine (Gln) $O=C(NH_2)—CH_2—CH_2—CH(NH_2)—COOH$

Derived amino acids. All the proteins are comprised of 20 amino acids. There are a number of other amino acids that are present in small quantities and in various organisms. If they are part of protein, however, they are derived from these 20 amino acids.

For example, **cystine** is a dimer of cysteine, formed by oxidizing the two. sulphahydral groups into a disulphide bond:

$$R_1-SH+HS-R_2 \xrightarrow{\frac{1}{2}O_2} R_1-S-S-R_2+H_2O$$

Cystine is widely distributed in proteins, as are the methyl derivatives of lysine, arginine, glutamate, and aspartate. Some other examples of such derived amino acids are as follows:

1. **β-Alanine** is a constituent of carnosine, anserine, panthothenic acid and muscle.
2. **Phosphoserine** and **phosphothreonine** are found in casein, and in a number of enzymes.
3. **Ergothionine** is found in ergot and blood.
4. **Hydroxylysine** is found in collagen and in calf embryo in the form of phosphate ester.
5. **Ornithine** is an intermediate in urea biosynthesis.
6. **Citrulline** is an intermediate in urea biosynthesis.
7. **Homocysteine** is an intermediate in methionine metabolism.
8. **Cystathionine** is an intermediate in methonine metabolism.
9. **γ-Aminobutyric acid** is found in bacteria, green plants, yeast and brain.
10. **β-Aminoisobutyric acid** is an intermediate of thymine metabolism.
11. **Dihydroxyphenylalanine** is an intermediate of phenyl-alanine metabolism.
12. **Creatine** is found in urea.
13. **Taurine** is found in bile salts.
14. **Hydroxyproline** makes up a major fraction of the connective tissue protein, collagen.
15. **Thyroxine** and **triiodothyronine** are iodine containing amino, acids which are synthesized from tyrosines of thyroglobulin, a thyroid protein and are freed into blood as hormones referred to as T4 and T3, respectively.

Formation of proteins. Because a molecule of the amino acid contains both amino (—NH_2) and acidic or carboxyl (—COOH) group, it can behave as an acid and base at a time. The molecules of such organic compounds which contains both acidic and basic properties, are known as **amphiteric molecules.** Due to amphiteric molecules, the amino acids unite with one another to form complex and large protein molecules. When two molecules of amino acids are combined then the basic group (—NH_2) of one amino acid molecule combines with the carboxylic (—COOH) group of other amino acid and the loss of a water molecule takes place. This short of condensation of two amino acid molecules by—NH—CO linkage or bond is known as **peptide linkage** or **peptide bond.** A combination of two

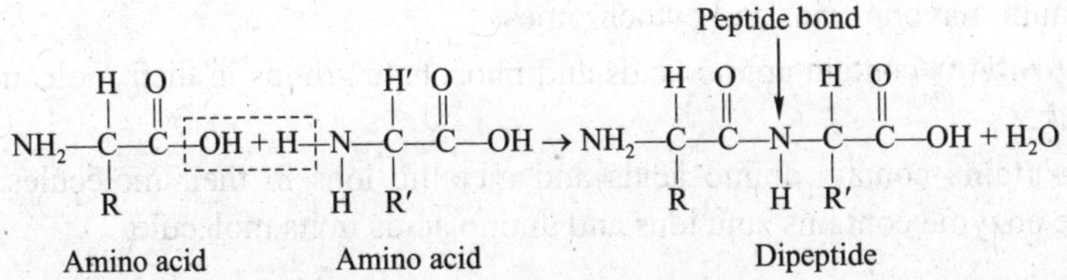

$$\underset{\text{Amino acid}}{NH_2-\overset{H}{\underset{R}{C}}-\overset{O}{\overset{\|}{C}}-OH} + \underset{\text{Amino acid}}{H-\underset{H}{N}-\overset{H'}{\underset{R'}{C}}-\overset{O}{\overset{\|}{C}}-OH} \rightarrow \underset{\text{Dipeptide}}{NH_2-\overset{H}{\underset{R}{C}}-\overset{O}{\overset{\|}{C}}-\underset{H}{N}-\overset{H}{\underset{R'}{C}}-\overset{O}{\overset{\|}{C}}-OH} + H_2O$$

(Peptide bond: the C—N bond of the dipeptide)

Fig. 5.20. A chemical reaction showing formation of a dipeptide.

amino acids by the peptide bond is known as **dipeptide**. When three amino acids are united by two peptide bonds, they form tripeptide. Likewise, by condensation of few or many amino acids by the peptide bonds the **oligopeptides** and **polypeptides** are formed respectively. The various molecules of polypeptides unite to form the **peptones, proteases** and **proteins**. Thus protein macromolecules are the polymers of many amino acid monomers. The macromolecules of proteins comparatively have high molecular weights. The molecular weight of certain animal proteins are given in the following Table 5.3.

Table 5.3. Molecular weight of some animal proteins.

S. No.	Name of the protein	Molecular weight (in daltons)*
1.	Insulin	12,000
2.	Cytochrome (Horse heart)	12,100
3.	Trypsin	23,800
4.	Pepsin	35,500
5.	Ovalbumin	44,000
6.	Serum albumin (Human)	65,000
7.	Haemoglobin (Human)	67,000
8.	Y-globulin (Human)	100,000
9.	Catalase	250,000
10.	Collagen	345,000
11.	Thyroglobin (Pig)	650,000

*One dalton being 1/16 the mass of an oxygen atom or about the mass of a hydrogen atom (Dyson, 1978).

Types of Proteins

The proteins are the organic compounds of immense biological significance. They are of following two types:

A. Simple proteins. The proteins which contain only amino acids in their molecules are known as simple proteins, *e.g.*, albumins, globulins, histones, prolamine and protamine.

B. Conjugated proteins. The proteins which contain amino acids and other chemical compounds in their molecules are known as conjugated proteins. Some important conjugated proteins are following:

1. **Glycoproteins** and **mucoproteins** contain carbohydrates and proteins in their molecules, *e.g.*, musin of saliva.
2. **Lipoproteins** contain amino acids and lipids in their molecules. *e.g.*, lipovitellin of egg yolk, serum, protein of brain and nerve tissues.
3. **Nucleoproteins** contain amino acids and nucleic acids in their molecules, *e.g.*, viruses and nucleic acid proteins.
4. **Chromoproteins** contain amino acids and pigments in their molecules, *e.g.*, haemoglobin, haemocyanin, fiavoproteins and cytochromes.
5. **Phosphoproteins** contain amino acids and phosphate groups in their molecules, *e.g.*, casein of the milk.
6. **Metalloproteins** contain amino acids and metallic ions in their molecules, *e.g.*, carbonic anhydrase enzyme contains zinc ions and amino acids in its molecule.

Protein Structure

Proteins are complex molecules not only in the number and sequence of amino acids present in them but also in their three-dimensional arrangements. For the sake of convenience, protein structure has been classified into four levels, known as primary, secondary, tertiary and quaternary levels of structure. Each level of structure has particular significance in protein functioning.

1. Primary protein structure. The primary protein structure is defined as the particular sequence of amino acids found in the protein. It is determined by the covalent peptide bondings between amino acids. Primary structure also includes other covalent linkages in proteins, for example the linkages that may exist between sulphur atoms of cysteine amino acids located in the chain of the protein, insulin. The first protein to have its primary structure determined was ox insulin, the pancreatic hormone that regulates glucose metabolism in mammals. Insulin has a molecular weight of 5,800 daltons and contains 51 amino acids. Insulin consists of two polypeptide chains of 21 and 30 amino acid residues, called the A and B chains, respectively. (An **amino acid residue** is that which is left when the elements of water are split out during polymerization). The linear sequence of amino acid residues within each chain was worked out by **Frederick Sanger** and his co-workers at Cambridge University in 1955 by using the techniques of hydrolysis (splitting) of proteins into smaller pep tides or free amino acids and of chromatography to separate and identify the amino acids and peptide fragments. Since the work of Sanger, more than 100 proteins have had their primary structure determined.

2. Secondary protein structure. Although primary protein structure is said to depend on covalent bondings, higher levels of protein structure are a result of weak secondary bonds formed between side groups of amino acids or between oxygen or nitrogen and hydrogen atoms of the polypeptide backbone structure. The nature of the amino acids present in a protein determines the nature and arrangement of the weaker bonds that can be formed. This, in turn, determines the particular three-dimensional shape of a protein molecule.

Secondary structure is any regular, repeating organization of the polypeptide chain. There are three types of secondary protein structure: The polypeptide chain may assume an **extended** configuration. This type of structure is found for example, when keratin, the protein of hair, is stretched. In some proteins, for example fibroin, the fibrous protein of silk, polypeptide chains are hydrogenbonded together, forming a **pleated sheet structure**. The general form of pleated sheet structure was first suggested by **W.T. Astbury** in the 1930's. The polypeptide chains of pleated sheet are stretched out and lie side by side, either parallel or antiparallel to one another. The bonded groups may be portions of the same chain folded back on itself, or they may be separate chains. Note how regularly arranged hydrogen bonds are formed between the oxygen of a carbonyl group (—C = O) on one chain and the hydrogen atom of an imino group (—NH) on another chain. Although each such bond is very weak, the large number of such bonds that can be formed leads to a strong, stable structure.

Linus Pauling and **R. B. Corey** predicted and then found in late 1940s another type of secondary structure, the **alpha helix**. Alpha helix is formed by a coiling of the polypeptide chain into a regularly ordered spiral. The result is a rigid, rod-like structure and is typical of many fibrous proteins. In this helix each hydrogen of an —NH group forms a hydrogen bond with the oxygen of a —C = O group lying three amino acids farther along the chain. Here also, the presence of many individually weak bonds results in a strong and very stable structure.

The helical and pleated sheet arrangements are known as the "**alpha**" and "**beta**" structures of proteins, respectively, because they were, first identified in α- and β-keratins. Keratin is a fibrous protein of the epidermis, and of hair, wool, fur, nails, beaks, feathers, hooves and so on.

The terms fibrous and globular proteins merit definition. **Fibrous proteins** have a length which is much greater than their diameter. They are usually characterized by the presence of a high degree of secondary structure. Secondary structure gives strength and rigidity to protein macromolecules, and fibrous proteins are usually found as structural components, where strength, elasticity, or rigidity are required in a cellular or an extra-cellular material. Fibrous protein molecules may aggregate to form fibrils that, in turn, may unite to form larger fibres. Important fibrous proteins include collagen (white connective tissue, tendons), elastin (yellow elastic connective tissue), keratin, fibrin (blood-clot proteins), and actin and myosin (muscle contractile proteins).

Globular proteins have a roughly spheroidal or ovoidal shape. Although they mayor may not have secondary structure, they are characterized by an irregular folding that is known as tertiary structure. Globular proteins are usually functional proteins. That is, globular proteins are usually enzymes, hormones, or immunological proteins. Globular proteins are usually water-soluble, where as many fibrous proteins are insoluble.

Collagen. Collagen, the fibrous protein of many connective tissues, is unusual in many respects and has an odd type of secondary structure. This protein has been found in all animals examined and often makes up 20 per cent or more of animal's dry weight, an unusual situation for a single protein. Alongwith mucopolysaccharides, it forms the bulk of the "glue" that holds cells together as tissues in most forms of animal life except arthropods. (The Greek root of the word collagen means "glue"). Collagen also supplies the matrix to which calcium salts are added to form bone and is the substance of scars and tendons, a function to which it is admirably suited by virtue of its enormous tensile strength—a 1 mm fibre can support a 10 kg mass.

The amino acid composition of collagen also differs from that of other proteins. About 30 per cent of its amino acids are in the group glycine, proline, hydroxyproline, and hydroxy lysine. In fact, hydroxyproline and hydroxylysine are amino acids found only in collagen.

The collagen fibre has a banded appearance, with a major repeat band period of 700 A°. The collagen fibre is formed from aligned collagen fibrils (called **tropocollagen subunits**) that are composed of three collagen polypeptide chains twined about one another in a spiral or helical secondary structure. The bands of the larger fibre appear because certain electron-dense groups of polypeptide chains, and also of the fibres, are aligned at regular intervals and, therefore, present the appearance of denser bands along the fibres. Tropocollagen subunits are synthesized and released by fibroblast cells. If collagen is boiled, the heat causes denaturation via strand separation. We then call it **gelatin**. (**Denaturation** refers to any change in a protein such that its normal biological properties are altered).

3. Tertiary protein structure. Most known proteins are more compact than secondary structure would permit. Their shape is roughly spherical, meaning that the protein polypeptide chain must be folded in same manner. **Tertiary structure** is defined as any irregular loops or bends in the polypeptide chain and is typical of globular protein structure. The polypeptide chain is held in position by weak secondary bonds. Whereas secondary structure is primarily the result of hydrogen bonding, tertiary structure results from hydrophobic bonds, weak electrostatic attractions between charged side groups of the polypeptide chain and other weak attractive forces. Thus, the bonds which stabilize tertiary structure are hydrogen bond, hydrophobic bond, disulphide bond, salt bridge (ionic interaction) and dipole interaction.

The complete tertiary structure of a protein can only be deducted by a laborious analysis of

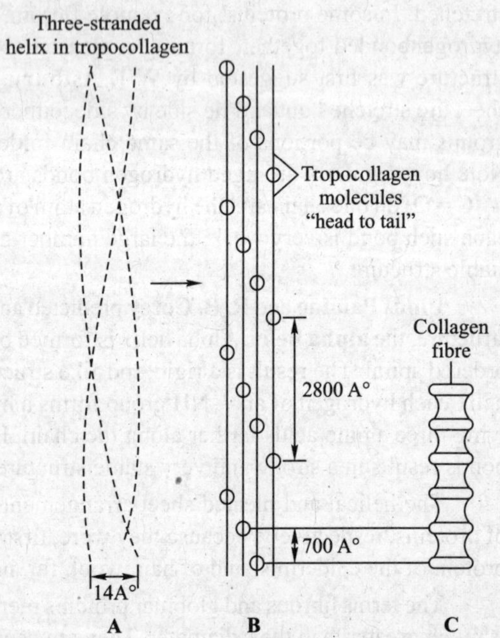

Fig. 5.21. Collagen. The polypeptide chains form a three-stranded helix in the tropocollagen subunit. Adjacent subunits overlap one another by three-quarter of their length, providing a 700 A° repeat distance to the fibrils, to give banded appearance (after Dyson, 1978).

X-ray scattering patterns from crystals. The first protein to have its secondary and tertiary structure determined was **myoglobin**, a 153-amino acid, oxygen-binding protein found primarily in red muscle and largely responsible for the colour of that tissue. The work was done at Cambridge under the direction of **J.C. Kendrew** (1961). Although at some points the polypeptide chain does have secondary structure (alpha-helical structure), the chain is mainly characterized by seemingly random loops and folds.

4. Quaternary protein structure. The highest level of protein structure, called quaternary, refers to the **subunit structure** of proteins. Proteins (*e.g.*, many globular proteins) that have more than one polypeptide chain may also have more than one independently folded unit, each of at least one chain. The independently folded units are called **subunits**. The manner in which subunits are arranged to form the intact functional protein is called the **quaternary structure**. Haemoglobin, for example, is composed of four polypeptide chains (Fig. 5.22). There are two pairs of identical chains. The members of one pair are almost identical with the polypeptide chain of myoglobin. The haemoglobin was the first protein to have the three-dimensional features of its quaternary structure determined by X-ray diffraction by **M.F. Perutz** at Cambridge, England.

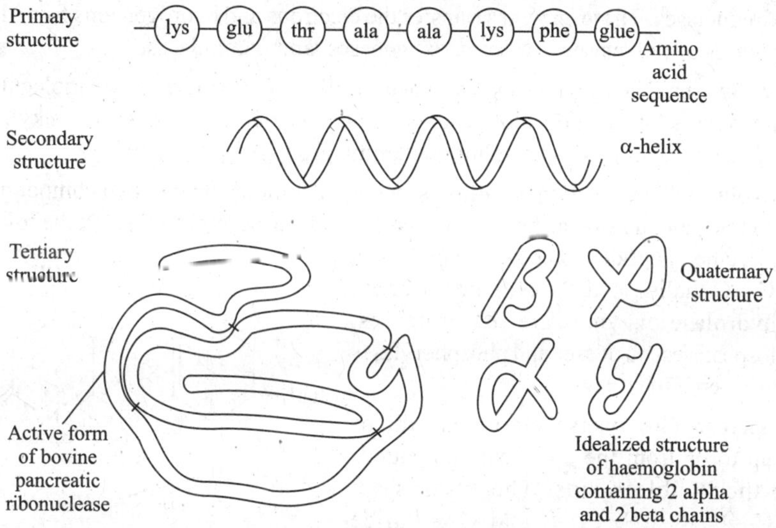

Fig. 5.22. The four levels of structural organisation in protein molecules (after Stansfield, 1969).

Certain Properties of Proteins

1. The proteins are amphiteric compound and, therefore, act as acids and bases. 2. The solubility of proteins depends on the pH value of the solvent. 3. The proteins can bind salts by forming ionic bonds. 4. The proteins are precipitated by salts of heavy metals and by high temperature. 5. Certain proteins are specific for a particular species and they have antigenic properties.

Uses of Proteins

According to functions following two types of proteins can be recognised:

1. The structural proteins which form various structures of the cell. **2. The functional proteins** or **enzymes** which function as specific catalysts in most biosynthetic and metabolic activities of the cell.

Enzymes

The cytoplasmic matrix and many cellular organelles contain very important organic compounds known as the **enzymes**. The word enzyme (Greek "in yeast") has been proposed by **Kuhne** in 1878.

The enzymes are the specialized proteins and they have capacity to act as catalysts in chemical reaction. Like the other catalysts of chemical world, the enzymes are the catalysts of the biological world and they influence the rate of a chemical reaction, while themselves remain quite unchanged at the end of the reaction. The substance on which the enzymes act is known as **substrate**. The enzymes play a vital role in various metabolic and biosynthetic activities of the cell such as synthesis of DNA, RNA and protein molecules and metabolism of carbohydrates, lipids, fats and other chemical substances.

Types of enzymes. Enzymes are divided into six major classes, according to the general type of chemical reaction they catalyze. All enzymes are named by adding the suffix—**ase** to the stem of the enzyme's name, which usually indicates either the major substrate or the type of reaction catalyzed by the enzyme. A few exceptions to this rule are found with the earlier known enzymes, such as pepsin, trypsin, chymotrypsin and papain: all digestive enzymes.

The major classes of enzymes are:

1. Oxireductases. The enzymes catalyzing the oxidation and reduction reactions of the cells are known as oxireductases. These enzymes transfer the electrons and hydrogen ions from the substrates, *e.g.*, hydrogenases or reductases, oxidases, oxygenases, and peroxidases.

2. Transferases. The enzymes which transfer following groups from one molecule to other are known as transferases: one carbon, aldehydic or ketonic residues, acyl, glycosyl, alkyl, nitrogenous; phosphorus containing groups and sulphur containing groups.

3. Hydrolases. These enzymes hydrolyse a complex molecule into two compounds by adding the element of the water across the bond which is cleaved. These enzymes act on the following bonds ester, glycosyl, ether, peptide, other C—N bonds acid anhydride, C—C, halide and P—N bonds. Certain important hydrolase enzymes are the proteases, esterases, phosphatases, nucleases and phosphorylases and all digestive enzymes.

4. Lysases. The Iysase enzymes add or remove group to or from the chemical compounds containing the double bonds. The lysases act on C—C, C—O, C—N, C—S and C— halide bonds.

5. Isomerases. These enzymes catalyze the reaction involving in the isomerization or intramolecular rearrangements in the substrates, *e.g.*, intramolecular oxidoreductases, intra-molecular transferases, intramolecular lysases, cis-trans-isomerases, racemerases and epimerases.

6. Ligases or synthetases. These enzymes catalyze the linkage of the molecules by splitting a phosphate bond. The synthetase enzymes form C—O, C—S, C—N and C—C bonds.

According to the chemical nature of the substrate the enzymes have also been classsified as follows:

1. Carbohydrases, 2. Proteases (endopeptidases and exopeptidases), 3. Amylases, 4. Esterases, 5. Dehydrogenases, 6. Oxidases 7. Decarboxylases, 8. Hydrases, 9. Transferases, and 10. Isomerases.

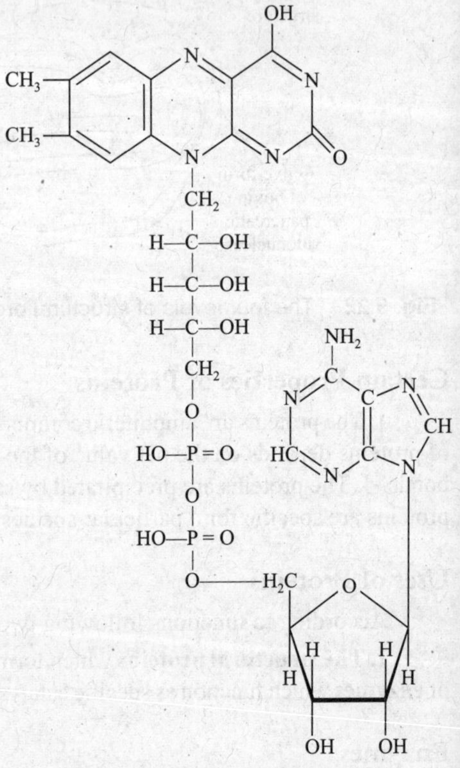

Fig. 5.23. Chemical formula of flavin adenine dinucleotide (FAD).

The enzymes are **specific** in action and many factors such as pH, temperature and concentration of the substrate effect the rate of the activity of enzymes. Certain enzymes, *viz.*, **zymogens**, occur in the inactive form and these are activated by other enzymes known as **kinases** to perform catalytic activities. Likewise, the enzyme **trypsinogen** of the pancreatic cells is activated in the intestine by the enzyme **enterokinase** and the enzyme **pepsinogen** of the Chief cells of the stomach is activated by the **hydrochloric acid** which is secreted by parietal cells.

Prosthetic Groups and Coenzymes

Many proteins contain organic or inorganic units that are the integral part of the molecule, but not composed of amino acids. These additions are called **prosthetic groups**; their presence defines a conjugated protein. For example, certian enzymes such as **cytochromes** are the conjugated proteins and contain prosthetic group as **metalloporphyrins** complex in their molecules.

Certain enzymes cannot function singly but they can function only by the addition with the small molecules of other chemical substance which are known as **coenzymes**. The inactive enzyme (which cannot function singly) is known as the **apoenzyme**. The apoenzyme and coenzyme are collectively known as **holoenzyme**. For instance, the enzyme **hydrogenases** is an apoenzyme which can function either with the coenzyme NAD^+ or NADP.

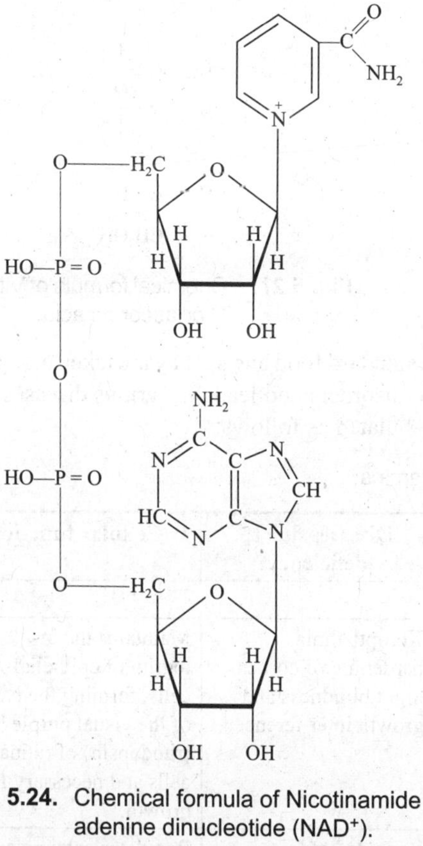

Fig. 5.24. Chemical formula of Nicotinamide adenine dinucleotide (NAD^+).

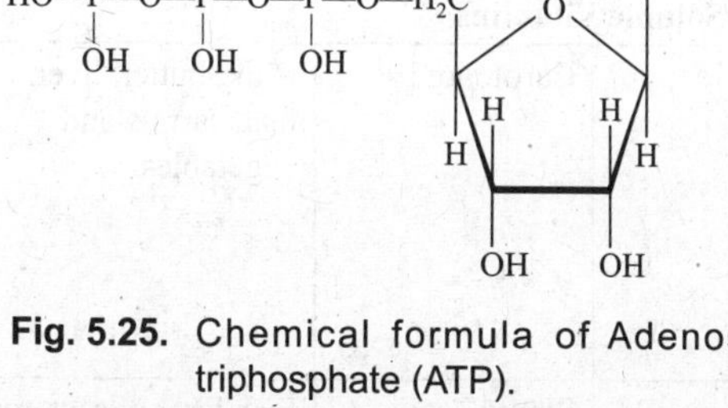

Fig. 5.25. Chemical formula of Adenosine triphosphate (ATP).

Some important coenzymes or cofactors are as follows:

1. Nicotinamide adenine dinucleotide (NAD) or Diphosphopyridine nucleotide (DPN), 2. Nicotinamide adenine dinucleotide phosphate (NADP) or Triphosphopyridine nucleotide (TPN), 3. Flavin adenine mononucleotide (FAM), 4. Flavin adenine dinucleotide (FAD), 5. Ubiquinone

(coenzyme Q or Q), 6. Lipoic acid (LIP or S_2), 7. Adenosine triphosphate (ATP), 8. Pyridoxyl phosphate (PALP), 9. Tetrahydrofolic acid (CoF), 10. Adenosylmethionine. 11. Biotin, 12. Coenzyme A (CoA), 13. Thiamine pyrophosphate (TPP), 14. Uridine diphosphate (UDP).

Isoenzymes

Recently, it has been investigated that some enzymes have similar activities and almost similar molecular structures. These enzymes are known as **isoenzymes**. The isoenzymes have relation with the heredity (**Latner** and **Skillen**, 1969, and **Weyer**, 1968). There are about 100 isoenzymes in the cell, *e.g.*, lactic dehydrogenase (LDH) occur in the form of five identical isoenzymes.

Vitamins

The vitamins are organic compounds of diverse chemical nature. They are required in minute amounts for normal growth, functioning and reproduction of cells. The vitamins play an important role in the cellular metabolism and act as the enzymes or other biological catalysts in the various chemical activities of the cell. Their importance for the animals has been reported by **Hopkins**, **Osborne**, **Mendal** and **McCollum** (1912–1913). **Funk** (1912) demonstrated the presence of basic nitrogen in them and give the name "vitamins" meaning vital amines to them.

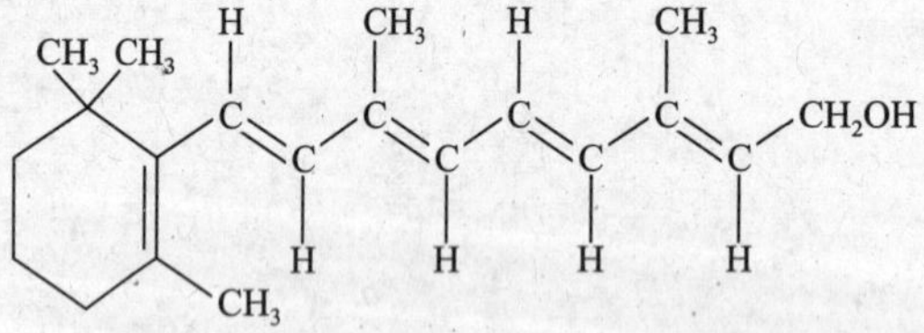

Fig. 5.26. Chemical formula of Vitamin A.

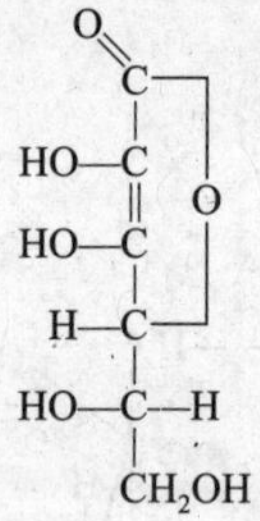

Fig. 5.27. Chemical formula of Vitamin C or ascorbic acid.

The cell cannot synthesize the vitamins from the standard food and so they are taken alongwith the food. Their deficiency in the cell causes metabolic disorders and leads to various diseases. The vitamins of utmost biological importance have been tabulated as follows:

Table 5.4. Classification and other characters of vitamins.

Vitamin	Chemical nature	Sources	Diseases due to deficiency	Cellular function
Fat Soluble Vitamins				
A	Carotenoid	Milk, butter, liver, fish, carrots and vegetables.	Xeropthalmia, hardening of cornea, night blindness and growth inter ference.	Maintains the integrity of epithelial cells, forming the part of the visual purple (rhodopsin) of retinal cells and necessary for growth.
D	Sterol	Fish liver oils, steroid containing food, ultraviolet light, butter, eggs.	Bone defects, *e.g.*, rickets and osteomalacia.	Regulates calcium and phosphorus metabolism.

Vitamin	Chemical nature	Sources	Diseases due to deficiency	Cellular function
E	Tocopherol	Green salad, vegetable oils, egg yolk and meat.	Sterility in male rats.	Rapid cell proliferation.
K	1-4 napin-thoquinone acetate	Green leafy vegetables, spinach, liver and eggs.	Haemorrhage	Forms prothrombin in the liver which is necessary for clotting of blood.
Water Soluble Vitamins				
B_1	Thiamine	Unpolished cereal grains, yeast, egg yolk, liver, nuts, and pork.	Beriberi and loss of appetite.	Coenzyme for pyruvate metabolism in cellular respiration and metabolism of carbohydrates. Promotes appetite.
B_2	Riboflavin	Liver, cheese, milk, egg-white, meat, kidney and green leaves.	Catract, form lesions in the mouth. tongue, nose, and eyes, cheiosis.	Cellular respiration and growth.
Niacin	Nicotinic acid	Milk, liver, kidney, meat legumes, coffee, tea, eggs, vegetables, etc.	Pellagra.	Part of dehydroge-nase coenzymes (NAD_2) and (NADA). Controls cellular functions.
B_6	Pyridoxine	Yeast, polished rice, cereal grains, egg-yolk, royal jelly (bee).	Anaemia, skin lesions.	Coenzyme in the metabolism of amino acids.
Pantothenic acid	Pantothenic acid	Yeast, liver, kidney, eggs, wheat, rice, bran, peanuts and peas.	Dermatitis and spectacle eye.	Part of coenzyme A.
Biotin (H)	Biotin	Egg-yolk, liver, kidney, milk, yeast and royal jelly (bee).	Dermatitis (Tat, pig, fowl), paralysis, muscle pain.	Coenzyme in CO_2 fixation.
Folic acid	Pteroylglutamic acid	Green leafy vegetables, yeast, beef, wheat and soyabean.	Anaemia.	Part of coenzymes of nucleic acid metabolism and essential for growth and formation of blood cells.
B_{12}	Cyanoco-balamin	Liver, eggs, milk, meat, and fish.	Pernicious anaemia	Coenzyme of an enzyme involved in methyl transfer and nucleic acid metabolism and red blood cell formation.
Protogen	Thioctic acid or α-Lipoic acid	Yeast and liver.	—	Coenzyme in pyruvate oxidation.

Vitamin	Chemical nature	Sources	Diseases due to deficiency	Cellular function
C	Ascorbic acid	Tomatoes, citrus fruits, green vegetables, flowers, and pepper.	Scurvy	Maintains optimal oxidation reduction potential, capillary walls and normal growth of bones and teeth.
P	Eriodictin, hesperidin, rutin	—	Capillary fragility.	Maintains cement of capillary walls.

Fig. 5.28. Chemical formula of vitamin D.

Fig. 5.29. Chemical formula of vitamin E (alphatocopherol).

Hormones

Hormones are the complex organic compounds which occur in traces in the cytoplasm and regulate the synthesis of mRNA, enzymes and various other intracellular physiological activities. The most important hormones are growth hormones, estrogen, androgen, insulin, thyroxine, cortisone, and adrenocortical hormones, etc. These hormones are synthesized by the ductless glands and transported to various cells of multicellular orginisms by blood vascular system. In cells they regulate various metabolic activities. For example, the ecdysone hormone has been found to form puffs (Balbiani rings) in the giant chromosomes of insects. The hormones activate or depress at the particular locus on the chromosome. Thus, hormones serve to coordinate the various activities concerned with a particular function, *e.g.*, the hormone ecdysone control moulting and metamorphosis in insects (**Beermann**, 1965).

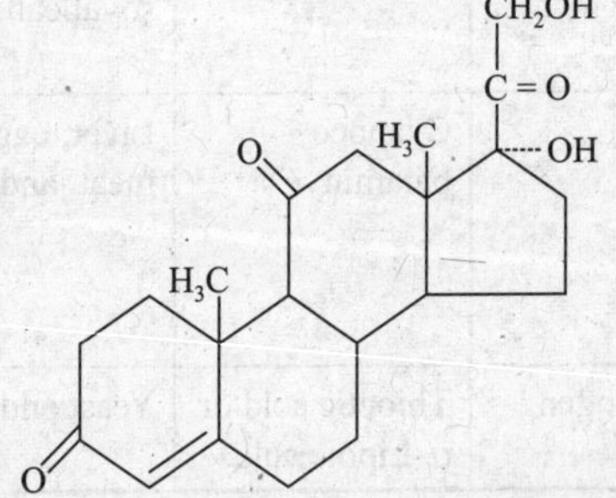

Fig. 5.30. Chemical formula of Cortisone.

In mammalian liver cells, the enzymes which convert glucose into glycogen are regulated by the hormone insulin which is synthesized by β-cells of the islets of Langerhans in the pancreas. Moreover, the hormone thyroxine, a secretion of thyroid gland, activates the enzyme phosphorylase to form glucose phosphate from the glycogen.

Nucleic Acids

The nucleic acids are the complex macromolecular organic compounds of immense biological importance. They control the important biosynthetic activities of the cell and carry hereditary informations from generation to generation. There occur two types of nucleic acids in living organisms, *viz.*, **ribonucleic acid (RNA)** and **deoxyribonucleic acid (DNA)**. Both types of nucleic acids are the polymers of the nucleotides. A nucleotide is composed of nucleoside and phosphoric acid. Even the nucleoside is composed of the pentose sugars (ribose or deoxyribose) and nitrogen bases (purines or pyrimidines). The **purines** are **adenine** and **guanine** and the **pyrimidines** are the **cytosine**, **thymine** and **uracil**. The cytoplasmic matrix contains only RNA, while DNA, exclusively remains concentrated in the nucleus.

Fig. 5.31. Chemical formula of ribose sugar.

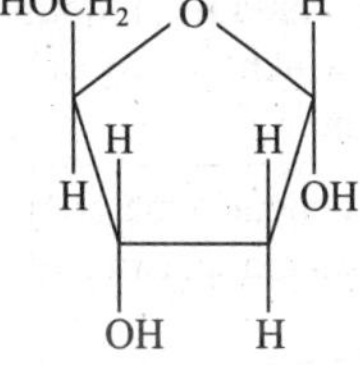

Fig. 5.32. Chemical formula of deoxyribose sugar.

Fig. 5.33. Chemical formula of Adenine.

Fig. 5.34. Chemical formula of Guanine.

Fig. 5.35. Chemical formula of Cytosine.

Fig. 5.36. Chemical formula of Uracil.

Fig. 5.37. Chemical formula of Thymine.

The DNA and RNA have almost similar chemical compositions except a few differences. Both can be compared as follows:

Table 5.5. Comparison of DNA and RNA

DNA	RNA
1. It contains pentose sugar known as deoxyribose.	1. It contains pentose sugar called the ribose.
2. The molecule contains the phosphoric acid (phosphate) molecule which connects various sugars with one another.	2. The molecule contains the phosphoric acid (phosphate) molecule which connects various sugars with one another.
3. The nitrogen bases are: (*i*) **Purines**—adenine and guanine; (*ii*) **Pyrimidines**—cytosine and thymine.	3. The molecule contains following nitrogen bases in its molecule: (*i*) **Purines**—adenine and guanine; (*ii*) **Pyrimidines**—cytosine and uracil.
4. Molecules have four nucleotides as deoxyadenosine monophosphate, deoxyguanosine monophosphate, deoxycytidine monophosphate and thymidine monophosphate.	4. Molecules have four nucleotides as adenosine monophosphate, guanosine monophosphate, cytidine monophosphate and uridine monophosphate.
5. The molecule contains a double stranded helix structure in which many nucleotides remain arranged in pair.	5. The molecules consist of singlechain of polynucleotides.
6. DNA is a genetic material and occurs in chromosomes, nucleoplasm and mitochondria, etc.	6. RNA is a carrier of genetic informations and it plays very significant role in the mechanism of protein synthesis. It mostly occurs in nucleolus, nucleoplasm and cytoplasm.

5.4 PROPERTIES OF CYTOPLASMIC MATRIX

The matrix is a living substance and it has following physical and biological properties:

Physical Properties. The most of the physical properties of the matrix are due to its colloidal nature and these are as follows:

1. Tyndall's effect. When a beam of strong light is passed through the colloidal system, of the matrix at right angles in the dark room, the small colloidal particles which remain suspended in the colloidal system reflect the light. The path of the light appears like a cone. This light cone is known as **Tyndall's cone** because, this phenomenon has been first of all reported by **Tyndall** (1820–1893) in colloids.

2. Brownian movement. The suspended colloidal particles of the matrix always move in zig-zag fashion. This movement of molecules is caused by moving water molecules which strike with the colloidal molecules to provide motion to them. This type of movement was first of all observed by Scottish botanist **Robert Brown** in 1827 in the colloidal solution. Therefore, such movements are known as **Brownian movement**. The Brownian movement is the peculiarity of all colloidal solutions and depends on the size of the particles and temperature.

3. Cyclosis and amoeboid movement. Due to the phase reversal property of the cytoplasmic matrix, the intracellular streaming or movement of the matrix takes place. This property of intra cellular movement of matrix is known as the **cyclosis**. The cyclosis usually occurs in the sol-phase of the matrix and is effected by the hydrostatic pressure, temperature, pH, viscosity, etc. The intracellular movements of the pinosomes, phagosomes and various cytoplasmic organelles such as the lysosomes, mitochondria, chromosomes, centrioles, etc., occur only due to cyclosis of the matrix. The cyclosis has been observed, in most animal and plant cells.

The amoeboid movement depends directly on the cyclosis. The amoeboid movement occurs in the protozoans, leucocytes, epithelia, mesenchymal and other cells. In the amoeboid movement the cell changes its shape actively and gives out cytoplasmic projections known as **pseudopodia**. Due to cyclosis matrix moves these pseudopodia and this causes forward motion of the cell.

4. Surface tension. The molecules in the interior of a homogeneous liquid are free to move and are attracted by surrounding molecules equally in all directions. At the surface of the liquid where it touches air or some other liquid, however, they are attracted downward and sideways or inward, more than upward; consequently they are subjected to unequal stress and are held together to form a membrane. The force by which the molecules are bound is called the **surface tension** of the liquid. The cytoplasmic matrix being a liquid possesses the property of surface tension. The proteins and lipids of matrix have less surface tension, therefore, occur at the surface and form the membrane, while the chemical substances such as NaCl have high surface tension, therefore, occur in deeper part of the matrix.

5. Adsorption. The increase in the concentration of a substance at the surface of a solution is known as adsorption (*L.*, *ad* = to, *sorbex* = to draw in). The phenomenon of adsorption helps the matrix to form protein boundaries.

6. Other mechanical or physical properties of matrix. Besides surface tension and adsorption, the matrix possesses other mechanical properties, *e.g.*, elasticity, contractility, rigidity and viscosity which provide to the matrix many physiological utilities.

7. Polarity of the egg. The colloidal system due to its stable phase determines the polarity of the cell matrix which cannot be altered by centrifugation of other mechanical means.

8. Buffers and pH. The matrix has a definite pH value and it does not tolerate significant variations in its pH balance. Yet various metabolic activities produce small amount of excess acids or bases. Therefore, to protect itself from such pH variation the matrix contains certain chemical compounds as carbonate-bicarbonate system known as **buffers** which mamtam a constant state of pH in the matrix.

Biological Properties

The matrix is a living substance and it has following biological properties:

1. **Irritability.** The irritability is the fundamental and inherent property of the matrix. It possesses a sensitivity to stimulation, an ability to transmission of excitation and ability to react according to stimuli. The heat, light, chemical substances and other factors stimulate the cytoplasmic matrix to contract.
2. **Conductivity.** The conductivity is the process of conduction or transmission of excitation from the place of its origin to the region of its reaction. The matrix of nerve cells possesses the property of the conductivity.
3. **Movement.** The cytoplasmic matrix can perform movement due to cyclosis. The cyclosis depends on the age, water contents, heredity factors and composition of the cells.
4. **Metabolism.** The matrix is the seat of various chemical activities. These activities may be either constructive or destructive in nature. The constructive processes such as biosynthesis of proteins, lipids, carbohydrates and nucleic acids are known as **anabolic processes,** while the destructive processes such as oxidation of foodstuffs, *etc.*, are known as **catabolic processes.** The anabolic and catabolic processes are collectively known as **metabolic process**.
5. **Growth.** Due to the secretory or anabolic activities (*Gr.*, *anabolism* = a throwing up) of the cell, new protoplasm continuously increases in its volume. The increase in the volume of the matrix causes into the growth of the cell which ultimately divides into daughter cells by the cell division.
6. **Reproduction.** The cytoplasm has the property of asexual and sexual reproduction.

REVISION QUESTIONS

1. What is cytoplasmic matrix? Describe various theories regarding the physical nature of the matrix. Also discuss various properties of the matrix.
2. How would you describe the importance to living systems of primary bonds and secondary bonds?
3. What is the structural basis for the unique properties of the water molecule? How do the properties of water make it of importance to living systems?
4. What are primary, secondary, tertiary, and quaternary levels of protein structure? What types of chemical bondings are responsible for each of these structural levels? Which of the structural levels play a fundamental direct role in protein functioning?
5. How would you define an enzyme? Describe some main types of enzymes.
6. How would you define carbohydrates? What are the major classes of carbohydrates? How do the polysaccharides differ trom the protein macromolecules?
7. What are the major classes of lipids and what types of functions are served by them?
8. Write short notes on the following:
   (*i*) Amino acids; (*ii*) ATP;
   (*iii*) Vitamins; (*iv*) Hormones;
   (*v*) Nucleic acids; (*vi*) Brownian movement; and
   (*vii*) Cofactor.

6

Chapter PLASMA MEMBRANE AND CELL WALL

The outer surface of all protoplasts is bounded by an exceedingly thin (*i.e.*, 70–100A° thick), elastic, semipermeable, trilaminar, lipoproteinous, living limiting membrane which separates the cellular protoplasm with their external environment. This membrane is called **cytoplasmic membrane, cell membrane, plasmalemma** or **plasma membrane**. The term cell membrane was coined by **C. Nageli** and **C. Cramer** in 1855 and the term plasmalemma has been given by **J.Q. Plowe** in 1931. Modern cytologists prefer the term plasma membrane for this membrane to avoid confusion (see **De Robertis** *et al.*, 1975). Plasma membrane lies between the cell wall and the cytoplasm in the bacterial and plant cells, and it is the outer limiting membrane of most animal cells.

The plasma membrane is present in most cell types and was the first membrane to develop during the evolution of living systems. The plasma membrane does not constitute a totally inert barrier between the cell and its environment. In fact, it is a delicately balanced, dynamic cellular organelle that determines the composition of cytoplasm by regulating which materials get in and out and the rate at which they do so. It thus permits the selective uptake of the solvents, solutes and particles (or water and nutrients) and secretion of waste products. Membranes found elsewhere in the cell, such as those around the nucleus, mitochondria, chloroplasts, various vacuoles, sacs, lysosomes, peroxisomes, etc., also represent highly selective barriers to the passage of materials. Though most membranes are quite similar in structure, their properties vary considerably.

6.1 METHODS OF ISOLATION AND ANALYSIS OF PLASMA MEMBRANE

W. Pfeffer (1890) was the first cytologist who established that the plasma membrane could not be differentiated from the inner cytoplasm with the light microscope. In fact, detailed structure of plasma membrane could be studied well, only after the improvement of microtechniques for isolation of pure and intact plasma membranes from the living cells and subsequent electron microscopy of such isolated plasma membranes. Several methods have been used to isolate plasma membrane from a variety of cells, *i.e.*, mammalian red blood cells (erythrocytes), medullated nerve fibres, Ehrlich mouse ascites tumour cells, liver cells, striated muscle, *Amoëba proteus*, sea urchin eggs and bacteria. The mammalian erythrocytes and the myelin sheath of the nerve fibre, however, have provided the bulk of information regarding the structure and properties of the plasma membrane. For such experiments, human red blood cells or erythrocytes have been selected by **E. Gorter** and **F. Grendel** (1925) for following advantages: these cells are easy to obtain and are known to be extremely simple. Since these cells contain no intracellular organelles or membrane, so the only membrane structure to be considered is almost entirely that of the cell surface. Lastly, the plasma membrane of erythrocytes is relatively tough and does not readily fragment (See **Lucy**, 1975).

To obtain plasma membrane from human erythrocytes, the cells are treated with hypotonic solutions that produce swelling and then loss of the haemoglobin content (*i.e.*, **hemolysis**) (**Waugh** and **Schmitt**, 1940; **Ponder**, 1940). The resulting membrane is generally called a **red cell 'ghost'**. Myelin was first isolated by **Robertson** (1958) and has been used as a source of plasma membrane. **Rajam** and **Jackson** (1958) isolated plasma membrane of Ehrlich mouse ascites tumour cells by disrupting the cells by ultrasonic methods and they reported the occurrence of antigens in their isolated material. **Wallach** and coworkers (1962) disintegrated Ehrlich ascites cells by suddenly releasing the pressure on cells supersaturated with nitrogen. Plasma membrane of liver cells of mouse and rat were isolated and studied by **Neville** (1960), **Emmelot** and **Bos**, 1962 and others. **O'Neill** and **Wolpert** (1961) prepared surface fractions from *Amoeba proteus* by a glycerol treatment which causes the cell contents to shrink away from the plasma membrane. **Mitchell** (1959) isolated and analysed the plasma membrane of a bacterium by first removing cell wall by enzyme treatment and then by bursting the cells in hypotonic solution. However, in most of these cases the purity of the fraction (*i.e.*, plasma membrane) has been controlled by electron microscopy, X-ray diffraction, enzyme analysis, the study of surface antigens, and other criteria (**Giese**, 1973; **De Pierre** and **Karnovsky**, 1973).

6.2 CHEMICAL COMPOSITION

The plasma membrane is composed mainly of protein, lipid, and a small percentage (1 to 5 per cent) of oligosaccharides that may be attached to either the lipids (glycolipids) or the proteins (glycoproteins). There is a wide variation in the lipid-protein ratio between different cell membranes, (see Table 6.1). Myelin is an exception in the sense that the lipid predominates, while in other cell membranes there is higher protein lipid/ratio (Table 6.1).

Table 6.1. Lipid and protein ratios in some cell membranes (**D. J. Triggle**, 1971).

	Species and Tissue		Protein (%)			Lipid (%)
1.	Human	CNS myelin	20			79
2.	Bovine	PNS myelin	23			76
3.	Rat	Muscle (skeletal)	65			35
4.	Rat	Liver	60			40
5.	Human	Erythrocyte	60			40
6.	Rat	Liver mitochondrion	70			27–29
			Molar ratio			Area ratio
		Amino acid	Phospholipid	Cholesterol		
7.	Myelin	264	111	75		0.43
8.	Erythrocyte	500	31	31		2.00

1. Lipid Fraction of Plasma Membranes

The plasma membrane contains about 20 to 79 per cent of lipids (see Table 6.1). The main lipid constituents of plasma membranes are phospholipids, cholesterol and galactolipids; their proportions varies in different cell membranes. The phospholipid components of plasma membrane are of following two kind—**neutral phospholipids** and **acidic phospholipids**. Neutral phospholipids such as phosphatidylcholine, phosphatidylethanolamine and sphingomyelin have no net charge at neutral pH and they tend to pack tightly in the bilayer. Acidic phospholipids such as phosphatidylinositol, phosphatidylserine, cardiolipin, phosphatidylglycerol, sulpholipids are negatively charged and in the membrane are associated principally with proteins by way of lipid-protein interactions (**Maddy**,1966). Acidic phospholipids form only 5 to 20 per cent fractions of the total phospholipids of plasma membrane.

A lipid molecule basically consists of two parts, a head (glycerol) which is water soluble or hydrophilic and two tails (fatty acids) which are water insoluble or hydrophobic. Different lipid molecules ef the plasma membrane of different cells are composed of a variety of fatty acids. For instance, red cell ghost of mammals contains the fatty acids, such as, palmitic, stearic, oleic, linoleic, and arachidonic acids.

2. Carbohydrate Fraction of Plasma Membranes

Bell (1962) has suggested the presence of carbohydrates in the plasma membrane. The most common oligosaccharides of plasma membranes of mammalian erythrocytes and liver cells are hexose, hexosamine, fucose and sialic acid. All of these usually remain bounded to proteins. Sialic acid is sensitive to neuraminidase and is attached to proteins by N-acetylgalactosamine on the outer surface of the membrane. A small amount of sialic acid exists in the form of **gangliosides** (*i.e.*, glycolipids) in the plasma membrane of liver cells.

3. Protein Fraction of Plasma Membranes

Proteins represent main and one of the most significant fractions of plasma membranes. They play an important role, not only in the mechanical structure of the membrane, but also as carriers or channels, serving for transport; they may also be involved in regulatory or ligand-recognition properties. Besides the structural proteins, there occur enzymatic proteins, and also the antigens and various kinds of receptor molecules, in the plasma membrane. Due to the diversity of proteins, different plasma membranes maintain their distinctive characteristics.

A. Peripheral and integral structural proteins. The structural proteins of plasma membranes have recently been classified into two groups: the **peripheral** or **extrinsic proteins** and the **integral** or **intrinsic proteins** (Table 6.2). The peripheral proteins are associated with membrane surface are, therefore, separated by mild treatment. They are soluble in aqueous solutions, and are usually free of lipids. The most common examples of peripheral proteins are *spectrin* found in erythrocytes; *ATPase* and *Cytochrome C*, found in mitochondria and acetylcholinesterase, in electroplax membranes. Spectrin includes in its molecular structure two polypeptides having molecular weights 2,55,000 and 2,20,000 and makes about 30 pet cent of the total proteins in this membrane. Mitochondrial AT Pase protein has a molecular weight of only 70,000.

Table 6.2. Criteria for distinguishing peripheral (extrinsic) and integral (intrinsic) proteins of plasma membrane (**Singer**, 1971).

Property	Peripheral protein	Integral protein
1. Requirement for dissociation from membrane.	Mild treatments sufficient: high ionic strength, metal ion chelating agents.	Hydrophobic bond-breaking agents required: detergents, organic solvents chaotropic agents.
2. Association with lipids when solubilized.	Usually soluble-free of lipids.	Usually associated with lipids when solubilized.
3. Solubility after dissociation from membrane.	Soluble and molecularly dispersed in natural aqueous buffers.	Usually insoluble or aggregated in natural aqueous buffers.
4. Examples	Cytochrome C and ATPase of mitochondria; spectrin of erythrocytes; acetylcholiesterse in electroplax membranes.	Most membranebound enzymes; histocompatibility antigens; drug and hormone receptors.

Integral or intrinsic proteins represent more than 70 per cent of the two protein types. They enter the lipid bilayer, extend all the way through it and require drastic procedures for isolation. Usually they are insoluble in water solutions and need the presence of detergents to be maintained in a non-aggregated form. The integral proteins may be attached to oligosaccharides to form glycoproteins or to special phospholipids to form lipoproteins (*i.e.*, proteolipids). The most common examples of integral proteins are *rhodopsin* found in retinal rod cells and *cytochrome oxidase* found in mitochondrial membrane.

Further, one of the major intrinisic proteins of erythrocyte ghosts has a molecular weight of 95,000 and is highly asymmetrical. **Knauf** and **Rothstein** have suggested that this protein is related to anion permeability. It is thought that this protein molecule has a roughly globular shape and spans the lipid bilayer. Each erythrocyte plasma membrane contains about 500,000 molecules of this type of protein. Using lithium diiodosalicylate which is a *chaotropic* (*i.e.*, water disordering) agent or phenol, an integral glycoprotein called **glycophorin** is released from the red cell ghost. Glycophorin has a molecular weight of 55,000 of which 60 per cent is carbohydrate. Near the COOH end of the molecule there is a region that is very hydrophobic and which interacts with the lipids of the membrane. The NH_2 end is more hydrophilic, is exposed to the external environment and has attached oligosaccharides that are at the outer surface of the membrane (**Marchesi** *et al.*, 1972). At the outer surface glycoproteins contain protein-bound **antigens** for the **ABO blood groups**, **H** and **Le blood groups** and others, such as **MN groups** reacting with rabbit antisera, the influenza virus, phytohemogglutinin, and wheat germ aglutinin. It has been calculated that there are about 700,000 copies of glycophorin protein per human red cells.

Among the most hydrophobic integral proteins of membrane the so-called **proteolipids** are characterized by their strong association with lipids and the fact that they are soluble in organic solvents. Proteolipids were first isolated by **Folch** and **Lees** (1951) from myelin, but they are found to present in all cell membranes and in many of them they represent receptor proteins either for synaptic transmitters or drugs (**De Robertis**, 1971). A bacterium containing permease system has a site of receptor proteins in its plasma membrane (**Geise**, 1973).

4. Enzymes of Plasma Membrane

In any cell in which active transport occurs, it is likely that enzymes occur in the surface of the cell. Perhaps part of the structural protein of a plasma membrane is enzymatic protein (**Chambers** and **Chambers**, 1961). About 30 enzymes have been reported from the isolated plasma membranes. Those most constantly found are 5-*nucleotidase*, *Mg^{2+}ATPase*, *Na^+—K^+ activated—Mg^+ ATPase*, *alkaline*, *phosphatase*, *adenyl cyclase*, *acid phosphomonoesterase* and *RNAse*. Some enzymes, have a preferential localization; for example, *alkaline phosphatase* and *ATPase* are more abundant at the bile capillaries, while *disaccharidases* are present in the microvilli of the intestine. Further, the plasma membrane of eukaryotes locks the enzymes for respiratory chain and glycolytic activity.

The enzyme Na^+—K^+ activated—Mg^+ *ATPase* is one of the most important enzyme of plasma membrane because of its role in ion transfer across the plasma membrane. This enzyme is dependent on the presence of lipid molecules (which influence the catalytic activities of other enzymes of plasma membrane; **Rothfield** *et al.*, 1966) and is inactivated when all lipids are extracted.

6.3 STRUCTURE OF THE PLASMA MEMBRANE

No technique exists as yet that permits direct observation of the molecular arrangments of proteins and lipids in the cell membrane. All information on membrane structure has been inferred from indirect evidence. Thus, certain experiments showed, that any damage to the surface of cell, such as a puncture or tear, resulted in a brief outflow of cytoplasm that stopped just as quickly as it began. It seemed that some sort of limiting barrier separated the cell from its environment. Likewise the swelling of cells, when placed in hypotonic solutions indicates the presence of a semi-permeable cell membrane which allows the passage of water into the cell while resisting the outflow of large molecules from cytoplasm. As the permeability of the cell membrane changes with changing conditions, this suggests that it is no passive barrier but exerts a selective action on which materials pass through it. From this, it is natural to conclude that for such selective permeability and active transport some regulating molecules like enzymes should be present in the plasma membrane.

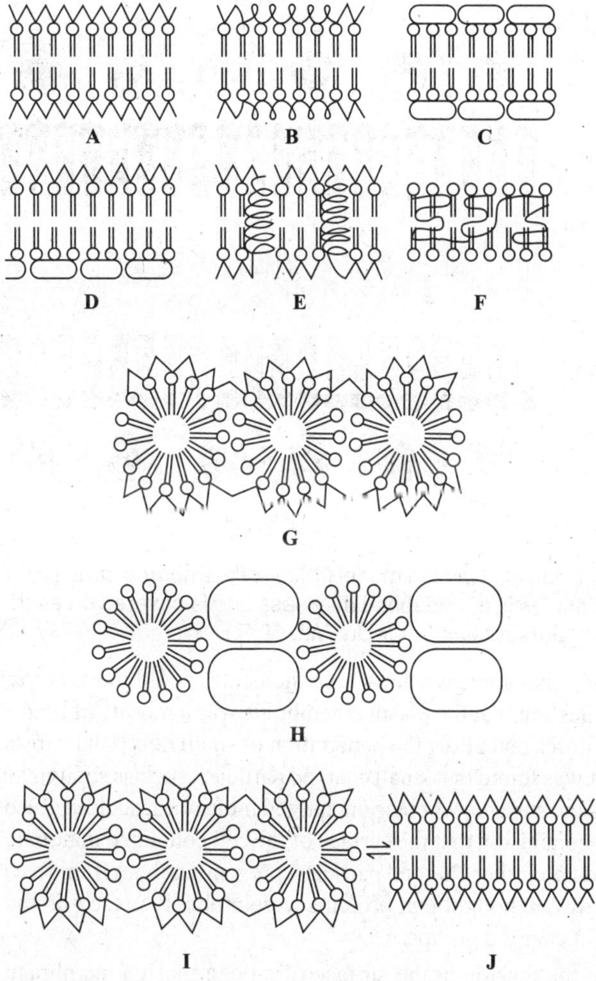

Fig. 6.1. A variety of molecular models proposed for the plasma membrane: A—F, models based on a lipid bilayer structure (*i.e.*, lamellar model); G—J, models based on globular arrangement (*i.e.*, micellar model). A, protein in β-form, B, α-helix: C, globular protein, D, asymmetry in the protein; E, partial penetration with protein channels or pores; F, protein within the lipid bilayer; G, lipid micelles with β-protein; H, lipid micelles with globular protein; I, and J., globular-bilayer transformation (after De Robertis *et al.*, 1975).

From similar kind of reasoning, early workers, specifically **Overton** (1902) concluded that the plasma membranes contained an important lipid component since fat solvents were found to destroy the membrane and fat-soluble substances were shown to pass across membranes much more readily than hydrated molecules. **Langmuir** had shown that fatty acid molecules at an interface stand at right angles to the surface of the water, and the same was thought to be likely in the plasma membrane.

When, in 1925, **Gorter** and **Grendel** showed that all the extracted lipids from red cell ghost occupy an area twice that for a single molecular film, it was thought that there was a membrane with a double layer of lipid molecules, each with its hydrophobic end to the other, standing at right angles to the surface (Fig. 6.2). This **lipid bilayer theory** was also supported by electrical measurements that indicated a high impedance at the plasma membrane. The high impedance is due to the fact that it is difficult for ions to penetrate a lipid layer.

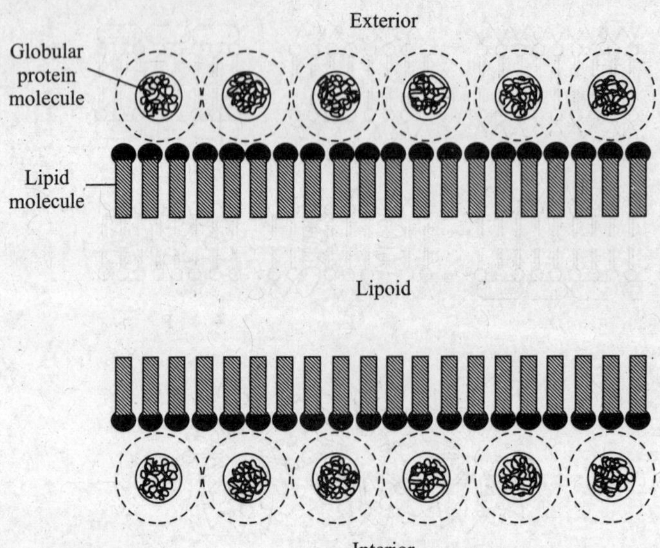

Fig. 6.2. The original Danielli-Davson model (1935) of membrane structure. The bimolecular layer of lipid molecules is of undefined thickness and is covered on each side by a continuous layer of globular proteins (after De Witt, 1977).

Later, it was found that some water-soluble molecules could move across the cell surface and this resulted in the suggestion that the plasma membrane was a mosaic of lipid and non-lipid patches and it contained small pores that allow the penetration of small non-polar substances (*e.g.*, water and methanol). However, it was found that small charged particles, such as sodium ions, showed relatively slow movement across the surface, whereas uncharged molecules, such as glucose, could move quite rapidly. This led to the conclusion that the surface of the cell contained materials with charged groups which could attract and hold other charged particles, preventing them from free movement across the surface. On this basis it was thought that proteins were probably present in the membrane, because these molecules contain charged groups.

Further, because the tension at the surface of an egg plasma membrane is much lower than that expected for a lipid, but approximately equal to the value for a lipid with a coating of proteins, it was postulated by many workers that proteins may cover, though not necessarily, completely the outer surface of the plasma membrane (**Davson** and **Danielli**, 1952; **Davson**, 1970). The elasticity of plasma membrane has also indicated towards the presence of protein molecules in it.

Certain experiments such as electrophoresis, immunological studies and electron microscopy have shown that some of the proteins present on the outer surface of the plasma membrane are glycoproteins containing carbohydrates attached by covalent linkages to the polypeptide chain (see **Lucy**, 1975).

There is, however, a dispute concerning the precise pattern of the molecular subunits (*i.e.*, lipids, proteins and carbohydrates) in the plasma membrane. The approach to the elucidation of membrane architecture has involved the construction of models of membrane structure that are able to account for observed functional characteristics of a particular membrane. Following models and hypotheses have been suggested by different cytologists for the possible molecular architecture of plasma membrane:

1. Lamellar Models

These include following two types of plasma membrane models:

A. Bimolecular leaflet model of Danielli and Davson. The first comprehensive model of membrane structure was formulated in an attempt to explain the observation by **Harvey**, **Cole** and others, in the early 1930s that the surface tension of the plasma membrane of a mammalian egg cell in aqueous medium is considerably lower than that of intra-cellular oil droplets. When it was subsequently shown by **E.N. Harvey** and **James Danielli** that protein adsorbed to the surface of lipid droplets had the effect of reducing the surface tension of the droplets. It seemed reasonable to conclude that plasma membranes consist not only of lipid, as proposed by **Overton** and by **Gorter** and **Grendel**, but also of adsorbed protein. This conclusion, reached by **J. Danielli** and **Hugh Davson** in 1934, formed the basis of what is now known as the **Danielli-Davson model** or **bimolecular leaflet model** of membrane structure. Their model of membrane structure, proposed in 1935, was the first significant attempt to describe the membrane in molecular terms and to relate the structure to observed biological and chemical properties.

In their model, **Danielli** and **Davson** proposed that the plasma membrane consists of two layers of lipid (phospholipid) molecules—**a bimolecular leaflet**—formed in such a way that the polar or hydrophilic part of the lipid molecules are in contact with the surrounding aqueous phase, where as the hydrophobic or non-polar hydrocarbon portions are associated in the central region of the leaflet, removed from the aqueous phase. They further envisioned the polar ends of the lipid molecules as being associated with a monomolecular layer of polar globular protein molecules. The entire structure would thus consist of a double layer of lipid molecules sandwiched between two essentially continuous layers of protein (Fig. 6.3). Subsequently, in 1956 the model was modified to include polar regions, presumably coated with protein, extending through the lipid bilayer and forming small pores 0.7 to 1.0 nm or 7 to 10A° thick (Fig. 6.4).

B. The unit membrane hypothesis. J. David Robertson studied the membranes of the cell from electron micrographs of sectioned materials. The preparations involved the usual steps of killing cells in fixing fluids such as solutions of osmium tetroxide and potassium permanganate, dehydrating in solvents such as acetone and alcohol, and embedding in plastics before sectioning. In the late 1950s, **Robertson** summarized a large amount of ultrastructural data obtained by himself and other workers and concluded that all cell membranes have a common molecular organization. **Robertson** noticed that plasma membranes of prokaryotes and eukaryotes and intracellular membranes from a wide variety of eukaryotic cells appear under the electron microscope as a three-layered (trilaminar) structure approximately 7.5 to 10.0 nm or 75 to 100A° in thickness, composed of two dark electrondense lines, each 2.0 to 2.5 nm (or 20 to 25A°) thick, separated by a light electron-transparent region of 3.5 to 5.0 nm (35 to 50A°). Robertson termed this structure a "**unit membrane**" and he concluded that all biological membranes had unit membrane construction—a generalization that became known as the **unit membrane hypothesis** (Fig. 6.3).

Robertson assumed that the dark lines of the trilaminar structure were proteins and polar groups of lipids and that the light central region consisted of non-polar groups (Fig. 6.4). This molecular organization is similar to that proposed by **Danielli** and **Davson**. However, he postulated a single layer of protein molecules over the inner and outer surfaces of the lipid bilayer, with extended (B-sheet) rather than globular protein conformations. This model fit the measurements of the three layers of a membrane that could be seen in electron micrographs, allowing 20A° each for the two protein coatings and 35A° for the interior lipid bilayer. Extended protein conformation fit the 20A° dimension fairly well, whereas globular proteins would generally be larger than 20A° in diameter.

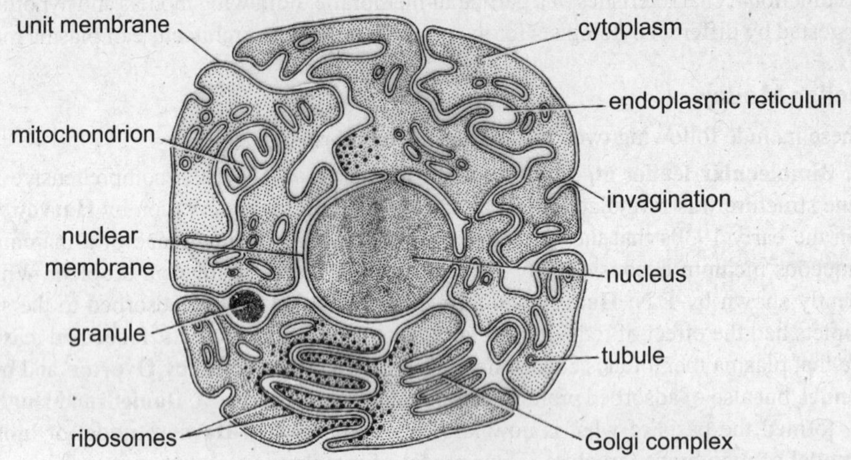

Fig. 6.3. Diagram showing the origin and development of membranous structures of cell from unit membrane.

Robertson's model was widely approved, but some cytologists showed their dissatisfaction with the model, mostly because these dynamic structures had been pictured as static and uniform elements. However, the unit membrane did account for a number of observed properties of cell membranes which are as follows:

1. The densely packed lipid bilayer easily accounted for the presence of 40 per cent lipid, by weight in membranes.
2. Hydrocarbons are poor electrical conductors, so the continuous hydrocarbon phase of the natural membrane would explain the known high electrical resistance of membranes.
3. High permeability of natural membranes to non-polar molecules could be explained by their ready solubility in the non-polar lipid phase, and at the same time account for relative impermeability to small ions which do not dissolve readily in this medium.
4. Phospholipids spontaneously form bilayer system *in vitro* when added to an aqueous environment, and there is no requirement for work input to maintain this minimum energy conformation of the artificial membrane.
5. The model accounted for the three-layered staining pattern of fixed membranes seen with the electron microscope.

Another positive feature of the unit membrane model was the asymmetry of the structure. **Robertson** based this in part on differences in appearance of the inner and outer stained layers of the unit membrane, and it fit well with known cellular membranes that contained saccharides and conjugated proteins (mucopolysaccharides or mucoproteins) on one surface and not on the other (see Fig. 6.4C). Due to this feature, unit membrane model is also known as **greater membrane model**.

Objections to unit membrane theory. Objections to the unit membrane model increased during the 1960s and this led to reexaminations of lipid-protein interactions and to new models. Studies of **F.S. Sjostrand** (1963), of smooth endoplasmic reticular, mitochondrial and chloroplast membranes underscored the differences between observed features of membranes and the uniformity that was required by the unit membrane concept. Mitochondrial and chloroplast membranes contain displays of particulate units in or on the membrane. The plasma membrane did not present the same appearance as mitochondrial or chloroplast membranes. It seemed that different models might be needed to describe different functional types. This unsuitable approach became unnecessary when a mosaic membrane model was proposed.

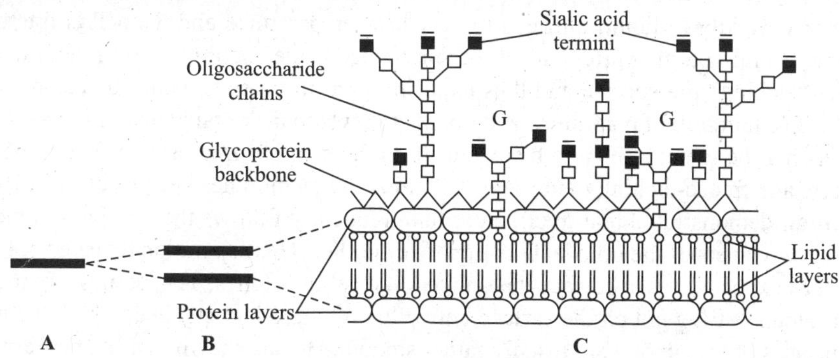

Fig. 6.4. The structure of plasma membrane as observed A—at low magnification of electron microscope, B—at high magnification of electron microscope, C—lamellar model of plasma membrane showing possible arrangment of the lipid, protein and oligosaccharide molecules in the plasma membrane (after De Robertis *et al.*, 1970).

2. Micellar Model

An alternative interpretation of molecular structure of plasma membrane (Fig. 6.1 g and h) has been postulated by **Hilleir** and **Hoffman** (1953). They have suggested that biological membranes may have a non-lamellar pattern, consisting instead of a mosaic of globular subunits known as **micelles** (see **Toner** and **Carr**, 1971), which have a lipid core and a hydrophilic shell of polar groups. Lipid micelles are possible building-blocks for membranes since they tend towards spontaneous association. In this model of membrane structure the protein components of the membrane may form a monolayer on either side of the plane of lipid micelles. Individual units of the micellar mosaic might be replaced by individual enzymes molecules or by arrays of enzymes with a precise-three dimensional organization, enabling specific functions to be 'built in' to the membrane structure.

The spaces between the globular micelles are thought to form water-filled pores 0.4 nm (4A°) in diameter, lined partly by the polar groups of the micelles and partly by the polar groups of associated protein molecules.

The appearance of membranes in high resolution electron micro-graphs lend some support both to the 'lamellar' and the 'micellar' theory of membrane structure, but do not provide convincing evidence for either which might resolve this controversy (see **Toner** and **Carr**, 1971; **Giese**, 1973). According to **De Robertis** *et al.*, (1975), some workers have postulated that intra-cellular membranes have micellar structures while plasma membrane has lamellar configuration and there occur a mutual transformation (*i.e.*, globular-bilayer transformation in Fig. 6.1 g and J) between the two.

3. Protein Crystal Model

The lamellar models and micellar models of plasma membranes were objected for their one or another shortcomings and in fact, in the middle 1960s, there were no models of membrane structure that were versatile enough to account adequately for the functional and compositional variation of cellular membranes. Much of the ultrastructural data on membranes was criticized during this period because of the possibility that methods of tissue preparation caused changes in the natural membrane structure. In order to overcome this criticism, cytologists turned to methods that allowed the examination of cellular membranes without treatment by the relatively harsh fixation and staining methods required for observing sectioned material in the electron microscope.

One method that avoids chemical fixatives is **freeze-fracture** and **freeze-etching**, both of which refer to a preparation procedure for electron microscopy. In this technique, cells or pieces of tissue are frozen rapidly in liquid nitrogen to very low temperatures and the cell is fractured by a sharp blow with a microtome knife. Part of the surface ice is then sublimed from the fracture faces in a vacuum, "etching" the surface and thus exposing part of the specimen. The etched surface is next coated with a thin film of platinum and carbon, after which the organic matter is dissolved away with acid, leaving the metal replica to be examined in the electron microscope. The importance of freeze-fracture and freeze-etching to the study of biological membranes became clear in 1966 when **Daniel Branton** demonstrated that the fracture line frequently follows the middle of a membrane, separating the two layers of the lipid leaflets from one another. This separation revealed not a smooth lipid surface, as expected, but a surface that looked like cobble-stones. The 'stones' are membrane-associated proteins, sitting not on the surface but within the lipid leaflets. In contrast, the true inner and outer surfaces of membrane are usually rather smooth. He has shown that 'stones' are globular proteins having diameter upto about 85A° and that the number, density and grouping of the particles (globular proteins) are dependent upon particular type of membrane studied. For example, the inner surfaces of myelin membranes are essentially free of such particles, whereas the inner surfaces of chloroplast thylakoid membranes appear highly particulate. Other types of membranes show intermediate degrees of particulate structures.

The demonstration of globular particles or proteins as components of a number of cell membranes has led to new models of membrane structure. **David Green** and his coworkers (1970) have proposed a **protein crystal model** which suggests that membrane proteins polymerize to form arrays of two layers of loosely packed globular proteins, 3.0 to 4.0 nm (or 30 to 40A°) in diameter. The proteins are envisioned as having extensive non-polar, as well as polar, regions on their surfaces. These non-polar regions may exhibit hydrophobic bonding with non-polar groups of phospholipid molecules that fill cavities between the globular protein units; the polar heads of phospholipid molecules remain at the membrane's surface.

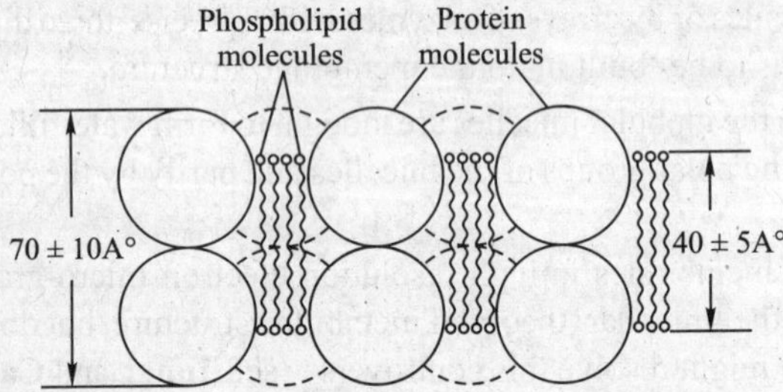

Fig. 6.5. The protein crystal model of membrane structure as proposed by **Vanderkooi** and **Green** (1970). Phospholipid molecules forming short regions of lipid bilayer fill cavities between protein molecules (large circles) (after De Witt, 1977).

The protein crystal model accounts for some of the observed chemical and functional characteristics of membranes. For example, isolated membrane proteins tend to be relatively compact structures often 40A° or more in diameter, not the flat sheets needed for some earlier models (*i.e.*, Robertson's unit membrane model). Membrane proteins also tend to be very insoluble in aqueous solution under mild conditions unless detergents are present, indicating the existence of a hydrophobic exterior unable to interact with the surrounding water. These features would be expected for proteins that are designed to be embedded in lipid membrane rather than situated on its surfaces.

Further, the existence of polar groups as well as non-polar groups on the surfaces of globular proteins could account for the permeability of many membranes to polar molecules. Such a membrane would be expected to show trilaminar structure in electron micrographs, as does a bilayer of phospholipid molecules, because both structures essentially have a non-polar core and a polar surface.

Green has recently modified the protein crystal model toward a more dynamic model in which the proteins and lipids are considered to move in the plane of the membrane. **Green** points out that a consequence of this modification is that the lipid bilayer forms essentially a continuum and any protein-protein interactions are temporary.

4. Fluid Mosaic Model

Another model of membrane structure was proposed by **S.J. Singer** and **G.L. Nicolson** in 1972 and has been widely accepted. **Singer** and **Nicolson** envisioned cell membranes as mosaics of lipids and proteins. The lipids are thought to be arranged primarily in a bilayer in which **peripheral** and **integral** proteins are embedded to varying degrees. During certain immunological experiments, the attachment of antibodies to surface-exposed integral membrane protein such as glycophorin led to the realization that membrane proteins are not fixed within the lipid bilayer but are free to move laterally, like icebergs floating submerged in a sea of lipid (Fig. 6.6). This picture inspired the name **fluid mosaic model**, coined by **Singer** and **Nicolson**. If this analogy of icebergs floating in a sea of lipid is valid, then it should be possible to freeze the proteins into place by solidifying the lipid sea in which they float. Indeed, that is readily accomplished, for as one lowers the temperature a point is reached at which a **phase transition** in the lipid sea occurs from a relatively liquid (called "**liquid crystal**") to a relatively solid (**crystalline**) state. At this point, mobility of the membrane proteins is greatly restricted.

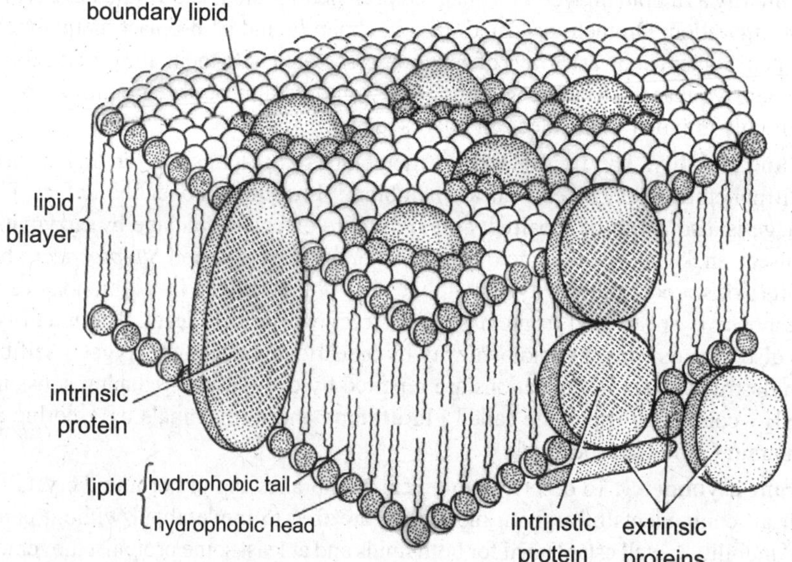

Fig. 6.6. Fluid-mosaic model of the plasma membrane. Proteins floating in a sea of lipid. Some proteins span the lipid bilayer, others are exposed only to one surface or the other (Modified after De Robertis *et al.*, 1975).

If this temperature (or phase) transition is really due to the freezing and melting of membrane lipids, then the temperature at which it occurs should vary with the fatty acid composition. Specifically, transition temperature should increase with chain length and decrease with degree of unsaturation. Since the fatty acid composition in both bacteria and eukaryotic membranes reflects to some degree the availability of fatty acids from outside sources (diet in the case of animals), it has been possible to verify the correlation between phase transition temperature and fatty acid composition. In fact, one of the mechanisms used by bacteria and fish to adapt to a very cold environments is alteration of their membrane lipids by using shorter, more unsaturated fatty acid chains, (**Dyson**, 1978).

Further, cholesterol drastically lowers or abolishes the apparent transition temperature by imposing a structure of its own on membrane lipids. It is because of their varying cholesterol content that animal cell membranes maintain a liquid crystalline state at body temperature inspite of having relatively long-chain (16 to 18 carbon) saturated fatty acids. The membranes of higher plants and bacteria, most of which do not contain cholesterol, maintain a liquid crystalline state by using shorter-chain fatty acids with more double bonds.

The mosaic nature of the membrane is favored by the results of freeze-etching techniques in which protein particles are shown at the plane of cleavage of the bilayer (**Pinto da Silva** and **Branton**, 1970; **Tillack** and **Marchesi**, 1970). The fluidity of the lipids is supported by many indirect studies based on X-ray diffraction, differential thermal analysis and electron spin techniques (**Hubbell** and **McConnell**, 1971; **Devaux** and **McConnell**, 1972). The fluidity of the integral proteins is supported by experiments on cell fusion (**Frye** and **Edidin**, 1970) and on those of clustering and 'capping' of surface antigens (**Taylor** *et al.*, 1971; **Edidin** and **Frambrough**, 1973).

The fluid mosaic model of membrane is now almost universally accepted. Though most of the work has been done on plasma membranes, the model is presumed to apply to membranes of all types, inspite of their varying and characteristic differences in lipid and protein composition. In fact, fluid mosaic model can account for the molecular organization and ultrastructure of membranes in terms of their chemical composition. Membranes such as myelin with little or no enzymatic activity would exist primarily as a lipid bilayer with attached peripheral protein and would have typical "unit membrane" configuration. On the other hand, in mitochondria and chloroplast membranes, which have a high protein content and vast arrays of enzymes associated with them, the protein components would be so extensive that the trilaminar framework would be almost obscured. Such membranes would appear highly granular in the electron microscope.

Membrane stability. The fluid nature of membranes is responsible for their resistance to damage. Small puncture wounds self-seal as membrane flows in to cover the defect. Localized chemical damage is also apt to be repaired, although more extensive damage by enzymatic attack from certain insect, snake and bacterial toxins (*e.g.*, of *Staphylococcus* and *Streptococcus* bacteria), or from **lymphotoxins** produced by T -type lymphocytes—the so called killer lymphocytes—during an immune response is apt to lead to membrane destruction and cell death. The integrity of cell membranes is also threatened in an unknown way by oxidations, molecular oxygen itself being the most common destructive agent. Oxidations are repaired by cytoplasmic reducing substances that include an—SH—containing tripeptide called **glutathione** and in mammals by ascorbic acid and tocopherol (vitamin C and E, respectively).

Membrane asymmetry. To describe biological membranes as fluid or liquid crystalline does not imply that all components of a given membrane are free to move about without constraints. Though lateral mobility is well established for both lipids and at least some proteins, movement is not necessarily random. Some membrane proteins are connected to underlying networks of microtubules and microfilaments, thus restricting and controlling their movements. This restriction may lead to marked differences in the protein content from one part of a membrane to another.

There is also marked asymmetry across membranes. Carbohydrate, which is primarily contributed by glycoproteins that are specific for cell and species type but also by glycopeptides and glycolipids, is found almost exclusively on the outer surface of plasma membranes. In cells lining the intestine, for example, carbohydrate produces a 0.1–5.0 μm thick branching network of fine filaments extending from the outer leaflet of the membrane. The inner surface of plasma membranes, in addition to its lack of carbohydrate, has typically a quite distinct set of antigenic determinants. Some of this asymmetry is due to integral proteins that extend from surface-to-surface such as erythrocyte glycophorin; some is also due to peripheral proteins which are confined to one side or the other, available, therefore, to chemical reagents or antibodies introduced from one side only.

Further, although lateral movement of some membrane protein is allowed, but there is very little tendency for them to flip, rotate or translocate to other side. However, lipids can move in and out of membranes. Lipid exchange between cytoplasmic lipoproteins and the inner surface of the cell membrane is readily demonstrated.

Membrane asymmetry is important to membrane function. The two sides of a membrane typically participate in very different activities. There is, for instance, a constant traffic of small molecules across the plasma membrane, in some cases made possible by highly directional transport systems contributed by membrane proteins. The membrane proteins thus serve specific functions as transport carriers, receptor sites, recognition molecules, and enzymes in energy transfer reactions.

Inter-cellular Space

In multicellular animals and plants, individual cells are found grouped together into **tissues**. Fat, bone and muscle are examples. The cells within a given tissue are not necessarily identical, but they cooperate to carry out a common task. In the tissues of multicellular animals, the plasma membrane of two adjacent cells usually remain separated by a space of 10 to 150A° wide. This inter-cellular space is uniform and contains a material of low electron density (mucopoly-saccharide) which can be considered as a cementing substance.

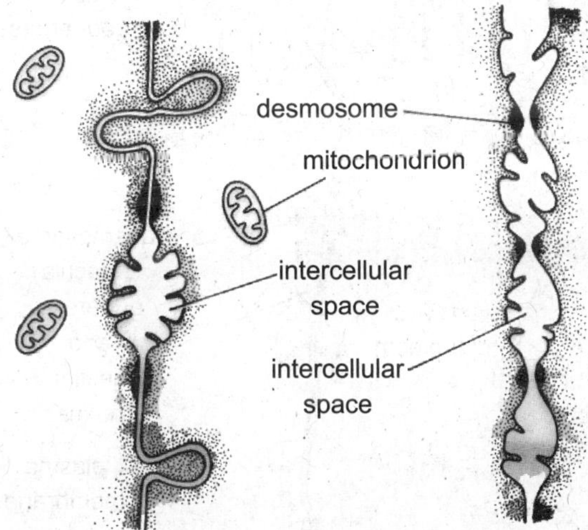

Fig. 6.7. Inter-cellular space.

6.4 SPECIALIZED STRUCTURES OF PLASMA MEMBRANE

The cell surface of certain cells performs various physiological activities such as absorption, secretion, transportation, etc. To perform such specialized functions certain modifications are inevitable in the plasma membrane of such cells. Certain most important specialized structurers of plasma membrane are following:

A. Specializations due to Outpushing or Evagination of Plasma Membrane

Microvilli. The columnar epithelial cells of intestinal epithelium have to perform active absorption of the digested food. The free surfaces of these epithelial cells give out many minute, fingerlike cytoplasmic processes of plasma membrane which are known as the **microvilli** (Fig. 6.8). These microvilli are 0.6 to 0.8 μm long and have the diameter of 0.1 μm (1000A°), represent cytoplasmic processes covered by the plasma membrane. Within the cytoplasmic core fine microfilaments along with α-actinin, myosin molecules and microtubules (Fig. 6.9) are observed which in the subjacent cytoplasm form a terminal web. The outer surface of the microvilli is covered by a coat of filamentous material (fuzzy coat) composed of glycoprotein macromolecules. A single cell may contain about 3000 microvilli. The narrow spaces between the microvilli form a kind of sieve through which substances may pass during the process of absorption. These microvilli increase the absorptive surface of the intestinal epithelial cell. Such microvilli also occur in comparatively low number in the hepatic cells, mesothelial cells of the convoluted tubules of the kidney and in the epithelial cells of gall bladder, uterus and yolk sac.

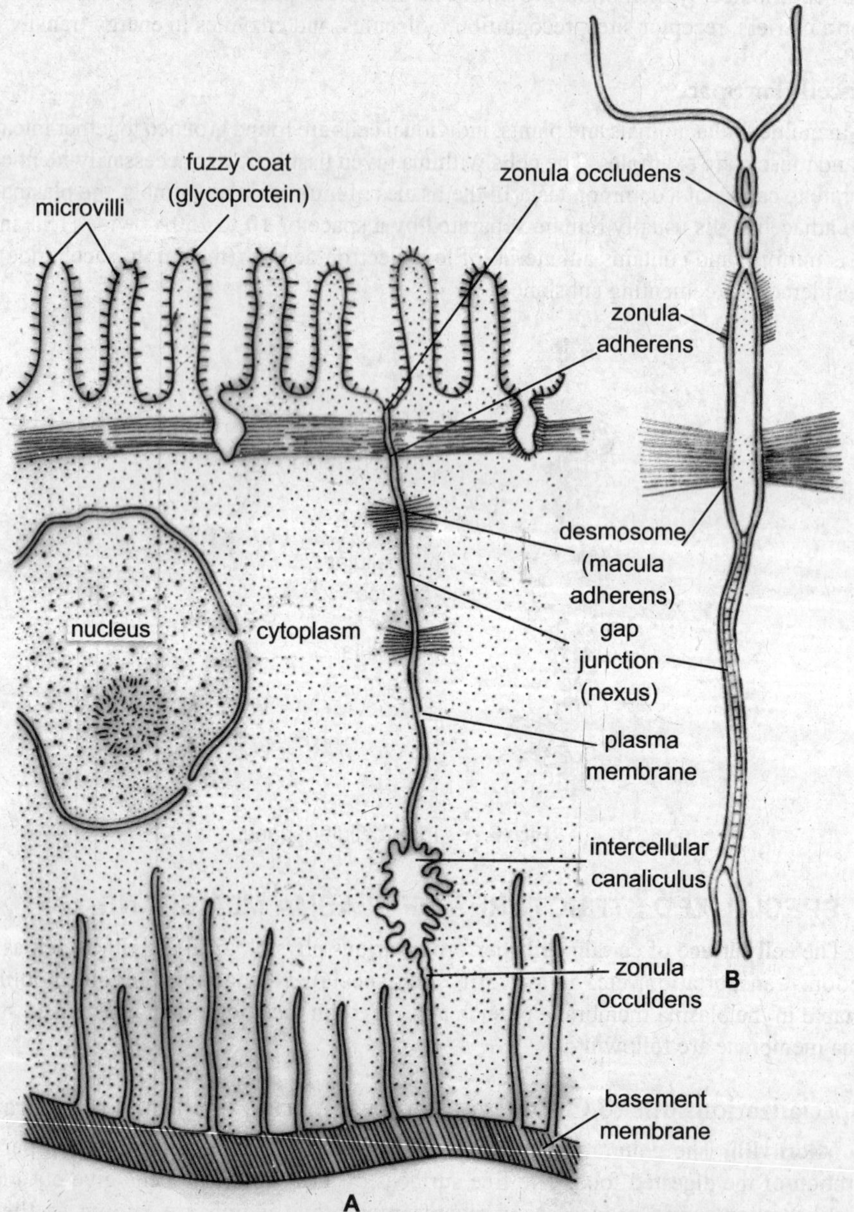

Fig. 6.8. A—A typical columnar epithelial cell showing the main differentiations of plasma membrane; B—Indicates the series of differentiations found between two epithelial cells (after De Robertis *et al.*, 1975).

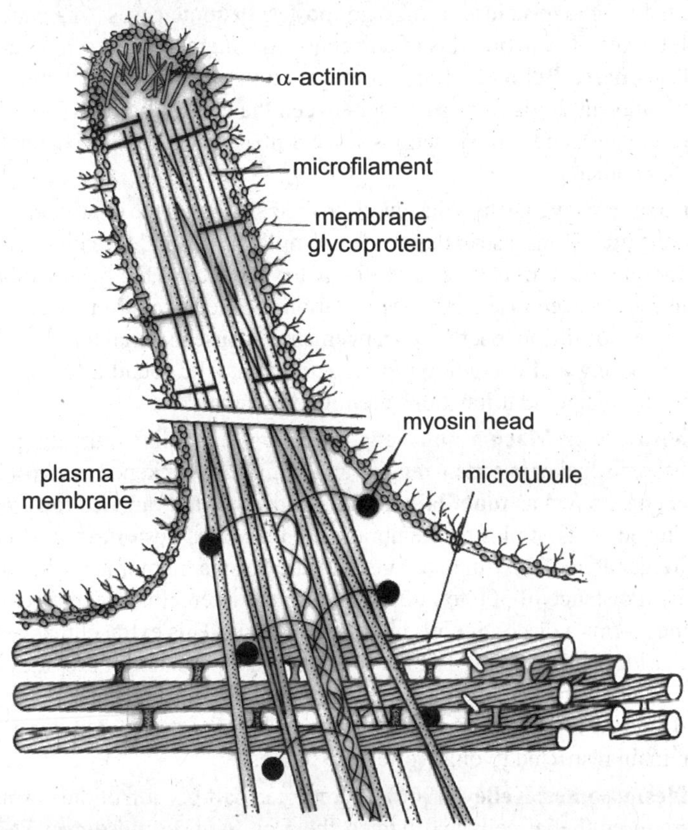

Fig. 6.9. Ultrastructure of a microvillus showing its different cytoskeleton components. Note glycoproteins embedded in the plasma membrane and connections between microfilaments and membrane proteins. Alpha actinin forms a non-muscle "Z line" to anchor the microfilaments. Myosin molecules are shown distributed along the base of microfilaments. Microtubules run parallel to the cell surface (after Dyson, 1978).

B. Specialization due to Inpushing or Invaginations of Plasma Membrane

The bases (inner ends) of certain cells perform active transportation like the cells of the kidney and contain many invaginations or infoldings of the plasma membrane. At the base of these folds there develops a septa and thus narrow compartments of basal cytoplasm are formed. These infoldings contain many mitochondria. These mitochondria along with the enzymes of plasma membrane possibly provide energy to the plasma membrane for the active transportation of solutes (Fig. 6.10).

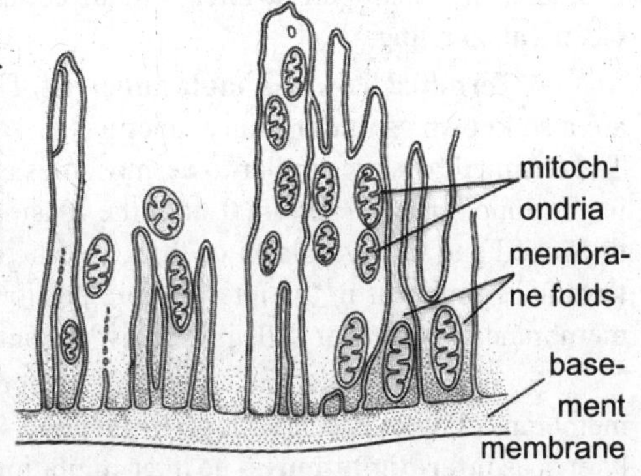

Fig. 6.10. Infoldings of plasma membrane.

C. Specialization in Plasma Membrane due to Contact

Though the plasma membrane of adjacent cells often remain separated by a uniform inter-cellular space but at certain places the plasma membrane of adjacent cells may come too close or may go too far. In some cases, this pattern is interrupted by areas in which the membrane proteins of adjacent cells interact with each other in a highly specific way to provide an **intercellular junction**. Some junctions are devices that glue cells together, others are barriers that prevent fluids from passing between the cells (*e.g.*, between cells lining fluid-filled cavities such as the gut), and some junctions serve primarily to establish channels of communication from one cell to another.

Cell junctions are given names that describe their shape and the relative closeness of cooperating membranes. If the junction is a strip that passes completely around the cell, it is called a **zonule**; if it is a spot, the appropriate term is **macule**. If the outer surfaces of the two membranes are very close together, in some cases even fused, the specialization is called **occludens** (*i.e.*, occluding) junction; a wider separation, filled with an indefinite arrangement of dense material forms an **adherens** (adhering) junction. Both adhering and occluding type junctions may be found as either macules or zonules. Following types of intercellular junctions are found in eukaryotes:

1. Desmosomes or Macula adherens. In certain epithelial cells, the plasma membrane of adjacent cells become thicker in certain regions and from these thickened areas (or intracellular plaque) many fine filaments known as **tonofilaments** or **tonofibrils** are radiated towards the interior of the cell. Such thickened areas of plasma membrane are known as **desomosomes**. The desmosomes are formed by a circular area of 0.5 μm in diameter of the plasma membranes of two adjacet cells which are separated by a distance of 300 to 500A°. Within the intercellular gap a coating material occurs which sometimes forms a discontinuous middle dense line. This extracellular material contains acid mucopolysaccharides and proteins. The extracellular coating material provides cellular adhesion at the desomosome and the tonofilaments provide intracellular mechanical support. Desmosomes thus, serve mainly to glue the cell together providing structural support. According to **J.P. Trinkaus** (1969), desmosomes remain restricted to only vertebrate tissues.

2. Hemidesmosomes. Kelley (1966) has reported half portion of the desmosomes at the basal surfaces of certain epithelial cells and named them as **hemidesmosomes**. The hemidesmosomes resemble with desmosomes in finer details but their outer side remain coated with collagen fibrils.

3. Septate desmosomes. Wood (1959), **Locke** (1965) and **Gauranten** (1967) have reported different types of desmosomes in the epithelia of invertebrates and named them as **septate desmosomes**. In septate desmosomes, the two plasma membrane remain separated by a distance of 150 to 200A° and both remain joined by many transverse parallel septa. These septa are found to be continuous upto outer proteinous layers of plasma membranes. The septate desmosomes lack the intercellular cementing substance and tonofilaments of the desmosomes. They act like attachment or adhesive devices of cells and they also permit inter-cellular communication and electrical coupling.

4. Terminal bars or Zonula adherens. The terminal bars are also known as intermediary junctions or zonula adherens. The terminal bars are similar to desmosomes except they lack in the tonofibrils. In terminal bars the plasma membrane is thickened and the cytoplasm of thickened area is dense. The terminal bars occur in the intermediate portion of the plasma membrane of columnar cells just below the surface.

5. Inter-digitations. At some places the plasma membrane of two adjacent cells gives out finger-like projections known as **inter-digitations**. The inter-digitations may become further complicated by the development of desmosomes and [illegible]l bars, etc.

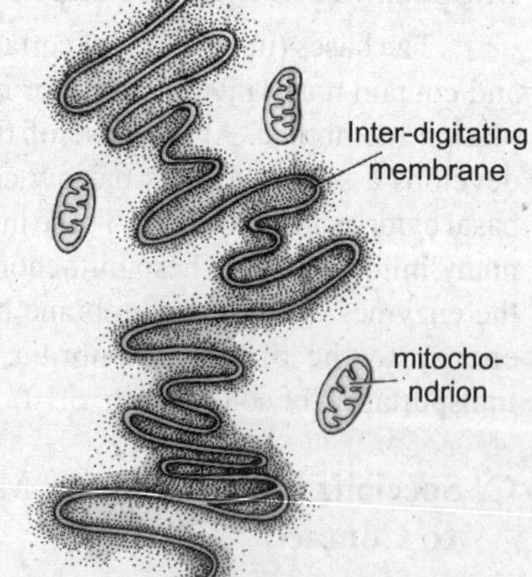

Fig. 6.11. Inter-digitation of plasma membrane.

6. Tight junctions or Zonula occludens. At certain places, the plasma membrane of two adjacent cells fuse so intimately that the inter-cellular space become wanting. Such fusions of the plasma membrane are known as tight junctions or zonula occludens. The tight junctions serve to seal the space between the cells and act as barriers for diffusion of the substances through these regions. The tight junctions occur in brain cells and acts as blood-brain barriers and the synaptic barriers. Tight junctions also occur in intestine cells and in cells lining cavities of gland, gall bladder, etc.

7. Gap junctions, macula occludens or nexus. The cells of myocardial tissue contain a inter-cellular gap of 20A° wide between their plasma membranes. These gaps are found to be hexagonal (70 to 75A° wide) in tangential sections. These hexagonal gaps are known as **gap junctions**. When the inter-cellular gap becomes 40–70A° wide, then such junctions are called **close junctions**. Gap junctions are found in a variety of embryonic and adult tissues such as muscles and invertebrate nerves. They provide intercellular communication by making possible direct passage of small molecules and ions between cells.

6.5 PHYSIOLOGY OF PLASMA MEMBRANE

The plasma membrane acts as a thin barrier which separates the intracellular fluid or the cytoplasm from the extracellular fluid in which the cell lives. In case of unicellular organisms (Protophyta and Protozoa) the extracellular fluid may be fresh, or marine water, while in multicellular organisms the extracellular fluid may be blood, lymph or interstitial fluid. Though the plasma membrane is a limiting barrier around the cell but it performs various important physiological functions which are as follows:

A. Permeability

The plasma membrane is a thin, elastic membrane around the cell which usually allows the movement of small ions and molecules of various substances through it. This nature of plasma membrane is termed as **permeability**. According to permeability following types of the plasma membranes have been recognized:

***(i)* Impermeable plasma membrane.** The plasma membrane of the unfertilized eggs of certain fishes allows nothing to pass through it except the gases. Such plasma membranes can be termed as impermeable plasma membranes.

***(ii)* Semi-permeable plasma membrane.** The membranes which allow only water but no solute particle to pass through them are known as semi-permeable membranes. Such membranes have not so far been recognized in animal cells.

***(iii)* Selective permeable plasma membrane.** The plasma membrane and other intracellular unit membranes are very selective in nature. Such membranes allow only certain selected ions and small molecules to pass through them. Once the membrane has been damaged or the cell has been killed, molecules move freely across the membrane and may reach equilibrium. Equilibrium is rarely achieved in living systems, so that the dynamic state of the living membrane acts as a regulatory barrier for entry and exit of molecules and particles.

***(iv)* Dialysing plasma membrane.** The plasma membrane having certain extraneous coats around it as the basement membranes of endothelial cells acts as a **dialyzer**. In these membranes the water molecules and crystalloids are forced through them by the hydrostatic pressure forces.

Permeability of the plasma membrane to water (osmosis). When molecules of two kinds are placed together they tend to mix with each other by a process known as the **diffusion**. Molecules diffuse from a region of greater concentration to a region of lesser concentration. The difference in the levels of the two concentrations is called the **concentration gradient**. The process by which the water molecules pass through a membrane from a region of higher water concentration to the region of lower water concentration is known as osmosis (Gr., *osmos*-pushing). The process in which the water molecules enter into the cell is known as **endosmosis**, while the reverse process which involves the exit of the water molecules from the cell is known as **exomosis**. In plant cells due to excessive exosmosis the cytoplasm along with the plasma membrane shrinks away from the cell wall. This process is known as **plasmolysis** (Gr., *plasma*-molded, *lysis*-loosing).

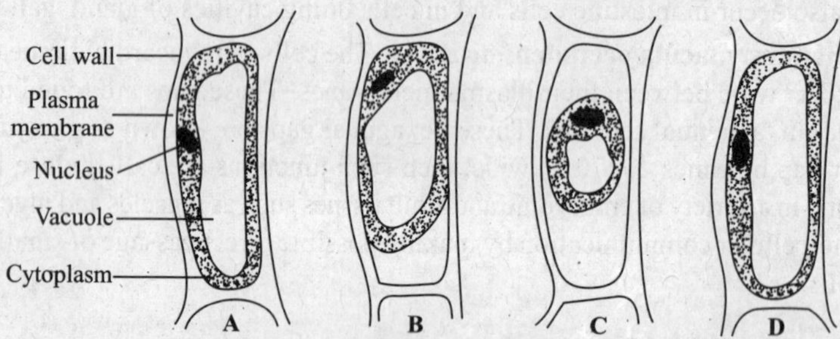

Fig. 6.12. Plasmolysis and deplasmolysis in plant cells. Plasmolysis occurs when a normal plant cell (A) is placed in a hypertonic solution. Water leaves the cell and the plasma membrane shrinks away from the cell wall (B, C). If solutes can penetrate the plasma membrane, the cell will eventually regain water—a process termed deplasmolysis (D) (after De Witt, 1977).

A cell contains a variety of solutes in it. For instance, the mammalian erythrocytes contain the ions of potassium (K^+), calcium (Ca^+), phosphate (PO_4^-), dissolved haemoglobin and many other substances. If the erythrocyte is placed in a 0.9% solution of sodium chloride (NaCl), then it neither shrinks nor swells. In such case because the intracellular and extracellular fluids contain same concentrations and no osmosis takes place. This type of extracellular solution or fluid is known as isotonic solution or fluid. If the concentration of NaCl solution is increased above 0.9% then the erythrocytes are shrinked due to excessive exosmosis. Such solutions which have higher concentrations of solutes than the intracellular fluids are known as **hypertonic solutions**. Further, if the concentration of NaCl solution decreases below 0.9% the erythrocytes will swell up due to endosmosis. The extracellular solutions which contain less concentration of the solutes than the cytoplasm are known as **hypotonic solutions**.

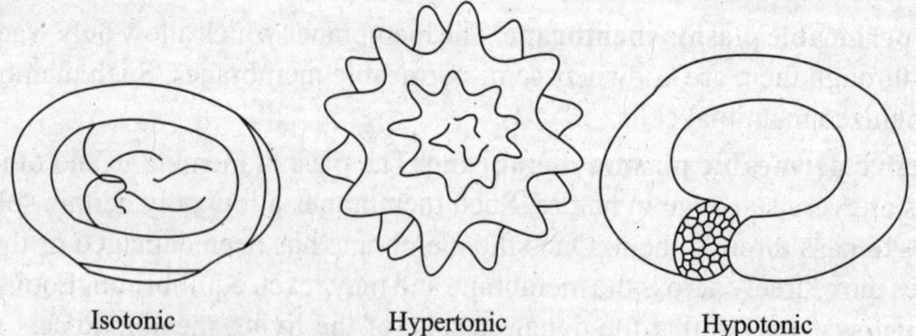

Fig. 6.13. The effects of isotonic, hypertonic and hypotonic solutions on erythrocytes. In isotonic solution erythrocytes maintain their normal shape. Hypertonic solutions cause water to leave erythrocytes, resulted in shrunken cells with a plasma membrane thrown into folds (crenated). Hypotonic solutions cause water influx and result in spherical cells that may eventually burst (**hemolyse**) (after Dyson, 1978).

Due to endosmosis or exosmosis the water molecules come in or go out of the cell. The amount of the water inside the cell causes a pressure known as **hydrostatic pressure**. The hydrostatic pressure hich is caused by the osmosis is known as osmotic pressure. The plasma membrane maintains a n between the osmotic pressure of the intracellular and intercellular fluids.

B. Transport Mechanism Across Membranes

There are three general routes and mechanisms by which substances cross the membrane barrier: (1) **free diffusion** or **passive diffusion** along a gradient going from higher to lower concentration of the molecule; (2) assisted passage or transport across the membrane either by a process of **facilitated** diffusion in which the substance moves as expected in the direction of its lower concentration, or by energy-expending active **transport** against a concentration gradient; and (3) enclosure in membranous vesicles to enter the cell by the process called **endocytosis** or be expelled from the cell in the reverse process of **exocytosis**.

1. Free diffusion. According to a large amount of evidences, many substances move through membranes at rates of free diffusion that are directly proportional to their solubility in lipid (Fig. 6.14).

Molecules of water, oxygen and carbon dioxide are notable exceptions to this rule since they freely diffuse through membranes regularly and rapidly. It has been suggested that membranes contain 8–10A° wide pores that are lined by hydrophilic residues (Fig. 6.14). Such openings would be large enough for water molecules but would hardly accommodate other water-soluble substances to pass through the narrow passage way. There exist no direct evidence to support this concept.

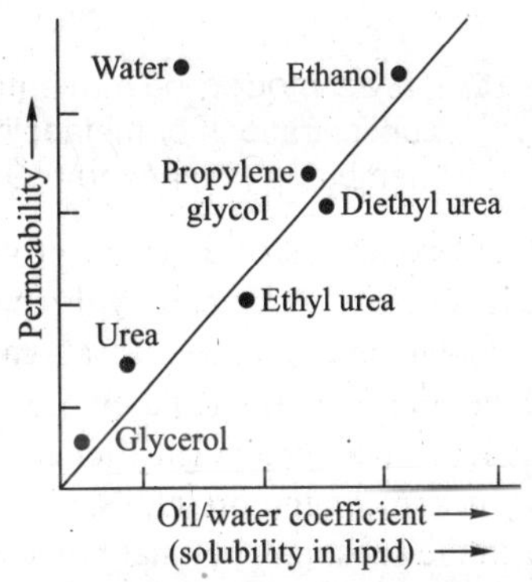

Fig. 6.14. Graph showing that the rate of free diffusion of chemicals through an oil/ water phase system (analogous to a membrane) is directly proportional to the solubility of the chemicals are an exception to this rule (after Avers, 1976).

Free diffusion is simplest type of transport mechanism. It requires no energy expenditure on the part of the cell, nor does it require any specific transport carrier molecule. As long as a favorable concentration gradient across the membrane is maintained, transport by free diffusion may occur; when the concentration gradient is dissipated, free diffusion stops. The rate of transport in free diffusion is strictly proportional to the concentration difference across the membrane; the greater the concentration difference, the greater the rate of passage.

A concentration gradient may be maintained by the cell in such a way that a substance will pass through a membrane essentially in one direction. For example, if molecules of a particular nutrient, entering the cell by free diffusion, are utilized in some metabolic process, additional molecules may continue to enter as long as an ample supply is readily available outside the cell. This occurs because the utilization of the nutrient keeps its intra-cellular concentration low and hence maintains the concentration gradient necessary for transport. In the same way, waste products may continue to leave the cell as long as they are washed away from the medium surrounding the outer surface of the plasma membrane.

2. Facilitated diffusion and active transport. Essential lipid-insoluble metabolites, such as sugars (glucose) and amino acids, enter and leave the cell or its compartments through processes involving reversible combination with membrane proteins, called **carriers**. These carriers are integral proteins that form part of the structure of the membrane. Carriers are highly specific. Each is assumed to have characteristic binding site which will bind one particular kind of molecule but not another that may be almost identical. The binding between carrier and metabolite is transient. After the bound molecule has been translocated to the other side of membrane, the carrier is freed and may recycle to assist other molecules of this substance to get across the membrane. The relative solubility of th metabolite in lipid is not significant since its interaction is with protein rather than lipid constituents of the membrane.

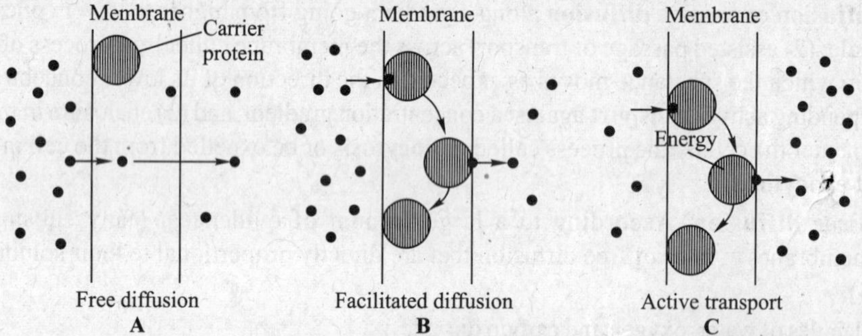

Fig. 6.15. Three modes of movement across the membrane by metabolites. The relative concentrations of metabolite are indicated by the number of dots on either side of the membrane (after Avers, 1976).

Certain carriers or transport proteins of bacterial systems are called **permeases**. The ending "—*ase*", normally associated with enzymes, was picked to emphasize certain analogies between carrier proteins and true enzymes: (1) carrier proteins accelerate the reaction being considered, namely membrane translocation; (2) they provide great selectivity; and (3) they are themselves unchanged in the process, being recycled after each assisted entry or exit. However, carrier proteins differ from the enzymes in one important respect: it is the function of an enzyme to bring about some chemical change in the substrate, but that process is not intrinsic to membrane transport.

Carriers may assist molecules across the membrane in the usual direction of the concentration gradient, from high to lower amounts of the metabolite, or against this usual "downhill" direction. Therefore, at least two carrier-mediated transport mechanisms must exist, one that sponsors facilitated diffusion and another that aids energy-requiring active transport in the "uphill" direction of a gradient. In **facilitated diffusion**, the carrier helps the molecule of metabolite along the direction in which that molecule ordinarily would move. Here, the diffusion is facilitated because the molecule cannot penetrate the selectively permeable membrane on its own by free diffusion movements. In **active transport**, a substance can continue to be accumulated in a region where it already exists in higher concentration only if energy from metabolism is continually supplied to the carrier system. Metabolic energy derives active transport. For example, glucose uptake by micro-organisms and by cells lining the intestines and kidney tubules of animals is typically active transport; in most other animal cells, it is achieved by facilitated diffusion.

Further, cells can accumulate substances in excess of expected amounts in at least three ways:

1. The substance can be precipitated from solution once it is inside the cell, effectively reducing the concentration of solute in water.
2. The molecule can be chemically changed after it has gone through the membrane, thus reducing the concentration of the specific molecule involved in the concentration gradient.
3. The transport of a metabolite can be coupled directly to a second reaction that is energetically favorable to driving the transport reaction "uphill".

The accumulation of Ca^{++} ions in cisternae of muscle endoplasmic reticulum operates by way of precipitation. Calcium phosphate is the precipitate in this case, and its formation maintains a favorable gradient of calcium ions. Sugars may accumulate inside the cell by a combination of ...ilitated diffusion and phosphorylation events, particularly in bacterial cells. If the entering sugar is ...ylated immediately, then the inside concentration of the non-phosphorylated sugar remains ... additional molecules will be transported into the cell along the usual "downhill" direction of the concentration gradient. Both of these situations differ from active transport in that their direction of metabolite movement is toward the region of lower concentration, whereas active transport leads to continued accumulation of a substance in the region where it occurs in its highest concentration.

Active transport and ion pumps. One unifying concept that has developed in recent years explains active transport on the basis of pumping actions. In particular, the active pumping of one substance out of a cell or compartment provides the driving force for active transport of various other substances inward. The pumping in of these metabolites is thus considered to be coupled to the outward transport of someone other material, but in a manner that provides the energy required to drive the needed materials inward, in the "uphill" direction of their concentration gradients. The pump is an economical as well as simple transport system since the outward movement of one kind of substance helps to drive in many kinds of metabolites.

The solutes that are most actively pumped into the cells are potassium (K^+) ions, sugars and amino acids. The driving force for this inward transport is believed to be a sodium (Na^+) gradient across the membrane, created by active transport of N^+ ions pumped out of the cell. The external Na^+ ion concentration remains high and the internal ion concentration remains low as Na^+ continues to be transported outside the cell. The energy required to pump Na^+ ions out of the cell is provided by *ATP*, which is hydrolyzed by a Mg^+ activated *ATPase* believed to be situated within the membrane. The free-energy difference between *ATP* and its *ADP* and inorganic phosphate products of hydrolysis is made available for active transport in the operation of the **primary sodium pump**. This pump acts in animal cells or of bacteria, neither of which requires Na^+ ions for its metabolism. **A hydrogen (H^+) pump** is active in bacterial cells; the pump in plant systems is not well understood (**Avers**, 1976).

The sodium pump was discovered by **A.L. Hodkin** and **R.D. Keynes** in 1955 and associated with *ATP hydrolysis in vitro* by **J.C. Skou** in 1957. It was the first documented instance of active transport. Further, it is readily demonstrated that the sodium pump requires metabolic energy and has the effect on volume regulation inside the cell, for when the cell is poisoned with cyanide, dinitrophenol, or cardiac glycosides such as Quabain and digitalis preparations, water influx takes place and swelling and lysis follows (see **Dyson**, 1978).

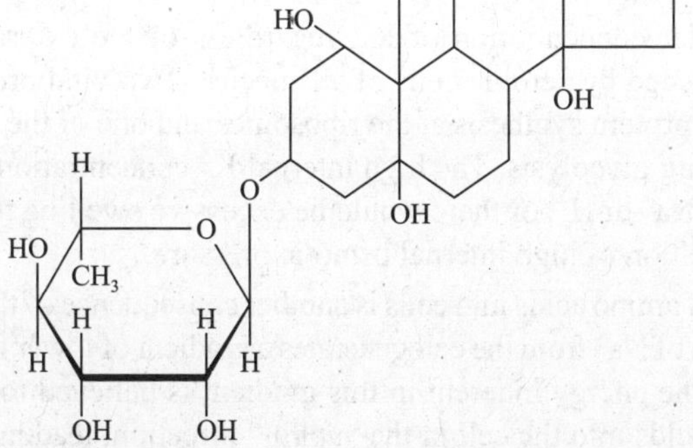

Fig. 6.16. Quabain (Strophanthin G).

Two distinct types of Na^+ pump have been described for animal cells which are as follows:

***(a)* Sodium/potassium exchange pump or coupled neutral pump.** In such a sodium pump, the outward pumping of Na^+ is tightly linked to the inward transport of K^+ ions. Since Na^+ and K^+ are exchanged in a compulsory way, outward movement of Na^+ is always accompanied by inward movement of K^+ (Fig. 6.17). This kind of pump occurs in nerve and muscle cells.

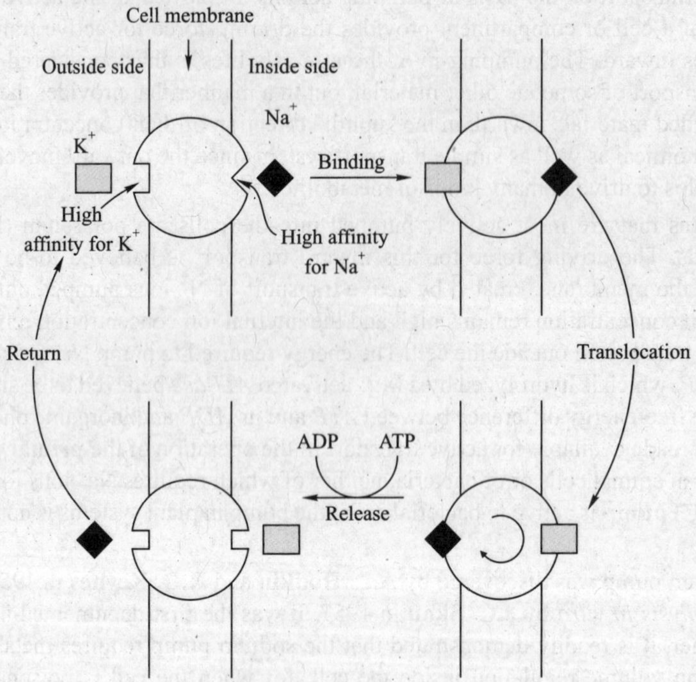

Fig. 6.17. Sodium-potassium exchange pump. Inward transport of K^+ ions is accompanied by compulsory outward transport of Na+ ions via carrier proteins situated within the membrane (after Dyson, 1978).

***(b)* Electrogenic sodium pump or sodium-coupled pump.** Inward transport of K^+ ions does not necessarily accompany outward extrusion of Na^+ in the electrogenic sodium pump. The electrogenic pump has been so named because a gradient of electrochemical potential may be generated when exit of Na^+ is not compensated by one-to-one entry of K^+. In most cells there is an accumulation of K^+ that exceeds the loss of Na^+ (or H^+ in bacteria), which is one of the indications that the electrogenic pump rather than the sodium/potassium exchange pump is operative.

A high intracellular concentration of K^+, regardless of the external concentrations of Na^+ and K^+, is especially needed by aerobic cells of all species. Two vital processes that require a high concentration of K^+ are protein synthesis at the ribosomes and one of the critical enzymatic steps in glucose processing during glycolysis. The high internal K^+ concentration must be balanced by loss of some cation, such as Na^+ or H^+, or there would be excessive swelling that would cause the cell to burst by creating a condition of high internal osmotic pressure.

Active transport of amino acids into cells is another consequence of the action of an electrogenic sodium pump. Extrusion of Na^+ from the cell generates a gradient of lower internal and higher external concentration of Na^+. The energy inherent in this gradient is believed to provide the driving force for transport of amino acids into the cell in the "uphill" direction, leading to accumulation of these essential compounds. The Na^+ gradient itself is formed at the expense of *ATP*. Specific carrier protein systems assist amino acids across the plasma membrane in these active transport events.

The capacity to accumulate sugars, like amino acids, is another feature of the cellular electrogenic sodium pump activity. Both sugar and amino acid active transport are accomplished under conditions in which the outside concentration of Na^+ is kept high enough to create an appropriate gradient whose energy drives metabolites into the cell from very dilute outside solutions of these substances. The accumulation of sugars is, therefore, coupled to Na^+ extrusion, as with amino acids, and is also assisted by specific active-transport (carrier) proteins (Fig. 6.18).

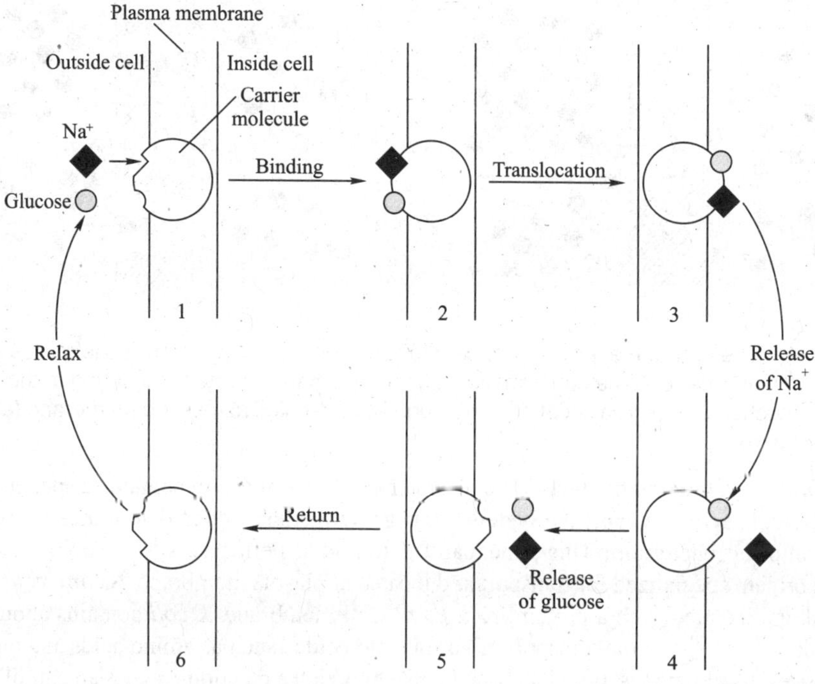

Fig. 6.18. Electrogenic sodium pump. Diagram showing the action of an electrogenic sodium pump through which sugars and other metabolites enter the cell along an electrical gradient generated by the energy-requiring extrusion of Na^+ ions (after Dyson, 1978).

(*c*) Translocation across the membrane. The carrier proteins assist hydrophilic molecules across a membrane thickness of 60 to 100A°. The metabolites are considerably smaller than 60A°, so it is important to know how these molecules are translocated across this relatively large distance by the carriers. Following two mechanisms have been proposed and accepted by many cytologists:

1. Carrier mechanism. This hypothesis postulates that the carrier binds with the hydrophilic molecules and then the entire transport protein rotates across the membrane and delivers its bound metabolite to the other side (Fig. 6.19A).

2. Fixed-pore mechanism. This hypothesis suggests that the carrier is fixed in place within the structure of the membrane and that the carrier molecule undergoes a conformational change that translocates the binding site across the membrane and bound metabolite along with it at the same time (Fig. 6.19B). Once the metabolite has been translocated the binding site is freed and restored to its original conformation, ready to bind another hydrophilic molecule in another transport event.

From the energetic standpoint fixed-pore mechanism expend less cellular energy than carrier mechanism. However, cytologists are still undecided about both of these transport mechanisms.

Lastly, the reasons for wide use of proteins as carriers in many types of membranes are the following: 1. Proteins are the direct products of genes: the production of a protein carrier may require only one gene, whereas establishing a biosynthetic pathway to produce any other kind of carrier might require several enzymes, and, therefore, several genee. 2. Proteins are specific in their capacity to bind other molecules. 3. Protein can alter their binding affinity for substrate. 4. Proteins, as catalysts, also make active transport possible by allowing an obligate coupling between two reactions, *e.g.*, sodium pump. Besides protein carrier, certain non-protein carriers also occur in the plasma membrane (see **Dyson**, 1978).

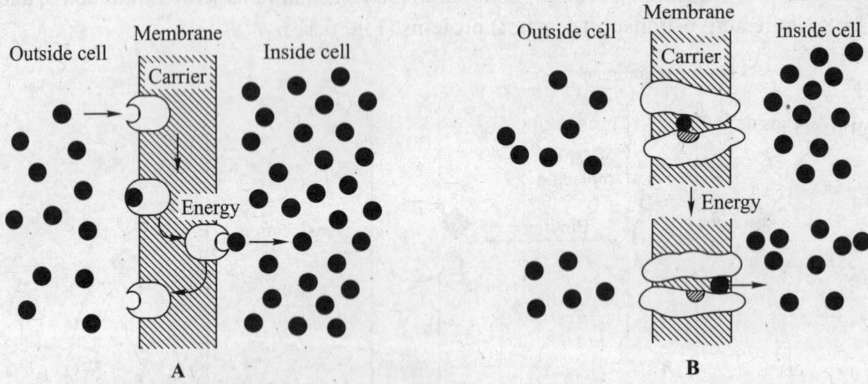

Fig. 6.19. A—The carrier mechanism concept for translocation of hydrophilic molecules across the membrane. B—The conformational change of carrier protein according to the fixed-pore mechanism for translocation of hydrophilic molecules across the membrane (after Avers, 1976).

Permease systems of bacteria. The plasma membrane of *E.coli* contains a specific chemical transport system such as, **permease system** for **β-galactosidase** which determines the penetration of lactose into the bacterium. This genetically determined permease system involves a specific membrane protein specialized for transport and located at plasma membrane. **Kennedy** *et al.* (1966) has labeled and isolated such a protein from *E.coli* cell membrane. *E.coli* contains about 30 to 60 such permease systems for the transport of various molecules such as amino acids and nucleotides. The permeases, like enzymes, only increase the rate at which a reaction reaches an equilibrium. The inner mitochondrial membrane also contains several permease systems (see **De Robertis** *et al.*, 1975).

3. Transport by vesicle formation (Endocytosis and exocytosis). Usually the cells of unicellular or multicellular organisms take their food in the form of solution. For instance, in a multicellular animal the food substances are digested by certain enzymes in the digestive tube, absorbed by and diffuse into the internal body fluids such as blood, lymph and interestitial fluid, in the molecular state. From the internal body fluids, the food which is now in molecular state, penetrates through the plasma membrane by the process of diffusion and active transport. This food is digested partially in the cytoplasm and completely oxidised by the mitochondria.

But some times the plasma membrane participates actively in the ingestion of certain large-sized foreign or food substances. The process by which the foreign substances are taken in and digested by the cell is known as *endocytosis* (Gr., *endon*-within + *kytos*-cell). The endocytosis differs with another process of the cell known as **exocytosis** (Gr., *exo*-outside + *kytos*-cell). In the process of exocytosis the cells which have secretory function such as pancreatic cells pass out their enzymatic secretions outside the cell. According to the nature of food or foreign substances, the endocytosis may be classified into two types, *viz.*, (*i*) **pinocytosis** and (*ii*) **phagocytosis**.

(*i*) Pinocytosis. When the ingestion of fluid material in bulk takes place by the cell through the plasma membrane the process is known as *pinocytosis* (Gr., *pinein*-to drink). The process of pinocytosis was first of all observed by **Edward** in *Amoeba* and by **Lewis** (1931) in the cultured cells.

In the process of pinocytosis, the particle free globules of fluid named as **pinosomes** by **Lewis** (1931) are surrounded and ultimately engulfed by the clasping folds of the cytoplasm. The plasma membrane forms membranous vacuoles around the pinosomes. In later stages the pinosomes are transported to the interior of the cell where they are fused with the lysosomes to form the digestive vacuoles. The digestion of food substances takes place in the food vacuoles and the digested food is diffused into the surrounding cytoplasm.

Micropinocytosis. Electron microscopic observations have been made on the pinocytosis process at subcellular or submicroscopic level in the cells. The pinocytosis which occurs at submicroscopic level is known as **micropinocytosis**. In the process of micropinocytosis the plasma membrane invaginates to form vesicles of 650A° diameter. These vesicles have opening on both outer and inner surface which suggest the possible transportation of fluids through these vesicles to the cell. The micropinocytosis has been observed in endothelial cells, Schawn and satellite cells of nerve ganglion, macrophages, muscle cells and reticular cells, etc.

***(ii)* Phagocytosis.** Sometimes the large-sized solid food or foreign particles are taken in by the cell through the plasma membrane. The process of ingestion of large-sized solid substance by the cell is known as **phagocytosis** (Gr., *phagien*-to eat, *kytos*-cell or hollow vessel). Thus, phagocytosis refers to enclosure of extracellular particles by the plasma membrane and the subsequent internalization of those particles without breaking the continuity of the membrane (**Dyson**, 1978).

Occurrence of phagocytosis. The process of phagocytosis occurs in most protozoans and certain cells of multicellular organisms. In multicellular organisms such as in mammals the phagocytosis occurs very actively in granular leucocytes and in the cells of mesoblastic origin (macrophage, neutrophil, etc.). The cells of the mesoblastic origin are collectively known as the cells of **macrophagic** or **reticuloendothelial system**. The cells of macrophagic system are histocytes of connective tissue, the reticular cells of the hematopoietic organs (bone marrow, lymph nodes and spleen) and the endothelial cells which form the lining of capillary sinusoid of the liver, adrenal gland and hypophysis. The cells of macrophagic system can ingest bacteria, Protozoa, cell debris or even colloidal particles by the process of phagocytosis.

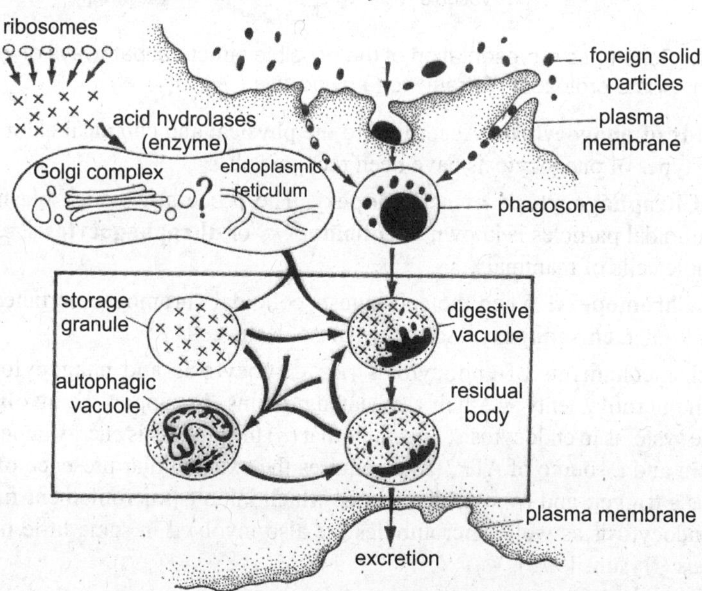

Fig. 6.20. Phagocytosis in the cell (after De Robertis *et al.*, 1970).

Process of phagocytosis. In Protozoa, phagocytosis is intimately linked to amoeboid motion. An amoeba ingests large particles, including micro-organisms, by surrounding them with pseudopodia to form a food vacuole within which the digestion of food takes place. In leucocytes and other phagocytic cells, phagocytosis may be carried out in immobile cells.

During the process of phagocytosis, first the particle **adheres** (is **adsorbed**) to the mass of the protoplasm, and then the particle actually penetrates the cell. This particle subsequently is surrounded by the plasma membrane which ultimately pinches off from the cell surface to form a vesicle or vacuole around the solid particle. The process of vacuole formation can be termed as **vacuolization**. The membrane bounded vesicles or vacuoles are known as **phagosomes**. The phagosomes migrate to the interior of the cell and fuse with the pre-existing lysosomes to form digestive vacuoles. The food is digested by the hydrolytic enzymes (acid hydrolase) of the lysosomes and the digested food is ultimately diffused from the digestive vacuoles to the surrounding cytoplasm. The undigested food is expelled from the plasma membrane by the process of **ephagy** or **egestion**.

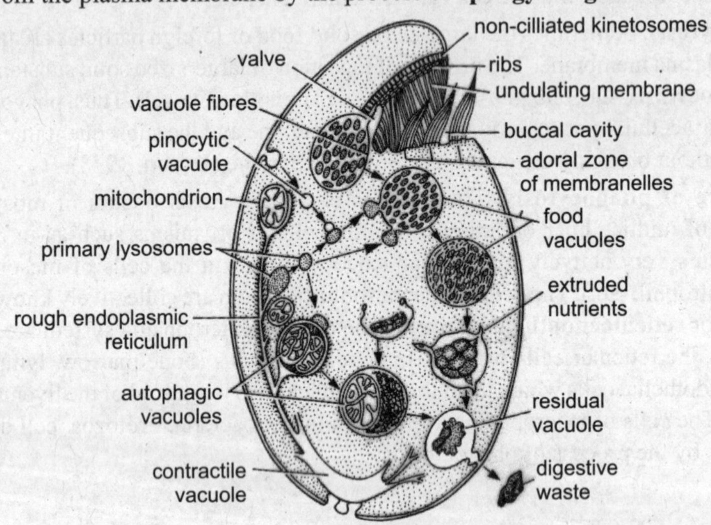

Fig. 6.21. Schematic representation of the possible structural pathways of intracellular digestion in ciliate protozoan *Tetrahymena pyriformis*.

Kinds of phagocytosis. According to the physical and chemical nature of foreign substance following types of phagocytosis have been recognized:

***(i)* Ultraphagocytosis or colloidopexy.** The process in which plasma membrane ingests smaller colloidal particles is known as **colloidopexy** or **ultraphagocytosis**, *e.g.*, leucocytes and the macrophagic cells of mammals.

***(ii)* Chromopexy.** When the cell ingests colloidal chromogen particles phagocytotically the process is known **chromopexy**, *e.g.*, some mesoblastic cells.

Both mechanisms of endocytosis (*i.e.*, pinocytosis and phagocytosis) depend on local changes in microfilaments and their associated proteins. To support the involvement of cytoplasmic contractile systems in endocytosis, one notes that (*a*) the process is energy dependent, requiring active metabolism and a source of ATP; (*b*) it requires the extracellular presence of Ca^{++}, entry of which may act as a trigger; and (*c*) cytochalasin B, which inhibits microfilament function, in many cases inhibits endocytosis as well. Microtubules are also involved in some little understood way during endocytosis (**Dyson**, 1978).

Emeiocytosis or Cell Vomiting

In certain cells as in the cells of pancreas, a process reverse to the endocytosis occurs. In such cells the vacuoles which have secretory products (enzymes) move from the interior of the cytoplasm towards the surface of the cytoplasm. At the surface these vacuoles fuse with the plasma membrane and discharge their stored products to the exterior of the cell. This process is known as **emeiocytosis** or **cell vomiting** or **exocytosis**.

6.6 ORIGIN OF PLASMA MEMBRANE

The problem of origin of plasma membrane is still little understood. Current view of origin of plasma membrane incorporates following two processes:

1. Turnover of membranes. Nothing in the cell is fixed or stable. There is constant movement, and there is constant turnover. The overall structure of the cell may not change visible, but with a molecule removed and replaced here, another removed and replaced there, it is only a matter of days before a typical cell—even a stable, long lived cell such as hepatocyte—is completely renewed. Thus, there is constant synthesis and turnover of all cell components, including the lipids and proteins of plasma membrane and other cellular membranes. The life time of various components differ markedly, however, including vast differences from one membrane protein to another, the destruction of which seems random for protein of a given type.

2. Plasma membrane synthesis. Plasma membrane is either derived directly from endoplasmic reticulum or ER or more commonly from ER via the Golgi apparatus. Most membrane-bound proteins are synthesized on membrane-bound ribosomes (*i.e.*, rough endoplasmic reticulum) and appear to be immediately incorporated into the membrane of the ER. Carbohydrate addition, if required, may occur on the cytoplasmic surface of the ER via transfer of the oligosaccharide chain from a lipid intermediate (a mechanism that appears to be different from the stepwise addition of sugars to secretory proteins that occurs within the cisternae of the ER, see chapter 8). From the site of synthesis there appears to be lateral movement to a segment of smooth-surface ER, taking advantage of the fluid nature of membranes and the multiple inter-connections of endoplasmic reticulum. From this point, however, there is by no means universal agreement among cytologists as to which path is followed.

If a membrane glycoprotein requires the addition of galactose, fucose or sialic acid it presumably must be transferred to the Golgi apparatus, for the enzymes capable of adding those sugars seem to be confined to Golgi cisternae. From there, the finished protein could be transferred to the plasma membrane or back to the endoplasmic reticulum in a Golgi-derived vesicle. A significant fraction of plasma membrane protein appears in some labelling studies to be rapidly transferred to the plasma membrane, possibly by direct transfer of vesicles derived from the endoplasmic reticulum.

Lipid components of membranes, like other lipids, are synthesized largely by enzymes associated with the smooth ER, though the Golgi apparatus is also implicated in some cases. Lipids may be transferred to cellular membranes either via lateral diffusion within ER or through the cytoplasm by way of cytoplasmic vesicles whose formation requires energy. A more rapid movement of lipid and one that requires no metabolic energy is thought to be catalyzed in many cells by specific cytoplasmic proteins. These **lipid exchange proteins** are capable of reversibly binding and releasing specific lipids. They diffuse about the cytoplasm, carrying lipid molecules from one membrane to another. The outer and inner membranes of mitochondria and chloroplasts appear to exchange lipids through lipid-linked proteins.

Further, there exists an extra-cellular lipid exchange method by lipid-linked proteins from cell to cell in mammalian erythrocytes. **Michael Brown** and **Joseph Goldstein** (1976) have established following mechanism in obtaining cholesterol by most mammalian cells outside liver: serum lipoproteins which carry almost all serum cholesterol are found to contribute lipids to membrane composition of mammalian erythrocytes. Cells of higher animals contain specific surface receptors for low density lipoprotein (LDL) of serum. Binding of LDL to receptors is followed by endocytosis and lysosomal digestion that breaks down the protein, freeing cholesterol and phospholipid to be used in membrane synthesis. These mechanisms of lipid-exchange are clearly known only for mammalian cells, however, they are suspected to occur in lower animals, especially in insects.

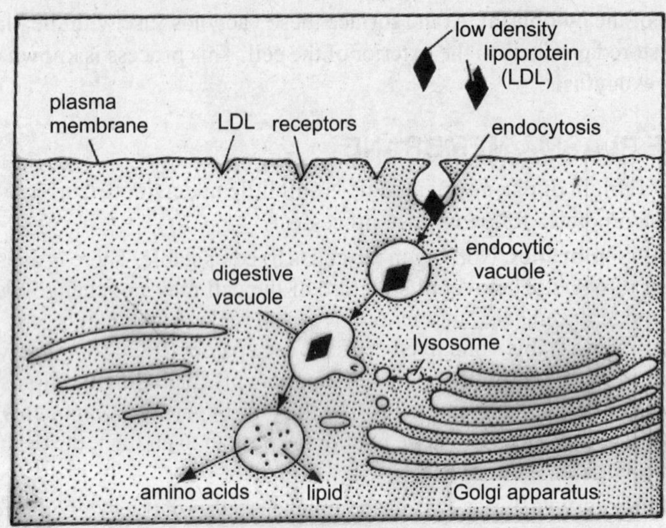

Fig. 6.22. Serum lipoprotein uptake. Cells of mammals get most or all of their cholesterol and much of their phospholipid from lipoproteins made by the liver. Specific receptors for low density lipoprotein (LDL) aid uptake (after Dyson, 1978).

6.7 EXTRANEOUS COATS OF PLASMA MEMBRANE

The plasma membrane of bacterial cells, plant cells and in some animal cells is remain covered by one or more thick protective layers of non-living substances. The outer protective layers around the plasma membrane are known as **extraneous coats**. The extraneous coats are very conspicuous in eggs of marine animals and in Amphibia. In them, a glycoprotein-like substance called **mucin** is the main constituent. Mucins also cover and protect the cell surface lining the gastrointestinal tract. Polysaccharides constitute the **pectin** and cellulose of plant cell walls and the chitin of Crustacea. Protein-lipid, polysaccharide complexes occur in the cell wall of bacteria. The extraneous coats of the cells of animals, plants and bacteria can be studied under separate headings as follows:

6.8 EXTRANEOUS COATS IN ANIMAL CELLS

The extraneous coats of the plasma membrane of animal cells are also known as basement membranes, basal laminae, boundary layer, glycoprotein mantle, external lamina and glycocalyx. Besides above discussed mucin, glycoproteins and polysaccharides, in the form of hyaluronic acid, are found at the base of most epithelial cells, in capillaries and also in many intercellular spaces. **Bennett** (1963) has coined the term **glycocalyx** for the glycoproteins and polysaccharide covering which surrounds many cells. The glycocalyx contains the oligosaccharide side-chains of the glycolipids and glycoproteins which are exposed to the outer surface of the membrane. In the so called greater membrane model (Fig. 6.3) of the plasma membrane both the cell coat and the liporprotein structure, are shown. The cell coat has negatively charged sialic acid termini, both on the glycoproteins and gangliosides, which may bind Ca^{2+} and Na^{+} ions.

Origin of Glycocalyx

The biosynthesis of the glycoproteins forming the glycocalyx takes place in the ribosomes of the endoplasmic reticulum. The final assembly of glycoproteins of glycocalyx with the oligosaccharide moiety is accomplished in the Golgi complex. The cell coat is thus a secretory product of the cell and it undergoes continuous renewal.

Functions of the Glycocalyx

Though glycocalyx is unnecessary for plasma membrane, but even then it performs some of the following significant functions for the cell:

1. Molecular recognition. Certain molecular entities which are used by the cell for specific recognition occur in the cell coat (*i.e.*, glycocalyx). The glycoproteins and glycolipids may possbily represent the molecular sites by which different cell types recognize one another, thus contributing to the formation of cell layers or compact tissues. This recognition also involves the important phenomenon of **contact inhibition** which refers to the *inhibition of cell motility and also of mitotic activity* in normal cells grown in tissue culture at the time they come into contact. It is evident that the function of molecular recognition reaches its maximum expression in the nervous system, where a neuron can make synaptic contact with numerous other neurons, thereby forming specific neuronal circuits of immense complexity. This property of molecular recognition of the cell membrane is dependent on the expression of genes located within the nucleus (**Singer** and **Rothfield**, 1973).

2. Filteration. The extraneous coats sometimes act as filters. For instance, the extraneous coats surrounding the blood capillaries of most vertebrates, especially the kidney glomerulus act as filter and regulate the passage of molecules through it. The extracellular coats of connective tissues contain the chemical compound **hyaluronate** which controls the diffusion.

3. Maintenance of the microenvironment of the cell. The extraneous coats of animal cells can affect the concentrations of different substances at the surface of the cell. For example, a muscle cell with its excitable plasma membrane which is surrounded by a glycocalyx is found to mainain the microenvironment of muscle cell by trapping the sodium ions.

4. Antigenicity. In the erythrocyte plasma membrane and other cell membranes there are specifically determined antigens for the A, B, and O blood groups and others that have been mentioned previously. Among the antigens are those of histocompatibility that permit the recognition of the cells of one organism and the rejection of other cells that are alien to it (*e.g.*, rejection of grafts or transplants from another organism).

6.9 EXTRANEOUS COATS OR CELL WALL OF PLANT CELLS

The extraneous coat of the plasma membrane of plant cells is known as **cell wall**. The cell wall is a rigid and protective layer around the plasma membrane which provides the mechanical support to the cell. The cell wall also determines the shape of plant cells. Due to the shape of cell walls many types of plant cells as the parenchymatous, collenchymatous, etc., have been recognized.

Chemical Nature of Cell Wall

The cell walls of plant cells are composed of carbohydrate known as **cellulose**. Beside the cellulose various chemical substances as **hemicellulose, pectin, liginin, cutin** and **chitin** also occur singly or along with the cellulose. The cell wall also contains certain minerals as Ca and Mg in the form of carbonates and silicates. The cellulose is a polysaccharide and it is most abundantly occurring chemical substance of most plant cell walls. The cellulose chemically consists of long chains of the molecules of glucose. The glucose is the structural unit of the cellulose and about 3000 glucose molecules are linked together to form the chains of cellulose molecules. X-ray diffraction reveals a crystalline pattern in cellulose, with a repeated period of 1.03 nm along the fiber axis. Many chains of cellulose molecules lie parallel to each other to form the bundles. A bundle of 100 chain molecules of cellulose forms the elementary fibril known as the **micelle**. The 20 micelles when get arranged parallely, form the fibrils of 25 nm or 250A° thick, known as **microfibrils**. These microfibrils form large-sized bundles (0.5 μ thick) of cellulose fibers to form the **macrofibrils**. The macrofibrils consisting of many cellulose fibrils form the main frame work of the cell wall. The **hemicellulose** is composed of monosaccharide units such as arabinose, xylose, mammose and galactose. It occurs sometimes in between the macrofibrils of the cellulose. The **pectin** chemically composed of glucuronic and galacturonic acids. The **liginin** chemically composed of coniferyl alcohols. The **cutin** composed of many fatty acids. The **chitin** is a polymer of glucosmine. The staining reactions and chemical constituents of different building blocks of cell walls can be summarized in following Table 6.3:

Table 6.3. Plant cell wall substances.

Substance	Chemical unit	Staining reaction
1. Cellulose	Glucose	Chlorzinc iodide (stains violet)
2. Hemicellulose	Arabinose, xylose, mannose, galactose	None specific
3. Pectin substances	Glucuronic and galactouronic acids	Ruthenium red
4. Lignin	Coniferyl	Phloroglucinol hydrochloride (stains rose)
5. Cuticular substances	Fatty acids	Sudan III (stains orange)
6. Mineral deposits	Calcium and magnesium in the form of carbonates or silic ates.	

Structure of Cell Wall

The Cell wall is complex in nature and remains differentiated in the following layers:

(*i*) Primary cell wall,

(*ii*) Secondary cell wall, and

(*iii*) Tertiary cell wall.

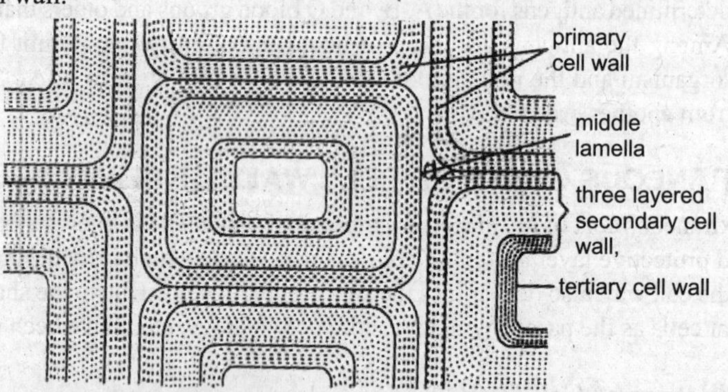

Fig. 6.23. Gross structure of a plant cell wall.

(*i*) Primary cell wall. The first formed cell wall is known as primary cell wall. It is the outer most layer of the cell and it forms the only cell wall in the immature meristamatic and parenchymatous cells. The primary cell wall is comparatively thin and permeable. Primary cell wall is composed mainly of the polysaccharide cellulose, but other substances may be incorporated in it. Lignin or suberin may be added to the primary cell wall and certain epidermal cells of the leaf and the stem also possesses the cutin and cutin waxes which make the primary cell wall impermeable. The primary cell wall of the yeast and the fungi is composed of the chitin.

(*ii*) Secondary cell wall. The primary cell wall is followed by secondary cell wall. The secondary cell wall is thick, permeable and lies near the plasma membrane or the tertiary cell wall, if the later occurs. It is composed of the three concentric layers which occur one after another. Chemically the secondary cell walls composed of compactly arranged macrofibrils of the cellulose in between which sometimes occurs lignin as a interfibrillar material.

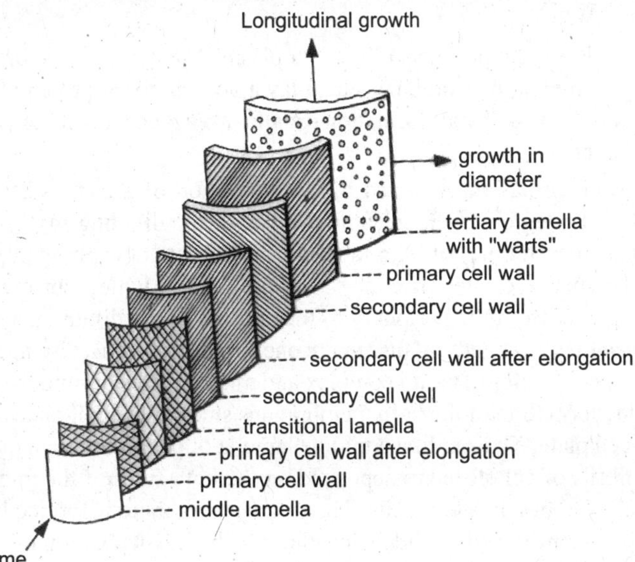

Fig. 6.24. Diagram showing the time sequence of the formation of the various types of cell wall layers in a tracheid of conifer plant. Arrangement of cellulose fibrils have been shown in different cell walls.

(*iii*) Tertiary cell wall. In certain plant cells, there occurs another cell wall beneath the secondary cell wall which is known as tertiary cell wall. The tertiary cell wall differs from the primary and secondary cell walls in its morphology, chemistry and staining properties. Besides the cellulose, the tertiary cell wall consists of another chemical substance known as the xylan.

Middle Lamella

The cells of plant tissues generally remain cemented together by an intercellular matrix known as the **middle lamella**. The middle lamella is mainly composed of the pectin, lignin and some proteins.

Ultrastructure of Cell Wall

Electron microscopic observations of cell walls of plant cell have revealed the fact that each cell wall is composed of two main parts—(*i*) the microfibrils of cellulose which are left if hemicellulose and pectic materials are removed and (*ii*) the ground substance or matrix in which fibrils are embedded. The amount and orientation of microfibrils may vary from cell wall to cell wall. Primary cell wall usually contains microfibrils which run in all planes of the wall and constitutes loose frame work; while secondary wall contains thicker microfibrils which remain parallel and more densely packed.

Plasmodesmata

The cell walls and the middle lamella of plant cells never occur in the form of continuous layers but have many minute apertures through which the cells of a tissue maintain cytoplasmic relations with each other. Such cytoplasmic junctions or bridges between the adjacent cells are known as **plasmodesmata**.

The plasmodesmatas of meristamatic cells have been found to be continuous with the plasmodesmatas of adjacent cells. Through these plasmodesmatas the cytoplasm and the endoplasmic reticulum remain continued to the adjacent cells. Most probably through the plasmodesmatas the intercellular circulation of solutions containing nutritional products, dissolved gases, ions or other substances takes place.

Origin of Cell Wall

The cell walls are the products of the cytoplasm. The cytoplasmic organelles as endoplasmic reticulum, Golgi complex, microtubules etc., play a very important role in the formation of the cell wall. The process of new cell wall formation usually takes place in a dividing cell immediately after the nuclear divisions.

The cell wall formation is started by the formation of a barrel-shaped plasma body called **phragmoplast** in the region of the equatorial plane of the dividing mother cell immediately after karyokinesis. The microtubules of mitotic spindle run through the phragmoplast. The phragmoplast is formed by the small vesicles of endoplasmic reticulum which cut off from the endoplasmic reticulum and migrate from the periphery to the equator of the dividing cell, where, these vesicles called **phragmosomes** arranged and fused with one another to form a discontinuous membranous **cell plate**. The secretory vesicles of Golgi complex and microtubules of mitotic spindle are recently held responsible in the formation of the both membranous sides of the cell plate and the pectic substance in the space of cell plate. Thus, at first a middle lamella of pectin forms in the centre of space of cell plate and then fibrils of cellulose are deposited on the both sides of the middle lamella to form the primary cell walls of both daughter cells. The plasma membrane is formed by the outer membranes of cell plate. The secondry cell wall deyelops later on by the deposition of cellulose, hemicellulose and pectin beneath the primary cell wall.

Growth of Cell Wall

In algae, the growth or expansion of a cell wall is marked by a tearing of the outer material and the addition of new materials on the inner surface. In higher plants, tearing is rare; instead there appear to be a loosening of the fibrils and a reorientation in the direction of elongation. The new fibrils forming on the inner surface become oriented in the same direction. According to **Cohn** (1969) the growth of plant cell wall is regulated by **auxins** or plant hormones.

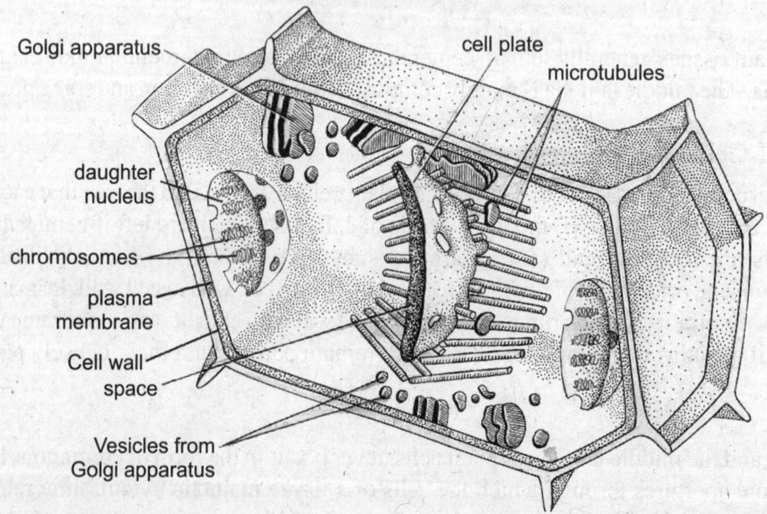

Fig. 6.25. Schematic representation of a cell of a higher plant as seen at telophase in mitosis. In the phragmoplast region, a region of membranes and microtubules, a cell plate forms and grows until it separates the cytoplasm into two daughter cells. The cell plate develops as a membrane- delimited structure enclosing a space in which new cell-wall will form. The Golgi complex contributes many vesicles to the phragmoplast membrane; the vesicle membranes apparently are incorporated into the membrane of the cell plate and the vesicle contents enter the forming cell wall (after Novikoff and Holtzman, 1970).

Lignification. The structure of cell wall is stabilized by the deposition of lignin in the cell wall matrix. Such a process of lignification was required in connection with the transition from aquatic to the terrestial plant life during organic evolution of plants. A lignified cell wall is composed of microfibrils of cellulose embedded in the matrix containing large amount of lignin. Usually the primary cell wall becomes more lignified than secondary cell wall.

Functions of Cell Wall

The chief function of cell wall in plant cells is that it provides mechanical strength to the latter. Like the exoskeleton or endoskeleton of animals, cell wall acts like a skeletal framework of plants. Particularly in vascular plants, the cell walls provide the main supporting framework.

6.10 BACTERIAL CELL WALL

The cell wall of a Gram-positive bacteria (*e.g., Bacillus subtilis*) is 150–200A° thick and appears to be attached to the plasma membrane along its entire length. While in Gram-negative bacteria (*e.g., E.coli*), the cell wall is thinner, 75–120A° and only makes intermittent contact with the plasma membrane. Bacterial cell walls are much more complex structures than the cellulose walls of plants. They contain a macromolecular compound that composed of two simple sugars and three or four amino acids. These molecules form the basal structure or **mucocomplex** which confers structural rigidity on the wall and is unique to bacterial cells. The two sugars are **N-acetylglucosamine** and **N-acetylmuramic acid**. The saccharide part of the wall consists of alternating units of these two amino sugars joined by glycosidic linkages. The amino acids are glutamic acid, alanine, glycine, and lysine or diaminopimelic acid. These few amino acids form short peptide chains which attach to the polysaccharide chains and cross-link to one another. Thus, a three-dimensional network of considerable toughness and mechanical strength is formed.

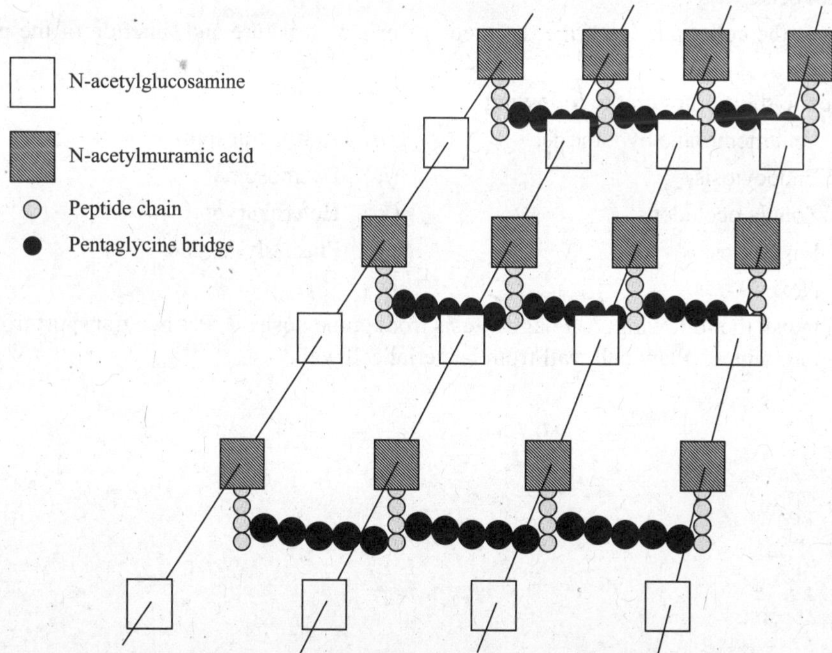

Fig. 6.26. Structure of the bacterial cell wall mucocomplex. The polysaccharide chains run from south-west to north-east. Attached to them are peptide chains linked to one another by pentaglycine bridges (after Ambrose and Easty, 1970).

Most Gram-positive bacteria are composed of large amounts of mucocomplex which is the only macromolecular constituent of their cell walls, but, in certain Gram-positive bacteria there are also simple polysaccharides and teichoic acids, which are polymers of glucose, alanine, and glycerol or ribitol (a five-carbon alcohol). In Gram-negative bacterial walls much less mucocomplex is present and there occur no teichoic acid. Tnere are, however, large amounts of lipid (20 to 30 per cent), proteins and polysaccharides. Electron microscopy indicates that there may be several different layers in Gram-negative walls, and *E.coli* has an outer layer of lipoprotein polysaccharide complex. Most bacterial cell walls contain antigenic specificity. Little is known about how bacterial walls increase in length, girth, and mass (see **Ambrose** and **Easty**, 1970).

Functions of Bacterial Cell Wall

The bacterial cell wall appears to be purely protective and mechanical, it plays no apparent part in permeability or in metabolism. The bacterial cell wall is also responsible for the characteristic shape of bacteria.

REVISION QUESTIONS

1. What is the nature of a biological membrane? Why do you think membranes are so important to all cells?
2. Describe the chemical composition of the plasma membrane.
3. What is meant by a "lipid bilayer"? Describe the fluid mosaic model and some of the more important observations that led to it.
4. Discuss in detail various functions of the plasma membrane.
5. What are the extraneous coats of the plasma membrane? Describe the extraneous coats of animal cells.
6. What is the cell wall? Describe the mode of origin, structure and function of the plant cell wall.
7. Write the short notes on the following:
   - (*i*) Unit membrane hypothesis;
   - (*ii*) Active transport;
   - (*iii*) Endocytosis;
   - (*iv*) Desmosome;
   - (*v*) Zonula occludens;
   - (*vi*) Heterokaryon;
   - (*vii*) Ion pumps;
   - (*viii*) Plasmolysis; and
   - (*ix*) Nexus.
8. Distinguish the following: A. Phagocytosis from pinocytosis; B. Passive transport from active transport; and, C. Plant cell wall from bacterial cell wall.

7 Chapter CYTOPLASMIC VACUOLAR SYSTEM

Through the cytologic evolution the cytoplasm of cell have been pervaded by numerous intracellular membranes which have subdivided it into numerous compartments and subcompartments. The membrane system forms a vast net-work of open cavities which subdivided the cytoplasm into two main compartments; one enclosed within the membrane; the other situated outside (the cytoplasmic matrix). The spaces which are enclosed by the intracellular membranes are known as vacuoles and these vacuoles often remain inter-communicated. This intracellular vacuolar and membrane bounded organization have been named as **cytoplasmic vacuolar system** by **Robertis**, **Nowinski** and **Saez** (1970) and **De Robertis** *et al.* (1975).

The cytoplasmic vacuolar system was observed first in cultured fibroblast cells by **Porter** in 1945. The vacuolar system of various animal and plant cells have been studied by various workers such as **Palade** (1956), **Sjostrand** (1956), **Haguenau** (1956), and **Porter** (1961).

The vacuolar system remains absent in bacteria, erythrocytes, eggs and undifferentiated embryonic cells. It becomes more and more developed with the differentiation of the cell. In the well differentiated animal and plant cells, the cytoplasmic vacuolar system usually has two types of membranes: agranular (*i.e.*, without ribosomes) and granular (*i.e.*, with attached ribosomes). The cytoplasmic vacuolar system is polymorphic and it includes following organelles: (1) Endoplasmic reticulum, (2) Golgi complex, (3) Nuclear envelope, (4) Vacuoles (*e.g.*, contractile vacuoles of the ciliate protozoan, *Paramecium* and vacuoles of other animal and plant cells) and (5) Vesicular components of the centrosphere. The different components of the cytoplasmic vacuolar system will be studied in more details in the forthcoming chapters.

Consequently, a cell can no longer be considered as a bag containing enzymes, ribonucleic acid (RNA), deoxyribonucleic acid (DNA), and solute surrounded by an outer membrane, as in the most primitive bacterium. Numerous membrane-bound compartments are responsible for vital cellular functions, among which are the separation and association of enzyme systems, the creation of diffusion barrier, the regulation of membrane potentials, ionic gradients, and different intracellular pH values, and other manifestations of cellular hydrogeneity. Furthermore, there is evidence that enzymes are spatially organized, forming multienzyme systems within the insoluble membranous framework of the cell.

7.1 FUNCTIONS OF CYTOPLASMIC VACUOLAR SYSTEM

The cytoplasmic vacuolar system performs following various vital functions of the cells:

1. **Mechanical support.** By dividing tbe fluid contents of the cell into compartments, the vacuolar system provides supplementary mechanical support for the colloidal structure of the cytoplasm.
2. **Exchange.** The membranes of the vacuolar system regulate the exchange between the compartments and the cytoplasmic matrix. Osmosis, diffusion and active transport may occur across the membranes of vacuolar system, as in the plasma membrane.

3. **Circulation.** The cytoplasmic vacuolar system act as a intracellular circulatory system and it circulates variety of substances inside and outside of cell. The flow of substances in the vacuolar system is supposed to be performed by its membranes.
4. **Synthesis and metabolism.** The membranes of vacuolar system have been found rich in variety of enzymes. Its membrane segregate the enzyme systems from the cytoplasm and keep them in it. The enzymes are used in the metabolism of steroids and phospholipids. Moreover, a variety of products such as glycogen, lipids, steroids, etc., are synthesized in the vacuolar system. Further, the proteins for export such as tropocollagen, etc., are secreted by the ribosomes of granular membranes of the vacuolar system.
5. **Storage.** The most important function of the cytoplasmic vacuolar system is the storage of its synthetic products. The vacuolar system in animal cells store the glycogen, enzymatic and structural proteins, etc. In plant cells the vacuoles of vacuolar system contain water, phenol, flavonols, anthocyanins, alkaloids, fats, sugars and proteins.
6. **Osmoregulation.** The vacuolar system in certain unicellular organisms such as *Paramecium* performs the function of regulation of internal osmotic pressure or osmoregulation of the cell.

REVISION QUESTIONS

1. What do you meant by cytoplasmic vacuolar system?
2. Describe various functions of the cytoplasmic vacuolar system.

8

Chapter ENDOPLASMIC RETICULUM (ER)

The cytoplasmic matrix is traversed by a complex network of inter-connecting membrane bound vacuoles or cavities. These vacuoles or cavities often remain concentrated in the endoplasmic portion of the cytoplasm; therefore, known as **endoplasmic reticulum**, a name derived from the fact that in the light microscope it looks like a "net in the cytoplasm." (Eighteenth-century European ladies carried purses of netting called **reticules**).

The name "endoplasmic reticulum" was coined in 1953 by **Porter**, who in 1945 had observed it in electron micrographs of liver cells. **Fawcett** and **Ito** (1958), **Thiery** (1958) and **Rose** and **Pomerat** (1960) have made various important contributions on the endoplasmic reticulum.

8.1 OCCURRENCE

The occurrence of the endoplasmic reticulum varies from cell to cell. The erythrocytes (RBC), egg and embryonic cells lack in endoplasmic reticulum. The spermatocytes have poorly developed endoplasmic reticulum. The adipose tissues, brown fat cells and adrenocortical cells of opossum's testis contain only smooth or agranular type of endoplasmic reticulum (**Christensen**, 1960). The cells of those organs which are actively engaged in the synthesis of proteins, as the pancreas and other endocrine glands are found to contain highly developed endoplasmic reticulum and most endoplasmic reticulum is of granular type. The liver cells possess both types of endoplasmic reticulum.

8.2 MORPHOLOGY

Morphologically, the endoplasmic reticulum may occur in the following three forms: 1. Lamellar form or cisternae (A closed, fluid-filled sac, vesicle or cavity is called **cisternae**); 2. Vesicular form or vesicle and 3. Tubular form or tubules.

1. Cisternae. The cisternae are long, flattened, sac-like, unbranched tubules having the diameter of 40 to 50 μm. They remain arranged parallely in bundles or stakes. RER usually exists as cisternae which occur in those cells which have synthetic roles as the cells of pancreas, notochord and brain.

2. Vesicles. The vesicles are oval, membrane-bound vacuolar structures having the diameter of 25 to 500 μm. They often remain isolated in the cytoplasm and occur in most cells but especially abundant in the SER.

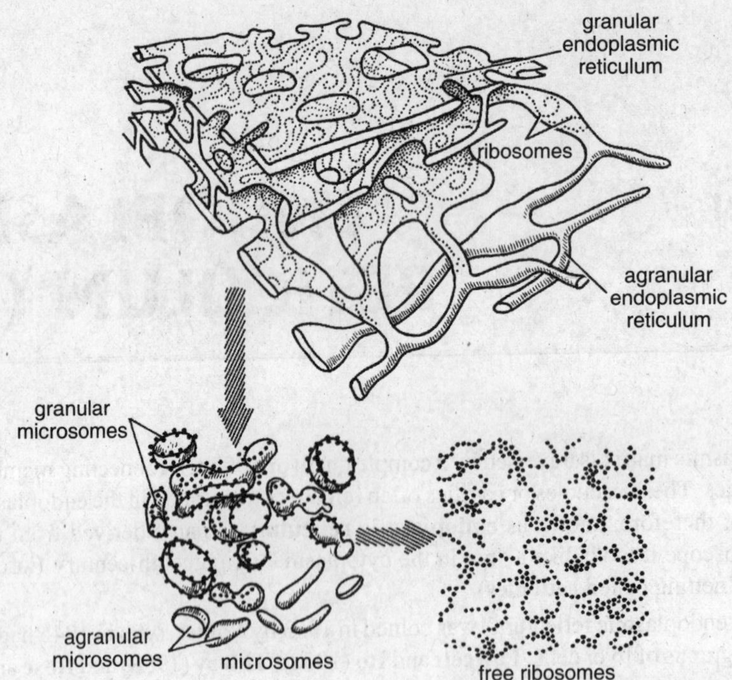

Fig. 8.1. Three dimensional structure of endoplasmic reticulum showing microsomes and ribosomes (after De Robertis *et al.*, 1970).

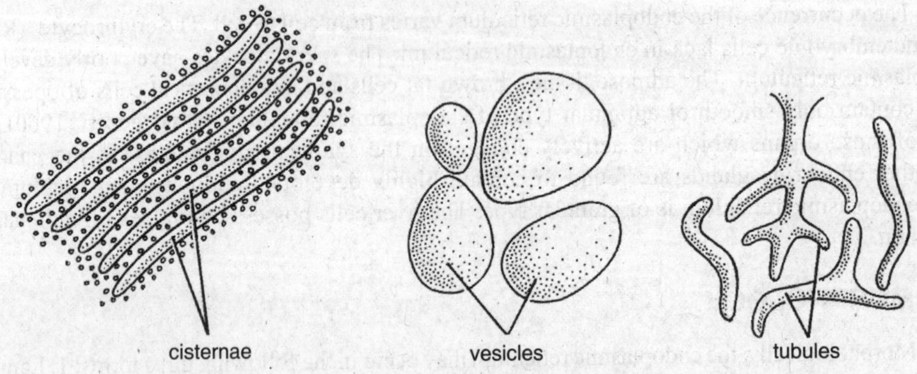

Fig. 8.2. Various components of the endoplasmic reticulum.

3. Tubules. The tubules are branched structures forming the reticular system along with the cisternae and vesicles. They usually have the diameter from 50 to 190 μm and occur almost in all the cells. Tubular form of ER is often found in SER and is dynamic in nature, *i.e.*, it is associated with membrane movements, fission and fusion between membranes of cytocavity network.

Ultrastructure

The cavities of cisternae, vesicles and tubules of the endoplasmic reticulum are bounded by a thin membrane of 50 to 60 Å thickness. The membrane of endoplasmic reticulum is fluid-mosaic like the unit membrane of the plasma membrane, nucleus, Golgi apparatus, etc. The membrane, thus, is composed of a bimolecular layer of phospholipids in which 'float' proteins of various sorts. The membrane of endoplasmic reticulum remains continuous with the membranes of plasma membrane, nuclear membrane and Golgi apparatus. The cavity of the endoplasmic reticulum is well developed and acts as a passage for the secretory products. **Palade** (1956) has observed secretory granules in the cavity of endoplasmic reticulum.

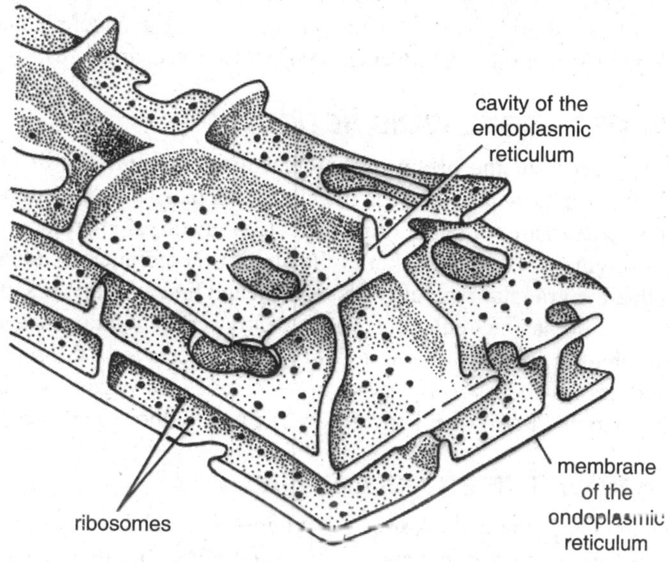

Fig. 8.3. Three dimensional structure of granular endoplasmic reticulum.

8.3 TYPES OF ENDOPLASMIC RETICULUM

Two types of endoplasmic reticulum have been observed in same or different types of cells which are as follows:

1. Agranular or Smooth Endoplasmic Reticulum

This type of endoplasmic reticulum possesses smooth walls because the ribosomes are not attached with its membranes. The smooth type of endoplasmic reticulum occurs mostly in those cells, which are involved in the metabolism of lipids (including steroids) and glycogen. The smooth endoplasmic reticulum is generally found in adipose cells, interstitial cells, glycogen storing cells of the liver, conduction fibres of heart, spermatocytes and leucocytes. The muscle cells are also rich in smooth type of endoplasmic reticulum and here it is known as **sarcoplasmic reticulum**. In the pigmented retinal cells it exists in the form of tightly packed vesicles and tubes known as **myeloid bodies**.

2. Granular or Rough Endoplasmic Reticulum

The granular or rough type of endoplasmic reticulum possesses rough walls because the ribosomes remain attached with its membranes. Ribosomes play a vital role in the process of protein synthesis. The granular or rough type of endoplasmic reticulum is found abundantly in those cells which are active in protein synthesis such as pancreatic cells, plasma cells, goblet cells, and liver cells. The granular type of endoplasmic reticulum takes basiophilic stain due to its RNA contents of ribosomes. The region of the matrix containing granular type of endoplasmic reticulum takes basiophilic stain and is named as **ergastoplasm, basiophilic bodies, chromophilic substances** or **Nissl bodies** by early cytologists.

3. Annulate Lamellae

Usually the endoplasmic reticulum has no pores or annuli in it but in certain cases the pores or annuli have been reported, *e.g.*, ER of invertebrates, ovocytes and spermatocytes of the vertebrates. These annuli resemble with the pores or annuli of the nuclear membranes. Like the annuli of nuclear membranes it contains a diaphragm across it and possesses an octagonal symmetry. The annulate lamellae (pores) of the ER arise by the evagination from the nuclear envelope and have their association with the ribosomes (**Merriam**, 1959; **Kessel**, 1963) (also see chapter 18).

8.4 ORIGIN OF ENDOPLASMIC RETICULUM

The exact process of the origin of endoplasmic reticulum is still unknown. But because membranes of ER resemble with the nuclear membrane and plasma membrane and also at the telophase stage the ER membranes are found to form the nuclear envelope. Therefore, it is normally assumed that the ER has originated by evagination of the nuclear membranes. **Seikevitz** and **Palade** (1960) have reported that the granular type of ER has originated first and later it synthesizes the agranular or smooth type of endoplasmic reticulum. Very recently certain worker such as **Leskes** *et al.* (1971) and **Eytan** and **Ohad** (1972) have suggested that one cell receives a full set of membranes from its ancestor cell and there is no *de novo* synthesis of membranes, they grow by expansion of pre-existing membranes. For details of turn-over and synthesis of membrane see chapter 6, plasma membrane.

8.5 ENZYMES OF THE ER MEMBRANES

The membranes of the endoplasmic reticulum are found to contain many kinds of enzymes which are needed for various important synthetic activities. The most important enzymes are the stearases, NADH-cytochrome C reductase, NADH diaphorase gluoose-6-phosphotase and-Mg^{++} activated ATPase. Certain enzymes of the endoplasmic reticulum such as nucleotide diphosphate are involved in the biosynthesis of phospholipid, ascorbic acid, glucuronide, steroids and hexose metabolism. The enzymes of the endoplasmic reticulum perform the following important functions:

1. Synthesis of glycerides, *e.g.*, triglycerides, phospholipids, glycolipids and plasmologens.
2. Metabolism of plasmologens.
3. Synthesis of fatty acids.
4. Biosynthesis of the steroids, *e.g.*, cholesterol biosynthesis, steroid hydrogenation of unsaturated bonds.
5. $NADPH_2 + O_2$—requiring steroid transformations: Aromatization and hydroxylation.
6. $NADPH_2 + O_2$—requiring steroid transformations: Aromatic hydroxylations side-chain oxidation, deamination, thio-ether oxidations, desulphuration.
7. L-ascorbic acid synthesis.
8. UDP-uronic acid metabolism.
9. UDP-glucose dephosphorylation.
10. Aryl-and steroid sulphates.

8.6 FUNCTIONS OF ENDOPLASMIC RETICULUM

The endoplasmic reticulum acts as secretory, storage, circulatory and nervous system for the cell. It performs following important functions:

A. Common Functions of Granular and Agranular Endoplasmic Reticulum

1. The endoplasmic reticulum provides an ultrastructural skeletal framework to the cell and gives mechanical support to the colloidal cytoplasmic martix.

2. The exchange of molecules by the process of osmosis, diffusion and active transport occurs through the membranes of endoplasmic reticulum. Like plasma membrane, the ER membrane has permeases and carriers.
3. The endoplasmic membranes contain many enzymes which perform various synthetic and metabolic activities. Further the endoplasmic reticulum provides increased surface for various enzymatic reactions.
4. The endoplasmic reticulum acts as an intracellular circulatory or transporting system. Various secretory products of granular endoplasmic reticulum are transported to various organelles as follows: Granular ER → agranular ER → Golgi membrane → lysosomes, transport vesicles or secretory granules. Membrane flow may also be an important mechanism for carrying particles, molecules and ions into and out of the cells. Export of RNA and nucleoproteins from nucleus to cytoplasm may also occur by this type of flow.
5. The ER membranes are found to conduct intra-cellular impulses. For example, the sarcoplasmic reticulum transmits impulses from the surface membrane into the deep region of the muscle fibres.
6. The ER membranes form the new nuclear envelope after each nuclear division.
7. The sarcoplasmic reticulum plays a role in releasing calcium when the muscle is stimulated and actively transporting calcium back into the sarcoplasmic reticulum when the stimulation stops and the muscle must be relaxed.

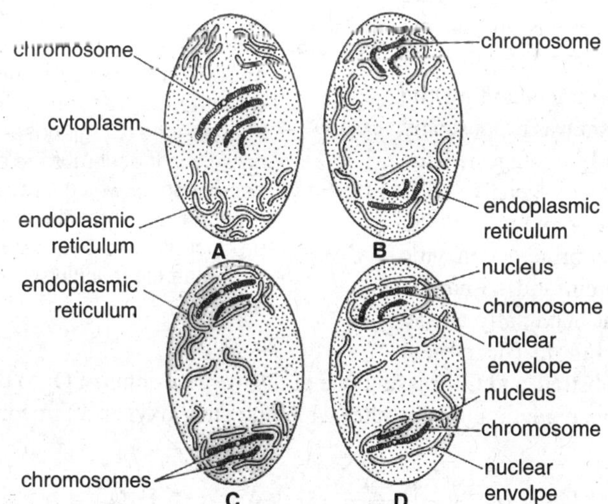

Fig. 8.4. Formation of nuclear envelope by the endoplasmic reticulum.

B. Functions of Smooth Endoplasmic Reticulum

The agranular or smooth type of endoplasmic reticulum synthesizes and stores various substances.

1. Synthesis of lipids. The cells in which active lipid metabolism takes place are found to contain large amount of the smooth type of endoplasmic reticulum. According to some workers such as **Christensen** (1961) and **Claude** (1968) the smooth type of endoplasmic reticulum is related with the synthesis and metabolism of the lipids and lipoproteins.

2. Glycogenolysis. The synthesis of glycogen is accomplished in the cytoplasmic matrix, but the smooth endoplasmic reticulum is involved in the glycogenolysis (break down of glycogen) through the action of glucose-6-phosphatase. Glycogenolysis by smooth ER occurs only in the cells of fasted animals.

3. Detoxification. Smooth ER plays an important role in detoxification in the liver. **Detoxification** involves those biochemical reactions by which harmful materials such as drugs like phenolorbitol, asparin (acetyl-salicylic acid), and pollutants are converted to harmless substances suitable for excretion by the cell. The reaction that detoxify substances consist of oxidations, reductions, hydrolyses, or a covalent linking (conjugation) to soluble small moleules, particularly conjugation to glucuronic acid, a sugar derivative. These changes either inactivate the substance or make it more soluble and hence more readily eliminated by the kidneys. These detoxification reactions of SER also handle various metabolic waste products like fatty acids, bile salts, steroids and haeme recovered from haemoglobin breakdown.

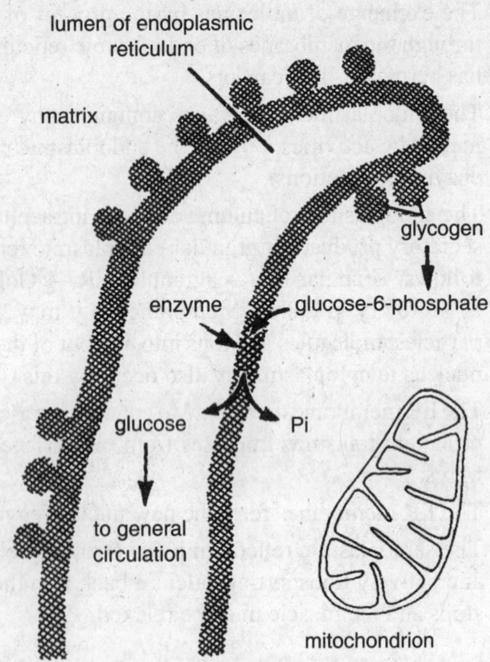

Fig. 8.5. Diagram of the intervention of the smooth endoplasmic reticulum in glycogenolysis with the consequent release of glucose. The enzyme (E), glucose-6-phosphatase, is present in the membrane and has a vectorial deposition by which it receives the glucose-6-phosphate from the matrix surface. The product-glucose-penetrates the lumen of the endoplasmic reticulum (after De Robertis *et al.*, 1975).

The first key to understanding the detoxification mechanism was proposed by **Howard S. Mason** and he suggested the involvement of molecular oxygen, NADPH and P 450 cytochrome enzyme in it. P 450 cytochrome enzyme is a principal enzyme which is a haeme protein and so named because it absorbs light maximally at 450 nm when in the reduced form. This protein is capable of binding substrate and O_2, passing one of the oxygen atoms of O_2 to the substrate in the form of an OH group (an oxidation of substrate) while the other oxygen atom combines with H^+ to form water:

$$S + P\,450\,(Fe^{3+}) \xrightarrow{02\,+\,2e^-} S - P\,450\,(Fe^{2+}) - O_2^-$$

$$\downarrow 2H^+$$

$$P\,450\,(Fe^{3+}) + S - OH + H_2O$$

Here, S is the substrate and Fe^{2+} the haeme-associated iron of P 450. The electrons are delivered to P 450 mostly from NADPH by smooth ER—associated electron transport chain involving flavoproteins and in some cases another cytochrome known as cytochrome b5. Cytochrome P 450 and other elements of the **microsomal electron chain** seem to be membrane bound proteins present mostly on the cytoplasmic surface of the smooth endoplasmic reticulum (**Dyson**, 1978).

4. Other synthetic functions. Smooth ER also plays a role in lipid and cholesterol metabolism in the liver; the secretion of chloride ions in the hydrochloric acid-secreting cells of the stomach lining; the synthesis of triglyceride in intestinal absorptive cells; and synthesis and secretion of steroid hormones by mammalian gonads and the adrenal gland (*i.e.*, adrenal cortex). Smooth ER of pigmented epithelial cells of the retina synthesizes certain visual pigments from vitamin A. In plant cells the smooth ER develop the surface where the cellulose walls are being formed.

C. Functions of Rough Endoplasmic Reticulum

The major function of the rough ER is the synthesis of protein. It has long been assumed that proteins destined for secretion (*i.e.*, export) from the cell or proteins to be used in the synthesis of cellular membranes are synthesized on rough ER-bound ribosomes, while cytoplasmic proteins are translated for the most part on free ribosomes. In fact, the array of the rough endoplasmic reticulum provides extensive surface area for the association of metabolically active enzymes, amino acids and ribosomes. There is more efficient functioning of these materials to synthesize proteins when oriented on a membrane surface than when they are simply in solution, mainly because chemical combinations between molecules can be accomplished in specific geometric patterns. Details of mechanism of protein synthesis will be discussed in chapter 24, "Biosynthesis of proteins", here, only specific involvement of RER into the synthesis and transportation of proteins will be discussed, as follows:

The membrane-bound ribosomes are attached with **specific binding sites** or **receptors** of rough ER membrane by their large 60S subunit, with small or 40S subunit sitting on top like a cap. These receptors are membrane proteins which extend well into and possibly through the lipid bilayer. The receptor proteins with bound ribosomes can float laterally like other membrane proteins and may facilitate formation of the polysome and probably translation which requires that the mRNA and ribosome move with respect to each other.

Likewise, membrane of rough ER appears to ensure translation of mRNA coding for secretory proteins according to following two recently discovered methods: 1. **David Sabatini** *et al.* (1975) have found that mRNA molecules coding for secretory proteins remain attached with rough ER membrane even after the removal of the ribosomes from the latter. They have suggested that 3′-end of such a mRNA may contain a coded sequence that binds specifically to rough ER or more likely to protein receptors within the rough ER. 2. **Gunter Blobel** *et al.* (1975) have reported an affinity between the nascent (incomplete) polypeptide chain of secretory protein and membrane of rough ER. They have suggested the occurrence of a segment of amino acids at the N-terminus of nascent polypeptide which being hydrophobic has strong affinity for RER membrane and which is later cleaved off from the chain by certain enzymes of rough ER.

Further, the secretory proteins, instead of passing into the cytoplasm, appears to pass instead into the cisternae of the rough ER and are thus protected from protease enzymes of cytoplasm. The passage of nascent polypeptide chain into the ER cisterna takes place during translation leaving only a small segment exposed to the cytoplasm at any one time.

How the polypeptide chain gets through the lipid bilayer is not so clear, but it is quite reasonable to propose that the membrane, proteins serving as ribosomal receptors also has a very fine channel through its core that opens into the cisterna of the rough ER. The chain may have great flexibility, permitting the amino acids to snake their way single file through the proposed pore. As soon as growing polypeptide chain reaches the cisterna, it folds into its secondary and tertiary structures and are thus trapped in the cisterna of the rough ER.

Glycosylation of secretory proteins. Nearly all proteins for secretion are glycoproteins (a notable exception is albumin). Glycosylation—that is, the addition of carbohydrate—begins even before the polypeptide chain is completed. The sugar molecules appear to be added one at a time, transferred usually from the nucleotide UDP, which serves as a carrier. Glycosylation is ordinarily still in progress when the polypeptide chain is completed and released into the cisterna of the rough ER. However, if the glycoprotein is to contain a terminal glucose, fucose or sialic acid, those sugars are added in the Golgi complex where the appropriate sugar transferases are localized.

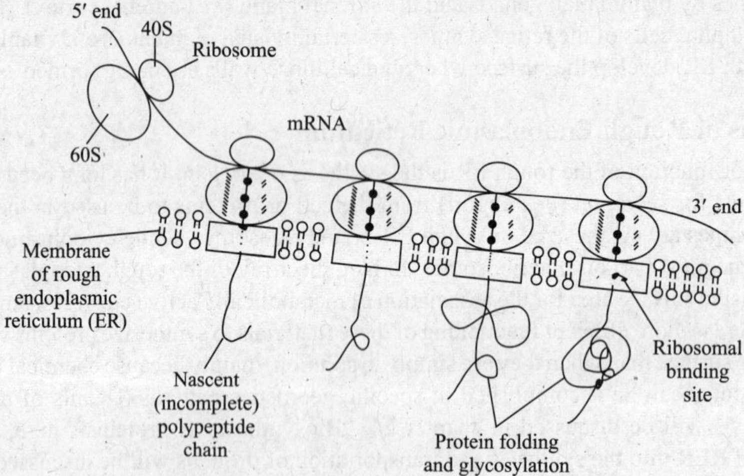

Fig. 8.6. Synthesis of secretory proteins on rough endoplasmic reticulum (after Dyson, 1978).

Recently, it has been reported that membrane proteins are glycosylated by a second entirely different method. In this method of glycosylation, the sugar chains are assembled in a stepwise manner from nucleotide sugars, but the assembly is not on the protein itself. Rather, it is on a lipid, either **retinol** (vitamin A) or one of a family of lipids called **dolichols**. Later on, the sugar chain is transferred intact to the protein. Thus, the oligosaccharide is transferred to protein intact from a lipid carrier (*e.g.*, dolichols) on which it was assembled. Such a lipid-linked glycosylation of membrane protein takes place on the cytoplasmic side of the membranes, rather than in the cisternae of rough ER. Although membrane proteins seem to be synthesized largely on membrane-bound ribosomes (one reason for the presence of rough ER in non-secretory cells), one can imagine that their hydrophobic nature causes them to become incorporated into the membranes of the endoplasmic reticulum rather than confined to the cisternae within. Transfer from lipid-carrier might then take place at the surface of the ER, which would also explain how membrane proteins come to be glycosylated in such an asymmetric way, *i.e.*, on only one side.

Lastly, from the rough ER, secreted proteins pass sequentially to smooth ER, Golgi complex, secretion vesicles and finally to the exterior of the cell. The membrane proteins follow similar path but they omit the formation of secretory vesicles.

REVISION QUESTIONS

1. What is endoplasmic reticulum? Describe the types, structure and functions of the endoplasmic reticulum.
2. What functions seem relegated mostly to smooth endoplasmic reticulum?
3. Proteins destined for secretion are translated primarily by the rough endoplasmic reticulum instead of by free ribosomes. What factors probably account for this selectivity?
4. If a polypeptide chain passes readily into the cisterna of the rough endoplasmic reticulum during synthesis, why does not it later leak out through the same passageway?
5. Describe the two systems of glycosylation for the proteins.

9 Chapter GOLGI APPARATUS (COMPLEX)

For the performance of certain important cellular functions such as biosynthesis of polysaccharides, packaging (compartmentalizing) of cellular synthetic products (proteins), production of exocytotic (secretory) vesicles and differentiation of cellular membranes, there occurs a complex organelle called **Golgi complex** or **Golgi apparatus** in the cytoplasm of animal and plant cells. The Golgi apparatus, like the endoplasmic reticulum, is a canalicular system with sacs, but unlike the endoplasmic reticulum it has parallely arranged, flattened, membrane-bounded vesicles which lack ribosomes and stainable by osmium tetraoxide and silver salts. It was by these staining reactions that **Camillo Golgi** (1898) first of all recognised it in the nerve cells of the barn owl and the cat, long before the discovery of endoplasmic reticulum. After the name of its discoverer Golgi apparatus was variously named as **Golgiosome**, **Golgi bodies**, **Golgi material**, **Golgi membrane**, etc. The Golgi apparatus of the cells of plants and lower invertebrates is usually referred as **Golgi body** or **dictyosome**.

9.1 OCCURRENCE

The Golgi apparatus occurs in all cells except the prokaryotic cells (*viz.*, mycoplasmas, bacteria and blue green algae) and eukaryotic cells of certain fungi, sperm cells of bryophytes and pteridiophytes, cells of mature sieve tubes of plants and mature sperm and red blood cells of animals. Their number per plant cell can vary from several hundred as in tissues of corn root and algal rhizoids (*i.e.*, more than 25,000 in algal rhizoids, Sievers, 1965), to a single organelle in some algae. In animal cells, there usually occurs a single Golgi apparatus, however, developing oocytes of chordates may contain many Golgi bodies.

9.2 DISTRIBUTION

In the cells of higher plants, the Golgi bodies or dictyosomes are usually found scattered throughout the cytoplasm and their distribution does not seem to be ordered or localized in any particular manner. However, in animal cells the Golgi apparatus is a localized organelle. For example, in the cells of ectodermal or endodermal origin, the Golgi apparatus remains polar and occurs in between the nucleus and the periphery (*e.g.*, thyroid cells, exocrine pancreatic cells and mucus producing goblet cells of intestinal epithelium) and in the nerve cells it occupies a circum-nuclear position.

9.3 MORPHOLOGY

The Golgi bodies of plant cells are about 1–3 μm in length and about 0.5 μm high. The Golgi bodies of plant cells and Golgi apparatus of animal cells basically have a similar morphology. Each type of organelle is disc-shaped and consists of central, flattened, plate-like compartments or **cisternae** (or **saccules** peripheral network of interconnecting **tubules**, and peripherally occurring **vesicles** and **Golgian vacuoles**.

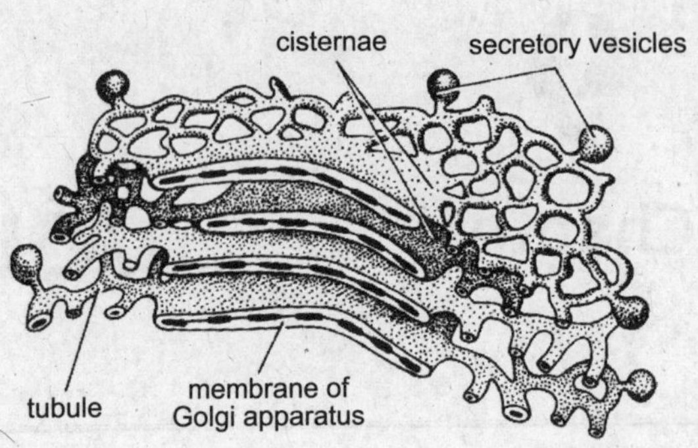

Fig. 9.1. Three dimensional view of Golgi apparatus.

1. Cisternae or Saccules

A cisterna is a sac or cavity filled with fluid contents within a cell or organism (**Morre** *et al.*, 1971). A Golgi body or Golgic apparatus usually consists of three to seven flat, tubular or filamentous cisternae which are closely held in parallel bundle or stack one above the other. The number of cisternae per Golgi body may exceed upto 30 or more in lower organisms (*e.g.*, insects). However, Golgi apparatus of some lower plants may contain only one saccule in it. All the cisternae of a stack of Golgi body or Golgi apparatus are slightly curved, so as to give a concave and a convex face to the whole stack.

Each cisterna of stack is enclosed by the usual three-layered and fluid mosaic unit membrane of 6 mμ thickness. In the stack, the cisternae are separated from each other by an inner-cisternal space of about 100–150 A° width. In some cells, a layer of parallel fibres, called **inter-cisternal elements** extends across each inter-cisternals space and may serve as strengthening elements maintaining the regular spacing between the individual lamellae (**Hall** *et al.*, 1974). Further, each cisterna consists of a central plate-like region of 0.5–1 μm diameter which is fenestrated at its peripheral margins due to its extension into network of tubules.

The cisternae have some definite polarity. One pole (convex surface) of each of them is associated with the nuclear envelope or with endoplasmic reticulum. This is **proximal pole** or **forming face**. The membranes of cisternae near this pole are developmentally youngest and morphologically and histochemically similar to endoplasmic reticulum. Toward the opposite pole (**distal pole** or **maturing face**), the cisternal membranes become progressively more like plasma membrane. The membrane of concave surface or distal pole is developmentally older. The secretory vesicles are formed from the distal poles of cisternae.

2. Tubules

From the peripheral area of cisternae arise a complex, anastomosing flat network of tubules of 300 to 500 A° diameter. **Clowes** and **Juniper** (1969) have compared this tubular network to a disc of lace.

3. Vesicles

The vesicles are small droplet-like sacs which remain attached to tubules at the periphery of the cisternae. They are of following two types:

1. Smooth vesicles. The smooth vesicles are of 20 to 80 mμ diameter. They contain secretory material (so often are called **secretory vesicles**) and are budded off from the ends of cisternal tubules within the net. Often more than one tubule connect to, and presumably fill, a single forming vesicle.

2. Coated vesicles. The coated vesicles are spherical protuberances, about 50 mμ in diameter and with a rough surface. They are found at the periphery of the organelle, usually at the ends of single tubules, and are morphologically quite distinct from the secretory vesicles. Their function is unknown.

4. Golgian Vacuoles

The Golgian vacuoles are large, spacious, rounded sac-like structures occurring at the distal ends of cisternae. They are produced by vesiculation of saccules of cisternae.

Zones of Exclusion

A Golgi body or Golgi apparatus is surrounded by a differentiated region of cytoplasm where ribosomes, glycogen, and organelles such as mitochondria and chloroplasts are scarce or absent. This is called **zone of exclusion** (**Morre** *et al.*, 1971) or **Golgi ground substance** (**Sjostrand** and **Hanzon**, 1954). Endoplasmic reticulum within the zone of exclusion has a smooth surface (lacking ribosomes), and coated vesicles of the Golgi apparatus are restricted to this region. Similar zones of exclusion are associated with microtubules (**Porter**, 1966), centrioles (**Bainton** and **Farquhar**, 1966) and regions of centriole formation (**Sorokin**, 1968).

9.4 CHEMICAL COMPOSITION

Chemical analysis of the membranes of the Golgi complex has shown that they have composition between that of the ER and of the plasma membrane (**Keenan** and **Morre**, 1970). The Golgi membranes are rich in phospholipids (*e.g.*, cephalin and lecithin), proteins and enzymes, as ADPase, ATPase, CTPase, thiamine pyrophosphatase, NADH-cytochrome C reductase, NADPH-cytochrome C reductase, UDP-N-acetyl glucosamine transferase, galactosyl transferase, glucose-6-phosphatase and other enzymes. The Golgi complex also contains some carotenoids, fatty acids and vitamin C.

Relationship of Golgi Apparatus with Endomembrane System

In conjunction with the endoplasmic reticulum, membranebounded vesicles and lysosomes, the Golgi apparatus forms an extensive inter-communicating membrane system called **endomembrane system** within the cell. The lumen enclosed by this membrane system is made up by that of the perinuclear space; the ER; the cisternae, tubules and vesicles of the Golgi apparatus; the lysosomes, the pinocytotic and autophagic vesicles; and in plant cells, the vacuole contained by the tonoplast. The region outside the plasma membrane is also included in the endomembrane system by **Northcote** (1973). All these spaces are connected either by a functional continuity or by a direct morphological connection, so that they together form a distinct channel which is separated from the rest of the cytoplasm and nucleoplasm of the cell and in which material can be synthesized, modified, and transported. The movement of material can take place either within the cell or from the inside to the outside of the cell and also from the exterior back into the vesicles and lysosomes. The Golgi apparatus occupies a key position in the functioning of this membrane system, since not only specific synthetic functions are carried out within the organelle and its associated vesicles, but also, as part of the transport route, it presents an irreversible connection between the perinuclear space and ER on the one hand and the vesicles and plasma membrane on the other (**De Duve**, 1969).

9.5 ORIGIN

Various cytological and biochemical evidences have established that the membranes of the Golgi apparatus are originated from the membranes of the smooth ER which in turn have originated from the rough ER. The proximal Golgi saccules are formed by fusion of ER-derived vesicles while distal saccules "give their all" to vesicle formation and disappear. Thus, Golgi saccules are constantly and rapidly renewed.

9.6 FUNCTIONS

The function of Golgi apparatus is to accept vesicles from the ER, to modify the vesicular membranes and their contents and then to distribute products to other parts of the cell. The modified and distributed vesicles may be identified as lysosomes, secretory vesicles or as isolation envelopes to support autophagy.

Mostly, secretory vesicles or lysosomes are derived from the distal saccules of Golgi apparatus. However, exceptions to this rule have been reported in certain cells such as, blood neutrophils and cells of corn root cap. For example, in blood neutrophils, for the process of phagocytosis, Golgi apparatus produces following two kinds of secretory vesicles: the large, "specific granules" that usually fuse first with the phagocytic vacuole are derived from proximal saccules, while lysosomes usually come from the distal saccules. Likewise, proximal saccules of Golgi complex of corn root cap produce secretory vesicles which secrete a polysaccharide mixture called **root cap slime**.

Some of the important functions of Golgi apparatus can be summarized as follows:

1. Processing of secretory and membrane proteins. The Golgi apparatus adds certain terminal sugars like sialic acid, fucose and galactose to the glycoproteins (both exportable proteins and membrane proteins) which are secreted by rough ER and thus, gives finishing touches to them. However, albumin which is synthesized and secreted by liver cells, has no carbohydrate yet is processed through the Golgi apparatus in the same sequence as exportable or membrane glycoproteins.

2. Secretion of polysaccharides. The Golgi apparatus has an important role in the secretion of polysaccharides. The polysaccharide scales found on some algae are assembled in the Golgi apparatus, as is a portion of cell wall of higher plants. The pectin and other mucilaginous substances of the plant cell wall are synthesized in the Golgi and are packaged in vesicles for secretion. Cellulose, however, is an exception, as its synthesis seems to take place extracellularly at the plasma membrane (see **Dyson**, 1978). The enzymes responsible for cellulose synthesis are membrane-bound and transported to the surface in Golgi-dervied vesicles.

3. Formation of plasma membrane. The Golgi apparatus may act as an one-way valve, controlling the modification of membranes from endoplasmic reticulum-like to plasma membrane-like. Continuity between the Golgi apparatus and plasma membrane probably occurs via secretory vesicles which compartmentalize materials destined for the cell surface. Carbohydrate residues present in the inside of the vesicle membrane could, on fusing with the existing plasma membrane, appear on the outside of the cell (see **Cook**, 1975).

4. Other functions. The Golgi apparatus also forms certain intra-cellular structures such as **acrosomes** of spermatozoa of animals, certain **yolk substances** and **cortical granules** of oocytes, the latter form the fertilization membrane around the plasma membrane of ovum after the entry of a sperm in the ovum during fertilization.

Lastly, the chief function of the Golgi apparatus, the secretion, can be discussed in detail as under:

9.7 GOLGI APPARATUS AND SECRETION

Secretion is an activity carried on by a great many different cells. For unicellular organisms, especially, it is a way of getting rid of waste products. For cells of higher plants and animals,it provides an extra-cellular matrix: the basement membrane on which many cells rest; the protein fibres on which the calcium salts of bone are deposited; root cap slime; the non-cellulose portion of plant cell walls and the enzymatic machinery for assembling the cellulose portion; and the protein components of arthropod cuticles, to name just a few. In addition, some cells are specialized for the purpose of secretion. **Exocrine** and **endocrine** glands secrete hormones, neurons secrete neurotransmitters, mucous cells lining the airways (respiratory organs) and gastrointestinal tract secrete protective polysaccharides and glycoproteins, etc. The basic mechanisms used for secretion by these cells are however, few.

Types of Secretion

Molecular transport and diffusion across membranes account for the transfer of some materials from cytoplasm to extra-cellular space. Cellular secretion may be of the following three types: holocrine, apocrine and merocrine.

(i) **Holocrine secretion.** In this kind of cellular secretion, the entire cell fills with secretory product and then is broken up and sacrificed. An example is the sebaceous gland, which secretes a fatty discharge onto adjacent hair and skin. It is this gland that, when overstimulated, gets plugged to form blackheads and ultimately the pimples of adolescent acne.

(ii) **Apocrine secretion.** In this kind of secretion, the secretion vesicle buds through the plasma membrane carrying with it a portion of that membrane and hence a thin layer of cytoplasm. The secretion vesicle is thus covered by two layers of membrane, its own plus the plasma membrane. Milk fat droplets (MFD) of the cells of the lactating mammary gland are released as apocrine secretion (Fig. 9.2).

(iii) **Merocrine or eccrine secretion.** It is a most common type of cellular secretion. This process is also called **exocytosis** because it is the function opposite of endocytosis. Thus, it involves the fusion of secretory vesicles with the plasma membrane and their opening to the exterior. It is the usual mode of secretion of most glands and of most other cells, both animal and plant. It is, for example, the mode of secretion of the **true sweat glands**, which are distributed over most of the human skin.

Pancreas which includes exocrine as well as endocrine cells has provided a best example of merocrine secretion.

A. The pancreatic aciner cells. The synthesis and secretion of digestive enzymes by the exocrine portion of the pancreas was the first secretory pathway to be investigated by modern methods. These cells secrete trypsin, chymotrypsin and other digestive enzymes in an inactive, or **zymogen**, form. The stimulus for secretion can come either from the nervous system or from hormones produced in the gastrointestinal system after a meal. **George Palade** and **Lucien Caro** took advantage of this fact and of the recent availability or radioactively labelled amino acids in a pioneering set of experiments during mid-1950s.

"Pulse-chase" experiments. Caro and **Palade** injected radioactive amino acids into fasted and re-fed guinea pigs. Injection was followed in three minutes by a much larger dose of unlabelled am ino acid in order to stop uptake of the radioactivity. Animals were then sacrificed at various times. Within a few minutes from the time of injection, radioactivity was found in the rough endoplasmic reticulum of the pancreatic cells; by 20 minutes it was found also in the Golgi apparatus and nearby vesicles; and by two hours it was localized to the secretory vesicles or zymogen granules. From such experiments following picture of secretion in an aciner pancreatic cell has emerged (**Palade**, 1975).

Secretory proteins are synthesized on membrane-bound ribosomes and pass immediately into the cisternae of the rough ER for proteolytic processing and carbohydrate addition. They then transfer to the contiguous smooth-surface ER; from there they travel, by ER-derived vesicles, to the Golgi saccules, where they may get their terminal carbohydrate. New Golgi saccules are formed from ER vesicles on one side and old ones yield their membrane to secretory vesicles on the other. The secretory vesicles fuse with the plasma membrane to empty themselves and complete the process (Fig. 9.2).

B. Mechanism of vesicle transport. The first requirement for a secreted material, once it has left the protection of the endoplasmic reticulum in vesicles derived therefrom, is to find the Golgi apparatus. That task would be easier if the vesicles formed only from a portion of the interconnected ER that happened to lie close to a Golgi saccule (*i.e.*, smooth-ER). In fact, **Michael Locke** and **P. Huie** (1976) have reported in several types of animal cells, the occurrence of rings of bead-like structures on the smooth-ER near the proximal face of the Golgi apparatus. These structures appear to mark a specialized region of the ER where vesicle formation and flow to the adjacent Golgi apparatus is permitted. This flow is dependent on a source of energy, though it is uncertain whether the requirement is for vesicle formation alone or for transport as well.

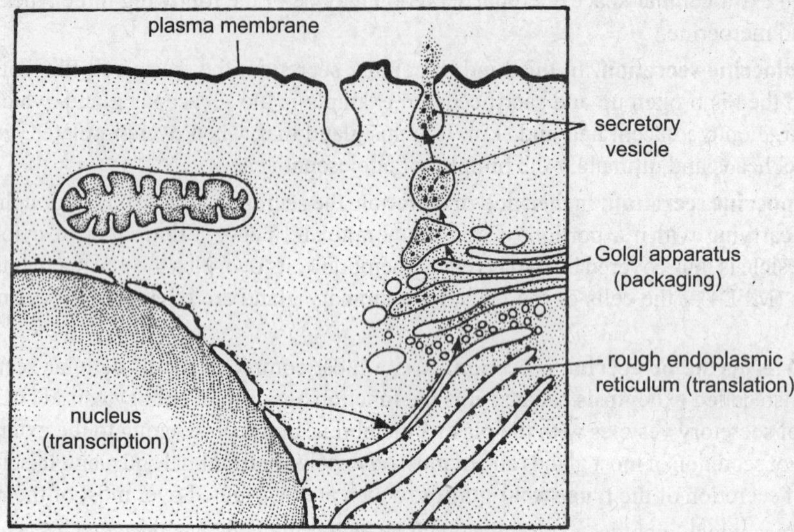

Fig. 9.2. A summary of the process of synthesis and secretion, including the path of mRNA from the nucleus to the rough endoplasmic reticulum, and progress of the polypeptide chains through the ER, transition vesicles, Golgi apparatus and secretory vesicles (after Dyson, 1978).

However, the trip of secretory vesicle from Golgi apparatus to plasma membrane is longer and demands a more definite travel plan. For example, exit from the cell is commonly permitted only in one specified region of the plasma membrane—at the lumen of an excretory duct in the case of exocrine glands or at the adjacent capillary in the case of endocrine glands. In fact, distance between vesicle formation and site of secretion can be very long. For example, in neurosecretory cells of the human brain, hormones oxytocin or vasopressin are packaged into secretory vesicles in the cell body, which resides in the hypothalamus at the lower part of the brain, but are secreted into the blood at the pituitary gland several centimetres away.

In all cases, secretory vesicles collect specifically at the membranes adiacent to where they will be emptied and in many cases microtubules are seen along the path of vesicle movement. Investigations of **W. Malaisse** *et. al.* (1975) on **insulin secretion** in β-cell of rat pancreas have confirmed that microtubules play a important role in the translocation of secretory vesicles and they have suggested following model for insulin secretion:

C. Insulin secretion. β-cells of pancreas of mammals are the endocrine cells that produce **insulin hormone** and release it into the blood stream. Release occurs at a low basal rate that is capable of being accelerated by the proper stimulus. An increase in blood glucose to high levels is an obvious choice of stimulus.

The secretory vesicles containing insulin are moved from the Golgi apparatus of a pancreatic β-cell toward a designated portion of the plasma membrane by microtubules. Movement stops when the microfilamentous web is reached. Changes in the web structure following glucose stimulation result in exocytosis of these vesicles, furnishing the early phase of the secretory response. Continued secretion requires the mobilization of more distant vesicles by microtubules and their energy-dependent transport to the secretory site. Similar mechanism is suspected to occur in all secretory cells.

D. Stimulus-secretion coupling. W.W. Douglas (1968) suggested that the coupling event between stimulus and secretion in a wide variety of cells is an increase in available Ca^{2+}. The Ca^{2+} ions pool may be extra-cellular (*e.g.*, nerve cells) or intracellular (*e.g.*, blood platelets). The level of Ca^{2+} may be changed directly by the stimulus (*e.g.*, by increased influx) or indirectly through cyclic adenosine monophosphate (cAMP) or cyclic guanosine monophosphate (cGMP).

E. Fate of secretory vesicles. The last step in the process of secretion is disposal of the secretory vesicle. With apocrine secretion, there is no problem, because the vesicle is gone. With merocrine secretion, there are two possibilities: the empty vesicle can detach from the plasma membrane and return to the cytoplasm for destruction or **recycling**, or the vesicle can merge with, and become part of the plasma membrane. The first option, returning the empty vesicle to the cytoplasm, is used by some cell types such as adrenal medulla where catecholamines are released and some insect cells. The second option, incorporation of vesicle into the plasma membrane, is most common for many secretory cells. In this case, however, the resulting increase in surface area must be compensated for by endocytic removal of plasma membrane in order to maintain a constant cell size (*e.g.*, nerve cells and other secretory cells).

One cell type has solved this problem in a very interesting way: the secretory cells of lactating mammary glands have two products, **casein** (the most abundant protein of milk) and **fat droplets**. Casein is ordinarily secreted by the merocrine mechanism, which adds membrane to the surface, whereas fat droplets are secreted in the apocrine fashion, which removes membrane from the surface (**W. Franke** *et. al.*, 1976). The two process can balance each other under some conditions to keep the cell size constant.

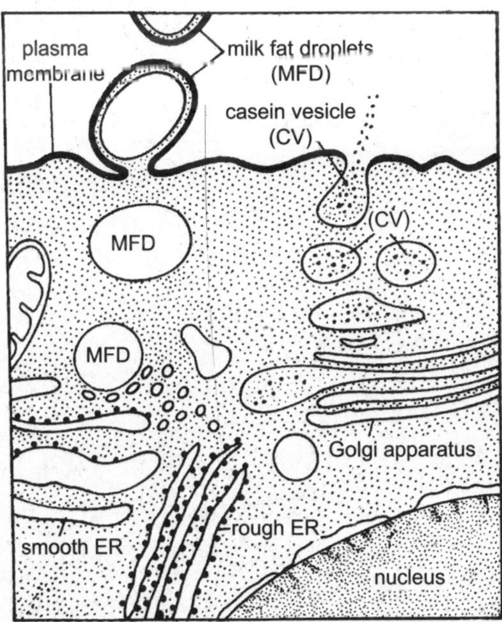

Fig. 9.3. Secretion in lactating mammary gland. Milk fat droplets are released by the apocrine mechanism, whereas casein vesicles normally release their protein by merocrine secretion. The former removes plasma membrane, the latter adds to it (after Dyson, 1978).

Lastly, while secretory cells that utilise exocytosis face the problem of removing excess plasma membrane, apocrine secretors and phagocytic cells have the opposite problem—that of adding new membrane to ever shrinking plasma membrane. For example, the phagocytically active soil amoeba, *Acanrhamoeba castellani*, is thought to ingest 5 to 50 times its surface area per hour, much of it by pinocytosis. It has been proposed that some of these small vesicles might be emptied and returned directly to the plasma membrane. However, phagocytic vacuoles probably are not. Thus, a human macrophage after ingesting a particularly large particle loses its surface microvilli, rounds up, and is thereafter phagocytically inactive 5–6 hours. Macrophages, like virtually all other cells can make and incorporate new plasma membrane. Hence, it gradually returns to its former shape and activity.

REVISION QUESTIONS

1. Describe the Golgi apparatus? Which is the proximal and which is the distal face? What types of vesicles arise from Golgi membranes?
2. Write an essay on "Golgi apparatus and secretion".
3. Describe various functions of Golgi apparatus in the cells.
4. There appears to be a regular turnover of Golgi membranes. According to the available evidence, where do the membranes comes from and what happens to them?
5. Describe the removal and replacement of plasma membrane. What is the likely explanation for the longer survival of plasma membrane proteins' compared to lipids? What is the significance of the lipid exchange proteins?

10
Chapter
LYSOSOMES

The lysosomes (*Gr., lyso* = digestive + *soma* = body) are tiny membrane-bound, vesicular structures of the cytoplasm which contain destructive enzymes called **hydrolases** capable of breaking down a wide variety of particulate materials (most macromolecules and some molecules) and thus, perform intra-cellular digestion of the cell. Lysosomes were first of all reported by **de Duve** in 1955.

10.1 OCCURRENCE

Usually the lysosomes occur in most animal cells except the mature mammalian red blood cell and many plant cells. The animal cells which are secretory in function such as the pancreatic cells, leucocytes, liver cells, spleen cells and kidney cells contain large number of the lysosomes. The lysosomes are particularly numerous and large in cells as macrophages which perform special digestive functions. The lysosomes often remain distributed evenly in the cytoplasm.

10.2 MORPHOLOGY

Shape and Size

The lysosomes, are generally spherical in shape but certain meristamatic cells of plant roots contain irregular-shaped lysosomes. The size of the lysosomes usually ranges from 0.2 to 0.8 μm but may be exceptionally large in the cells of mamamlian kidney, *i.e.*, upon 5 μm and even more in phagocytes and leucocytes.

Structure

The lysosomes are round vacuolar structure which remain filled with dense material and acid phosphatase enzymes. The lysosomes are bounded by a unit membrane of the lipoprotein. The space or vacuole of the lysosome contains dense, granular, vacuolated and homogeneous material.

10.3 CHEMICAL COMPOSITION

The lysosomes have been found to contain molecules of about 40 different enzymes or hydrolases. The one most often used as a "marker", because of the ease with which its activity can be localized in electron microscopy, is acid phosphatase. Some important lysosomal hydrolases are β-glucuronidase, β-galactosidase, β-N-acetyl-glucosaminidase, α-glucosidase, α-mannosidase; cathepsin A (Acid protease), cathepsin B (Acid protease), aryl sulphatase A, aryl sulphatase B, acid ribonuclease, acid deoxyribonuclease, acid phosphatase, acid lipase, phospholipase A, phosphotidic acid phosphatase, hyaluronidase, phosphoprotein phosphatase, amino peptidase A, dextrnase, saccharase, lysozyme (muramidase), Mg^{++} activated ATPase, indoxylacetate, esterase and plasminogen activator. All these enzymes of the lysosomes are enclosed within the single lipoprotein membrane which can be ruptured easily by progesterone, endotoxins, testosterone, vitamin A and E, proteases digitonin, X-irridation. ultra-violet irridation and bile salts. But the lysosomes remain stable in living cells. The stability to the lysosomes is provided by certain chemical substances such as cholesterol, cortisone, cortisol and chloroquine. These substances stabilize the membrane of the lysosomes.

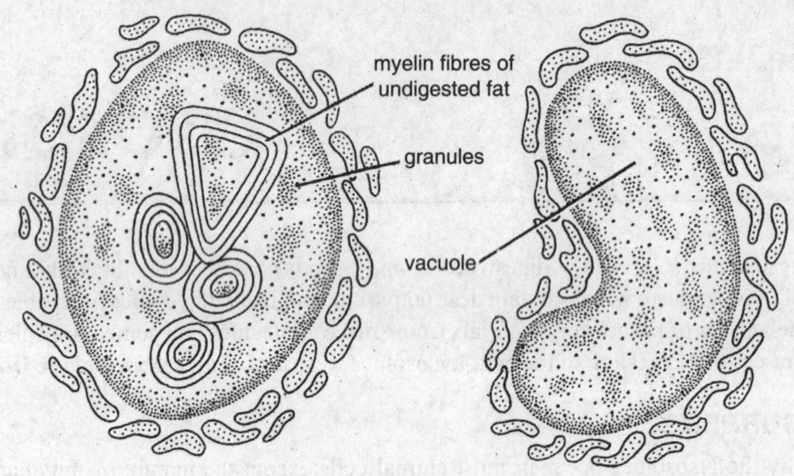

Fig. 10.1. Two different kinds of lysosomes of the kidney cells of rat.

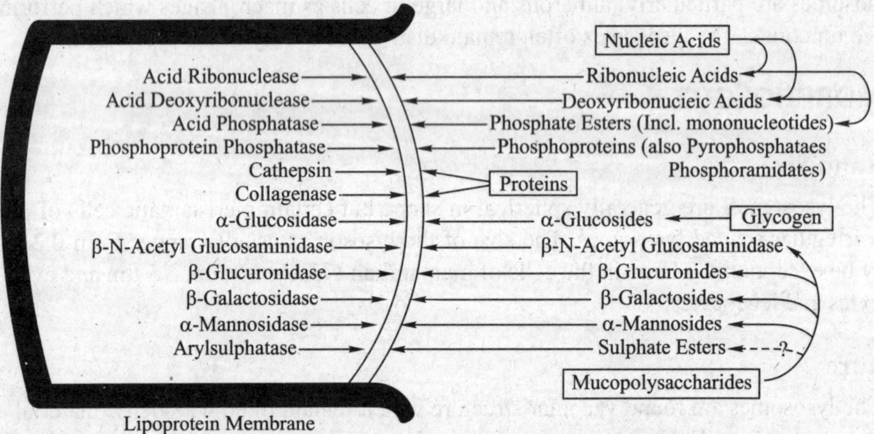

Fig. 10.2. The enzymes of lysosomes and their substances (De Robertis *et. al.*, 1970).

10.4 KINDS OF LYSOSOMES (POLYMORPHISM IN LYSOSOMES)

In different types of cells and at different times in a same cell four types of lysosomes have been observed which are as follows:

1. Primary lysosomes,
2. Secondary lysosomes,
3. Residual bodies, and
4. Autophagic vacuoles or cytolysosomes.

1. Primary Lysosomes

Newly formed lysosomes are called primary lysosomes. They ate formed principally as vesicles pinched off from Golgi membranes but in some cells a specialized portion of endoplasmic reticulum called **GERL** (Golgi-associated ER from which lysosomes arise) is probably also involved (see **Dyson**, 1978).

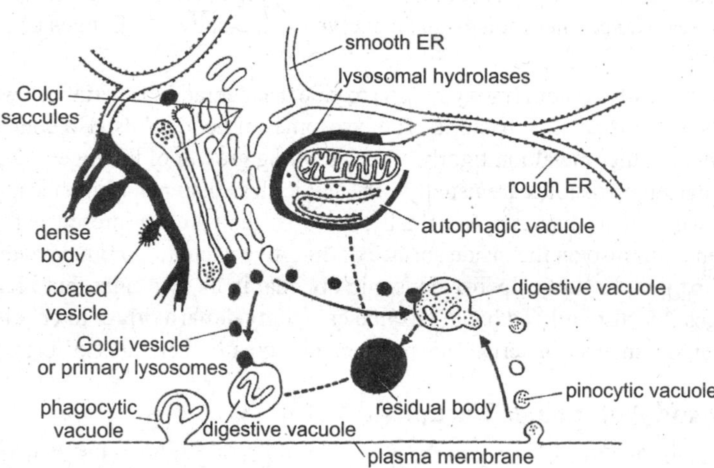

Fig. 10.3. Diagram suggesting probable inter-relations of some organelles in the transport of lysosomal hydrolases and the formation of lysosomes (after Novikoff and Holtzman, 1970).

2. Secondary Lysosomes

The secondary lysosomes are also known as **heterophagosomes** or **digestive vacuoles**. When the cells feed on foreign or exogenous or extracellulur substances by the process of phagocytosis or pinocytosis (heterophagy), then the plasma membrane forms the membranebound vesicles known as **pinosomes** or **phagosomes** around these substances. The pinosomes or phagosomes ultimately fuse with the pre-existing primary lysosomes and form the **seqondary lysosomes** or **heterophagosomes**. In neutrophils (and eosinophils) this step is preceded by fusion of specific granules with the phagocytic vacuole, so that a digestive vacuole in these cells contains enzymes from two sources.

The objective of secondary lysosome formation is to mix lysosomal hydrolases with the ingested material so that breakdown of the latter can occur. The digestion products (amino acids, nucleotides) has low molecular weight and readily pass through the lysosomal membrane to become sources of energy or raw materials for biosynthetic pathway. As products leave, the lysosome often diminishes in size. This change requires a loss of surface area, which can be achieved by an inward budding of the limiting membrane in much the same way as pinocytic vesicles are formed. The internalized membrane is then digested. This process, which is particularly prominent in the digestion or pinocytic vesicles, leads to an electron micrographic picture of a vacuole (the secondary lysosome) containing numerous small vesicles and fragments, a structure known as **multivesicular body** (**J. Braaten** *et. al.*, 1975).

The fusion of a lysosome with an endocytic vacuole is a selective process. The vacuoles do not fuse with endoplasmic reticulum, mitochondria, etc. Nor do the lysosomes fuse with plasma membrane under ordinary circumstances, even though plasma membrane and phagocytic vacuole are made of the same stuff. However, in the presence of cytochalasin B, extra-cellular release of lysosomal enzymes does occur readily, indicating that perhaps the microfilamentous web beneath the plasma membrane normally protects it from fusion with lysosomes.

There is some evidence also for involvement of microtubules in guiding endocytic vacuoles, lysosomes and specific granules, and there is evidence for regulation by cyclic nucleotides *i.e.*, cAMP and cGMP, probably via their effect on microtubules. In certain cells, at least, colchicine and cAMP seem to inhibit and cGMP to promote digestive vacuole formation.

Killing in secondary lysosomes. Simple enzymatic digestion by hydrolases is not the only process that occurs in secondary lysosomes. Many microorganisms, while they are viable, resist attack by hydrolases. Hence, mechanisms have evolved specifically to kill ingested organisms prior to their breakdown.

Lysosomes typically contain **lysozyme**, an enzyme that degrades bacterial cell walls, especially the simpler walls of gram-positive bacteria. The lysosomes of neutrophils also contain **lactoferrin**, which binds iron and other metal ion tightly, thus inhibiting growth of the ingested organisms. The contents of the digestive vacuoles are usually very acidic (less than pH 4 in neutrophils), which by itself inhibits growth of many bacteria. And finally, oxidases, thought to be present at the surface of the cell membrane and thus also on the inside surface of digestive vacuoles, produce hydrogen peroxide from molecular oxygen. Hydrogen peroxide is microbicidal in its own right, but in neutrophils and most macrophages it is also utilized by an enzyme called **myeloperoxidase** to covalently fix Cl^- or I^- onto organic targets such as bacteria. This halogenation greatly facilitates killing of the organism.

3. Autophagy and Autophagic Vacuoles

Lysosomes are involved not only in the process of digesting extra-cellular material, known as **heterophagy**, but also in the digestion of intra-cellular substances, an activity known as **autophagy**. In autophagy, lysosomes are responsible for turnover of organelles of animal cells, a process that is accelerated during involutional states—in a muscle that is not being used, during starvation, after injury, or during the remodelling that occurs with cellular differentiation. Even in unstressed normal cells, the turnover of organelles by autophagy is relatively rapid. The half life of liver cell mitochondria, for example, is five to six days, for peroxisomes it is one to two days and for ribosomes about five days.

The autophagy of cytoplasmic organelles start with an **isolation envelope** (Fig. 10.3), which is a sack of smooth-surfaced membrane that wraps around the material to be removed and separates into a sort of phagocytic vacuole known as an **isolation body**. The source of the isolation membrane, at least in damaged liver and kidney seem to be the endoplasmic reticulum. However, recent work of **Michal Locke** and his associates (1975) indicates that the isolation membrane in insect cells during metamorphosis and in some other animal cells, is derived from the Golgi complex. In any case, lysosomes can fuse with the isolation body to create an **autophagic digestive vacuole** and release breakdown products to the cytoplasm to be used as an emergency source of food or as raw material for cellular remodelling.

4. Residual Bodies

Although killing and breakdown (digestion) in the lysosomes are efficient, some materials are simply not digestible. These substances may be relelsed from the cell by fusion of the digestive vacuole with the plasma membrane (exocytosis). This process is very efficient in Protozoa, but not so efficient in higher animals. Hence, inactive digestive vacuoles containing debris may accumulate.

These debris-filled organelles, called **residual bodies**, are of no consequence to cells like macrophages or neutrophils, because the cells do not live long enough for significant amounts to accumulate. In cells that do not divide, and are not replaced, substantial quantities of this material may accumulate. In neurons and muscle cells, especially, there is a steady increase in the number of these bodies, which are called in this context **lipofuscin granules**. The age of an animal can often be estimated from their concentration and residual bodies play important role in the process of aging.

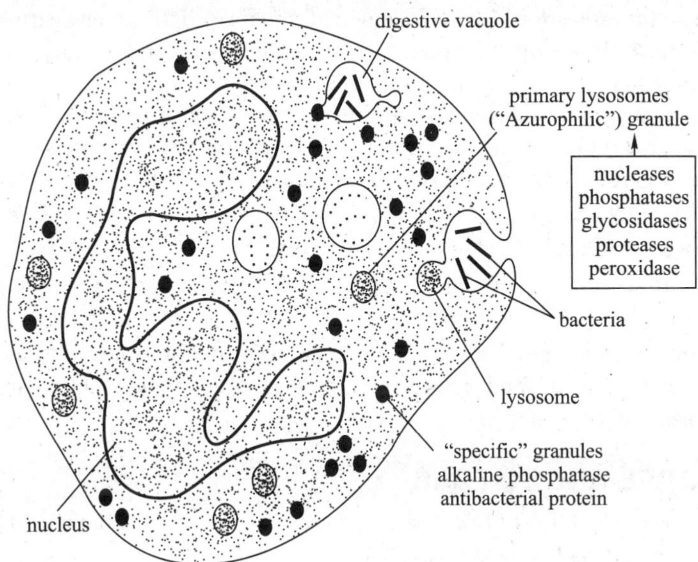

Fig. 10.4. Diagram of a white blood cell (neutrophil) ingesting bacteria. Two types of granules fuse with the phagocytic vacuoles and contribute digestive enzymes and other components (after Novikoff and Holtzman, 1970).

10.5 ORIGIN OF LYSOSOMES

The origin of lysosomes is not known with any amount of certainty. Some workers have suggested that the lysosomes have originated from the pinocytic vacuoles (pinosomes) which in their turn originate from the plasma membrane. Others believe that because the acrosome of the sperm (which contains a high concentration of acid phosphatase) is formed by the secretory activity of the Golgi complex, the lysosomes have Golgi origin. Still others consider the lysosomes as inclusions containing digested material. It seems likely that the membran part of a lysosome is derived from Golgi membranes and the enzymes part from secretory products of Golgi complex. **Novikoff** (1965) has shown that the lysosomes originated directly from the granular endoplasmic reticulum.

10.6 FUNCTIONS OF LYSOSOMES

The important functions of lysosomes are as follows:

1. Digestion of large extracellular particles. The lysosomes digest the food contents of the phagosomes or pinosomes. The lysosomes of leucocytes enable the latter to devour the foreign proteins, bacteria and viruses.

2. Digestion of intracellular substances. During the starvation, the lysosomes digest the stored food contents, *viz.*, proteins, lipids and carbohydrates (glycogen) of the cytoplasm and supply to the cell necessary amount of energy.

3. Autolysis. In certain pathological conditions the lysosomes start to digest the various organelles of the cells and this process is known as **autolysis** or **cellular autophagy**. When a cell dies, the lysosome membrane ruptures and enzymes are liberated. These enzymes digest the dead cells. In the process of metamorphosis of amphibians and tunicates many embryonic tissues, *e.g.*, gills, fins, tail, etc., are digested by the lysosomes and utilized by the other cells.

4. Extracellular digestion. The lysosomes of certain cells such as sperms discharge their enzymes outside the cell during the process of fertilization. The lysosomal enzymes digest the limiting membranes of the ovum and form penetration path in ovum for the sperms. Acid hydrolases are released from **osteoclasts** and break down bone for the reabsorption; these cells also secrete lactic acid which makes the local pH enough for optimal enzyme activity. Likewise, preceding ossification (bone formation), **fibroblasts** release cathepsin D enzyme to break down the connective tissue.

5. The lysosomes are supposed to initate the mitosis in cells.

6. Allison and Mallueci (1964) have suggested that lysosomes and the release of lysosomal enzymes may be involved in carcinogensis.

7. The lysosomes form a built-in mechanism of the cell and enable the cell to adopt metabolically rapidly changing conditions of food supply, oxygen concentration and other environmental factors which occur in many living systems.

10.7 LYSOSOMES AND DISEASE

Defects in normal function of lysosomes often cause a variety of pathological conditions in the animals including man, which are discussed as under:

The importance of hydrogen peroxide in phagocytic killing of micro-organisms is illustrated in humans by a X-linked recessive condition called **chronic granulomatous disease**. A **granuloma** is a collection of dead and dying macrophages. The disease is a deficiency of the oxidase enzyme that produces hydrogen peroxide in the digestive vacuole. The macrophages and neutrophils of these individuals are unable to kill effectively even common bacteria, which may live and multiply inside the cell, eventually killing it instead. Such people are prone to all sorts of fungal and bacterial infections, in spite of an immune system that is otherwise normal.

Other types of defects in lysosomal function include failure to fuse with the endocytic vacuole and failure to digest certain classes of chemical substances due to lack of one or more critical enzymes. For example, fusion of lysosome and phagocytic vacuole is sometimes inhibited, for reasons that are not understood, when the vacuole contains live bacteria responsible for **tuberculosis** or **leprosy**, or when it contains live **toxoplasma**, a common protozoan parasite contracted from raw meat or cat faeces. Lack of fusion permits these organisms to live within the phagocytic cells and often to destroy them and to establish active disease. Algae that live symbiotically in Protoza seem to be similarly protected. The only clue how fusion might be avoided in these cases comes from the observation that concanavalin A-induced endocytosis also results in vacuoles that frequently fail to fuse with lysosomes. (**Note. Concanavalin A** or **con A** is a **lectin**, the plant protein that behaves very much like antibodies in their ability to bind to specific chemical configurations such as α-D-mannose or α-D-glucose of plasma membrane and thus, cause cellular adhesion in plant cells. Con A is found to cause activation (DNA synthesis, cell division, etc.) of lymphocytes by cross-linking with receptors of lymphocyte plasma membrane, the latter get anchored to the underlying cytoskeleton. However, high dose of con A immobilizes many receptors of lymphocyte and prevents activation, (see **Dyson**, 1978). Hence the distribution of membrane glycoprotein and the effect this has on underlying filaments and tubules may be involved in some way.

Fusion of phagocytic vacuoles with lysosomes and specific granules may also come too soon. If fusion occurs before the plasma membrane has closed over the forming vacuole, contents somes and specific granules may **regurgitate** through the vacuole and into the extra-cellular space. Because of the destructive character of these enzymes, a **local inflammation** (redness, swelling, tenderness, etc.) may result. This process, especially common with neutrophils, is important in localizing an infection and hence not always undesirable. However, it is probably also responsible for some of the **degenerative joint changes in rheumatoid** and **gouty types of arthritis**. The effectiveness of colchicine in the treatment of gout is probably due to its inhibition of lysosomes and granule movement and fusion, which are processes that involve microtubules.

Another type of defect in lysosomal function occurs if an essential hydrolase is missing. Because there are many hydrolases, there are many (more than 24) of these **lysosomal storage diseases**. They are almost always inherited as autosomal recessive traits because one good gene out of the two alleles inherited from the two parents is usually enough to prevent symptoms. The diseases have names like **Tay-Sachs**, **Hunter's**, **Hurler's**, **Niemann-Pick**, and so on, because they were described long before lysosomal function was understood. Most of these diseases result in accumulation of undigested lipids or polysaccharides, which eventually fill the cell and thus compromise its function. The type of cell most affected will be determined by which enzyme is faulty, but the central nervous system is commonly affected, resulting in progressive lack of body control and loss of mental function leading to a slow death.

10.8 LYSOSOMES IN PLANTS

It has become clear now that plant cells though have no lysosome exactly similar to lysosomes of animal cells, but many membrane bounded storage granules of them are found to contain certain digestive enzymes and these granules are considered as lysosomes of plant cell (**Gahan**, 1972). According to **Matile** (1969) the plant lysosomes can be defined as membrane-bounded cell compartments containing hydrolytic digestive enzymes. Following storage granules of plant cells are found to possess lysosome-like activittes:

1. Spherosomes,
2. Alcurone grain, and
3. Vacuoles.

1. Spherosomes

The spherosomes are membrane-bounded, spherical particles of 0.5 to 2.5 μm diameter, occurring in most plant cells. They have a fine granular structure internally which is rich in lipids and proteins. They originate from the endoplasmic reticulum (ER). Oil accumulates at the end of a strand of ER and a small vesicle is then cut off by constriction to form particles, called **prospherosomes**. The prospherosomes grow in size to form spherosomes. Basically, the spherosomes are involved in lipid synthesis and storage. But, the spherosomes of maize root tips and spherosomes of tobacco endosperm tissue have been found rich in hydrolytic digestive enzymes and so have been considered as lysosomes. Like lysosomes they are not only responsible for the accumulation and mobilization of reserve lipids, but also for the digestion of other cytoplasmic components incorporated by phagocytosis.

3. Aleurone Grain

The aleurone grains or protein bodies are spherical membrane-bounded storage particles occurring in the cells of endosperm and cotyledons of seeds. They are formed during the later stages of seed ripening and disappear in the early stages of germination. They store protein (*e.g.*, globulins) and phosphate in the form of phytin. **Matile** (1968) has demonstrated that aleurone grains from pea seed contain a wide range of hydrolytic enzymes including protease and phosphatase which are required for the mobilization of stored protein and phosphate, although the presence of other enzymes such as β-amylase and RNAase suggest that other cell constituents may also be digested. Thus, like spherosomes, aleurone grains store reserve materials, mobilize them during germination and in addition form a compartment for the digestion of other cell components. The aleurone grains are derived from the strands of the endoplasmic reticulum.

3. Vacuoles

The plant cells also contain particles called **vacuoles** that are approximately spherical and bounded by a single unit membrane usually show little internal structure, contain a variety of hydrolytic enzymes and may show some degree of polymorphism. The vacuoles are derived from endoplasmic reticulum which gives out **provacuoles**. The provacuoles are analogous to the primary lysosomes of animal cells and develop by fusion to form larger vacuoles.

REVISION QUESTIONS

1. What are the lysosomes? Describe their origin, structure and function.
2. Describe the digestive events that usually follow phagocytosis. What mechanism assist in the killing of micro-organisms after phagocytosis?
3. Describe the process of autophagy. What is the ultimate fate of the digestive vacuole?
4. Write the short notes on the following:
   (*i*) Polymorphism in lysosomes;
   (*ii*) Lysosomes and disease;
   (*iii*) Lysosomal enzymes; and
   (*iv*) Lysosomes of plants.

11 Chapter

MITOCHONDRIA

The mitochondria (Gr., *mito* = thread, *chondrion* = granule) are filamentous or granular cytoplasmic organelles of all aerobic cells of higher animals, plants and also of certain microorganisms including Algae, Protozoa and Fungi. These are absent in bacterial cells. The mitochondria have lipoprotein framework which contains many enzymes and coenzymes required for energy metabolism. They also contain a specific DNA for the cytoplasmic inheritance and ribosomes for the protein synthesis.

11.1 OXIDATIVE ORGANELLES

Mitochondria, chloroplasts and peroxisomes (microbodies) form **oxidative organelles** of eukaryotic cells. A typical eukaryotic cell depends on mitochondria or chloroplasts to supply most of its energy. Chloroplasts, found only in plant cells, capture light energy and transform it to chemical energy in the form of ATP and reduced coenzymes, a process called **photosynthesis**. Mitochondria, found in both animal and plant cells, oxidize reduced coenzymes and certain other organic molecules, using molecular oxygen from the air as an electron acceptor. **Oxidation** release energy, a portion of which is captured by mitochondria and used to form ATP. In spite of a few exceptions, mitochondria and chloroplasts are the "power houses" of most eukaryotic cells. Peroxisomes are another type of oxidative organelles of cells which use molecular oxygen, but produce no ATP molecule for the cell.

In this chapter, the most significant oxidative cellular organelle of plants and animals, the mitochondria, will be discussed. Remaining oxidative organelles have been discussed in forthcoming chapters.

11.2 HISTORICAL

The mitochondria were first of all observed in 1857 by **A. Kolliker** in muscles and he described them as the "sarcosomes". In 1888 **Kolliker** teased mitochondria out of muscle cells of insects and he showed that they were individual entities and not connected directly to other parts of the cell. In 1882, **Flemming** named them as **fila**. Later on **Altmann** (1890) developed a specific stain for mitochondria. named them as **bioblasts** and suggested that they were autonomous organelles. The present name **mitochondria** was assigned by **Benda** (1897, 1898) to them. He stained mitochondria with alizarin and crystal violet. **Michaelis** (1900) stained mitochondria by janus green. In 1912, **B.F. Kingsbury** proposed that they might be sites of cellular respiration—that is the site of oxygen utilization. **Kennedy** and **Lehninger** (1948–1950) showed that the citric acid cycle (Krebs cycle), oxidative phosphorylation and fatty acid oxidation took place in the mitochondria. In 1951, **Lehninger** proved that oxidative phosphorylation requires electron transport. **Palade** (1954) described the *cristae mitochondriales*, or crista membrane. **Nass** (1963) observed and proved the presence of the DNA molecule in the mitochondria.

Previously the mitochondria have been known by various, names such as **fuchsinophilic granules**, **parabasal bodies**, **plasmosomes**, **plastosomes**, **fila**, **vermicules**, **bioblasts** and **chondriosomes**.

11.3 DISTRIBUTION OR LOCALIZATION

The mitochondria move autonomously in the cytoplasm, so they generally have uniform distribution in the cytoplasm, but in many cells their distribution is very restricted to an area of particularly heavy utilization of ATP. Thus, they are often found in rows adjacent to the contractile elements of muscle, wrapped about the base of a sperm flagellum and adjacent to lipid droplet of fat cells. Likewise, in the rod and cone cells of the retina all the mitochondria are located in a portion of the inner segment, in certain muscles of the diaphragm the mitochondria are concentrated around the I band of the myofibril and forming a ring, and in the cells of renal distal tubules the mitochondria lie near and perpendicularly to the cell membranes. The concentration of the mitochondria in such cells has suggested their utility in providing more energy to these cells for active metabolic functions.

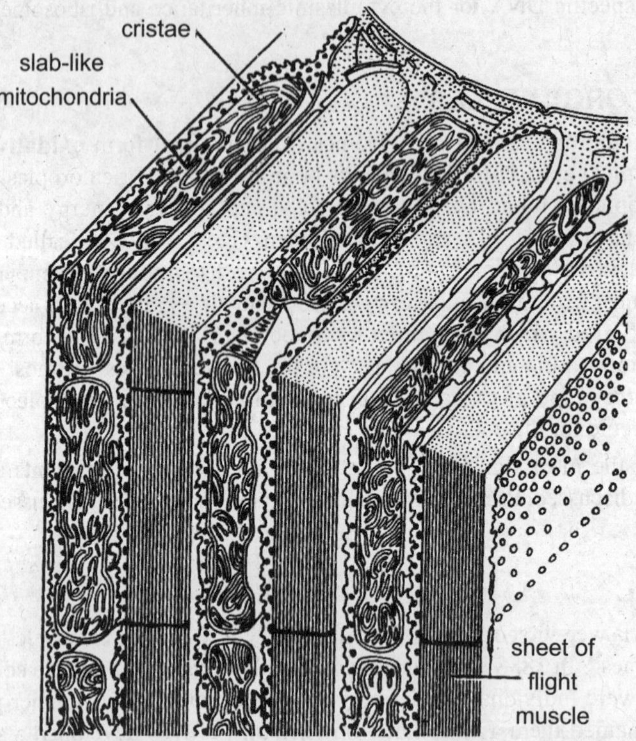

Fig. 11.1. Mitochondria of the flight muscle of a dragon fly, showing profuse cristae.

In some cells, the mitochondria are concentrated in the peripheral cytoplasm or cytoplasm just beneath the plasma membrane as in *Paramecium*, pancreatic cells, cells of the Malpighian tubules of the insects and young spermatids of the rat. While in certain cells the mitochondria remain concentrated around the nucleus. During the cell division (mitosis and meiosis) the mitochondria get concentrated around the spindle.

11.4 ORIENTATION

The mitochondria have definite orientation. For example, in cylindrical cells the mitochondria usually remain orientated in basal apical direction and lie parallel to the main axis. In leucocytes, the mitochondria remain arranged radially with respect to the centrioles. The orientation of the mitochondria is said to depend on the nature of the cytoplasmic matrix, vacuolar system and the direction of the diffusion currents of the cell.

11.5 MORPHOLOGY

Number. The number of mitochondria in a cell depends on the type and functional state of the cell. It varies from cell to cell and from species to species. Certain cells contain exceptionally large number of the mitochondria, *e.g.*, the *Amoeba*, *Chaos chaos*, contain 50,000; eggs of sea urchin contain 140,000 to 150,000 and oocytes of amphibians contain 300,000 mitochondria. Certain cells, *viz.*, liver cells of rat contain only 500 to 1600 mitochondria. The cells of green plants contain less number of mitochondria in comparison to animal cells because in plant cells the function of mitochondria is taken over by the chloroplasts. Some algal cells may contain only one mitochondrion. However, red blood cells (erythrocytes) of mammals and other higher animals contain no mitochondria. Mature red blood cells obtain energy from glycolysis.

Shape

The mitochondria may be filamentous or granular in shape and may change from one form to another depending upon the physiological conditions of the cells. Thus, they may be of club, racket, vesicular, ring or round-shape.

Size

The size of the mitochondria may vary from cell to cell. The diameter of the mitochondria ranges from 0.2 μm to 2 μm and the length may range from 0.3 μm to 40 μm. The pancreatic cells of mammals contain mitochondria of 10 μm length and the oocytes of amphibian *Rana pipens* contain 20 to 40 μm long mitochondria.

11.6 STRUCTURE

The mitochondria are bounded by a double membrane envelope which provides good tensile strength, stability and flexibility to them. The outer and inner mitochondrial membranes are 60–70 A° thick and trilaminar fluid-mosaic in nature. Each of them is composed of an outer and inner dense, osmiophilic layer of protein molecules of 20 to 25 A° thickness and a middle 25 A° thick biomolecular layer of lipids. The two mitochondrial membranes are separated by an intermembrane space called **outer compartment** or **perimitochondrial space** of 60–80 A° width (**Tyler**, 1973).

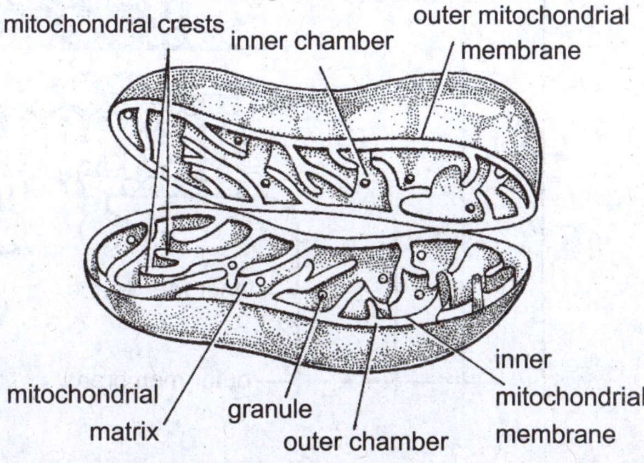

Fig. 11.2. Detailed structure of a typical mitochondrion.

The inner mitochondrial membrane lines the innermost compartment which remains filled with **matrix**. The mitochondrial matrix contains lipids, proteins, circular DNA molecules, 70S ribosomes and certain **granules** which are related to the ability of mitochondria to accumulate ions. Granules are prominent in the mitochondria of cells concerned with the transport of ions and water, including kidney, tubule cells, epithelial cells of the small intestine, and the osteoblasts of bone-forming cells. Further, the inner membrane has an outer **cytosol** or **C face** toward the perimitochondrial space and an inner **matrix** or **M face** toward matrix.

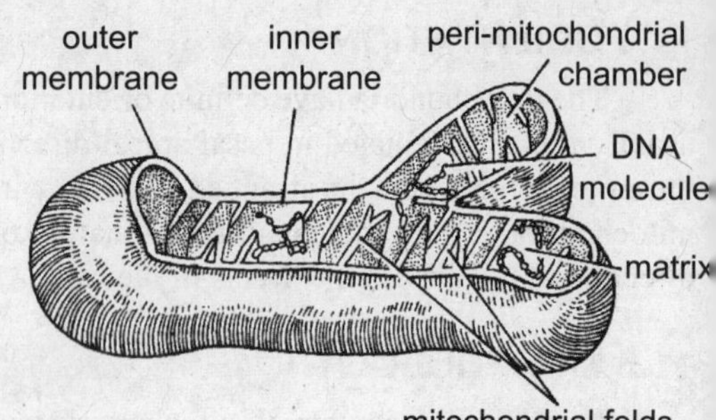

Fig. 11.3. A mitochondrion showing its various components and the position of DNA molecules inside it.

The inner mitochondrial membrane increases its surface area by giving out plate-like or tubular invagination called **mitochondrial crests** or **cristae mitochondriales**, which penetrate the mitochondrial matrix. In general, the cristae of plant mitochondria are tubular, while those of animal mitochondria are lamellar or plate-like (**Hall**, **Flowers** and **Roberts**, 1974), but, in many Protozoa and in steroid synthesizing tissues including the adernal cortex and corpus luteum, they occur as regularly packed tubules (**Tyler**, 1973). The space within the cristae which is continuous with the perimitochondrial space is known as **intracristal space**.

Inner membrane subunits or **elementary particles**. Under high resolving power of the electron microscope the inner membrane of the mitochondria appears to be studded with tennis-racket-like or mushroom-like projections pointing toward the mitochondrial matrix. Each projection is part of a respiratory assembly consisting of a cluster of membrane proteins, a 80–100 A° head piece (or inner membrane sphere) and a stalk some 30–40 A° in diameter. These projections are regularly placed at a distance of 100 A° and may be 10^4 to 10^5 in number in each mitochondrion and are known as **elementary particles**, **F_1 particles** or **inner membrane subunits**. Usually the inner membrane subunits occur in the thickness of inner mitochondrial membrane but in certain special conditions of mounting only these particles are coming out of the membrane.

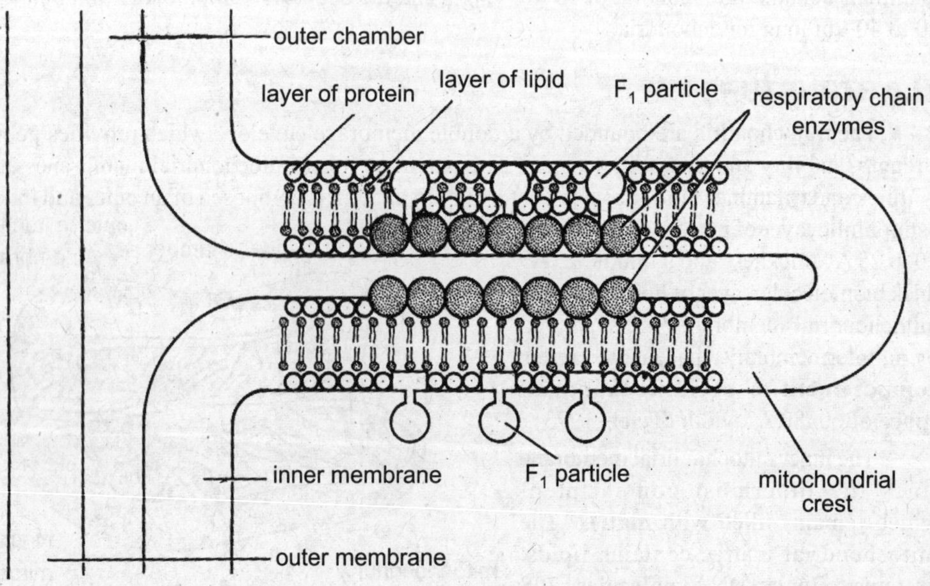

Fig. 11.4. Ultrastructure of a mitochondrial crest.

Previously the inner membrane subunits were thought to contain all the enzymes for electron transport system and for oxidative phosphorylation and, therefore, named as **electron transport particles** or **ETP** (**Parons**, 1963). But recently **Racker** (1967) has shown that the F_1 particles represent a special ATPase or ATPsynthetase and are involved in the process of oxidation and phosphorylation.

11.7 STRUCTURAL VARIATIONS

There exists great structural variability among the mitochondria from protozoans to mammals and from algae to angiosperms. The structural variations in the mitochondria take place usually due to the difference in number, size, shape and arrangement of **cristae** in the mitochondria which are as follows:

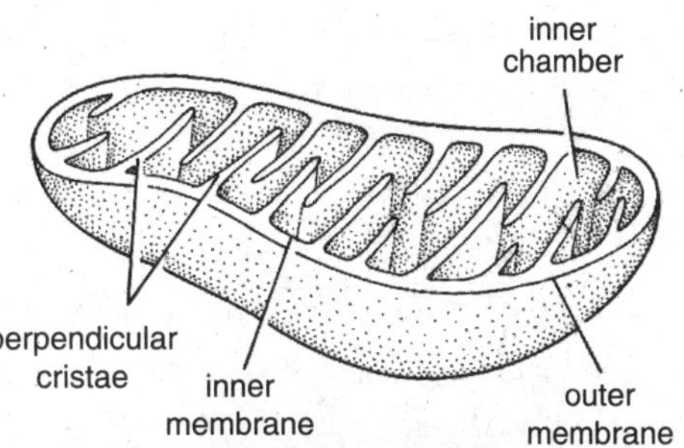

Fig. 11.5. Mitochondrion with perpendicular cristae.

1. Variation due to number of cristae. Among mitochondria of most animal and plant cells, the number of cristae per unit volume is variable. For example, the mitochondria of liver and germinal cells contain few cristae and great amount of the mitochondrial matrix, while the mitochondria of active cells such as kidney cells and muscle cells contain comparatively large number of cristae. Further, the mitochondria of the flight muscles of the insects contain greatest concentration of cristae in it. The number of cristae of the mitochondria seems to be correlated with its oxidative activity.

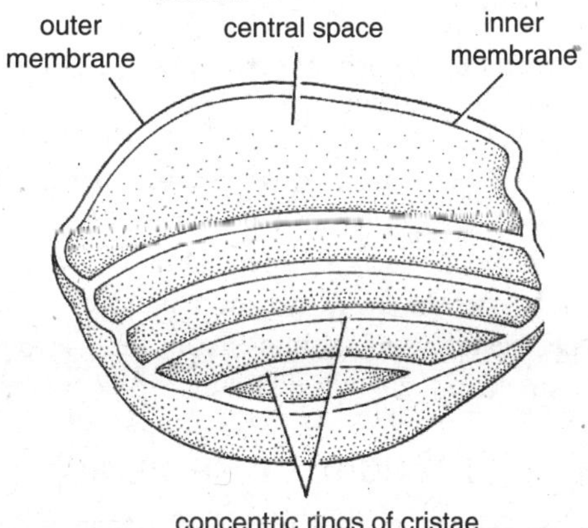

Fig. 11.6. Mitochondrion showing parallel cristae.

2. Variation due to the structure and arrangement of the cristae. Normally the cristae occur perpendicularly to the long axis of the mitochondria but various arrangements and shapes of cristae have been observed in the mitochondria of the different cells which are as follows:

(*i*) The mitochondrial cristae may be arranged longitudinal and parallel to the main axis of the mitochondria, *e.g.*, neurons and striated muscles (Fig. 11.6).

(*ii*) The mitochondrial cristae may be arranged in concentric rings which lie parallel to the main axis of the mitochondria, *e.g.*, spermatogonia of oppossum and humans.

(*iii*) The mitochondrial cristae may be small, branched and anastomosingly arranged in the mitochondria, *e.g.*, human leucocytes, parathyroid gland cells.

(*iv*) The mitochondrial cristae may be haphazardly distributed in the mitochondria, *e.g.*, *Chaos chaos*, the multinucleate amoeba (Fig. 11.7).

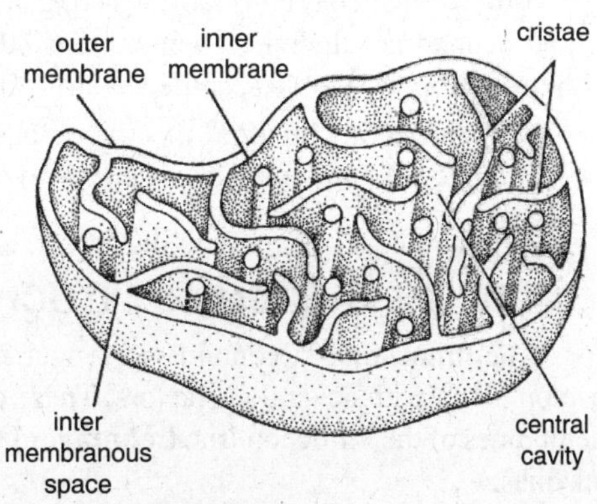

Fig. 11.7. Mitochondrion showing haphazardly distributed cristae.

(*v*) The mitochondrial cristae may be regular in shape instead of lamellar in shape and they may be arranged perpendicularly, *e.g.*, Protozoa

(*Paramecium*), flight muscles of insects (Fig. 11.5) and adrenal cells.

(*vi*) The mitochondrial cristae may be spherical in shape, *e.g.*, spermatocytes (Fig. 11.8).

(*vii*) The mitochondrial cristae may be extremely reduced and irregular, *e.g.*, interstitial cells of oppossum testis (Fig. 11.9).

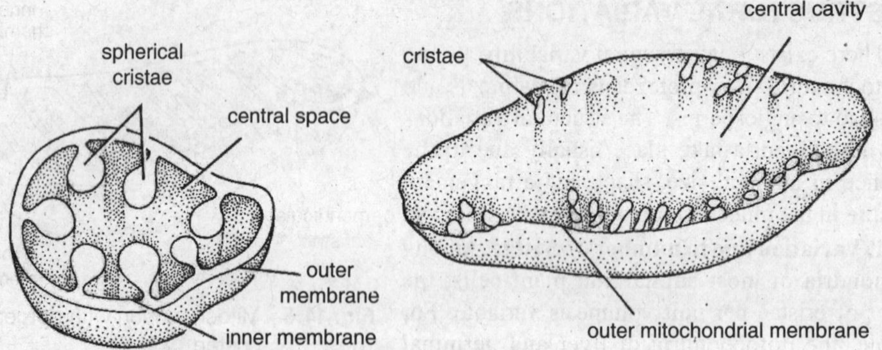

Fig. 11.8. Mitochondrion showing spherical cristae.

Fig. 11.9. Mitochondrion showing reduced cristae.

3. Variation due to the fusion. De Robertis (1957) has reported a peculiar type of behaviour in the mitochondria of spermatids of certain insects. In early spermatids all the mitochondria of the cytoplasm aggregate around the nucleus and all fuse together to form a single mitochondrial body.

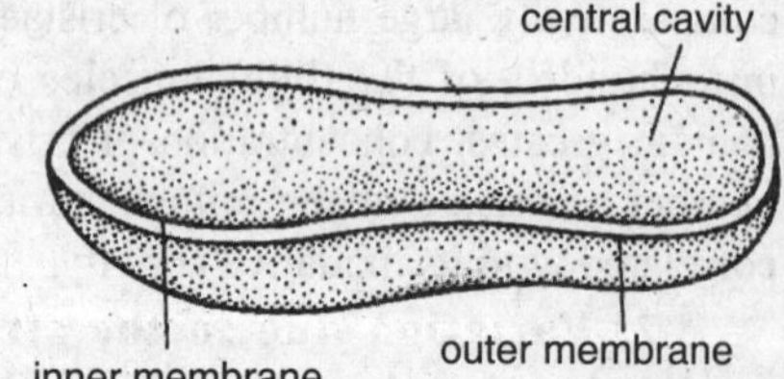

Fig. 11.10. Mitochondrion without cristae.

11.8 CHEMICAL COMPOSITION

The gross chemical composition of the mitochondria varies in different animal and plant cells. However, the mitochondria are found to contain 65 to 70 per cent proteins, 25 to 30 per cent lipids, 0.5 per cent RNA and small amount of the DNA. The lipid contents of the mitochondria are composed of 90 per cent phospholipids (lecithin and cephalin), 5 per cent or less cholesterol and 5 per cent free fatty acids and triglycerides. The inner mitochondrial membrane also contain phospholipids, the composition of which is unusual, consisting of about 20 per cent *cardiolipin*. In many cases (*e.g.*, liver cell mitochondria), the inner membrane is 80 per cent protein : most of the proteins are associated with respiratory assemblies, some are structural proteins.

The outer mitochondrial membrane has typical ratio of 50 per cent proteins and 50 per cent phospholipids of 'unit membrane'. However, it contains more unsaturated fatty acids and less cholesterol.

11.9 ENZYME SYSTEM OF MITOCHONDRIA

The mitochondria contain more than 70 enzymes and co-enzymes which act in an orderly fashion along with several co-factors. These enzymes are distributed in the matrix, outer and inner membranes of the mitochondria. **Lehninger** (1969) has tabulated following important mitochondrial enzymes:

A. The enzymes of outer mitochondrial membrane are monoamine oxidase, rotenone insensitive NADH-cytochrome-C-reductase, kynurenine hydroxyalase, and fattty acid CoA ligase.

B. The enzymes of outer mitochondrial chamber are adenylate kinase and nucleoside diphosphokinase.

C. The enzymes of inner mitochondrial membrane are the enzymes of electron transport pathways, *viz.*, nicotinamide adenine dinucleotide (NAD), flavin adenine dinucleotide (FAD), diphosphopyridine nucleotide (DPN) dehydrogenase, four cytochromes (Cyt. b, Cyt. c, Cyt. a and Cyt. a_3), ubiquinone Q_{10} or Coenzyme Q_{10}, non-heme copper and iron, succinic dehydrogenase, ATP synthetase, succinate dehydrogenase: β-hydroxybutyrate dehydrogenase; carnitive fatty acid acyl transferase.

D. The enzymes of the mitochondrial matrix are malate dehydrogenase, isocitrate dehydrogenase, fumarase, aconitase, citrate synthetase, α-keto acid dehydrogenase, β-oxidation enzymes. Moreover, the mitochondrial matrix contains different nucleotides, nucleotide coenzymes and inorganic electrolytes—K^+, HPO_4^-, Mg^{++}, Cl^- and SO_4^-.

11.10 FUNCTIONS

The mitochondria perform most important functions such as oxidation, dehydrogenation, oxidative phosphorylation and respiratory chain of the cell. Their structure and enzymatic system are fully adopted for their different functions. They are the actual respiratory organs of the cells where the foodstuffs *i.e.*, carbohydrates and fats are completely oxidised into CO_2 and H_2O. During the biological oxidation of the carbohydrates and fats large amount of energy is released which is utilized by the mitochondria for synthesis of the energy rich compound known as **adenosine triphosphate** or **ATP**. Because mitochondria synthesize energy rich compound ATP, they are also known as "**power houses**" of the cell.

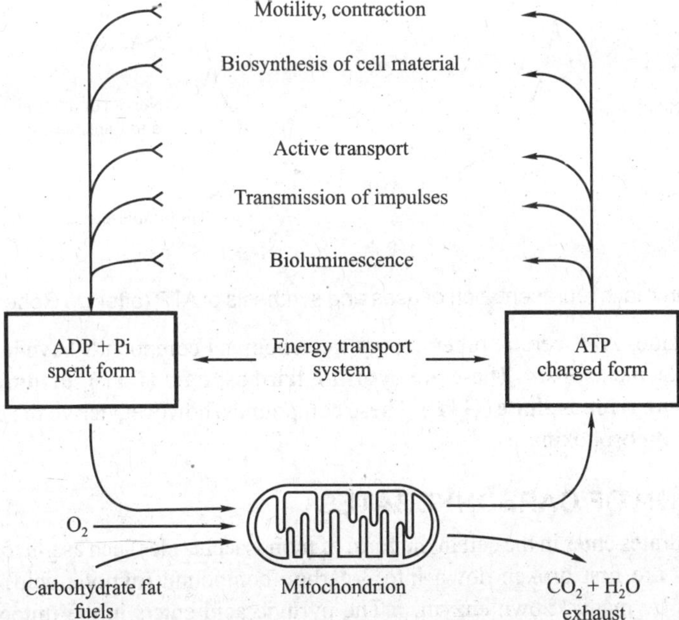

Fig. 11.11. Diagrammatic representation of the energy liberation in mitochondrion and its utilization in various cellular functions (after De Robertis *et al.*, 1970).

Adenosine tripbospbate or **ATP**. The ATP consists of a purine base **adenine**, a pentose sugar **ribose** and three molecules of the **phosphoric acids**. The adenine and ribose sugar collectively constitute the nucleoside **adenosine** which by having one, two or three phosphate groups forms the adenosine monophosphate (AMP), adenosine diphosphate (ADP) and adenosine triphosphate (ATP) respectively. In ATP the last phosphate group is linked with ADP by a special bond known as "**energy rich bond**" because when the last phosphate group of the ATP is released the large amount of energy is released as shown by the following reaction.

$$\underset{\text{(ATP)}}{A - P \sim P \sim P} = \underset{\text{ADP}}{AP \sim P} + \underset{\text{Phosphate group}}{P_1} + 7000 \text{ calories}$$

In the above reaction, we have seen that by the breaking of the energy rich bond about 7000 calories of energy is released, while the common chemical bond releases only 300 calories of energy. The chemical reactions which synthesize the energy rich bond or ~P bond require great amount of energy which is supplied by the oxidation of the food stuffs in the mitochondria. The utility of energy rich phosphate bond (~P) of the ATP is that great amount of energy is kept stored in the ready state in a very limited space of the cell. The stored chemical energy is disposed off very quickly at the time of the need in various cellular functions such as respiratory cycle, protein and nucleic acid synthesis, nervous transmission, cell division, transportation and bioluminescence, etc.

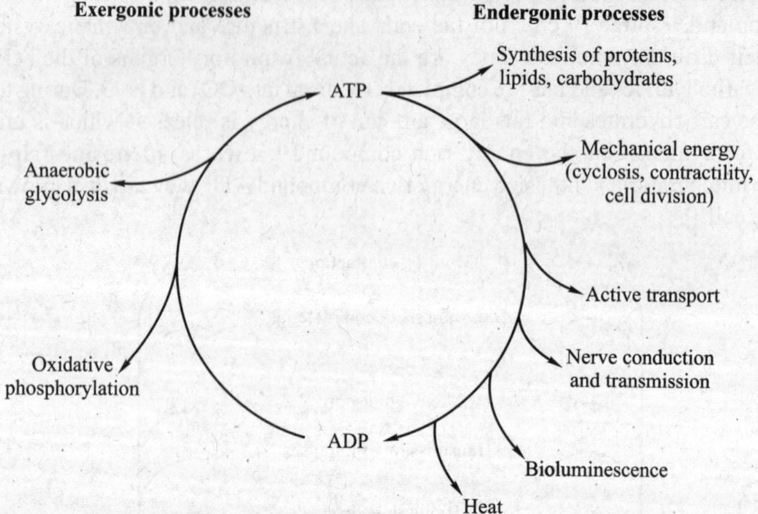

Fig. 11.12. Diagrammatic representation of uses and synthesis of ATP (after De Robertis *et al.*, 1970).

Recently, besides ATP, certain other energy rich chemical compounds have been found to be active in the cellular metabolism. These are **cytosine triphosphate (CTP), uridine triphosphate (UTP)** and **guanosine triphosphate (GTP)**. These compounds, however, derive the energy from the ATP by nucleoside diposphokinases.

11.11 OXIDATION OF CARBOHYDRATES

The carbohydrates enter in the cell in the form of monosaccharides such as glucose or glycogen. The hexose sugars are first broken down into 3-carbon compound (pyruvic acid) by a series of chemical reactions by many known enzymes. The pyruvic acid enters in the mitochondria for its complete oxidation into CO_2 and water. The reactions which involve in the oxidation of glucose in to known CO_2 and water are known to form the **metabolic pathways**. Metabolism includes two kinds of reactions anabolic and catabolic. Reactions that require energy and that result in the biosynthesis of needed compounds are called **anabolic**. Reactions that provide this energy at the expense of the degradation of food molecules are called **catabolic**. These catabolic reactions can be grouped under the following heads:

1. Glycolysis or Embden-Meyerhof pathways (EMP) or Embden-Meyerhof Parnas pathways (EMPP);
2. Oxidative decarboxylation;
3. Krebs cycle; citric acid cycle or tricarboxylic acid cycle;
4. Respiratory chain and oxidative phosphorylation.

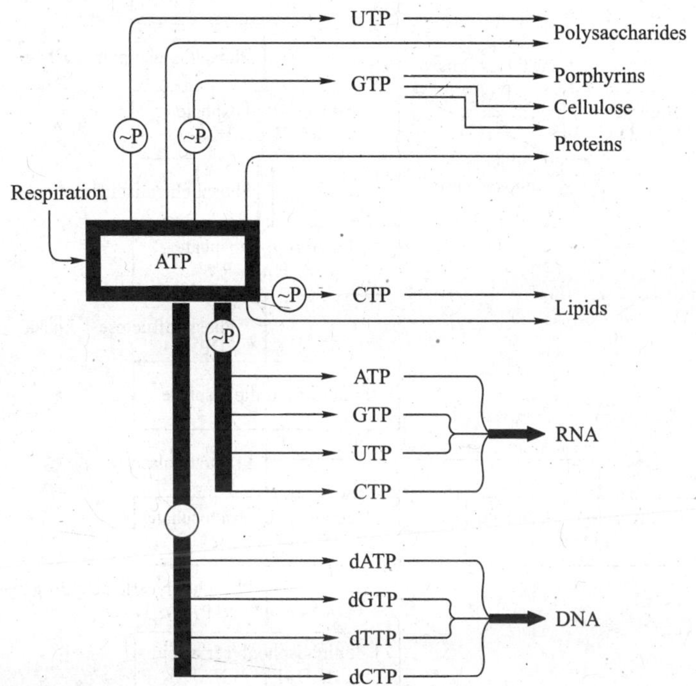

Fig. 11.13. Channelling of phosphate bond energy by ATP into specific biosynthetic routes of the cell (after De Robertis *et al.*, 1970).

(*i*) Glycolysis or Embden-Meyerhof Pathways

In the process of glycolysis (Gr., *glykys*-sweet, *lysis*-destroy) the six carbon chain glucose or glycogen molecule is hydrolysed into two molecules of 3 carbon chain pyruvic acid molecules. The hydrolysis of glucose takes place in various steps and each step is catalyzed by a specific enzyme. These steps have been worked out by two German biochemists, **Embden** and **Meyerbof** and, therefore, known as **Embden-Meyerhof pathways** after the name of its discoverers. The Embden-Meyerhof pathways takes place in the cytoplasm and it does not require any amount of oxygen. The various steps of anaerobic degradation or hydrolysis of glucose have been shown in the Fig. 11.14.

Thus, during the Embden-Meyerhof pathways the glucose molecule is broken into molecules of pyruvic acid and it releases the energy which is sufficient to synthesize two molecules of ATP. The pyruvic acid is either converted into ethyl alcohol or lactic acid in anaerobic cells such as yeast and muscle cells or enter in the mitochondria of the aerobic cells and oxidized into CO_2 and water. The conversion of pyruvic acid into ethyl alcohol or lactic acid in the yeast and muscle cells have been shown by following reactions:

(In yeast cells) Pyruvic acid $\xrightarrow{-CO_2}$ Acetaldehyde $\rightarrow$ Ethyl alcohol + Energy

(In muscle cells) Pyruvic acid $\xrightarrow[\text{+NADH}]{\text{Lactic dehydrogenase}}$ Lactic acid + NAD + Energy

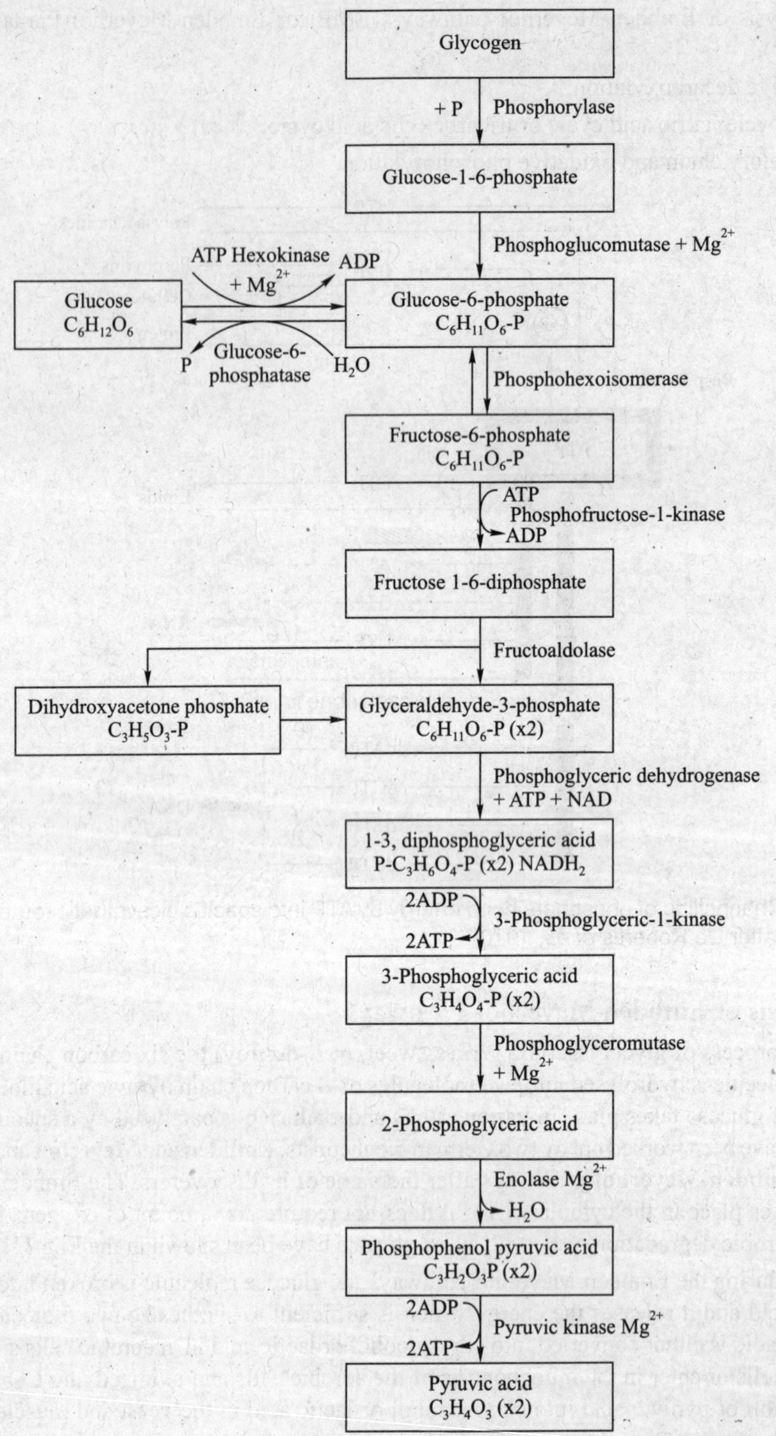

Fig. 11.14. Glycolysis or Embden-Meyerhof pathway showing the step-wise degradation of glucose to pyruvic acid.

(*ii*) Oxidative Decarboxylation

In the aerobic cells the pyruvic acid enters in the mitochondria where it is converted into acetyl coenzyme. The over all reaction in which both molecules of pyruvic acid are converted into two molecules of acetyl coenzyme is called **oxidative decarboxylation** since, it involves both oxidation and loss of carboxyl group as CO_2, of pyruvic acid. The oxidative decarboxylation process involves a complex system of three enzymes, *viz.*, pyruvic acid decarboxylase, dihydroxylipoyl transacetylase, and dihydroxylipoyl dehydrogenase and five co-factors- coenzyme A, NAD, lipoic acid, Mg^{++}, and thiamine pyrophosphate. Acetyl CoA is formed as the acetyl moiety of pyruvic acid, is transferred to coenzyme A; concomitantly, the carbon of the carboxyl group is liberated as carbon dioxide. Two hydrogen atoms remain; one from the pyruvate carboxyl group and other from the sulphhydryl coenzyme A. These hydrogen molecules are transferred to NAD. The reactions of oxidative decarboxylation have been shown in Fig. 11.15.

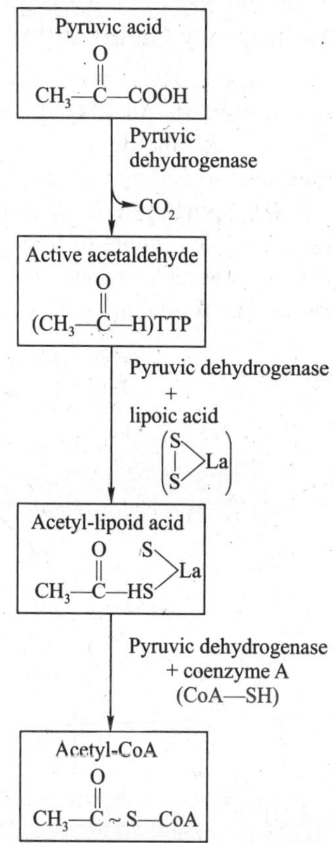

Fig. 11.15. The oxidative decarboxylation of pyrurvic acid to acetyl coenzyme A.

(*iii*) Krebs Cycle

The acetyl coenzyme A enters in a cycle of biochemical reactions in the course of which it is degraded to CO_2 and water and one molecule or flavoprotein (FAD) and three molecules of nicotinamide adenine dinucleotide (NAD) are reduced. This cycle is called **Krebs cycle** after the name of it discoverer **Sir Hans Krebs** (1837). It is called cycle because citrate or citric acid which is the nominal starting point of reaction, is produced again at the end of the pathway from oxaloacetate, utilizing acetyl CoA. The Krebs cycle occurs in the mitochondrial matrix and it is also known as **citric acid cycle** or **tricarboxylic acid cycle** and involves many enzymes and coenzymes. The Krebs cycle first begins to turn properly when the acetyl CoA gives its acetyl group to oxaloacetic acid to form citric acid. Citrate synthetase catalyzes this reaction which is also called condensing enzyme. The citric acid passes through various stages involving a variety of enzymes and coenzymes and ultimately oxidised into oxaloacetate as shown in the Fig. 11.16.

The structure of mitochondria is most important in relation to their function. Glycolysis takes place in the cell cytoplasm because the product of one reaction merely needs to be passed on to the next enzyme. Glycolysis can equally well occur in the test tube. But an examination of Krebs cycle shows that it leads to gross production of NADH and succinate $—OOC—CH_2—CH_2—COO^-$. The molecules of NADH and succinate are small and in a reduced state and these must be protected from the oxidative conditions in the cytoplasm. So these molecule pass through the space between the two mitochondrial membrane to reach the F_1 particles which carry out respiration. The compartment between the two mitochondrial membranes is, therefore, in a reduced state and large potential difference exists between this space and the cell cytoplasm. This can only be maintained by protective action of the lipid membranes. Because the series of reactions is a cyclic process there are clear advantages in having an organized group of enzymes in which the products can be passed from one enzyme to another. This is achieved in the outer mitochondrial membrane.

(*iv*) Respiratory Chain and Oxidative Phosphorylation

During the oxidation of one molecule of acetyl coenzyme A by the Krebs cycle occurring in the mitochondrial matrix, one molecule of flavoprotein (FP or FAD) and three molecules of nicotinamide adenine dinucleotide (NAD) are reduced. These reduced coenzymes are oxidized by molecular oxygen by way of a system of enzymes and coenzymes called **respiratory chain** or **electron transport system** occurring in the inner mitochondrial membrane. During this, oxidation process enormous amount of free energy is released, some of which is utilized by inner membrane subunits or F_1 particles containing three **coupling factors** ATPase enzyme, in the synthesis of ATP molecules. The formation of ATP molecules during oxidation is called **oxidative phosphorylation**.

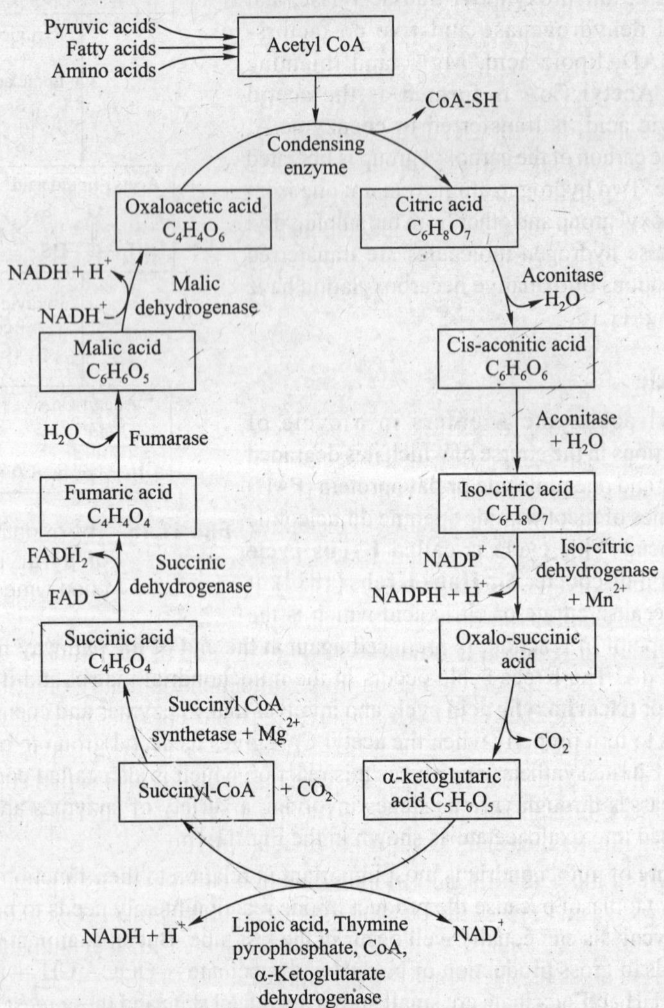

Fig. 11.16. Krebs cycle or tricarboxylic acid cycle.

According to the widely accepted **chemi-osmotic hypothesis** of oxidative phosphorylation of **Mitchell** (1968), various components of respiratory chain or electron transport system are arranged in the inner mitochondrial membrane in the following sequence—succinic dehydrogenase (SOH) which remain associated with coenzyme NAD; flavoprotein (FP or FAD), non-haem iron protein or iron-sulphur protein, flavoprotein (FP or FAD), cytochrome b, ubiquinone or coenzyme Q_{10}, cytochrome c_1, cytochrome c, cytochromé a, cytochrome a_3 and three coupling sites (the sites where phosphorylation is coupled oxidation in the presence of ATPase enzyme, **Hall** *et al.*, 1974). The respiratory chain manufactures the ATP molecules during the oxidation of reduced coenzymes in the following steps:

1. The dehydrogenase enzyme removes the hydrogen from the substrate. The hydrogen atom becomes ionized into protons (+) and electrons (e^-):

$$2H \rightarrow \underset{\text{Protons}}{2H^+} + \underset{\text{Electrons}}{2e}$$

The protons or hydrogen ions reduce the coenzyme NAD:

$$NAD + 2H^+ \rightarrow NADH + H^+$$

The NADH molecule passes through the M-side of inner mitochondrial membrane and enters in the respiratory chain system.

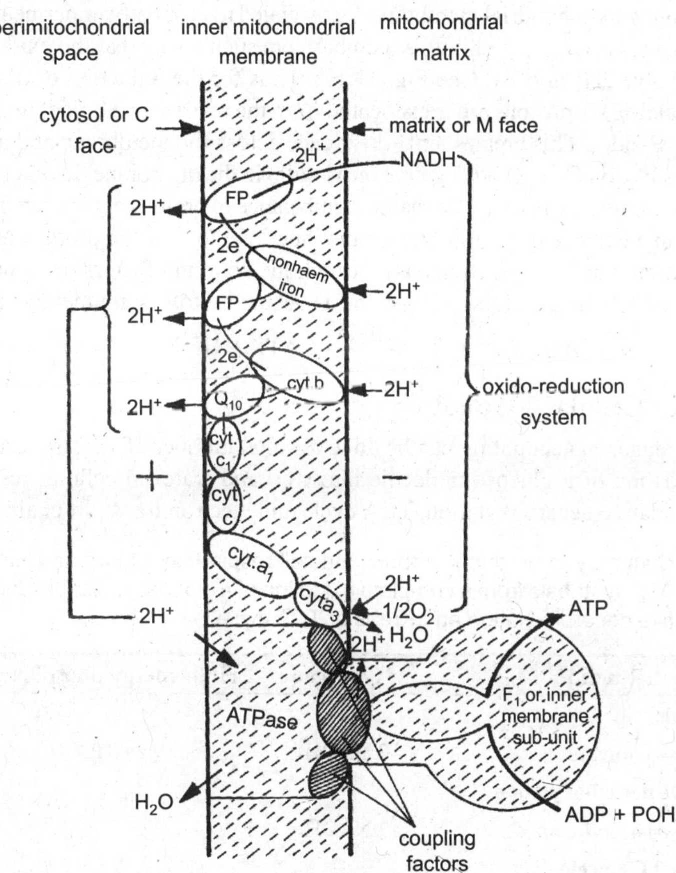

Fig. 11.17. Diagram showing the possible arrangement of respiratory chain enzymes and coenzymes in the inner mitochondrial membrane according to the chemi-osmotic hypothesis of oxidative phosphorylation and process of oxidative phosphorylation [Mitchell (1968) and Racker (1972)].

2. The NADH is oxidized into NAD^+ by transferring its proton (hydrogen ion) to the flavoprotein (FP or FAD) which act as a hydrogen carrier. From the flavoproteins each proton or hydrogen ion is discharged into perimitochondrial space through the C-side of inner mitochondrial membrane and electrons are passed on to non-haem iron protein, from which they cycle through different components of respiratory chain and ultimately form the water molecules.

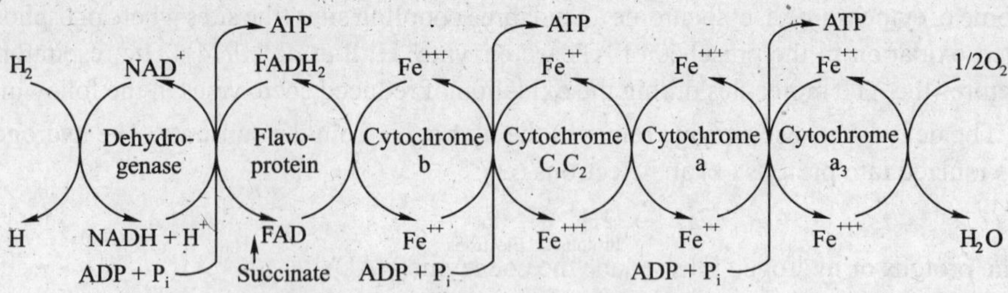

Fig. 11.18. Diagram showing cycle of electrons through respiratory chain and synthesis of ATP molecules, (A) is oxidized substrate.

3. The inner mitochondrial membrane is postulated to be mostly impermeable to protons and the respiratory chain is arranged within this membrane in such a way that the oxido-reduction reactions alternately involve $2H^+$ and $2e^-$ (see Fig. 11.17). Thus for the reduction of one atom of oxygen by malic acid (malate), six protons are translocated from the matrix (or M-side) to the perimitochondrial space side (or C-side). This creates a pH difference across the membrane and an electrical potential difference (positive on C-side and negative on M-side) in the membrane. In other words, when protons or electrons pass down the respiratory chain, an imbalance of protons occurs across the inner membrane and to maintain a balance of protons across the ihner membrane, the protons tend to return towards the mitochondrial matrix, they often pass through the coupling factors or F_1 particles. During their passage through coupling factors, ATP synthesis occurs by following method:

$$\text{ADP} + \text{POH} \xrightarrow{\text{ATPase}} \text{ATP} + \text{H}^+$$

Energetics of Cellular Respiration

At this stage, an accounting can be done for total number of ATP molecules produced during complete oxidation of a glucose molecule into CO_2 and water in cellular respiration (*i.e.*, during glycolysis, oxidative decarboxylation, TCA cycle and electron transport chain (See Table 11.1).

Table 11.1. Summary of products produced in cell respiration and an accounting of net amount of ATP synthesis from a complete oxidation of a glucose molecule during glycolysis, oxidative decarboxylation and Krebs or TCA cycle.

Reaction	Hydrogen	High-energy phosphate	Carbon dioxide
1. **Glycolysis**			
glucose → pyruvate	2 $NADH_2$	2 ATP	
2. **Oxidative decarboxylation**			
pyruvate → acetyl-CoA	2 $NADH_2$		2 CO_2
3. **Krebs or TCA cycle**			
isocitrate → α-ketoglutarate	2 $NADH_2$		2 CO_2
α-ketoglutarate → succinate	2 $NADH_2$	2 GTP	2 CO_2
succinate → fumarate	2 $FADH_2$		
malate → oxaloacetate	2 $NADH_2$		
	10 H_2 or 12 $NADH_2$ 2 $FADH_2$	4 ~ P	6 CO_2

(i) Since a single $NADH_2$ produces three ATP molecules by passing through the electron transport chain, so that a total of $10 \times 3 = 30$ ATP molecules are produced by 10 $NADH_2$.

(ii) Since a single $FADH_2$ produces two ATP molecules by passing through the electron transport chain, so a total of $2 \times 2 = 4$ ATP molecules are produced by 2 $FADH_2$.

(iii) 2 GTP molecules may be used directly in many reactions or are use to phosphorylate 2 ADP via a mixed nucleotide kinase:

$$2\,GTP + 2\,ADP \rightleftharpoons 2\,ATP + 2\,GDP$$

Thus, in total 30 + 4 + 4 = 38 ATP molecules are produced from complete oxidation of a glucose molecule into CO_2 and H_2O, such as is summarized in following reaction:

$$C_6H_{12}O_6 + 6H_2O + 38ADP + 38Pi \xrightarrow[\text{enzymes}]{\text{respiratory}} 6CO_2 + 12H_2O + 38ATP$$

We can estimate the efficiency of this respiratory process in capturing the energy released from glucose: 1 mole of glucose (180 grams) will release about 690,000 calories when it is oxidized completely to CO_2 and H_2O. Knowing that it requires roughly 10,000 calories (10 Kcal.) to form the high-energy phosphate bond in one mole of ATP, we can calculate that 38 moles of ATP will trap 380,000 calories or approximately 45 per cent of the total released energy from the glucose. The other 55 per cent of the energy is released immediately as heat.

Functional Organization of Mitochondrion

What is the arrangement of the more than 70 enzymes, co-enzymes and cofactors within the mitochondria to provide for the organized production of ATP molecules for cellular metabolism? This question has been partially answered by recent cytological and biochemical investigations. Now, the mitochondrion is seen as a **compartmentalized system**: specific enzymes are located within the outer membrane, others are located within the inner membrane and still others are restricted to the fluid space between the outer and inner membranes or are located within the central matrix of the organelle. Moreover, there is considerable evidence that the enzymes within these areas are organized in particular regions and in particular patterns.

The matrix of the mitochondrion contains all the enzymes of Krebs or TCA cycle. Also the enzymes for the oxidation of fatty acids (β-oxidation) are localized; in the inner compartment as well as are DNA, ribosomes, and RNA necessary for protein synthesis. Substrates to be used by the TCA cycle must pass from the cytoplasm through the mitochondrial membranes and spaces to reach the matrix before they are oxidized. End products of metabolism must pass out in the reverse direction.

On the inner membrane are located both the cytochrome system, the dehydrogenase enzymes which remove hydrogen from TCA substrates, and the enzymes involved in ATP production. The latter molecules are bound to F_1 particles.

11.12 OXIDATION OF FATS

Although carbohydrates are the major energy source for immediate use in the cell, fats are extremely important as an energy reserve. The energy in a gram of fat is more than twice that of a gram of starch; consequently, lipids are a convenient form of energy storage. Hibernating, migrating, or starving animals depend almost totally upon fats for energy. Fats can be stored in cells in a precipitated form, usually as fat droplets, and do not require water for their solution.

Fat molecules in cells are primarily neutral fats (triglycerides) or their products. A neutral fat consists of a glycerol molecule connected to three fatty acids. Lipase enzymes within the cell split the three fatty acids away from glycerol with the introduction of three water molecules, similar to the hydrolysis reaction occurring during digestion of fats in the small intestine. Glycerol and fatty acids are oxidized by different routes such as follows:

Glycerol is a 3-carbon compound and by addition of a phosphate from ATP and the removal of two hydrogens by NAD it is readily converted to dihydroxyacetone phosphate (DHAP):

$$\text{Glycerol} \xrightarrow[\text{NAD}\rightarrow\text{NADH}_2]{\text{ATP}\rightarrow\text{ADP(H)}} \text{Dihydroxyacetone phosphate (DHAP)}$$

Figure 11.14, shows that this DHAP is routinely converted into 3-phosphoglyceraldehyde. when it enters the mainstream of glycolytic pathway. Complete oxidation of one glycerol molecule produces a net gain of 22 ATP molecules.

Most fatty acids in cells have an even number of carbons (commonly 16 or 18) joined in a chain. The fatty acid molecules of various types are oxidized in a similar manner. In general, coenzyme A attaches to the carboxyl end of the fatty acid. This costs one ATP molecule. In a series of reactions where water is added, four hydrogen atoms are removed (two by NAD and two by FAD) from the two carbon atoms nearest to CoA. The 2-carbon fragment with CoA attachcd is split away from the rest of the fatty acid as another coenzyme A is introduced to the new end of the fatty acid. The resulting 2-carbon unit is acetyl-CoA. In a similar way other 2-carbon segments are chopped off the fatty acid, becoming acetyl-CoA (Fig. 11.19). The resultant acetyl-CoA molecules enter the Krebs cycle or TCA cycle for complete oxidation (Fig. 11.16). The process of fatty acid oxidation is called **beta oxidation**, because the fatty acid is progressively severed at the second or beta carbon. Beta oxidation occurs within the cytoplasm of the cell and the acetyl-CoA molecules are transported across the mitochondrial membranes into the matrix where the oxidative process continues.

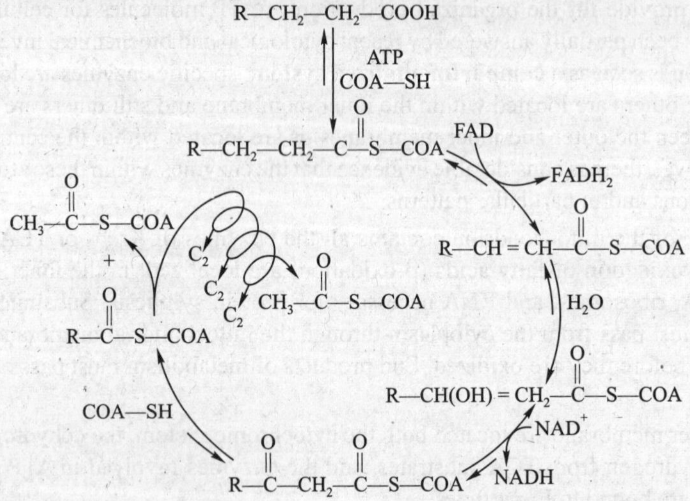

R—CH_2—CH_2—COOH
ATP
COA—SH
R—CH_2—CH_2—C(=O)—S—COA
FAD
$FADH_2$
R—CH = CH—C(=O)—S—COA
H_2O
R—CH(OH) = CH_2—C(=O)—S—COA
NAD^+
NADH
R—C(=O)—CH_2—C(=O)—S—COA
COA—SH
CH_3—C(=O)—S—COA
+
R—C(=O)—S—COA
C_2
C_2
C_2
C_2
CH_3—C(=O)—S—COA

Fig. 11.19. The oxidation of fatty acids by the β-oxidation helical scheme.

To calculate the energy derived from the total oxidation of a fatty acid, one must know the structure of the molecule. Suppose that the fatty acid had 18 carbons; the β-oxidation would cost an initial ATP molecule but would produce 9 acetyl-CoA molecules and 16 hydrogen pairs attached to coenzymes. The 9 acetyl-CoA molecules passing through the Krebs cycle would produce 12 ATP molecules each, for a total of 108 ATPs. Passage of 16 H_2 through the cytochrome system would yield 40 ATPs: 8 pairs would be handled via NAD and give 3 ATP molecules per hydrogen pair ($8 \times 3 = 24$ ATP) and 8 pairs would be handled via FAD and give 2 ATP molecules per hydrogen pair ($8 \times 2 = 16$ ATP). Thus adding 108 ATP from the oxidation of acetyl-CoA to 40 ATP generated by the passage of H_2 via the cytochrome system and substracting the initial ATP used in the first phosphorylation, we find that 147 ATP are produced for one 18-carbon fatty acid. Considering that each neutral fat has three such fatty acids along with one glycerol, we can estimate that 463 molecules of ATP are developed per triglyceride. This is over 12 times as much energy as that produced from one molecule of glucose. However, since the fat is a considerably larger molecule than glucose; energetic comparison is best based on the number of ATPs resulting per gram of nutrient "burned". On this basis, fat produces more than twice as many ATP molecules as the same weight of starch.

11.13 OXIDATION OF PROTEINS

Proteins are not stored within the cell in significant quantities. Those proteins present are either in the form of enzymes or an integral part of the cellular structure such as in the cell membrane. Therefore, proteins are not typically broken down and used as an energy source except in cases of starvation. Catabolism of proteins is also required for other cellular activities.

Before proteins can be introduced into the mainstream of metabolism (catabolism) they must be split into amino acids. The process is accomplished by protease enzymes similar to the process occurs in digestion. Each peptide bond is severed with the introduction of a water molecule, a hydrolytic reaction. Next, nitrogen is removed from amino acids by anyone following two processes: oxidative deamination and transamination.

During **oxidative deamination**, the amino group of the amino acid is split off from the rest of the molecule, forming ammonia (NH_3). The remainder of the amino acid then enters the main metabolic stream as a keto acid. Water is required for this process and two hydrogens are removed by coenzyme NAD. The ammonia formed during deamination may be immediately excreted or organized into another molecule before excretion; for example, in human beings the ammonia is converted into urea molecules by the liver cells before being sent via the blood to the kidney. The energy derived from oxidative deamination depends upon the amino acid involved. For example, oxidative deamination of glutamic acid involves its conversion into α-ketoglutaric acid, which is oxidized by the Krebs cycle:

$$\underset{\text{(amino acid)}}{\text{Glutamic acid}} \xrightarrow[\swarrow H_2O \qquad \searrow NH_3]{NAD \rightarrow NADH_2} \underset{\text{(keto acid)}}{\alpha\text{-ketoglutaric acid}}$$

In this case, high-energy phosphates would be created by the transfer of hydrogen from $NADH_2$ (formed in deamination) through the cytochrome system.

Transamination reaction consists of an amino group being shifted from one molecule to another in exchange for an oxygen. For example, due to transamination amino acid glutamic acid being converted into α-ketoglutaric acid, as is shown by following reaction:

$$\underset{\text{(amino acid)}}{\text{Glutamic acid}} + \underset{\text{(keto acid)}}{\text{Oxaloacetic acid}} \rightarrow \underset{\text{(keto acid)}}{\alpha\text{-ketoglutaric acid}} + \underset{\text{(amino acid)}}{\text{aspartic acid}}$$

In this case, the amino group is not lost completely but is transferred to one of the substrate of Krebs cycle. Oxaloacetic acid loses its oxygen and picks up the NH_2 group and becomes the amino acid, aspartic acid. Thus one amino acid is converted into keto acid while another keto acid is transformed into an amino acid. The usual purpose of such reactions is to maintain a particular balance among amino acids and substrates rather than providing grist for the metabolic mill.

Further, amino acids have different structures, and they are fed into the main metabolic pathway at different points depending upon the number of carbons they possess. Amino acids with three carbons (*e.g.*, serine, cysteine, alanine, valine) are converted into 3-carbon pyruvic acid or pyruvate. The 2-carbon amino acid glycine is converted to acetyl-CoA; the 5-carbon glutamic acid is transformed into α-ketoglutaric acid; the 4-carbon aspartic acid is converted to oxaloacetic acid, and so on.

11.14 OTHER FUNCTIONS OF MITOCHONDRIA

Besides the ATP productions, mitochondria serve the following important functions in animals:

1. Heat production or thermiogenesis. As we have already discussed earlier that only 45 per cent of the energy released during the oxidation of glucose is captured in the form of ATP, the rest 55 per cent is either lost as heat or used to regulate body temperature of warm-blooded animals. In some mammals, especially young animals and hibernating species, there is a specialized tissue called **brown fat**. This tissue, typically located between the shoulder blades, is especially important in temperature regulation; it produces large quantities of body heat necessary for arousal from hibernation.

The colour of brown fat comes from its high concentration of mitochondria, which are sparse in ordinary fat cells. The mitochondria appear to catalyze electron transport in the usual way but are much less efficient at producing ATP. Hence, a higher than usual fraction of the oxidatively released energy is converted directly to heat (called **non-shivering thermiogenesis**). Measurements made on isolated mitochondria from these cells reveal a relatively leaky inner membrane. Thus much of the electrochemical gradient produced by electron transport is dissipated without generating ATP—the mitochondria are uncoupled.

2. Biosynthetic or anabolic activities. Mitochondria also perform certain biosynthetic or anabolic functions. Mitochondria contain DNA and the machinery needed for protein synthesis. Therefore they can make less than a dozen different proteins. The proteins so far identified are subunits of the ATPase, portions of the reductase responsible for transfer of electrons from CoQ to the iron of Cyt C, and three of the seven subunits in cytochrome oxidase. Altogether, no more than 5–10 per cent of mitochondrial components can be attributed to mitochondrial genes. The majority of mitochondrial components are specified by nuclear genes and transported to the mitochondrion after synthesis.

Some biosynthetic functions of mitochondria are of primary benefit to the rest of the cell. For example, the synthesis of **haeme** (needed for cytochromes, myoglobin and haemoglobin) begins with a mitochondrial reaction catalyzed by the enzyme, delta or δ-aminolevulinic acid synthetase. Likewise, some of the early steps in the conversion of cholesterol to steroid hormones in the adrenal cortex are also catalyzed by mitochondrial enzymes. The tubulovesicular cristae of these mitochondria resemble the smooth ER and contain many enzymes of steroid pathway.

3. Transport properties. The outer mitochondrial membrane is relatively permeable to a variety of substances. However, the inner mitochondrial membrane is impermeable to all but selected metabolites. It contains transport systems to control passage in and out. ADP and ATP, for example, are exchanged one for the other by a specific carrier. There is also a phosphate-hydroxyl exchange (the **glycerol-phosphate shuttle**) and additional carriers for certain of the carboxylic acids (**malate shuttle**). Besides these **facilitated diffusion** transport systems, mitochondria have many active transport systems, mostly driven by electrochemical gradients. The most important is **calcium pump**. Ca^{2+} uptake by mitochondria can occur against significant gradients and at the expense of electron transport. In fact, active transport of Ca^{2+} suppresses ADP phosphorylation.

Mitochondria of animal cells can accumulate very large amounts of Ca^{2+} and can store it in part as a calcium phosphate gel. Most of the Ca^{2+} in a typical cell is sequestered in this way and can be released in response apropriate stimuli.

11.15 MITOCHONDRIAL DNA AND RIBOSOMES

The mitochondria contain one or two molecule s of DNA according to its size. The mitochondrial DNA molecule is highly twisted, double-stranded and circular in snape. The length of mitochondrial DNA molecule has been measured as 5 μm and it resembles with the bacterial DNA which also contains circular molecules. Mitochondrial DNA, besides its circular shape, differs from the nuclear DNA in many respects. **Rabinowitch** (1968) has shown that the mitochondrial DNA contains more guanine and cytosine (GC) contents than the nuclear DNA. The mitochondrial DNA is shorter than the nuclear DNA, therefore, cotains few coded informations.

The mitochondrial DNA behaves like a chromosome and duplicates in the usual manner. **Parson** and **Simpson** (1967) have shown that the mitochondria contain the enzyme **DNA polymerase** which helps in the duplication of mitochondrial DNA themselves. Due to DNA molecule the mitochondria are capable to undergo self-reproduction by the division and they may carry biological informations to exhibit a type of cytoplasmic inheritance.

The mitochondria also contain small-sized 55S ribosomes similar to the bacteria in their matrix and they are called mitoribosomes. The mitochondria thus contain several components required for protein synthesis, including DNA, DNA-dependent RNA polymerase, RNA, ribosomes and amino acid-activating enzymes (**Ashwell** and **Work**, 1970).

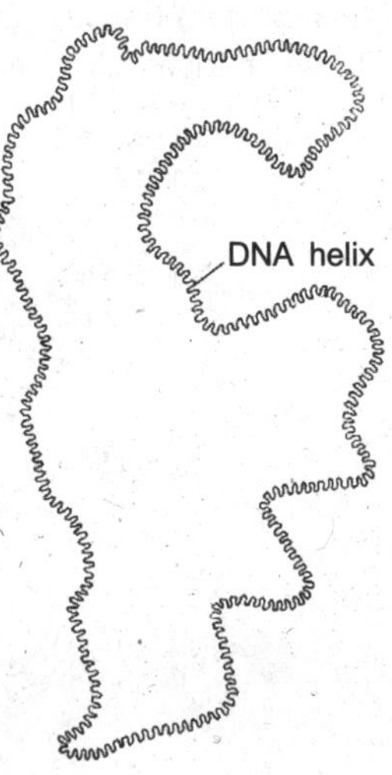

Fig. 11.20. Mitochondrial DNA molecule.

11.16 ORIGIN OR BIOGENESIS OF MITOCHONDRIA

Regarding the origin of the mitochondria, several hypotheses have been postulated which are as follows:

1. "de novo" origin.
2. Origin from the endoplasmic reticulum or plasma membrane.
3. Origin by division of pre-existing mitochondria.
4. Prokaryotic origin.

1. "de novo" origin. According to this hypothesis, the mitochondria are originated "de novo" (L. anew) from the simple building blocks such as amino acids and lipids. But, there is no direct evidence in support of "de novo" hypothesis for the origin of the mitochondria, therefore, it is discarded now.

2. Origin from the endoplasmic reticulum or plasma membrane. According to **Morrison** (1966) the new mitochondria might have been originated from the endoplasmic reticulum or plasma membrane. This hypothesis also could not provide direct evidences, therefore, it is not well accepted at present time.

3. Origin by division of pre-existing mitochondria. The electron microscopic and radio autographic observations of the culture cells have shown clearly that the new mitochondria are originated by the division of the pre-existing mitochondria. It has been observed that the mitochondria sometimes become elongated and fragmented into small pieces. Each fragment forms a new mitochondria in later stages. Moreover, during the cell division, the mitochondrion divides transversely into two and each daughter mitochondrion develops into a mature mitochondrion.

4. Prokaryotic origin or symbiont hypothesis. Early cytologists such as **Altmann** and **Schimber** (1890) have suggested the possibility of origin of the mitochondria from the prokaryotic cells. According to their hypothesis. the mitochondria and chloroplasts may be considered as intra-cellular parasites of the cells which have entered in the cytoplasm of eukaryotic cells in early evolutionary days, and have maintained the symbiotic relations with the eukaryotic cells. The mitochondria are supposed to be derived from the bacterial cells, while chloroplasts are supposed to be originated from the blue green algae. Due to these reasons **Altmann** suggested the name "**bio-blast**" to the mitochondria and he also hinted about their self-duplicating nature.

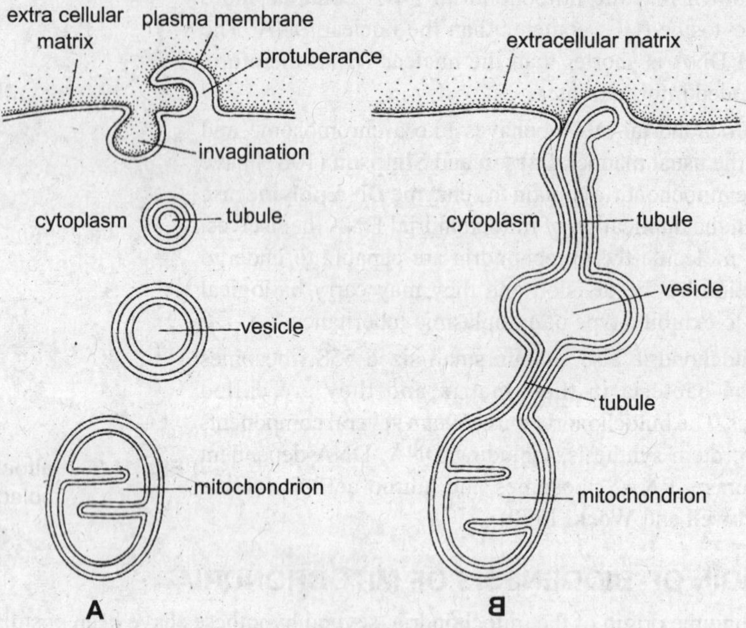

Fig. 11.21. Hypothetical diagrams showing the origin of mitochondria from plasma membrane.

Recent cytological findings have also suggested many homologies between the mitochondria and the bacterial cells. The similarities between the two can be summarised as follows:

1. Similarity in inner mitochondrial membrane and bacterial plasma membrane. (*i*) In the mitochondria the enzymes of the respiratory chain are localized on the inner mitochondrial membrane like the bacteria in which they remain localized in the plasma membrane. The bacterial plasma membrane resembles with the inner mitochondrial membrane in certain respects.

(*ii*) The plasma membrane of certain bacterial cells gives out finger-like projections in the cytoplasm known as mesosomes. The mesosomes can be compared with mitochondria crests. **Salton** (1962) has reported respiratory chain enzymes in the mesosomes.

(*iii*) Because the outer mitochondrial membrane resembles with the plasma membrane, therefore, it may be assumed that the mitochondrial matrix and the inner mitochondrial membrane represent the symbiont which might be enclosed by the membrane of the cellular origin (outer mitochondrial membrane).

2. Similarity in DNA molecule. The DNA molecule of the mitochondria is circular like the DNA molecule of the bacterial cells. Further the replication process of the mitochondrial DNA is also similar to bacterial DNA.

3. Similarity in ribosomes. The mitochondrial ribosomes are small in size and resemble the ribosomes of the bacteria.

4. Similarity in the process of protein synthesis. The process of protein synthesis of both mitochondria and bacteria is fundamentally same because in both, the process of protein synthesis can be inhibited by same inhibitor known as chloramphenicol.

Further, the mitochondria for the process of protein synthesis depend partially on the mitochondrial matrix and DNA and partially on the nucleus and cytoplasm of the eukaryotic cells. This shows the symbiotic nature of the mitochondria.

Due to the above mentioned similarities between the bacteria and mitochondria, the symbiont hypothesis postulated that the host cell (eukaryotic cell) represented an anaerobic organism which derived the required energy from the oxidations of food by the process of glycolysis. While the mitochondria represent the symbionts which respire **aerobically** and contain the enzymes of **Krebs cycle** and **respiratory chain**. The symbionts seem to be capable to get the energy by **oxidative phosphorylation** from the partially oxidised food (pyruvic acid) of the host cell.

REVISION QUESTIONS

1. What are the characteristic structural features of mitochondria that aid in their identification?
2. Why are mitochondria termed as the "power houses" of the eukaryotic cells?
3. What is the major function of mitochondria?
4. What differences exist in structure and function between the inner and outer membranes of the mitochondria?
5. Would you expect plant cells to have the Embden-Meyerof glycolytic pathway? Explain your answer.
6. What is the significance of acetyl-coenzyme A and where does it come from?
7. What is an oxidative decarboxylation? Give an example.
8. Of what value to the cell is a cyclic process such as the Krebs cycle?
9. Analyze the statement: The glycolytic pathway probably evolved very early in the history of living organisms.
10. Define the following: electron transport; respiratory chain; oxidative phosphorylation ; cytochrome oxidase. Summarize various schemes for coupling electron transport to ADP phosphorylation.
11. What is a fermentation, and why is it needed by some cells? Often the products of a fermentation are useless to the organism that produces them, but people find various uses for some of these? As an example, why is yeast fermentation of such commercial importance?
12. What is the special function of brown fat mitochondria and how is it carried out?
13. Describe the β-oxidation of fats.
14. Describe the biogenesis of the mitochondria.

12 Chapter

PLASTIDS

The plastids are the cytoplasmic organelles of the cells of plants and some protozoans such as *Euglena*. Plastids are enclosed by double trilaminate membranes. They are self-replicating and contain DNA and a protein-synthesizing capacity comparable to that of mitochondria. They perform most important biological activities as the synthesis of food and storage of carbohydrates, lipids and proteins. The plastids occur in most plant cells and few protozoans except the cells of the bacteria, blue green algae, fungi and animals which contain chromatophores instead of the plastids.

12.1 CHROMATOPHORES

The chromatophores (Gr., *chrom*-colour, *phor*-to bear) are the plastid-like colouring bodies of the cells of the bacteria, blue green algae and fungi. In chromatophores the pigments are arranged in concentric rings or plates. The chromatophores are of various types and are as follows:

***(i)* Bacterial chromatophores.** Certain bacteria such as purple sulphur bacteria have the chromatophores which contain the pigment bacterio-chlorophyll. The pigment bacterio-chlorophyll absorbs the infra-red portion of the light. The green sulphur bacteria contain the pigment bacterio-viridin in its chromatophores.

***(ii)* Blue-green chromatophores.** The blue-green algae contain the blue-green chromatophores which have the pigment phycocyanin and pnycoerfthrin. Both the pigments perform photosynthetic process.

***(iii)* Carotenoids.** Certain bacteria, fungi and red-coloured ripe tomato, pepper or flower contain the carotenoids. The carotenoid pigment lycopene gives red colour to the ripe tomato and ripe pepper. The bacteria and fungi contain the pigment capsanthin in their carotenoids. The other carotenoid pigments as **fucoxanthin**, **xanthophyll** and **carotene**, etc., occur singly or along with the chlorophyll in the algae and other plant cells.

12.2 CLASSIFICATION OF THE PLASTIDS

The term 'plastid' is derived from the Greek word "*plastikas*" (=formed or moulded) and was used by **A.F.W. Schimper** in 1885. **Schimper** classified the plastids into following types according to their structure, pigments and the functions:

A. Chromoplasts. The chromoplasts (Gr., *chroma*-colour, *plast*-living) are the coloured plastids of the plant cells. The chromoplasts contain variety of pigments and synthesize the food by the process of photosynthesis. The most common chromoplasts of micro-organisms and plant cells are as follows:

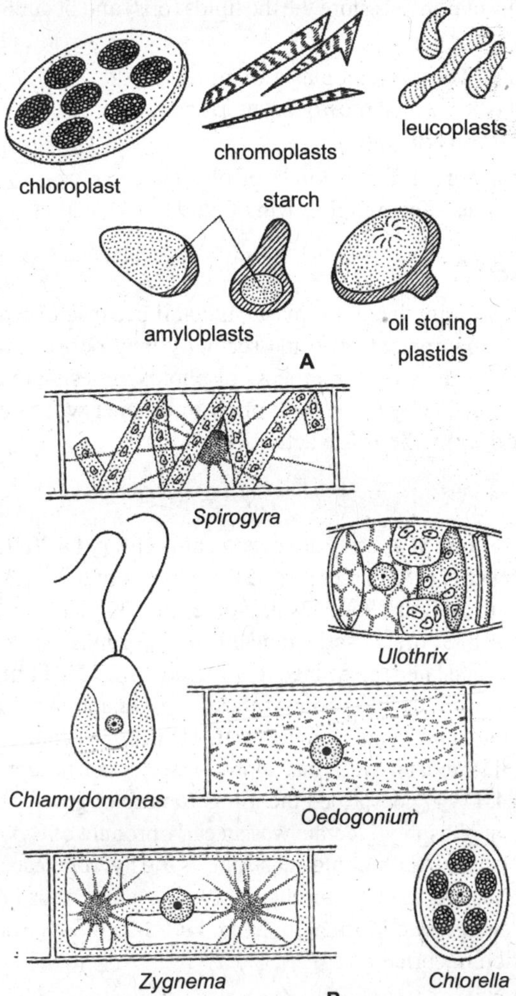

Fig. 12.1. A—Different kinds of plastids; B—Various types of choloroplast found in Algae.

***(i)* Chloroplast.** The chloroplast (Gr., *chlor*-green, *plast*-living) is most widely occurring chromoplast of the plants. It occurs mostly in the green algae and higher plants. The chloroplast contains the pigment chlorophyll *a* and chlorophyll *b* and DNA and RNA.

***(ii)* Phaeoplast.** The phaeoplast (Gr., *phaeo*-dark or brown, *plast*-living) contains the pigment **fucoxanthin** which absorbs the light. The phaeoplasts occur in the diatoms, dinoflagellates and brown algae.

***(iii)* Rhodoplast.** The rhodoplast (Gr., *rhode*-red, *plast*-living) contain the pigment phaeoerythrin which absorbs the light. The rhodoplast occur in the red algae.

B. Leucoplasts. The leucoplasts (Gr., *leuco*-white, *plast*-living) are the colourless plastids which store the food material as carbohydrates, lipids and proteins. The leucoplasts are rod-like or spheroid in shape and occur in the embryonic cells, sex cells and meristematic cells. The most common leucoplasts of the plant cells are as follows:

***(i)* Amyloplasts.** The amyloplasts (L., *amyl*-starch; Gr., *plast*-living) are those leucoplasts which synthesize and store the starch. The amyloplasts occur in those cells which store the starch.

***(ii)* Elaioplasts.** The elaioplasts store the the lipids (oils) and occur in seeds of monocotyledons and dicotyledons.

***(iii)* Proteinoplasts.** The proteinoplasts or proteoplasts are the protein storing plastids which mostly occur in seeds and contain few thylakoids (**Heinrich**, 1966).

According to **Schimper**, different kinds of plastids can transform into one another, as shown in following figure:

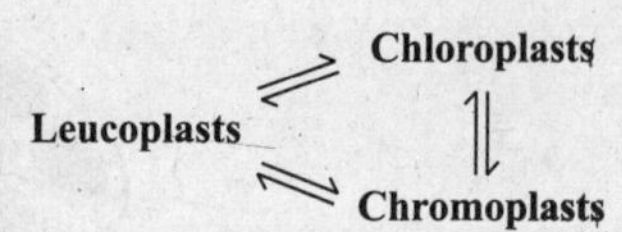

Fig. 12.2. Interconversion of three kinds of plastids.

12.3 CHLOROPLASTS

We will describe here only the chloroplasts in detail because of two reasons. Firstly they are most common plastids of many plant cells and secondly they perform the photosynthetic activity of greatest biological importance. By the process of photosynthesis the chloroplast synthesize the carbohydrates which contain energy in the form of chemical energy. The chemical energy is utilized by all living beings to perform various life activities.

12.4 HISTORICAL

Chloroplasts were described as early as seventeenth century by **Nehemiah Grew** and **Antonie van Leeuwenhoek**. **Dutrochet** (1837) recognized that chlorophyll was essential to oxgen evolution by plants. In 1862, **Sachs** proved that starch was synthesized by plants in a light-dependent reaction (photosynthesis). **Meyer** (1883) first described details of chloroplast structure. **Wilstatter** and **Stoll** (1913) isolated chlorophyll and later determined its structure. In 1923, **Thunberg** recognized that CO_2 was reduced and water oxidized during photosynthesis. **Wood** and **Werkman** (1936) distinguished between the "light reaction" and "dark reaction". **R. Hill** (1938) found that isolated chloroplasts evolved oxygen when illuminated, provided that appropriate electron acceptor was also made available. **K. Porter** and **S. Granick** (1947) described the ultrastructure of grana of chloroplasts. **Calvin** and **Benson** (1948) showed that phosphoglycerate was an early product of CO_2 fixation. **S. Ochoa** and **R. Vishniac** showed in 1950 that $NADP^+$ could substitute as the hydrogen acceptor in the, Hill reaction. **R. Emerson** *et al.* (1956) suggested the presence of two different traps in chloroplasts, each with a pigment system feeding energy into it. In 1966, **M.D. Hatch** and **S.R. Slack** suggested an alternate pathway for carbon fixation in corn.

12.5 DISTRIBUTION

The chloroplasts remain distributed homogeneously in the cytoplasm of plant cells. But in certain cells, the chloroplasts become concentrated around the nucleus or just beneath the plasma membrane. The chloroplasts have a definite orientation in the cell cytoplasm.

12.6 MORPHOLOGY

Shape

Higher plant chloroplasts are generally biconvex or plano-convex. However, in different plant cells, chloroplast may have various shapes, *viz.*, filamentous, saucer-shaped, spheroid, ovoid, discoid or club-shaped (see Fig. 12.1). They are vesicular and have a colourless centre.

Size

The size of the chloroplasts varies from species to species. The chloroplasts generally measure 2–3 μm in thickness and 5–10 μm in diameter (**Hall** *et al.*, 1974). The chloroplasts of polyploid plant cells are comparatively larger than the chloroplasts of the diploid plant cells. Chloroplast size is generally dependent upon sunlight availability; plants grown in the shade have large chloroplasts with more chlorophyll than those grown in sunlight.

Number

The number of the chloroplasts varies from cell to cell and from species to species and is related with the physiological state of the cell, but it usually remains constant for a particular plant cell. The algae usualy have a single huge chloroplast. The cells of the higher plants have 20 to 40 or upto 1,000 chloroplasts.

12.7 CHEMICAL COMPOSITION

The chloroplasts are composed of the carbohydrates, lipids, proteins, chlorophyll, carotenoids (carotene and xanthophylls), DNA, RNA and certain enzymes and coenzymes. The chloroplasts also contain some metallic atoms as Fe, Cu, Mn and Zn.

The carbohydrates occur in very low percentage in the chloroplasts. The most common carbohydrates of the chloroplasts are the starch and sugar phosphates.

The chloroplasts contain 20–30 per cent lipids of its dry weight. The lipids are composed of 50 per cent fats, 20 per cent sterols, 16 per cent waxes and 7 to 20 per cent phospholipids. The most common alcohols of the lipids are the choline, inositol, glycerol, ethanolamine.

The proteins constitute 35 to 55 per cent of the chloroplast. About 80 per cent proteins are insoluble and forming the unit membranes of the chloroplasts along with the lipids. The 20 per cent proteins are soluble and occur in the form of the enzymes.

The chlorophyll is a green pigment of the chloroplasts. The chlorophyll contains an assymetrical molecule which has hydrophilic head of four rings of the pyrols and hydrophobic tail of the phytol chain. Chemically the chlorophyll is a porphyrin like the animal pigment haemoglobin and cytochromes except besides, the iron (Fe), it contains Mg atom in between the rings of the pyrols which remain connected with each other by the methyl groups. The chlorophyll consists of 75 per cent **chlorophyll a** and 25 per cent **chlorophyll b**.

The carotenoids are carotenes and xanthophylls, both of which are related to vitamin A. The carotenes have hydrophobic chains of unsaturated hydrocarbons in their molecules. The xanthophylls contain many hydroxy groups in their molecules.

12.8 ULTRASTRUCTURE

The chloroplasts are bounded by two unit membranes like the mitochondria. Each membrane of the chloroplast is trilaminar, lipo-proteinous and 50A° thick. Both unit membranes of plastids are separated by one another by a distinct space known as the "**peri-plastidial space**". In *Nicotiana*, this *periplastidial space* is 100A°–300A° wide. The inner contents of the chloroplasts are heterogeneous and composed of following structures:

1. The matrix or stroma,
2. The grana.

1. The matrix or stroma. The inner periplastidial space of the chloroplasts is filled with a watery, proteinaceous and transparent substance known as the **matrix** or the **stroma**. The dark reaction of photosynthesis occurs in the matrix or stroma of chloroplast and the stroma contains the multienzyme complex for the dark reaction. The stroma also contains 25A°-wide fibrils of DNA, 70S ribosomes about 150–200 A° in diameter and RuDP carboxylase molecules which tend to be found along the outer face of the thylakoid. In the matrix of the chloroplasts the unit structures of the chloroplasts, the grana and intergrana connecting membrane remain embedded.

2. The grana. The chloroplasts consist of many lamellar or membranous, granular and chlorophyll bearing bodies, known as the **grana**. Grana are the structures of chloroplast where light reaction of photosynthesis takes place. The size of grana may range from 0.3 to 2.7 μm. The chloroplasts may contain 40 to 80 grana in their matrix.

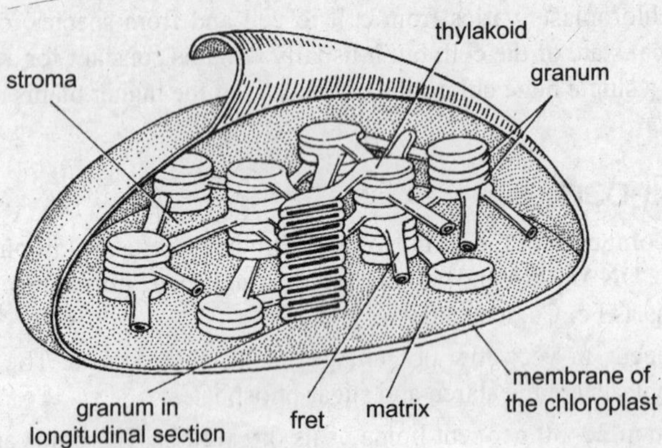

Fig. 12.3. Submicroscopic structure of the chloroplast.

Each granum of the chloroplast of a higher plant cell is composed of 10 to 100 disc-like, superimposed, membranous compartments known as **thylacoids** or **thylakoids** (thylacoid-sac-like), 0.25 to 0.8 μm in diameter with membranes about 0.01 μm (10A°) thick. However, in the chloroplasts of different plant species, the number of thylakoids per granum varies. Thus, there may be single thylakoids (*e.g.*, red alga), paired thylakoids (*e.g.*, Chrysophyta), triple thylakoids and multiple thylakoids (*e.g.*, green algae and higher plants) (Fig. 12.4). Each thylakoid remains separated from the stroma or the matrix of chloroplast by its unit membranes. In a granum these thylakoids remain arranged parallely to form the stack.

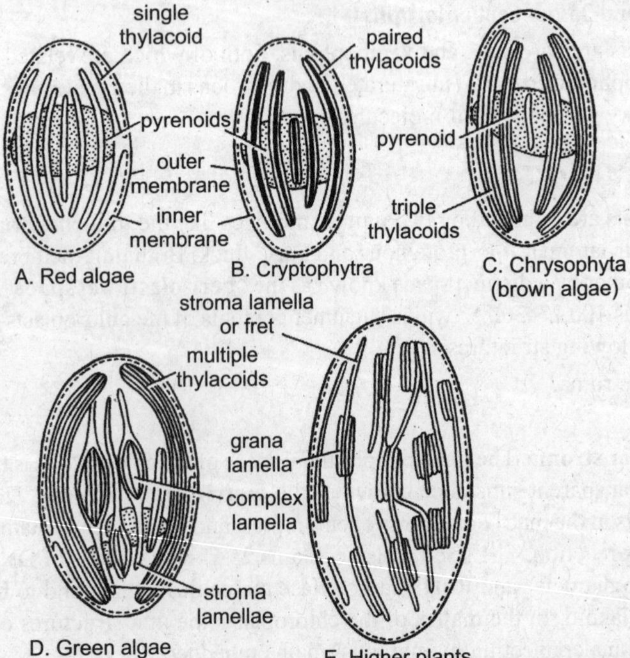

Fig. 12.4. Different kinds of chloroplasts contianing variable number of thylakoids per granum.

The grana of the chloroplasts are interconnected by a network of membranous tubules which are given out by the membranes of certain thylakoids into the matrix. These interconnecting membranes of the grana are known as the **stromal lamellae** or **frets**. The chlorophyll occurring in the membranes of thylakoids and frets often remain associated with their lipidous layers.

12.9 QUANTOSOME CONCEPT

Electron microscopic studies of the inner surface of the thylakoid. or compartment forming the grana, has established the existence of a paracrystalline array of spheroid particles of 200 × 100A°, called **quantosomes (Park** and **Pon**, 1963). When the fine structure of chloroplasts is studied by the freeze-etching technique by **Park** and associates (1964, 1967), quantosomes and some other particles were found to lie within the membrane of the thylakoid. Quantosomes were interpreted as photosynthetic units within thylakoid membrane each of which was capable of carrying out the photochemical reaction.

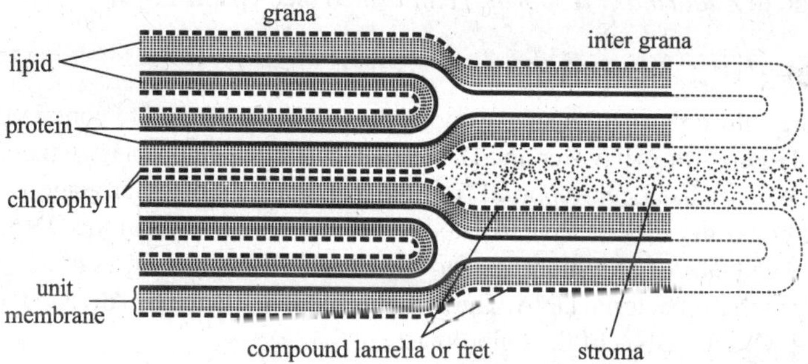

Fig. 12.5. Macromolecular structure of grana of a chloroplast.

According to recent freeze-fracture studies of chloroplast membranes by **Peter Satir** (1970s) and **C.J. Arntzen** and **P. Armond** (1977), the following four kinds of membrane particles occur in thylakoid membrane: 1. The larger, more widely spaced particles associated with exoplasmic or E leaflets (or that is on the interior of the thylakoids), have **pigment system II** or **PS II**. The 'quantosomes' appear to be an unusual array of these ES or PS II particles that protrude above the exoplasmic surface (ES) of thylakoid membrane. 2. The smaller, closely spaced particles associated with protoplasmic (P) leaflets (or that half of membrane bilayer that is on the outside of the thylakoid) have **pigment system I** or **PS I**. 3. **Coupling factor I** or **CF I** are spherical particles, some 90A° in diameter and occur on the outside of the thylakoid rather than on the inside of the membrane as in the mitochondria; CF1 has been identified as chloroplast ATPase. 4. RuDP carboxylase or **ribulose diphosphate carboxylase** is an enzyme that is found in aggregates loosely bound to membrane surface (outside thylakoid membrane) (see **Avers**, 1976; **Dyson**, 1978).

Mutation and Chloroplast Structure

The organization of chloroplasts and other plastids is often modified due to mutations. **D. Von Wettstein** (1956) reported that the plastids of normal barley plant have a well organized system of grana and stroma. But the plastids of an albino mutant of barley, fail to develop beyond a particular stage and there occurs no differentiation of grana and stroma. Further, plastids of a yellow-green mutant of barley develop somewhat further than plastids of an albino plant.

12.10 PYRENOIDS AND STIGMA

In contrast to the chloroplastids of typical cells of higher plants, chloroplastids of protozoan flagellates (*e.g.*, *Euglena*) and algae contain **pyrenoids** and **stigmata (eye spots)**. The pyrenoids are characterized by the prevalence of a densely granular or fibrillar ground substance. In the most simple cases, *e.g.*, in the chrysomonod *Olisthodiscus*, there is only a wider spacing of the lamella in the region of the pyrenoid. Usually, however, the ground substance is so extensive that it is traversed only by a few lamellae whose course is no longer parallel. In addition, the lamellae of the pyrenoid are usually reduced to one or two thylakoids only, which though continuous with those of the plastid, are more or less inflated and transformed into tube-like structures within the pyrenoid. The fact that polysaccharides are condensed either as starch orparamylon granules in the vicinity of the pyrenoid serves as an indication of its function. Thus, pyrenoids are the structures of chloroplasts for the storage of polysaccharides (see **Grell**, 1973).

The stigmata or eye spots are the photoreceptor organelles. They have a yellow or red colour in life. This is due to an accumulation of pigment granules of carotenoid of equal size, arranged as a single layer or in several layers on top of each other. The layers may be bent like a dish and are separated by membranes evidently connected with thylakoids of chloroplast. Such chloroplastid stigmata are found in *Eudorina* (*Pleodorina*) *californica* (see **Grell**, 1973).

12.11 DNA OF CHLOROPLAST

Recently the chloroplasts of the algae and higher plants are found to contain DNA molecules. First of all **Ris** and **Plant** (1962) have reported DNA molecule in the chloroplast of the *Chlamydomonas*. Later on DNA molecule has been reported from the chloroplasts of other alage and higher plants. **Woodcock** and **Fernandez** (1968) have isolated 150 μm long segments of the DNA molecules from the chloroplasts. The DNA of the chloroplasts differs from the nuclear DNA in many respects and it resembles closely with the bacterial DNA. The cytoplasmic inheritance and division of the chloroplast have been related with the DNA of the chloroplast.

12.12 RIBOSOMES OF CHLOROPLAST

The chloroplasts contain the ribosomes which are smaller than the cytoplasmic ribosomes. The ribosomes of the chloroplast are of 70S type and resemble with the bacterial ribosomes. The ribosomes of the chloroplasts consist of two ribosomal RNAs, 23S rRNA and 16S rRNA (**Stutz** and **Noll**, 1967, **Bager** and **Hamilton**, 1967). **Lyttleton** (1962) has also separated polyribosomes or'polysomes from the chloroplasts. The chloroplasts also contain aminoacyl—tRNAs, aminoacyl—tRNA synthetases, methionyl—tRNA.

12.13 PHOTOSYNTHETIC PIGMENTS OF CHLOROPLAST

There are three classes of photosynthetic pigments in the photosynthetic cells : **chlorophylls**, **carotenoids** and **phycobilins**. One or more kinds of chlorophylls and carotenoids occur in all photosynthetic species, but phycobilins are found in red algae and blue-green algae. Most photosynthetic species contain chlorophylls and carotenoids in tightly bound association with thylakoid membranes. However, phycobilins are loosely associated with these membranes and can be separated very easily from other photosensitive pigments. Phycobilins are concentrated in granules called **phycobilisomes** which look like amorphous particles in the electron micrographs of these algal cells (*e.g.*, red alga, *Porphyridium cruentum*). Photosynthetic pigments are thus concentrated and localized in some fashion in all cells and are not dispersed at random in either stroma or cytosol.

1. Chlorophylls. Chlorophylls are most important and lipid-soluble photosynthetic pigments. A chlorophyll molecule consists of four rings of carbon and nitrogen bound together into what is called a **porphyrin ring**. A magnesium atom is nestled in the centre of this structure. A long chain of carbon and hydrogen atoms (**phytol chain**) trails off one side of the chlorophyll molecule.

There are several kinds of chlorophylls which vary in structure only slightly. Higher plants and algae, including prokaryotia blue-green algae, all contain **chlorophyll a**. Eukaryotes also contain a second chlorophyll. which varies according to the species group. The sccond chlorophyll may be **chlorophyll b** (higher plants and most green algae), **chlorophyn c** (diatoms, dinoflagellates and brown algae), or **chloropbyll d** (red algae).

2. Carotenoids. Carotenoids also participate in photosynthesis in all organisms. These yellow or orange pigments are usually masked by the green colour of chlorophyll and are not commonly visible in leaves until autumn when the chlorophyll disintegrates. Carotenoids consist of a chain of carbon atoms connecting two six carbon rings. Two classes of carotenoids are important in photosynthesis : **carotenes** and **carotenols.**

3. Phycobilins. Phycobilins are accessory pigments found in eukaryotic red algae and prokaryotic blue-green algae. They are conjugated to specific protein. The protein conjugate of the pigment phycoerythrobilin in most red algae is called **phycoerythrin** and its analog in almost all blue-green algae is **phycocyanin**. In. contrast to cyclic porphyrin component in chlorophyll, phycobilins are open chain porphyrin type.

12.14 FUNCTIONS OF CHLOROPLASTS

The chloroplasts are anabolic (biosynthetic) organelles of plant cells and they perform the following anabolic functions for the cells.

1. Photosynthesis

The photosynthesis is vital to the survival of most organisms on earth. Not only are the organic molecules manufactured during photosynthesis used by plants to build leaves, stems., roots, flowers, and the like, but plant products are eaten by many animals and microbes. The photosynthetic activities of chloroplasts include the following two reactions: the **light reaction** and the **dark reaction**. In the light reaction, light energy is used to oxidize water to oxygen, passing the electrons to $NADP^+$ to create NADPH and, at the same time, generating some ATP. The light reaction seems to be concentrated in the membranes of thylakoids and frets. The dark reaction, which is catalyzed by soluble enzymes found in the stroma, consists of those steps by which the "reducing power" of NADPH is used to turn CO_2 into carbohydrate.

A. Photosynthetic light reaction. The photosynthetic light reaction is completed by passing through the following processes.

***(i)* Light absorption by photosynthetic pigments. Einstein** suggested in 1905 that light and other electromagnetic radiations travel in discrete packets called **quanta** or **photons** and that when light interacts with matter it does so by annihilating complete photons, never a part of one. Further, according to Einstein's, pbotoelectric theory, it takes one photon to eject one electron. Increasing the intensity of light, or flux of photons, only increases the number of electrons ejected, not their velocities. On the other hand, changing the wavelength of light does change the velocity of ejected electrons, implying that the energy of a photon must be related to its wavelength.

When a molecule absorbs a photon of light, it is absorbing a **quantum** of energy. Several things can happen to this energy: *(i)* It can be dissipated in molecular motion. manifest as heat. *(ii)* It can be reemitted as a new photon of light at a longer wavelength, with the shift representing losses to other processes—if remission occurs very quickly, it is called **fluorescence**; if there is a long lag (milli-seconds to seconds) between absorption and remission, the process is called **phosphorescence**. *(iii)* The energy of light can cause a chemical change in the compound that absorbs it. It is this latter possibility that can happen when a molecule of chlorophyll absorbs a photon. In fact, chloroplast acts as an energy transducer, *i.e.*, it can convert light energy to chemical energy, much as a solar battery uses light to run a transistor radio.

Visible light is only one small part of an immense spectrum of electromagnetic waves, which includes X-rays, ultraviolet radiations, visible light, infrared radiation and radio and television frequencies. The waves act as particles (quanta or photons) of variable energy content. Short wavelengths carry the most energy and can cause damage to living systems. Long wavelengths carry so little energy that they do not appear to affect cellular activities. Light waves in the visible range are most important in photosynthesis and have intermediate energy content.

Light energy must be absorbed by photosynthetic pigments in order to be useful for photosynthesis. Each pigment absorbs different wavelengths. The absorption characteristics of a pigment can be found by using a **spectrophotometer**. Light of a particular wavelength is passed through a sample of pigment and the relative absorption of light is determined. After this process is repeated with different wavelengths, a graph showing the absorption spectrum can be drawn. An **absorption spectrum** is a plot of degree of absorption of different wavelengths of a spectrum by a test substance. Chlorophyll absorbs both long (red and orange) and short (blue and violet) wavelengths well, leaving the intermediate wavelengths (yellow and green). The latter are not absorbed to any extent by plants; this light is reflected back to our eyes and we see the plants as green. In a comparable way the phycoerythrin of red algae absorbs blue and green wavelengths and reflects yellow and red light ; the phycocyanin of blue green algae absorbs long wavelengths and reflects blue light.

Within a fraction of a second after light is absorbed by a photosynthetic pigment, the molecule is altered; some electrons associated with the pigment are raised to new energetic heights, changing their spin or modifying their position. If enough energy is absorbed, an electron may even be ejected and thus oxidation occurs. When these events happen, we say that the molecule is in an **excited state**. In fact, the presence of a conjugated bond structure (alternating double and single bonds) in the photosynthetic pigments (*e.g.*, chlorophyll) greatly increases the number of possible electronic configurations. Each double bond adds a pair of electrons that are shared by the whole pigment molecule. These are the electrons that are vulnerable to, excitement.

Thus,chlorophyll *a* is altered within 10^{-15} second after being struck by a photon. The excitement lasts only for a fraction of a second before the energy is given up and the molecule returns to its initial unexcited state.

Photosynthetic units. The basic photosynthetic units seem to be groups of roughly 300 pigment molecules located in the chloroplast membranes (thylakoid disc). Although all the pigment molecules in the unit (carotenoids, chlorophyll *b*, etc.) are capable of capturing light energy, they must transfer it to a single key chlorophyll *a*, molecule called the **reaction centre**. The latter then loses an electron to a series of electron carrier molecules. Thus the other 299 accessory pigment molecules are referred to as **antenna molecules** or **antenna pigments**, to designate their role in the capture of light energy. Energy is not passed randomly through these molecules but follows a definite pattern. In green plants excitation energy captured by the carotenoids is first passed to chlorophyll *b* and then through a sequence of chlorophyll *a* molecules with slightly different absorption characteristics, to ultimately rest in the reaction centre. At various stages of transfer among pigments, small amounts of energy are lost, so all, the energy funneling into the reaction centre is ultimately at the same level.

We do not know the structural arrangement of the antenna pigments and the reaction-centre chlorophyll. Some investigators think that reaction-centres are positioned randomly throughout a mass of pigment molecules. A photon would be absorbed by any of the pigments and then the excitation energy would be transferred at random throughout the system until it reached a reaction-centre or reemitted as fluorescent light. This concept is known as the "**lake model**". An alternative view, called the "**puddle model**" suggests that the various photosynthetic units are separated from one another, as puddles dotted around the landscape; each unit has its own reaction centre surrounded by antenna pigments. Thus excitation energy cannot be transferred between units. Actually both models appear to have validity, and a hybrid model, called the "**connected puddle model**" has been proposed which suggests that although photosynthetic units are somewhat isolated functionally, some transference of energy does occur between them.

Dual pigment systems. Higher plants are found to have two types of photosynthetic units, associated with two different pigment systems, which absorb light of different wavelengths. **Pigment system I** or **photosystem I (PS I)** units occur in the thylakoid membrane in the form of small and densely packed particles. Each PS I unit consists of about 200 molecules of chlorophyll *a* and 50 carotene molecules. The reaction centre (chlorophyll *a* molecule) is called **P 700** because it has a maximum light absorption at 700 nanometers. Energy funneling into P 700 is responsible for the ejection of an electron from the chlorophyll. **Pigment system II** or **photosystem II (PS II)** units occur in the thylakoid membrane in the form or larger, more widely spaced particles or ES particles (or quantosomes). Each PS II unit consists of approximately 200 molecules of chlorophyll *a*, 200 molecules of carotenols, chlorophyll *b*, and chlorophyll *c* or *d*, depending upon the species. Its reaction-centre chlorophyll *a* is designated **P 690** or **shorter-wavelength trap**. In the thylakoid membrane PS I and PS II are, probably arranged near one another because they are functionally related ; excitation energy originating in one can be shunted to the other system. However, two photosystems are coupled chemically rather than through direct energy transfer.

***(ii)* Electron transport systems and oxidation of water.** The reaction-centre of both photosystems I and II eject electrons when they become excited. As these electrons are passed from molecule to molecule of electron transport systems associated with both photosystems of the ehloroplast, energy is sequentially released and some of it is trapped in chemical bonds during endergonic reactions. All carrier molecules needed for electron transport are found to occur in the thylakoid membranes. The following scheme of electron transport and roles of PS I and PS II in the oxidation of water is based on a model, proposed by **R. Hill** and **F. Bendall**, called the **Hill-Bendall model**.

(*a*) Photosystem II. P 690 captures light energy and uses it to oxidizc water. When PS II absorbs two quanta (2 hv) of light, it removes two electrons (2 e^-) from one molecule of water (H_2O), liberating a molecule of oxygen (½ O_2) gas and two hydrogen ions (2 H^+), such as follows

$$H_2O \xrightarrow{2\,hv} \frac{1}{2}O_2 + 2H^+ + 2e^- \qquad ...(12.1)$$

These two electrons are passed to an electron transport chain at some **electron acceptor**, Q, from which they cyclically oxidize and reduce four types of **electron carriers**, namely, **plastoquinone**, **cytochrome-559**, **cytochrome-553** (or cytochrome f) and **plastocyanin**, before being passed to PS I (Fig. 12.6). The compound Q has got its name from the fact that chemically it is a quinone and also because it quenches fluorescence. When the electrons are passed through the chain of carrier molecules each at a lower energy level, at each stage energy released and at one or two points energy is harvested. Every electron traversing the electron transport chain produces one ATP from ADP and inorganic phosphate (Pi). This process of ATP synthesis involves **cytochrome b6** and is accomplished by coupling factor 1 or CF I occurring at the outerside of a thylakoid membrane and is called **photophosphorylation** and it resembles with that of mitochondria. Thus, during light reaction occurring in PS I two ATP molecules are produced.

(*b*) Photosystem I. Earlier we said that when P 700 becomes excited by a photon, it ejects an electron. The electron is replaced by one from photosystem II; consequently, there is a steady flow of electrons from photosystem II to photosystem I as long as light is available. The electrons that are lost from P 700 are first passed to an electron acceplor molecule called X and through a series of electron transport molecules such as **ferredoxin**, **ferredoxin NADP-reductase**, etc., at successively lower energy levels (Fig. 12.6). Energy is lost along the way. The last electron carrier molecule in the chain is coenzyme NADP. When it receives an electron, it picks up a H^+ from the cellular fluids to form NADPH. The readers will recall two H^+ were tormed when one water molecule fed their electrons into photosystem II. These H^+ rejoin their electrons as two NADPH molecules are formed. Thus, an additional photon input, trapped by P 700, "boosts" the electrons to a level. from which $NADP^+$ can be reduced into NADPH. The light reaction I, catalyzed by PS I, can be summarized as follows:

$$2e^- + 2H^+ + 2NADP^+ \xrightarrow{2\,hv} 2NADPH \qquad ...(12.2)$$

The total light reaction, including ATP synthesis can be shown such as follows:

$$H_2O + 2NADP + 2ADP + 2\,Pi \xrightarrow{4\,hv} \frac{1}{2}O_2 + 2NADPH + 2ATP \qquad ...(12.3)$$

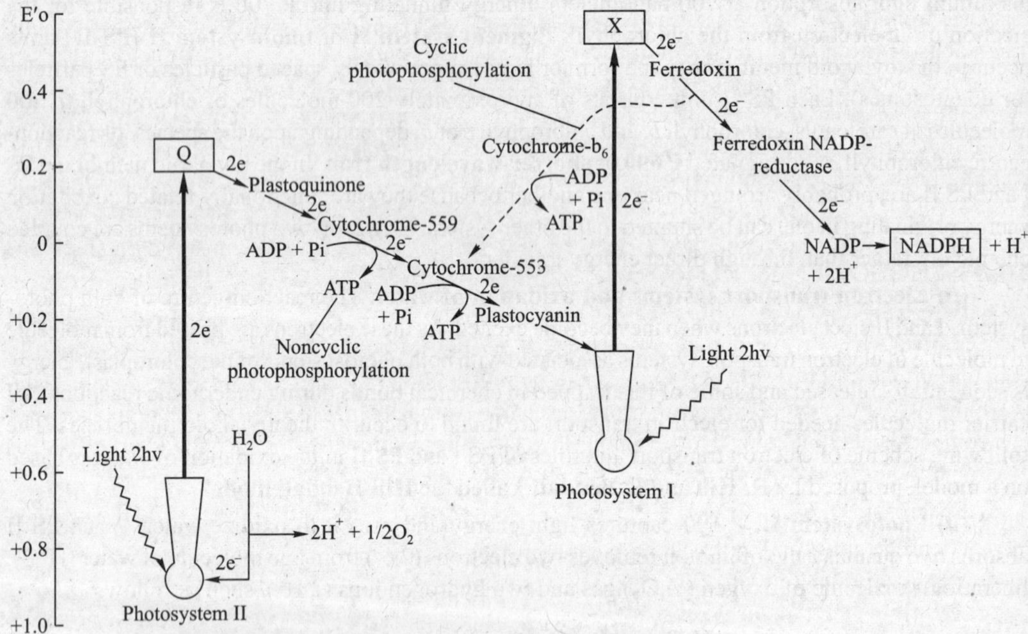

Fig. 12.6. Photosynthetic light reaction showing major events occurring in photosystem I and photosystem II of chloroplasts.

Cyclic photophosphorylation. The scheme just outlined includes both NADPH and ATP production. ATP production can occur by itself, however, when the bulk of available $NADP^+$ is already in the reduced form, electrons can be shunted from the PS I receptor back to the main electron chain (*i.e.*, the electron transport chain linking two photosystems). The result is additional ATP production via photophosphorylation but without the release of oxygen and without reduction of $NADP^+$. This process, called **cyclic photophosphorylation**, is purely a light-driven ATP synthesizer.

B. Photosynthetic dark reaction: CO_2 fixation. The light reaction just described accounts for the capture of radiant energy and explains how this energy is made available for biosynthesis in the form of NADPH and ATP, evolving oxygen in the process. The biosynthetic reaction most often associated with photosynthesis is, of course, the production of glucose from CO_2 and water. Since glucose synthesis can occur without light, as long as NADPH and ATP are available, it is termed the "**dark reaction**". The light reaction is centered in the thylakoid membranes, while the dark reaction is enzymatically catalyzed within the stroma (Fig. 12.7).

During the dark reaction, CO_2 from the environment is formed into sugar and other organic molecules. This is known as **CO_2 fixation**. For every CO_2 converted into carbohydrate, three ATP and two NADPH molecules are required. We can summarize the process:

$$6CO_2 + 12NADPH + 18ATP \rightarrow C_6H_{12}O_6 + 12NADP^+ + 18ADP + 18\,Pi$$

This simple equation masks an extremely complex process, the basic details of which were worked out in the 1940s and 1950s by **Melvin Calvin** and his coworkers **James Bassham** and **Andrew Benson** of the University of California, at Berkeley. The cycle of reactions is today called the **Calvin-Benson-Bassham** cycle or simply **Calvin** cycle. The enzymes involved in the Calvin cycle were identified later by **E. Racker** and **B. Horecker** (see **Avers,** 1976).

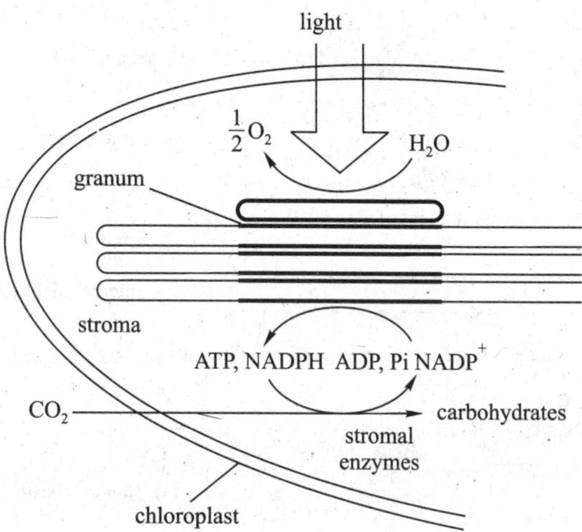

Fig. 12.7. Localization of the light and dark reactions of photosynthesis. The light reaction is catalyzed by chloroplast lamellae, especially in the grana. The dark reaction is catalyzed by enzymes of the stroma (after **Dyson**, 1978).

Calvin cycle. Using the single-celled alga *Chlorella*, Calvin and his colleagues tracked the fate of the CO_2 absorbed from the water by using radioactively labelled CO_2 (*i.e.*, $^{14}CO_2$). By exposing the algae to $^{14}CO_2$ for brief periods of time, the investigators subsequently ground up the algae and biochemically analyzed the organic products that showed radioactivity. They note that CO_2 was first joined to a 5-carbon sugar (ribulose 1, 5-diphosphate) to form a 6-carbon compound which immediately broke into two 3-carbon molecules of 3-phosohoglycerate (PGA), an intermediate in glycolysis from which any other chemical constituent of the cell can be made.

After two molecules of PGA are formed in the dark reactions, a phosphate from ATP is added to each molecule, forming two molecules of 1, 3-diphosphoglycerate. This step is followed by the addition of the hydrogen carried by coenzyme NADPH and the loss of phosphate, thus producing two molecules of 3-phosphoglyceraldehyde (PGAL). The two PGAL molecules join together to form the 6-carbon sugar fructose 1, 6-diphosphate, which then losses, a phosphate and becomes fructose 6-phosphate and then glucose 6-phosphate. All these steps are thus a reversal of the first six steps of glycolysis.

After glucose has been formed, it can join with other glucose units to form the polysaccharides **starch** or **cellulose**, or it can join with a fructose molecule to form the disaccharide sugar **sucrose**. All the above steps are of course catalyzed by particular enzymes. The ribulose 5-phosphate is provided by **pentose phosphate pathway**.

The Hatch Slack pathway. The Calvin cycle just described is not the only carbon-fixing reaction sequence. In 1966 **M.D. Hatch** and **C.R. Slack** suggested an alternate pathway for carbon fixation in corn and certain other hot-weather plants. In this pathway, CO_2 diffuses into the leaf through stomata and then is organically fixed in mesophyll cells by being added to phosphoenolpyruvate (PEP). The product is a four-carbon,compound, normally an intermediate in the Krebs cycle, called oxaloacetate (OAA). Oxaloacetate is transferred to another cell where it gives up its new carbon to the Calvin cycle. A major advantage is the highly favourable corboxylation step, which permits partial closure of stomata and hence water conservation (Fig. 12.8).

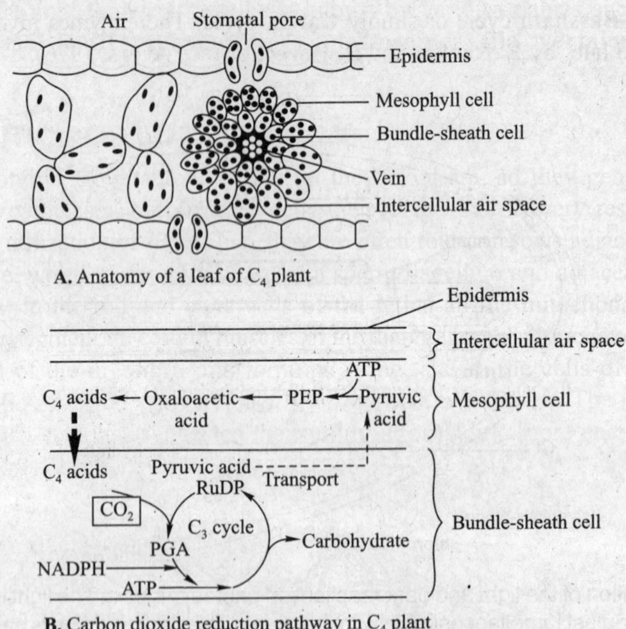

Fig. 12.8. Hatch-Slack pathway or C_4 cycle (After Avers, 1976).

2. Protein Synthesis

According to most recent studies (see **Hall** *et al.*, 1974). the DNA of chloroplast codes for chloroplast mRNA, rRNA, tRNA, and ribosomal proteins. It also codes for certain structural proteins of thylakoid membranes. The synthesis of other chloroplast components as chlorophyll, carotenoids, lipids and photosynthetic and starch synthesizing enzymes, is controlled by nuclear genes. The 70S ribosomes of *Euglena* chloroplast are found to require Mg^{++} for their stability and also have a requirement for N-formyl methionyl—tRNA in chain initiation process of protein synthesis like the bacteria. The protein synthetic mechanism of chloroplasts is inhibited by chloram phenicollike that of mitochondria and bacteria (**Ellis**, 1969).

12.15 ORIGIN AND DEVELOPMENT

The chloroplasts are never originated *de novo*. About the origin of chloroplasts following concepts have been postulated:

1. The origin from the mature chloroplast.
2. The origin from the proplastid.
3. Nuclear origin.
4. Monotropic development.
5. Symbiotic origin.

1. The origin from the mature chloroplast. In algae and ferns the new chloroplast originates by the division of the mature chloroplast. Under certain abnormal conditions (*viz.*, regeneration of plant from dissected leaves) the new chloroplasts originate by **budding** from the mature plastids.

2. The origin of chloroplast from the protoplastids. In higher plants, the new chloroplast develops from the proplastids. The protoplastids are the spheroid structures of 0.5 µm diameter and each remains bounded by two unit membranes and contains dense stroma. The development of the thylakoids and frets takes place according to the synthesis of the chlorophyll in the sunlight. The inner membrane of the chloroplast gives off vesicles which arrange themselves parallely in the matrix. These vesicles fuse together to form large discs or lamellae. At certain places the discs or lamellae vesicles arrange themselves in closely packed bundles of thylakoids to form a grana. Some thylakoids, however, remain connected with each other by the tubules or stromal lamellae or frets in the mature chloroplast. This lamellation takes place only in the presence of light (Fig. 12.9). In the absence of light these structure start disorganizing (Fig. 12.10).

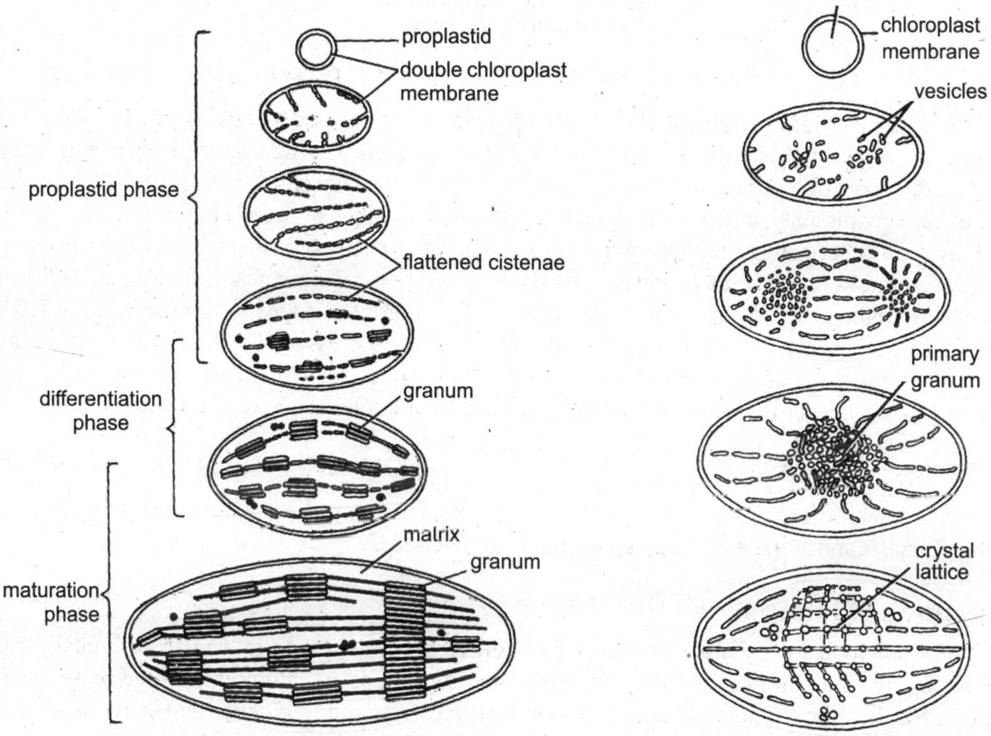

Fig. 12.9. Development of a chloroplast from a submicroscopic proplastid in the presence of light.

Fig. 12.10. Development of a chloroplast from submicroscopic proplastid in dark.

3. Nuclear origin. A large number of building blocks (membranes, etc.) or initials of proplastids have been observed under special conditions around the nucleus. This suggested that the initials originated due to evagination of the double nuclear membrane and give rise to mitochondria and proplastids.

4. Monotropic development. According to the theory of monotropic development of chloroplast, the plastids are autonomous structures, which can change from one form to another but can never be originated *de novo*. Although in certain cases the change from one form to the other is reversible, at other times irreversible changes can also be brought about. For example, if chloroplasts become sufficiently yellow due to absence of light, they may not become green again and will therefore only degenerate. Similarly, in the transformation of chloroplasts into chromoplasts, the chlorophyll disappears and this change may be irreversible. It is for this reason that the chromoplasts are considered as degenerating forms of plastids (chloroplasts). The mode of monotropic development of plastid can be illustrated by following Fig. 12.11:

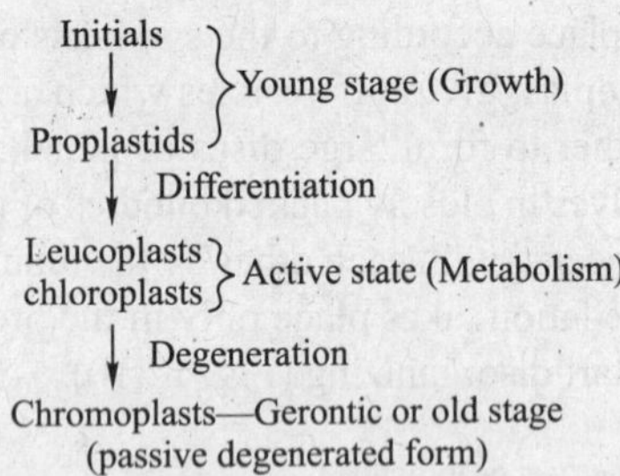

Fig. 12.11. Monotropic development of plastids.

5. The symbiotic origin of the chloroplast. In certain characeristics, the chloroplasts are comparable with that of as semi-autonomous or symbiotic organism living within the plant cells. They divide, grow and differentiate, they contain circular DNA, ribosomal RNA, messenger RNA and are able to conduct protein synthesis. By visualizing these similarities between chloroplast and micro-organism, it has been suggested that chloroplasts might have resulted from a symbiotic relationship between an autotrophic micro-organism, one which is able to transform radiant energy from sunlight and heterotrophic host cell. The symbiotic origin of the chloroplast appears very justified but **Kirk** (1966) has shown that certain important enzymes which are necessary for the develoment of the chlorophyll and for the photosynthetic mechanism are synthesized according to the codes of the nuclear DNA. There still exists certain doubts about the symbiotic origin of the chloroplast.

12.16 AMYLOPLASTS

Amyloplasts or starch granules are leucoplasts which lack any visible pigment and are involved in the synthesis and storage of various kinds of carbohydrates.

Structure and Function

The amyloplasts resemble proplastids and differ from them only in size. They contain less number of lamellae, but, can build up thylakoid structure found in chloroplast, in the presence of light. In the dark they synthesize and store starch. The conversion of glucose into starch is a chief characteristic of amyloplasts. However, chloroplasts can also synthesize starch and store it in stroma region. But, this starch in chloroplasts disappears quickly and is, therefore, known as **transitory starch**. The starch of amyloplasts on the other hand can be stored for longer periods and is, therefore, called reserve starch.

Origin of Amyloplasts

The starch development begins with the formation of a particle in the stroma. This particle consists of several tubuli and thylakoids and is surrounded by additional rings of starch. It grows till the amyloplast is filled with starch. Ultimately, the tubuli are pressed against the wall and gradually, starch granule exceeds the size of amyloplast. Finally, the membranous wall of amyloplasts ruptures and withers away, so that the starch granules can be seen.

12.17 CHROMOPLASTS

The plastids which contain pigments other than chlorophyll are the chromoplasts. They can be originated from chloroplasts and also from leucoplasts. The common example of their derivation from chloroplasts can be observed in the petals which are green initially but become coloured subsequently. Similarly in carrot roots, chromoplasts are derived from leucoplasts as is clear from the fact that the roots have no colour in the beginning but become coloured at a later stage.

Structure and Function

Chromoplasts appear to be products of degeneration or disintegration of chloroplasts or leucoplasts. Their specific functions in plant cell are still little understood. However, their presence in flowers definitely serves in attracting insects for pollination and propagation.

Origin of Chromoplasts

The chromoplasts can originate either from chloroplasts or from leucoplasts:

(*i*) When a chloroplast transforms into a chromoplast, it has been observed that some yellow coloured droplets called **globulins** appear in the former. In the course of development chlorophyll and starch of chloroplasts gradually decrease, large globuli are formed, the lamellar structure breaks down and stroma is disorganized. Ultimately, globuli are arranged along plastid membrane and the centre of the plastid appears empty due to disintegration of stroma.

(*ii*) During the transformation of leucoplasts into chromoplasts, certain fibrils appear which give rise to crystals filling up the whole plastids. These crystals are normally found in the form of sheet like structures containing large quantities of carotenoids.

REVISION QUESTIONS

1. What is the chloroplast? Describe the ultrastructure of the chloroplast. What are some of the more obvious similarities and differences between chloroplasts and mitochondria?
2. Define the following: granum, thylakoid, chromoplast, leukoplast, proplastid.
3. What part of chloroplast is associated with the light reaction? Where dark reaction takes place?
4. Define the following: photon; a quantum of energy; fluorescence; photoelectric effect. What are the possible fates of an absorbed photon?
5. What is the Calvin cycle, and what is its purpose? Describe it.
6. Write an essay on "chloroplasts and photosynthesis".
7. Write short notes on tbe following:
   (*i*) Chromatophores;
   (*ii*) Quantosome concept:
   (*iii*) Pyrenoid;
   (*iv*) Photosynthetic pigments of chloroplasts;
   (*v*) Dark reaction; and
   (*vi*) Origin of chloroplasts.

13 Chapter MICROBODIES-PEROXISOMES AND GLYOXYSOMES

The cells of Protozoa, fungi, plants, liver and kidney of vertebrates contain certain membrane-bounded, spherical bodies of 0.2 to 1.5 μm diameter in close association of endoplasmic reticulum, and mitochondria or chloroplast, or both. These organelles have a central granular or crystalloid core containing some enzymes and are called **microbodies**. Microbodies use molecular oxygen like mitochondria, but instead of having cytochromes and capacity of **ATP** synthesis like them, they contain flavin-linked oxidases and catalases for the hydrogen peroxide metabolism and also enzymes for fatty acid metabolism.

13.1 TYPES OF MICROBODIES

Recent biochemical studies have distinguished two types of microbodies, namely **peroxisomes** and **glyoxysomes**. These two organelles differ both in their enzyme complement and in the type of tissue in which they are found. **Peroxisomes** are found in animal cells and in the leaves of higher plants. In both they participate in the oxidation of substrates, producing hydrogen peroxide which is subsequently destroyed by catalase activity:

1. Reduced substrate → Oxidized substrate, coupled with $FAD \to FADH_2$, coupled with $O_2 \to H_2O$ (cyclic arrows as printed: Reduced substrate / Oxidized substrate ⟲ $FADH_2$ / FAD ⟲ H_2O / O_2)
2. $H_2O_2 \rightarrow H_2O + \frac{1}{2}O_2$

In plant cells, peroxisomes remain associated with ER, chloroplasts and mitochondria and are involved in photorespiration. **Glyoxysomes** occur only in plant cells and are particularly abundant in germinating seeds which store fats as a reserve food material. They remain intimately associated with lipid bodies, the spherosomes and contain enzymes for fatty acid metabolism and glyconeogenesis (*i.e.*, fermentation of glucose from various non-carbohydrate precursors as succinate in this case). Apart from peroxisomes and glyoxysomes, a number of other terms have been used to describe microbodies, including **cytosomes**, **phragmosomes** and **crystal-containing bodies**. A detailed discussion of each type of microbody can be made as follows:

13.2 PEROXISOMES

Peroxisomes occur in many animal cells and in a wide range of plants. They are present in all photosynthetic cells of higher plants in etiolated leaf tissue, in caleoptiles and hypocotyls, in tobacco stem and callus, in ripening pear fruits and also in Euglenophyta, Protozoa, brown algae, fungi, liverworts, mosses and ferns.

Structure

Peroxisomes are variable in size and shape, but usually appear circular in cross section having diameter between 0.2 and 1.5 μm. They have a single limiting membrane of lipid and protein molecules, which encloses their granular matrix. In some cases (*e.g.*, in the festucoid grasses) the matrix contains numerous threads or fibrils, while in others they are observed to contain either an amorphous nucleoid or a dense inner core which in many, species shows a regular crystalloid structure (*e.g.*, tobacco leaf cell, **Newcomb** and **Frederick**, 1971). Little is known about the function of the core, except that it is the site of the enzyme urate oxidase in rat liver peroxisomes and much of the catalase in some plants (see, **Hall** *et al.*, 1974).

Biochemical Activity

Peroxisomes are found to perform following two types of biochemical activities:

A. Hydrogen peroxide metabolism. Peroxisomes contain catlase enzyme together with one or more enzymes which produce hydrogen peroxide. The primary electron donor for these latter enzymes is usually glycolate, L-Iactate or another L-hydroxy acid, and one mole of hydrogen peroxide is produced with the uptake of one mole of oxygen. Subsequently, the action of catalase causes peroxidations such as that of ethanol to acetaldehyde ($CH_3CH_2OH + H_2O_2 \rightarrow CH_3CHO + 2H_2O$), formic acid to carbon dioxide and water ($HCOOH + H_2O_2 \rightarrow CO_2 + 2H_2O$) or of a further mole of peroxide to oxygen and water ($2H_2O_2 \rightarrow 2H_2O + O_2$). In every case there is a net uptake of oxygen.

B. Glycolate cycle. Peroxisomes of plant leaves contain catalase together with the enzymes of **glycolate pathway**, as glycolate oxidase, glutamate glyoxylate, serine-glyoxylate and aspartate-α-ketoglutarate aminotransferases, hydroxy pyruvate reductase and malic dehydrogenase. They also contain FAD, NAD and NADP coenzymes. The glycolate cycle is thought to bring about the formation of the amino acids glycine and serine from the non-phosphorylated intermediates of photosynthetic carbon reduction cycle, *i.e.*, glycerate to serine, or glycolate to glycine and serine in a sequence of reactions which involve chloroplasts, peroxisomes and mitochondria (**Tolbert**, 1971, **Bird** *et al.*, 1972). There is a net uptake of oxygen and evolution of CO_2 during the operation of the glycolate cycle ; this is known physiologically as **photorespiration** since it is stimulated in the light.

Photorespiration may be a wasteful evolutionary accident caused by increasing atmospheric concentrations of oxygen and the sensitivity of ribulose diphosphate carboxylase to it. It is avoided in some of the more advanced plants that feature C_4 metabolism because enzymes of the Calvin cycle are in interior cells of these plants, further away from outside air and its high concentrations of oxygen.

Comparison between Peroxisomes and Mitochondria

Peroxisomes resemble with mitochondria only in one respect that they use molecular oxygen, otherwise, they differ with them in following two objects:

(*i*) The rate of peroxisomal oxygen uptake is almost directly proportional to the oxygen concentration, while mitochondrial oxygen uptake is almost independent of oxygen concentration (above about 5%) due to extremely high affinity of cytochrome oxidase for oxygen.

(*ii*) In mitochondria the respiration is involved in ATP synthesis, but the peroxisomal respiration in animals is not involved in ATP synthesis and in this respect it appears to be a wasteful process.

Functions

The peroxisomes have following functions:

(*i*) In plants, they are involved in the synthesis of glycine and serine and possibly of C—1 donor from the primary products of photosynthesis.

(*ii*) They protect the cellular organelles from the toxic effect of hydrogen peroxide.

13.3 GLYOXYSOMES

Glyoxysomes are found to occur in the cells of yeast, *Neurospora*, and oil rich seeds of many higher plants. They resemble with peroxisomes in morphological details, except that, their crystalloid core consists of dense rods of 6.0 µm diameter. They have enzymes for fatty acid metabolism and gluconeogenesis, *i.e.*, conversion of stored lipid molecules of spherosomes of germinating seeds into the molecules of carbohydrates.

Biochemical Activities

Glyoxysomes puform following biochemical activities of plant cells.

1. Fatty acid metabolism. During germination of oily seeds, the stored lipid molecules of spherosomes are hydrolysed by the enzyme lipase (glycerol ester hydrolase) to glycerol and fatty acids. The phospholipid molecules are hydrolysed by the enzyme phospholipase. The long chain fatty acids which are released by the hydrolysis are then broken down by the successive removal of two carbon or C_2 fragments in the process of **β-oxidation**.

β-Oxidation. During β-oxidation process, the fatty acid is first activated by enzyme fatty acid thiokinase or **fatty acyl-CoA** which is oxidized by a FAD-linked enzyme fatty acyl-CoA dehydrogenase into **trans-2-enoyl-CoA**. Trans-2-enoyl-CoA is hydrated by an enzyme enoyl hydratase or crotonase to produce the **L-3-hydroxyacyl-CoA**, which is oxidized by a NAD-linked L-3-hydroxyacyl-CoA dehydrogenase to produce **3-keto acyl-CoA**. The 3-keto acyl-CoA looses a two carbon fragment under the action of the enzyme thiolase or β-keto thiolase to generate an **acetyl-CoA** and a new **fatty acyl-CoA** with two less carbon atoms than the original. This new fatty acyl-CoA is then recycled through the same series of reactions until the final two molecules of acetyl-CoA are produced. The complete β-oxidation chain can be represented as follows:

Fatty acid —(Activation; Fatty acid thiokinase + CoA)→ **Fatty acyl-CoA** —(Oxidation; Fatty acyl-CoA dehydrogenase + FAD)→ **trans-2-Enoyl-CoA**

trans-2-Enoyl-CoA —(Hydration (Enoyl-hydratase))→ **L—3-hydroxy-acyl-CoA**

L—3-hydroxy-acyl-CoA —(Oxidation; L-3-hydroxyacyl-CoA dehydrogenase + NAD)→ **3-keto acyl-CoA** —(Thiolytic cleavage; β-keto thiolase)→ **Fatty acid-CoA** + **Acetyl-CoA**

In plant seeds β-oxidation occurs in glyoxysomes (**Cooper** and **Beevers**, 1969). But in other plant cells β-oxidation occur in glyoxysomes and mitochondria. The glyoxysomal β-oxidation requires oxygen for oxidation of reduced flavoprotein produced as a result of the fatty-acyl-COA dehydrogenase activity. In animal cells β-oxidation occurs in mitochondria.

In plant cells the acetyl-CoA, the product of β-oxidation chain is not oxidized by Krebs cycle, because it remains spatially separated from the enzymes of Krebs cycle, instead of it, acetyl-CoA undergoes the **glyoxylate cycle** to be converted into succinate.

Glyoxylate cycle. The glyoxylate pathway occurs in glyoxisomes and it involves some of the reactions of the Krebs cycle in that **citrate** is formed from **oxaloacetate** and **acetyl-CoA** under the action of citrate synthetase enzyme. The citrate is subsequently converted into **isocitrate** by aconitase enzyme. The cycle then involves the enzymatic conversion of isocitrate to **glyoxylate** and **succinate** by isocitratase enzyme:

$$\textbf{Isocitrate} \xrightarrow{\text{Isocitratase}} \textbf{Glyoxylate + Succinate}$$

The glyoxylate and another mole of acetyl-CoA form a mole of **malate** by malate synthetase:

$$\textbf{Acetyl-CoA + Glyoxylate} \xrightarrow{\text{Malate synthetase}} \textbf{Malate}$$

This malate is converted to oxaloacetate by malate dehydroenase for the cycle to be completed. Thus, overall, the glyoxylate pathway involves:

$$\textbf{2 Acetyl-CoA} + NAD^+ \rightarrow \textbf{Succinate} + NADH + H^+$$

Succinate is the end product of the glyoxysomal metabolism of fatty acid and is not further metabolized within this organelle.

The synthesis of hexose or gluconeogenesis involves the conversion of succinate to oxaloacetate, which presumably takes place in the mitochondria, since the glyoxysomes do not contain the enzymes fumarase and succinic dehydrogenase. Two molecules of **oxaloacetate** are formed from four molecules of acetyl-CoA without carbon loss. This oxaloacetate is converted to **phosphoenol pyruvate** in the phosphoenol pyruvate carboxykinase reaction with the loss of two molecules of CO_2:

$$\textbf{2 Oxaloacetate + 2ATP} \rightleftharpoons \textbf{2 Phosphoenol pyruyate} + 2CO_2 + \textbf{2ADP}$$

The phosphoenol pyruvate is converted into monosaccharides (*e.g.*, glucose, fructose), disaccharide (sucrose) and polysaccharide (starch) by following reaction:

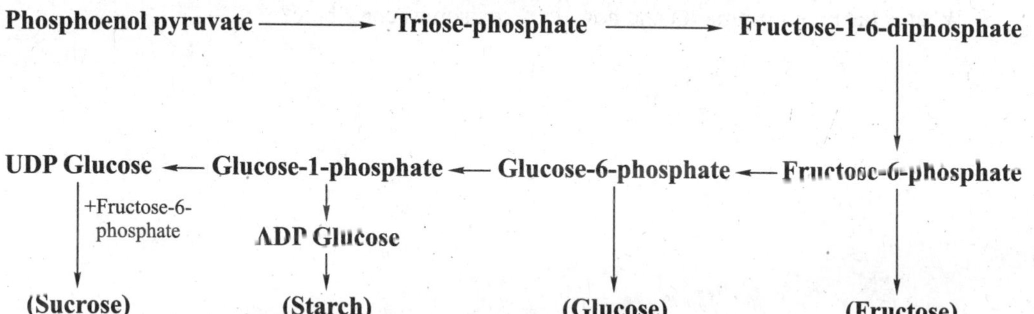

Other Biochemical Activities of Glyoxysomes

Glyoxysomes are found to contain enzyme **urate oxidase** and **allantoinase**. Urate oxidase (uricase) converts uric acid to allantoin and allantoillase hydrates allantoin to allantoic acid during the degradation of purines.

13.4 ORIGIN OF MICROBODIES

The microbodies or peroxisomes and glyoxysomes lack ribosomes and nucleic acids. Little is known about their origin. Their close association with the rough ER had led to the speculation that they are produced from that membrane. According to **Trelease** *et al.* (1971), the glyoxysomes appear first during germination of seed and later on, are converted into peroxisomes by changing their enzymal complement. However, **Kagawa** and **Beevers** (1970) and **Vigil** (1970) have found that the glyoxysomes are destroyed following fat utilization, so, there arises no question of conversion of glyoxysomes into peroxisomes. Further, because Trelease *et al.* (1971) could not provide electron micrographic evidence to support their hypothesis, so, the controversy is still awaiting resoultion (see **Hall** *et al.*, 1974).

Symbiotic Origin of Microbodies

It has been proposed that modern microbodies are the evolutionary remnants of an ancient precursor that was the major site of oxidative metabolism in eukaryotes prior to the appearance of mitochondria. Thus, **De Duve** (1969) speculated that microbodies arose as respiratory particles during the increase in oxygen levels occurring in the earth's atmosphere. This oxygen was and still is able to react with certain metabolic intermediates to produce toxic amounts of hydrogen peroxide. The peroxisomes could, therefore, have served a dual role both in destroying the peroxide and also acting as a terminal oxidase for the products of fermentation, thus providing a sink for electrons which would otherwise produce a pool of reduced metabolites. Mitochondria were envisaged as having originated from parasitic bacteria which had since evolved to a state of symbiosis with the host cell. Once both mitochondria and microbodies were established in the cell, competition between the two must have taken place. The fact that the microbodies have survived such competition indicates that they may well have function in addition to those already postulated, particularly in animal cell.

REVISION QUESTIONS

1. What are the microbodies? Describe the symbiotic origin theory of the microbodies.
2. Define the terms peroxisome and glyoxysome.
3. What would be the most likely role of peroxisomes in cells lacking mitochondria?
4. What is the function of the glyoxylate cycle?
5. What is the photorespiration and how do peroxisomes contribute?

14 Chapter MICROTUBULES AND MICROFILAMENTS

If anything is characteristic of living things, it is movement: movement of cells or organisms from one place to another; the continual shuffling of cellular organelles within the cytoplasm referred to as **cytoplasmic streaming**; the separation of chromosomes and pinching of a cell in two during division; changes in cell shape; the beating of cilia or flagella, and so on. These and certain other functions such as the production and maintenance of cell shape are performed by activities of two basic systems, one of them involving **microtubules** and the other involving **microfilaments**, the structure and function of which can be discussed such as follows:

14.1 MICROTUBULES

Microtubules (MTs) were first of all observed in the axoplasm of the myelinated nerve fibres by **Robertis** and **Franchi** (1953). They called them **neurotubules**. The exact nature of microtubules was brought into light when **Sabatini**, **Bensch** and **Barnett** (1963) made use of the glutarldehyde fixative in the electron microscopy. Microtubules of plant cells were first described in detail by **Ledbetter** and **Porter** (1963).

Occurrence

Microtubules are widely distributed cell components, but they are apparently absent from certain cells, such as amoebae, slime molds, mature mammalian erythrocytes and a few others. In the cytoplasm of animal and plant cells, microtubules occur at following seven sites: 1. Cilia and flagella, 2. Centrioles and basal bodies, 3. Nerve processes, 4. The mitotic apparatus, 5. The cortex of meristematic plant cells, 6. Elongating cells such as during the formation of the lens or during spermatogenesis of certain insects. 7. Selected structures in Protozoa such as the axostyle of parasitic flagellates, the axoneme of *Echinosphaerium*, the fibre system of *Stentor*, and the cytopharyngeal basket of *Nassula*.

Structure

A microtubule consists of a long, unbranched, hollow tube of several microns length and 210 to 250A° (or 21–25 mμ) diameter. Its wall is composed of globular subunits, each 40A° or 4 mμ in diameter, and the subunits are aligned in 13 longitudinal strands, called **protofilaments**.

Although the cytoplasmic microtubules are usually isolated from each other, there are examples of precise associations of several tubules into more or less permanent structures. The axonemata of cilia and flagella, for example, have a characteristic 9 + 2 arrangement of modified tubules. On occasions, thin thread-like bridges have also been observed between microtubules of cilia and flagella; axostyle of flagellates; spermatids of fowl; mitotic apparatus; axons; axonemes of *Echinosphaerium*; *Stentor* and *Nassula*; and cell plate of dividing plant cells. The function of these bridges is still unknown, however, there is evidence, that they give pattern to clusters of microtubules as well as playing a major role in motility (**Tilney**, 1971).

Chemical Composition

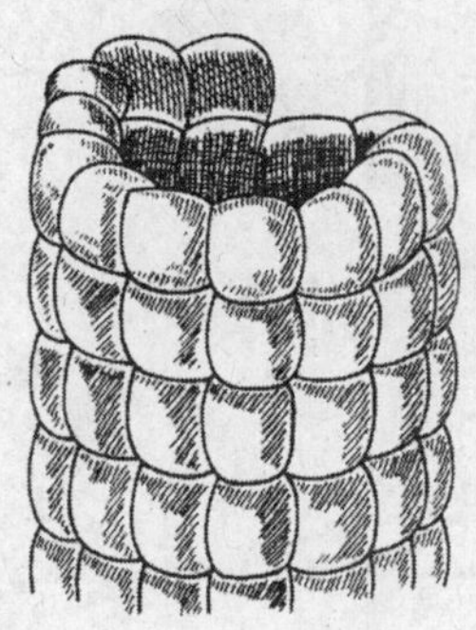

Fig. 14.1. Microtubule: the microtubule is a hollow unbranched cylindrical structure formed by 13 adjacent rows of protofilaments which themselves are linear arrays of the globular protein called tubulin.

The protein chemistry of microtubules of animal cells has been worked out by the help of drugs called **colchicine** and its derivative **colcemide**, and **vincristine**, **vinblastine** and **podophyllotoxin** which inhibit microtubule assembly, because they bind tightly to the subunit proteins and preventing their polymerization. Each microtubule subunit has a sedimentation cofficient of about 6S and consists of two globular polypeptides called α and **β-tubulin**, each with a molecular weight of about 60,000 daltons and with an amino acid composition quite similar to that of the muscle protein actin. These two polypeptide molecules form a dimeric protein, called **tubulin** and having molecular weight 110,000 to 120,000 daltons. Some enzymatic activity have been reported for tubulin, for example, it has a protein kinase activity and ATPase activity (see **De Robertis** *et al.*, 1975). Further the subunits will bind a single molecule of GTP, suggesting that this nucleotide might play some role in the assembly of the microtubules.

Assembly and Disassembly of Microtubules

The microtubules of cilia, flagella and axostyle are stable and under normal conditions, they do not break down and reassemble. But the microtubules of cytoplasm are labile, and they readily undergo reversible assembly and disassembly. It has been observed that during mitosis, a constant flux between the polymer and subunits (monomers) occurs at the tip of each microtubule of cytoplasm of dividing cells. Further, there exists a delicate equilibrium between subunits (monomers) and polymers of microtubules. Colchicine influences this equilibrium by binding monomers and removing them from the system so that the microtubules dissociate by a mass action effect. It has also become evident that the same monomeric units can be assembled into different forms depending upon local conditions of pH, cation concentration and temperature and this may account for the diversity of fibril dimensions that has been noted in different organisms. For example, tubulin polymerizes spontaneously at body temperature (37°C) to form the 13-protofilament structure seen *in vivo* (Fig. 14.2). This reversible process has been used to permit tubulin isolation—centrifugation at 37°C brings down microtubules, leaving behind small molecular weight debris, while centrifugation at O°C brings down large particles, leaving behind tubulin dimers. Repeated cycles result in a preparation containing tubulin and a small amount of **microtubule-associated protein (MAP)**. When the MAPs are removed, purified tubulin still polymerizes at 37°C but only very slowly. Readdition of a small amount of MAP results in rapid polymerization, implying a nucleation function for the MAPs. Other factors required for the assembly are the nucleotide GTP and the divalent ions Mg^{2+} and Ca^{2+}.

Nucleating centres. The microtubules are not found helter-skelter about the cell, but are organized in specific patterns designed to carry out specific functions. Spontaneous nucleation, as seen *in vitro* (Fig. 14.2), probably does not occur *in vivo*. Rather, initiation of assembly occurs at **microtubule organizing centres (MTOC)**. MTOCs exist in basal bodies (*e.g.*, *Chlamydomonas*); in centrioles (*e.g.*, most animal cells); at the poles of mitotic spindles in dividing cells that do not have centrioles (*e.g.*, most plant cells); on chromosomes (*i.e.*, **kinetochore**); in membranes and probably many other places as well. Turning on and off of these organizing centres for microtubule assembly at different times in the cell's life are probably regulated by one or all the following factors: changes in nucleation centres, changes in Ca^{2+} concentration and involvement of MAPs.

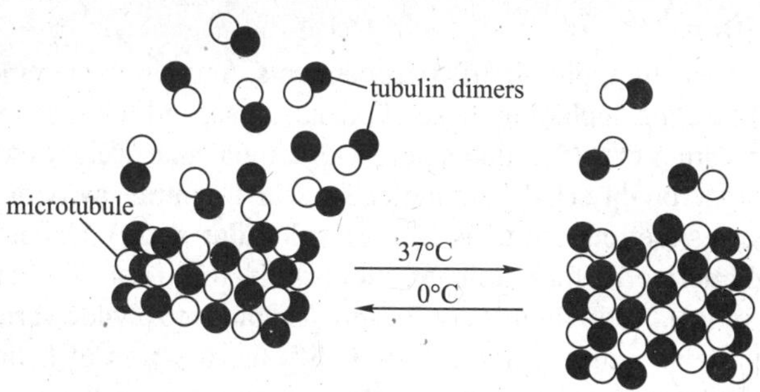

Fig. 14.2. Assembly of microtubules. The microtubules elongate spontaneously at higher temperature by addition of tubulin dimers. Lowering the temperature cause dissociation again (after Dyson, 1978).

Functions

Microtubules perform following important functions of cells:

1. Microtubules are specifically related with movement such as, undulation of cilia, flagella and axostyle.
2. Microtubules form the mitotic apparatus (or spindle) during cell division and get attached with the kinetochore of the chromosomes. Their contraction causes the movement of the chromosomes toward the opposite poles of the cells.
3. In the protozoan *Nassula*, microtubules drive the food in the gullet.
4. Microtubules are also associated with cytoplasmic streaming (cyclosis) in plant cells, the mitotic apparatus, and the axopodia of *Echinosphaerium*.
5. They serve as **cytoskeletal** agents of some kind, maintaining local areas of stress and rigidity and defining cytoplasmic channels.
6. Microtubules also function like a **microcirculatory system** for the intracellular transport of small molecules of water and inorganic ions.
7. During embryonic development, microtubules play a vital role in the process of differentiation.

14.2 MICROFILAMENTS

Thin, solid **microfilaments** of actin protein, ranging between 5 to 7 nm in diameter and indeterminate length; represent the active or motile part of the cytoskeleton. They appear to play major role in cyclosis and amoeboid motion. With high voltage electron microscopy a three-dimensional view of microfilaments has been obtained (*i.e.*, an image of **microtrabecular lattice**). These microfilaments are sensitive to **cytochalasin-B**, an alkaloid that also impairs many cell activities such as beat of heart cell, cell migration, cytokinesis, endocytosis and exocytosis. It is generally assumed that the cytochalasin-B-sensitive microfilaments are the contractile machinery of non-muscle cells.

Distribution

Microfilaments are generally distributed in the cortical regions of the cell just beneath the plasma membrane. In contrast, intermediate filaments and microtubules are found in subcortical and deeper regions of the cell. Microfilaments also extend into cell processes, especially where there is movement. Thus, they are found in the microvilli of the brush border of intestinal epitheliun and in cell types where amoeboid movement and cytoplasmic streaming are prominent.

Chemical Composition

Actin is the main structural protein of microfilaments. Actin is an extremely abundant protein in virtually all eukaryotic cells, including those of plants, algae, and fungi. Actin is synthesized as a single polypeptide consisting of 375 amino acids, with a molecular weight of about 42 kDa. Once synthesized, it folds into a roughly U-shaped molecule, with a central cavity that binds ATP or ADP. Individual actin molecules are referred to as **G-actin (globular actin)**. Under the right conditions, G-actin molecule polymerize to form **microfilaments**; in this form the actin is referred to as **F-actin (filamentous actin)**. Actin in the G or F form also binds to a wide variety of other proteins. These actin-binding proteins either regulate and modify the function of actin, or are themselves regulated or organized by their association with actin.

Of the three types of cytoskeletal proteins, actin is the most highly conserved. In functional assays, all actins appear to be identical and actins from diverse organisms will copolymerize into filaments. Despite this high degree of sequence similarity, actins do differ among different organisms. Based on sequence similarity, actins can be broadly divided into two major groups: 1. The **muscle-specific actins** (*e.g.*, **α-actin**) and 2. **Non-muscle actins** (*e.g.*, **β-actin** and **γ-actin**).

In addition to the various types of actin, another class of protein known as **actin-related proteins (Arps)** show recognizable sequence similarity to actin Arp 2 and Arp 3 are found to be involved in nucleating assembly of new microfilaments in migrating cells.

Polymerization of G actins. Like tubulin dimers, monomers of G-actin polymerize into long filaments of F-actin with a diameter of about 7 nm (Fig. 14.3). In F-actin, a full turn of the helix occurs every 36–37 nm, with about 13.5 monomers required for a full turn. The addition of each G-actin monomer is usually followed by hydrolysis of ATP molecules so that it is tightly bound to the monomer, although the energy of ATP hydrolysis is not required to drive the polymerization reactin.

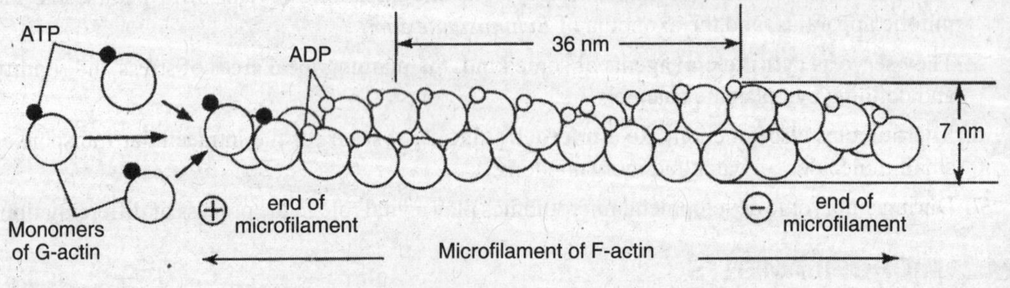

Fig. 14.3. A model for microfilament assembly *in vitro* (after Becker *et al.*, 2007)

Within a microfilament, all the actin monomers are oriented in the same direction, so that an MF, like a microtubule, has an inherent polarity, with one end differing chemically and structurally from the other end. This polarity can be readily demonstrated by incubating MFs with **heavy myosin (HMM)** or **myosin subfragment (S1)**, a proteolytic fragment of myosin (Fig. 14.4). HMM/S1 fragments bind to, or "decorate" the actin MFs to give a distinctive arrowhead pattern, the term **pointed end** and **barbed end** are commonly used to identify the **minus** and **plus ends** of a MF, respectively. The polarity of the microfilament is important, because it allows for independent regulation of actin assembly or disassembly of each end of the filament. Normally, plus end grows faster than the minus end.

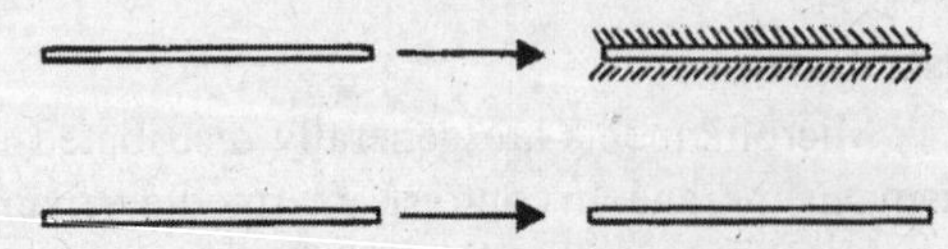

Fig. 14.4. Mode of "decoration" of actin filaments by heavy myosin or HMM. Intermediate filaments are not decorated by HMM. (after Thorpe, 1984).

Capping of MFs. Whether microfilament ends are available for further growth depends on whether or not the filament end is **capped**. Capping occurs when a **capping protein** binds the end of a filament and prevents further addition or loss of subunits, thereby stabilize it. One such protein that acts as a cap for the plus end of microfilament is appropriately named **Cap Z** (see **Becker** *et al*., 2007).

Function

Microfilaments are found to be involved in movement associated with furrow formation in cell division, cytoplasmic streaming in plant cells (*e.g.*, *Nitella* and *Chara*) and cell migration during embryonic development.

14.3 INTERMEDIATE FILAMENTS

Intermediate filaments (IFs) are tough and durable protein fibres in the cytoplasm of most higher eukaryotic cells. Constructed like woven ropes, they are typically between 8 nm to 10 nm in diameter, which is "intermediate" between the thin and thick filaments in muscle cells, where they were first described; their diameter is also between microfilaments (actin filaments) and microtubules. IFs are found resistant to colchicine and cytochalasin B and are sensitive to proteolysis.

In most animal cells IFs form a "basket" around the nucleus and extend out in gentle curving arrays to the cell periphery. IFs are particularly prominent where cells are subjected to mechanical stress, such as in epithelia, where they are linked from cell to cell at desmosomal junctions, along the length of axons, and throughout the cytoplasm of smooth muscle cells. Various names have been attached to the intermediate filaments that have a basis in the cell type in which they are observed. Thus, IFs in epidermal cells are called **tonofilaments**, in nerve cells they are referred to as **neurofilaments** and in neuroglial cells they are designated as **glial filaments**.

In cross-section, intermediate filaments have a tubular appearance. Each tubule appears to be made up of 4 or 5 protofilaments arranged in parallel fashion (**Thorpe**, 1984). IFs are composed of polypeptides of a surprisingly wide range of sizes (from about 40,000 to 240,000 daltons).

Types of Intermediate Filaments

Intermediate filaments are only found in multicellular organisms, in contrast to MTs and MFs, differ markedly in amino acid composition from tissue to tissue. Based on cell type in which they are found, IFs and their proteins can be grouped into six classes.

Class I and II IFs comprise the **keratins**, proteins that make up the **tonofilaments** found in the epithelial cells that cover the body surfaces and line its cavities (the IFs visible beneath the terminal web in the intestinal mucosa cell consists of keratin). Class I keratins are **acidic keratins**, whereas class II are **basic** or **neutral keratins**.

Class III IFs include vimentin, desmin, synemin and glial fibrillarly acidic protein. **Vimentin** is present in connective tissue and other cells derived from non-epithelial cells. Vimentin-containing filaments are often prominent features, in cultured fibroblast cells. **Desmin** is found in muscle cells. **Synemin** is a protein of 230,000 daltons, which is also present in the intermediate filaments of muscle, together with desmin and vimentin. Vimentin and synemin containing IFs can be observed in the chicken erythrocytes. **Glial fibrillary acidic (GFA) protein** is characteristic of the glial cells that surround and insulate nerve cells.

Class IV IFs are the **neurofilaments** (NF) **proteins** found in the neurofilaments of nerve cells.

Class V IFs are the **nuclear lamins** A, B and C, which form a filamentous scaffold along the inner surface of the nuclear membrane of virtually all eukaryotic cells.

Neurofilaments found in cells in the embryonic nervous system are made of **nestin** protein, which constitute class VI IFs.

Each of these IF proteins tends to assemble spontaneously *in vitro* to form homopolymers and will also co-assemble with the other Types III IF proteins to form **co-polymers** and **hetero-polymers**. In fact co-polymers of vimentin and desmin, or of vimentin and glial fibrillary acidic protein, are found in some type of cells. For example, desmin remains concentrated in the Z-lines and T-tubule system of striated or skeletal system, together with vimentin, synemin and α-actinin. Since desmin links actin to plasma membrane, from this fact the name of desmin has been derived by **Lazarides** and coworkers in 1976 (in Greek desmin means link or bond).

General Structure of IFs

All six types of intermediate filaments (IFs) contain proteins which have a central rod like domain consisting of four **helical segments**. The central domain is highly conserved in size, secondary structure, and sequence, though sequence homologies are confined to the helical regions. In types I-IV, the helical segments contain a total of 276 amino acids and the linker segments are non-helical (Fig. 14.5). In type V, the helical segments contain 318 amino acids and their linker segments are also helical. The N- and C-terminal domains that flank the central section are non-helical and are much more variable in size and sequence.

Assembly of IFs

A popular model of assembly of a intermediate filament includes the following steps: 1. Two identical **monomers** pair to form a **dimer** in which the conserved helical central regions are aligned in parallel and are wound together into a coiled coil. 2. Two dimers then line up side-by-side to form a 48 nm by 3 nm **protofilament** containing four polypeptide chains. 3. These protofilaments then

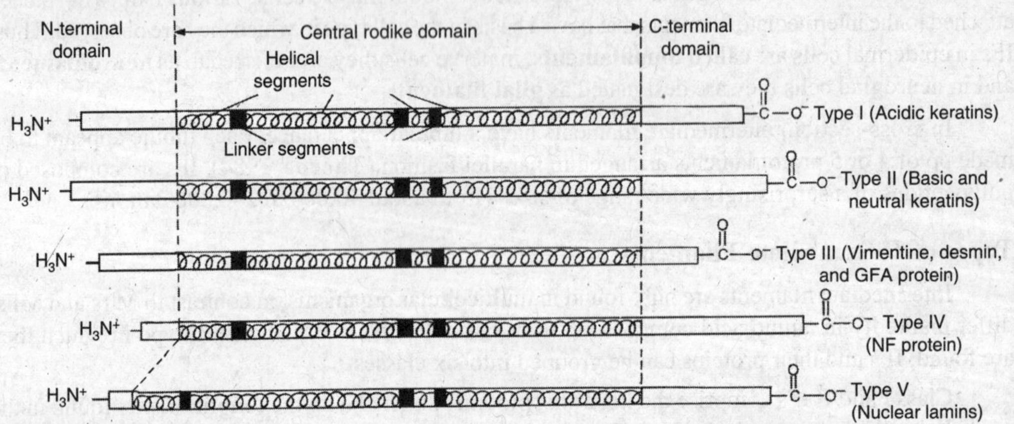

Fig. 14.5. Structural similarities of intermediate filament protein. Except VI or nestin, all the five IFs are shown (after Becker *et al.*, 2007).

associate in a staggered manner to form successively larger structures. 4. The final 10 nm diameter of the intermediate filament is thought to be composed of 8-protofilaments (*i.e.*, 32 polypeptide chains) joined end on end to neighbours by staggered overlap to form the long rope-like filaments. It is still not known whether IFs are polar structures (like actin and tubulin) or non-polar (like the DNA double helix).

IFs During Mitosis

Mitosis of cultured epithelial cells shows striking changes in intermediate filaments of cytokeratin and vimentin. During prophase the 10 nm filaments unwind into threads of 2 to 4 nm and into spheroidal aggregates containing both types of proteins. At metaphase and anaphase most vimentin and cytokeratin appear as spheroid bodies, while at telophase the filamentous cytoskeleton become gradually reestablished. From these experimental studies, **Franke** (1982) has concluded that the living cells contain factors that promote the reversible disintegration and restoration of intermediate filaments during mitosis.

Functions of IFs

The main function of most intermediate filaments is to provide mechanical support to the cell and its nucleus. IFs in epithelia form a transcellular network that seems designed to resist external forces. The neurofilaments in the nerve cell axons probably resist stresses caused by the motion of the animal, which would otherwise break these long, thin cylinders of cytoplasm. Desmin filaments provide mechanical support for the sarcomeres in muscle cells, and vimentin filaments surround and probably support the large fat droplets in the fat cells.

Comparison of Microtubules, Intermediate Filaments and Microfilaments

The three components of the cytoskeleton, namely microtubules, intermediate filaments and microfilaments have been compared in Table 14.1

Table 14.1. Comparison of some properties of microtubules, intermediate filaments and microfilaments (*Source:* Thorpe, 1984).

Property	*Microtubules*	*Intermediate filaments*	*Microfilaments*
1. Structure	Hollow with walls made up of 13 protofilaments	Hollow with walls made up of 4 to 5 protofilaments	Solid made up of polymerized actin (F-actin)
2. Diameter (nm)	24–25	10	7–9
3. Monomer units	α- and β-tubulin	Six types of protein defining six major classes	G-actin
4. ATPase activity	Present in dynein arms	None	None
5. Functions	1. Motility of eukaryotes	1. Integrate contractile units in muscle	1. Muscle contraction
	2. Chromosome movement	2. Cytoskeletal structural function in cytoplasm	2. Cell shape changes
	3. Movements of intracellular materials		3. Protoplasmic streaming
	4. Contribute toward maintaining cell shape		4. Cytokinesis

REVISION QUESTIONS

1. What are the microtubules? Describe their structure and functions in the cell.
2. What are the contractile filaments? Describe the structure and functions of contractile filaments of muscle cells and non-muscle cells.
3. Define the terms myofilament, myofibril, sarcomere, actomyosin and actin.
4. What are the major elements of the so-called cytoskeleton and in what kinds of movements are each thought to be involved?
5. What systems appear to determine shape in mammalian and non-mammalian erythrocytes, respectively?

15 Chapter CENTRIOLES AND BASAL BODIES

Cytoplasm of some eukaryotic cells contains two cylindrical, rod-shaped, microtubular structures, called **centrioles**, near the nucleus. The portion of the cytoplasm in which centriole formation takes place is called **centrosome**. Centrioles lack limiting membrane and DNA or RNA and form a spindle of microtubules, the mitotic apparatus during mitosis or meiosis and sometimes get arranged just beneath the plasma membrane to form and bear flagella or cilia in flagellated or ciliated cells (**Fulton**, 1971). When a centriole bears a flagellum or cilium, it is called **basal body**. There are many synonyms for basal body, including kinetosome, kinetoplast, blepharoplast, basal granule, basal corpuscle, and proximal centriole.

15.1 OCCURRENCE

Centrioles occur in algae, fungi, bryophytes, terns, gymnosperms, protozoans (ciliates and flagellates) and most of the multicellular animals. They are absent in prokaryotes, diatoms, yeast and most higher plants (conifers and angiosperms). Centrioles are most often found associated in pairs and a pair of centrioles is called **diplosome**. Usually during interphase these are next to the nuclear envelope, though in some cell types they are near the cell surface (**Fawcett**, 1966). Sometimes these pairs are arranged end to end, but more commonly they come together to form a right angle. Often the area in which a centriole or a diplosome lies is relatively devoid of cellular constituents as mitochondria, chloroplasts, ribosomes and glycogen granules. This area has different appearance than the surrounding cytoplasm and contains a fine fibrous material and is called **centrosphere** (**Robbins** *et al.*, 1968; **Kalnius** and **Porter**, 1969).

15.2 STRUCTURE

Centrioles and basal bodies are cylindrical structures which are 0.15–0.25 μm in diameter usually 0.3–0.7 μm in length, though, some are as short as 0.16 μm and others are as long as 8 μm (see **Fulton**, 1971). Both have following ultrastructural components:

1. Cylinder wall. The most striking and regular ultrastructural feature of centrioles and basal bodies is the array of nine triplet microtubules equally spaced around the perimeter of an imaginary cylinder (Fig. 15.1). The space between and immediately around the triplet is filled with an amorphous, electron-dense material (see Chapter 46). In transverse section the triplets are arranged like vanes or blades of pinwheel or turbine. Each triplet or blade is tilted inward to the central axis at an angle of about 450 to the circumference; within each blade the tubules twist from one end to the other or describe a helical course. Since centrioles have no outer membrane, the triplets are considered to form the wall of the cylinder, and arbitrarily define the inside and outside of the centriole.

2. Triplets. The nine triplets that make up the wall are basically similar in centrioles and basal bodies. The three subunit microtubules have been designated A, B, and C, with the innermost tubule being A (Fig. 15.2). Individual tubules are 200–260 Å in diameter. Only the A tubule is round; the others are incomplete, C-shaped and share their wall with the preceding tubule. At both ends the C tubule often terminates before the A and B tubules.

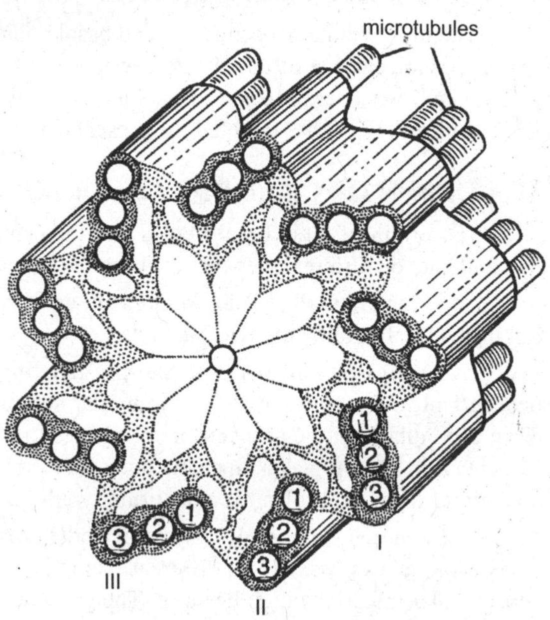

Fig. 15.1. Cross-sectional structure of a centriole. There are nine groups of three microtubules (after De Witt, 1977).

The substructure of A, B and C tubules, is similar to the structure of other microtubules (**Stephens**, 1970). The A tubule has 13, 40–45 Å globular subunits around its perimeter. Three or four of these subunits are shared with the B tubules, which in turn share several of its subunits with the C tubules.

Often the triplets are thought to run parallel to one another and to the long axis of the cylinder, but this is not always the case. In the basal bodies of some organisms, the triplets get closer toward, the proximal end, so the diameter of the cylinder gets smaller. In some centrioles the triplets are parallel to one another but turn in a long-pitched helix with respect to the cylinder axis (**Fulton**, 1971).

3. Linkers. The A tubule of each triplet is linked with C tubule of neighbouring triplet by protein **linkers** at intervals along their entire length. These linkers hold the cylindrical array of the microtubules and maintain the typical radial tilt of the triplets.

4. Feet and Cartwheel. There are dense condensations from the A tubules toward the centre of the cylinder, forming a series of 'feet'. Further, at the proximal ends of centrioles and basal bodies, occur connections between tubules in the form hub-spokes cartwheel. The cartwheel consists of a central hub and 9 radial spokes which run toward the A tubules. These spokes end in the dense "feet".

5. Ciliary Rootlets. In some cells, from the basal ends of the basal bodies originate the ciliary rootlets which are of following two types:

***(i)* Striated root fibrils.** Striated root fibrils contain regular cross bands, each of which remain separated by a distance of 550 to 700A°.

***(ii)* Tubular root fibrils.** The tubular root fibrils have the diameter of 200Å.

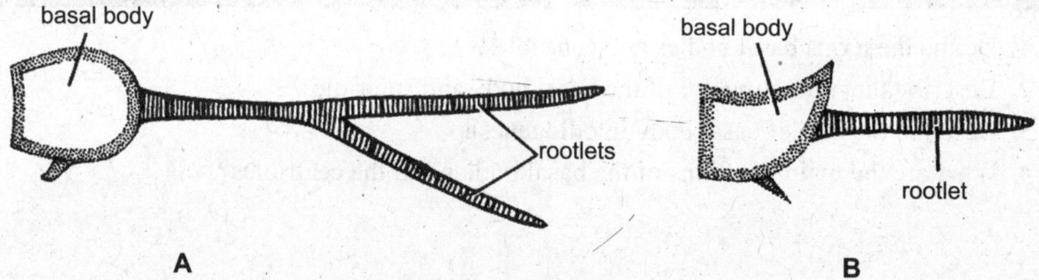

Fig. 15.2. Relation of rootlets with the basal body.

15.3 CHEMICAL COMPOSITION

The microtubules of centrioles and basal bodies contain the structural protein, **tubulin**, along with lipid molecules (**Fulton**, 1971). The centrioles and basal bodies contain a high concentration of ATPase enzyme. There exists a controversy that whether centrioles and basal bodies have DNA and RNA. **Fulton** (1971) has doubted the presence of nucleic acids in these organelles.

15.4 ORIGIN OF CILIA, BASAL BODIES AND CENTRIOLES

The origin of cilia, basal bodies and the centrioles is inter-related. The centriole originates first and later on differentiates into the basal bodies which ultimately give rise to the cilia or flagella.

According to **Gall** (1961), **Mizukanni** and **Gall** (1966) and **Sorokin** (1968) centriole may be originated by the following two methods:

1. During the cell division the pre-existing centrioles give rise daughter centrioles or **procentrioles**. Procentrioles arise as annular structures which become lengthened into cylinders. From each tubule of the procentriole originates three subfibrils and the maturation of the centriole takes place in the cytoplasm. Such method of centriole formation occurs only during the cell division. Sometimes these centrioles form the primary cilia which are transitory and are short-lived.

2. When centriole is to form basal bodies of kinetosomes and cilia or flagella, then origin of centriole takes place by the different methods. In this method the centriole originates from the fibrogranular material which lies in it. The granules are formed, increased in size and aggregate to form the spheroid bodies. These spheroid bodies give rise to the procentrioles. Procentrioles after maturation form centrioles which get arranged in rows just beneath the plasma membrane. Each centriole produces other procentrioles from its lateral side and itself converted into the basal bodies. Basal bodies produce the ciliary rootlets from their basal ends and the cilia or flagella from their apical ends. Such sort of differentiation occurs in the ciliary epithelium. The portion of the cytoplasm in which centriole formation takes place lies near the nucleus and is known as **centrosomes**.

The formation of the cilia from the basal bodies is started by the formation of a vesicle-like structure of the cytoplasm towards the distal end of the basal bodies. The walls of the vesicle are invaginated due to rapid growth of ciliary shaft. The walls of the vesicle are temporary and are replaced by the new and permanent ciliary sheaths.

15.5 FUNCTIONS

Centrioles and basal bodies have following functions:

(*i*) Centrioles serve as foci for the production of new centrioles and basal bodies.

(*ii*) Centrioles are foci at the poles of the mitotic apparatus, where they are surrounded by microtubules.

(*iii*) The microtubules of cilia and flagella originate and bear by basal bodies.

REVISION QUESTIONS

1. Define the terms basal bodies and centrioles.
2. Describe the ultra-structure of the basal body and centrioles.
3. Describe the role of basal body in ciliogenesis.
4. What are the main functions of the basal bodies and the centrioles?

16 Chapter CILIA AND FLAGELLA

The cilia (*L.,cili*=eye lash) and flagella (*L.*, little whip) are microscopic, contractile and filamentous processes of the cytoplasm which create food currents, act as sensory organs and perform many mechanical functions of the cell. Morphologically and physiologically, the cilia and flagella are identical structures but even then both can be distinguished from each other by their number, size and functions. Their distinguishing features are as follows:

1. The flagella are less (1 or 2) in number than the cilia which may be numerous (3000 to 14000 or more) in number.
2. The flagella occur at one end of the cell, while the cilia may occur throughout the surface of the cell.
3. The flagella are longer (up to 150 μm) processes, while the cilia are short (5 to 10 μm) appendages of the cytoplasm.
4. The flagella usually beat independently, while the cilia tend to beat in a coordinated rhythm.
5. The flagella exhibit undulatory motion, while the cilia move in a sweeping or pendular stroke.

16.1 STEREOCILIA AND KINOCILIA

The cell sometimes gives out immobile cytoplasmic extensions known as **stereocilia**. The sterocilia differ from the true cilia which are known as **kinocilia**. The sterocilia occur in most epithelial cells of the epididymis and macula and crista of the internal ear.

16.2 DISTRIBUTION OF THE CILIA AND FLAGELLA

The flagella occur in the protozoans of the class Flagellata, choanocyte cells of the sponges, spermatozoa of the Metazoa and among plants in the algae and gamete cells. The cilia occur in the protozoans of the class Ciliata and members of other classes and ciliated epithelium of the Metazoa. The cilia may occur on external body surface and may help in the locomotion of such animals as the larvae of certain Platyhelminthes, Nemertines, Echinodermata, Mollusca and Annelida. The cilia may line the internal cavities or passages of the metazoan bodies as air passage of the respiratory system and reproductive tracts. The nematode worms and arthropods have no cilia.

16.3 STRUCTURE OF THE CILIA AND FLAGELLA

The ciliary apparatus is composed of following basic components: 1. The **shaft** or **cilium**, which is the slender cylindroid process that projects from the free surface of the cell; 2. The **basal body** or granule, a centriole like cellular organelle from which the cilium originates; and 3. In some cells fine fibrils—called **ciliary rootlets**. Basal body remains separated from cilium by a **ciliary** or **basal plate** which has two functions: termination of the C tubule of each triplet of basal body; and beginning of two central microtubules. The cilia and flagella are extremely delicate, permanently formed, thread-like extension of cytoplasm and their thickness is often at the limit of the resolving power of light microscope.

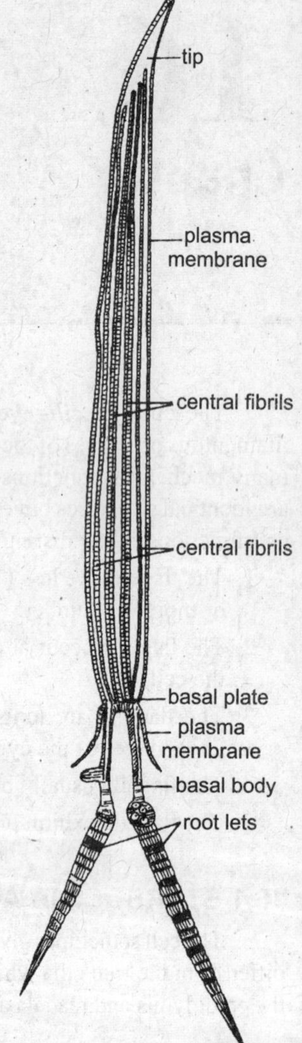

Fig. 16.1. A ciliary apparatus in L.S. showing fundamental structure of cilium or shaft, basal bodies and ciliary rootlets.

Although the fine structure of cilia and flagella has been described with accuracy only recently, there were intimations of their structure as early as 1887, when **Jensen** observed a fraying of the end of sperm flagellum. Later, similar observations were made on the cilia and flagllea of Protozoa. There were also suggestions that the component fibrils of a flagellum had contractile properties. More detailed analyses of fine structure came in the 1950's, with the studies of **Grigg** and **Hodge** (1949) on the flagella of spermatozoa and **Manton** *et al.* (1952) on the cilia of higher plants. In each instance the structures appeared to consist of 11 fibrils, two of which were centrally located with the outer nine arranged around them. **Fawcett** and **Porter** (1954) confirmed the 9 + 2 fibrilar arrangement of cilia and flagella and found this to be universally occurred fundamental pattern. Later on, it was found that the nine peripheral fibrils were thick and consisted of **doublet** or **pairs** of **microtubules**, whereas, the two central fibrils were small and contained **single microtubules**. The basic microtubular frame work of cilia and flagella is termed as **axial complex** or **axoneme** and it is thought to be the essential motile element. The component microtubules of axoneme run longitudinally within the shaft or cilium, perpendicular to the surface of the cell. Further, in various flagella **accessory** structures made of fibres, microtubules, crystalline bodies or mitochondrial derivatives are found along with the axoneme but these are not considered to be an integral part of the motile mechanism.

Fine Structure of Axoneme

Electron microscopic studies revealed the same basic plan of fine structure in the flagella and cilia of all eukaryotes (Protozoa, Metazoa and plants). This is indication not only of phylogenetic relationship but also of similar mode of action (see **Grell**, 1973).

The axoneme of a cilium or flagellum may range from a few microns to 1 to 2 millimeters in length, but the outside diameter is about 0.2 μm to 2000 A° at the base, which may be upto 10 μm above the cell surface. The axoneme is generally surrounded by a 95A° thick, trilaminar, lipoproteinous **outer ciliary membrane**, which is continuous with the plasma membrane. All the components of the axoneme are embedded within the **ciliary ground substance** or **matrix** (Fig. 16.1).

Typically the axoneme of most cilia and flagella has a 9 + 2 microtubular pattern which has been shown in Fig. 16.3. However, the central or core microtubules exhibit some variation in different species (**Warner**, 1972). Recently, it has been observed that a plane perpendicular to the line joining the two central microtubules divides the axoneme into a right and a left symmetrical half. It is well evident now that the plane of the ciliary beat remains perpendicular to this plane of symmetry (see **De Robertis** *et al.*, 1975).

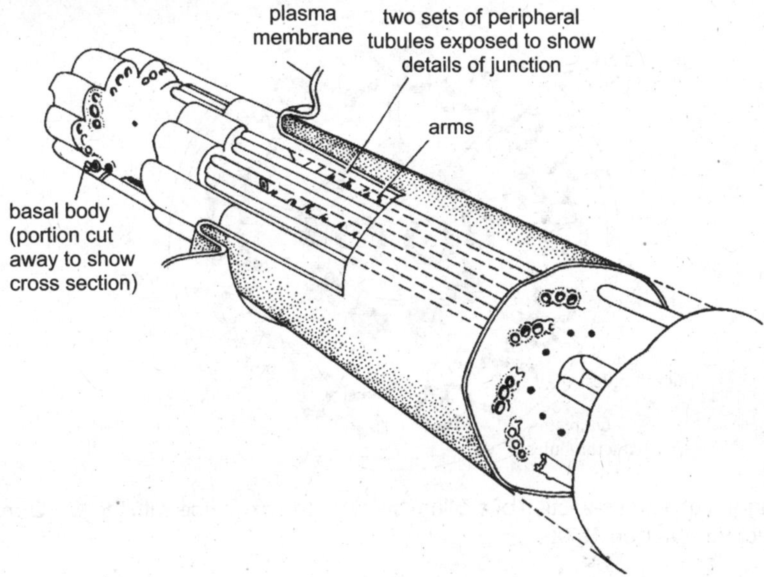

Fig. 16.2. Three-dimensional structure of a flagellum (after De Witt, 1977).

The nine pairs of peripheral microtubules an ellipsoidal configuration, whereas, the central ones are circular. Each of the nine peripheral fibrils is 360A° in diameter and composed of two microtubules of 180 to 250A° diameter. The two microtubules of each peripheral pair or **doublet** remain morphologically distinguishable. In the cylinder of nine doublets, each doublet remains separated with other by a distance of 200A° and each doublet is approximately 250A° away from the outer ciliary membrane. Further, the doublets are skewed at about 10 degrees, so that one tubule, designated **subfibre A** lies closer to the axis than the other (*i.e.*, **subfibre B**). The microtubule of subfibre A is smaller, but complete, whereas that of subfibre B is larger and incomplete, since it lacks the wall adjacent to subfibre A.

From subfibre A two types of projections called **arms** arise. The **outer arm** terminates in a hook-like bend, whereas, the **inner arm** has no terminal hook. A fine linkage, termed the **peripheral link** or **interdoublet link** appears to connect the end of the inner arm to the adjacent subfibre B (**Allen**, 1967; **Kiefer**, 1970). In longitudinal sections the arms appear as regularly spaced projections along subfibre A, with a period ranging from 160 to 220A°. The arms of subfibre A are oriented in the same direction in all A microtubules. This orientation is clockwise when the axoneme is viewed from base to tip. In many cells, the arms of doublet number 5 are permanently attached to doublet number 6. In Fig. 16.3 the nine doublets are numbered, starting from the one lying in the plane of symmetry, and continuing in the clockwise direction.

On the other hand, each central fibril has a diameter of about 250A° and is composed of 60A° thick wall. Both central fibrils are separated by a space of 350A° and remain enveloped in a common **central sheath**. In certain axonemes, the central sheath contains a helically wound fibre with a space of 160A° (**Warner**, 1970).

Radial linkage. Each peripheral doublet remains connected to the central sheath of two central microtubules by spoke-like, radially oriented cross bridges or links. These nine links are about 360A° long. Each of them remains attached to subfibre A on one side (**Gibbons**, 1967; **Allen**, 1968), and ends in a dense **knob** or **head** which may have a fork-like structure. In longitudinal sections the radial links are spaced alternately at 320, 560 or 640 A°. The heads of all radial links join the central sheath by way of **transitional junction**.

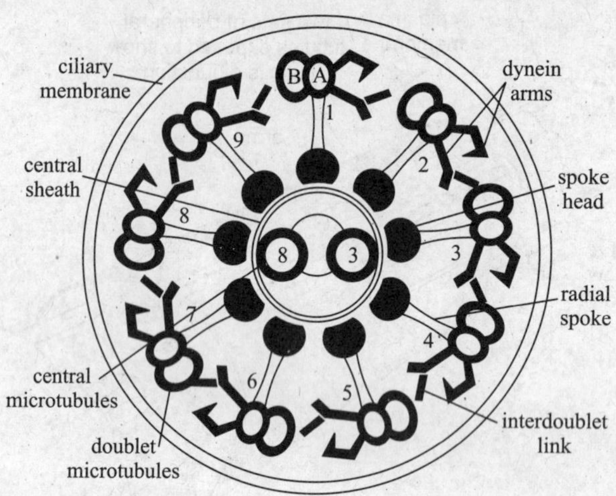

Fig. 16.3. Diagram of a cross-section of a cilium showing the axoneme with the '9 + 2' microtubular structure (Warner, 1972).

Biochemistry of Axoneme

For biochemical analysis of axoneme, first the cilia or flagella are isolated by various procedures (**Gibbons**, 1967; **Rosenbaum** and **Child**, 1967), then, the ciliary membrane is removed in a calcium free medium or by detergents (**Witman** *et al.*, 1972) and relatively clear axonemes lacking only the soluble proteins of the matrix, are obtained (**Gibbons** and **Gibbons**, 1969). Finally, the axonemes are treated with detergents to solubilize selectively the structural components or they are treated with trypsin, which disrupt the linkages between the microtubules (**Summers** and **Gibbons**, 1971). The isolated ciliary microtubules and arms of subfibre A are found to contain following chemistry:

1. Tubulins. Renaud *et al.* (1968) have isolated two distinct proteins from the ciliary peripheral microtubules (*i.e.*, doublets) by gel electrophoresis. These proteins have 'been termed **tubulin A** and **B** and have a molecular weight of 55,000 to 60,000 (**Stephens**, 1970). **Stephens** (1970) thought that tubulin A corresponded to the subfibre A, and tubulin B, to the subfibre B; however, further studies of **Witman** *et al.* (1972) in *Chlamydomonas* indicated that both tubulins are present in the various microtubules of the axonema. Besides tubulins, axonemes of flagella are found to contain about ten soluble, structural secondary proteins (see **De Robertis** *et al.*, 1975).

2. Dynein. The arms of subfibre A, radial linkages and their attachment to the core surface are found to contain a myosin-like protein called **dynein**. This protein has a ATPase activity (**Gibbons** and **Rowe**, 1965). Dynein is found to be a dimeric protein containing two fractions which sedimenting at 30S and 14S. The 14S polypeptide chain has a molecular weight of about 600,000 and is probably a monomer of the 30S (molecular weight of 5×10^6 daltons).

Molecular Structure of Microtubules of Cilia and Flagella

The high resolution microscopy has revealed that the microtubules of each of the subfibre A and central fibrils of the cilia and flagella are composed of 13 filamentous subunits, the **protofilaments**, of 40A° thickness, in their walls. Each subfibre B of doublets is incomplete and have either 10 or 11 protofilaments. Protofilaments are polymerized α and β tubulin proteins (Fig. 16.4).

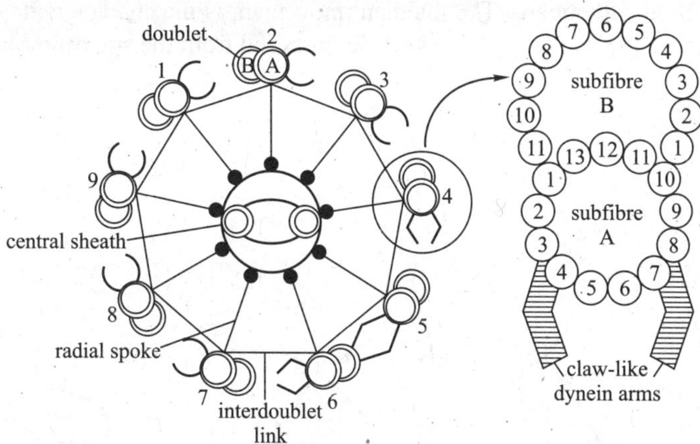

Fig. 16.4. A detailed structure of the axoneme. Note the nine outer doublets, each with two claw-like dynein arms on the A subfibre and a radial spoke connecting the doublet to the central sheath. Note also the fine interdoublet links and the bridge between doublets 5 and 6 and between the two central microtubules. The detail shows the protofilament substructure (after Dyson, 1978).

16.4 PHYSIOLOGY OF CILIARY MOVEMENT

The cilia and flagella serve many purposes and their movements propel the organism. The cilia are contractile structures and in them two types of rhythms known as **metachronic** and **isochronic** or **synchronic rhythms** produce the wave of contractions in the cilia. In the **metachronic** type of rhythm the cilia of a row beat one after the other, while in the **synchronous** or isochronic rhythm, all the cilia of a row beat simultaneously. In contrast to the cilia, the flagella exhibit undulant motion and beat independently.

The beating of cilia or flagella is caused by the intraciliary excitation which is followed by the interciliary conduction. **Hayashi** (1961) has reported that the two inner filaments of a cilium transmit excitation and the nine outer filaments are the seat of ATP splitting. The movement of cilia may be under nervous or cytoplasmic control. In a few invertebrate embryos the cilia are probably under nervous control since their movement may be stopped upon stimulation of the embryo. In ciliates they are thought to be coordinated by a neuromotor centre near the mouth since destruction of the fibres connecting the centre to the cilia results in uncoordinated movements (**Taylor**, 1920). However, **Okajima** (1966) reported coordinated movements in *Euplotes* even after complete dissection of the neuro-motor fibres. Recent studies have shown that cytoplasm is necessary for the ciliary movements. The ATP provides necessary amount of energy for the motion of the cilia and flagella. Four types of ciliary movements have been recognized which are as follows:

1. The pendulus ciliary movement. The pendulus type of ciliary movement is carried out in a single plane. It occurs in the ciliated protozoans which have rigid cilia. In such cases the movement of the cilia is carried out by a flexion at its base.

2. The unciform ciliary movement. The unciform (hook-like) ciliary movement occurs commonly in the metazoan cells. In such type of movement, when the cilia contract it becomes double and acquires a hook-like shape.

3. The infundibuliform ciliary movement. The infundibuliform ciliary movement occurs due to the rotary movement of the cilium and flagellum. In this case, the cilium or flagellum is passed through three mutually perpendicular planes in the space and makes conical or funnel-shaped shape.

4. The undulant movement. The undulant movement is the characteristic of the flagellum. In undulant movement the waves of the contraction proceed from the site of implantation and pass to the border.

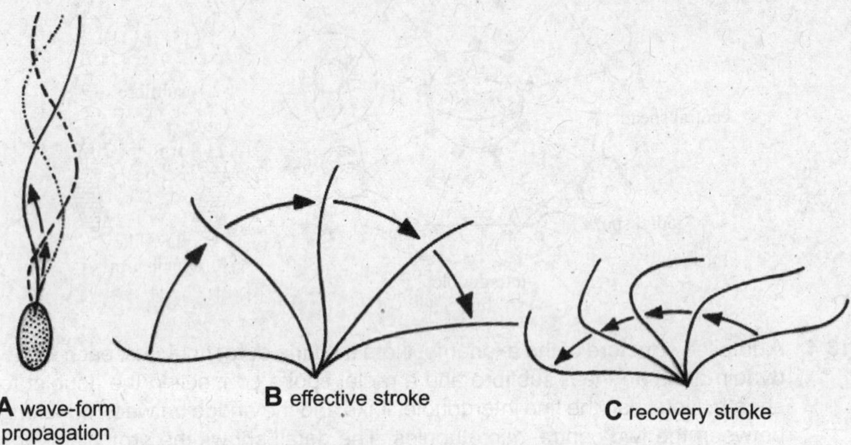

Fig. 16.5. Movement of cilia and flagella. A—Typical wave-form propagation of a flagellum, such as that found in sperm; B—Effective stroke common with cilia of all types; C—Recovery of cilium prior to the next effective stroke (after Dyson, 1978).

During ciliary or flagellar movement, initiation and propagation of contraction remains apparently a property of the entire flagellum. The plane of beat of cilium is perpendicular to the plane passing through the central microtubules. In Fig. 16.3, this plane passes through Doublet 1 and between Doublets 5 and 6. However, there are many indications that there is a three-dimensional movement during the beat. Thus, one cycle of beat includes following three phases—rest position, effective stroke and recovery phase. Although the effective stroke is in a single plane, thé cilium moves away from the original plane during the recovery phase. **Tamm** and **Horridge** (1970) have demonstrated by scanning electron microscopy that during ciliary movement either the whole cilium rotates at its base or that the central microtubules rotate.

Macromolecular Mechanisms Involved in Ciliary Motion

Since the last century, ciliary and flagellar motion have been compared to that of muscle. However, the complex structure of the axonemes suggests that this motion may be more complex than the planer sliding of myofilaments in muscle. Following two main theories have been postulated for ciliary and flagellar motion:

1. Localized contraction theory,
2. Sliding mechanism theory.

1. Localized contraction theory. Localized contraction theory of ciliary motion is proposed by **Bradfield** (1955) and it states that the movement of a cilium or flagellum depends on unequal contractions or localized shortenings of the longitudinal fibrils. This theory is based on several assumptions, namely, that the nine outer fibrils are able to contract and send wave of contraction from the base to the tip of the flagellum, that the central fibrils are not contractile, and that the origin of the impulse causing contraction is in the basal body beneath one of the outer fibrils. In the initial movement or beat a wave of contraction starts in the first fibril (which can be called number 1) and spreads to fibrils 2, 9, 10 and 11 (the central pair) (Fig. 16.6). From fibrils of 10 and 11, waves of contraction move up and stimulate fibrils 2, 3, 8, and 9 so that they contract simultaneously. The shortening of the fibrils resulting from the contractions makes the cilium bend in a forwarded direction as if it were a rigid body. On the return beat, the fibrils participating in the initial movement relax, and contractions occur at a slower rate in fibrils 4, 5, 6, and 7, to pull the cilium back to its original upright position. The cycle is repeated when a new impulse arises under fibril number 1.

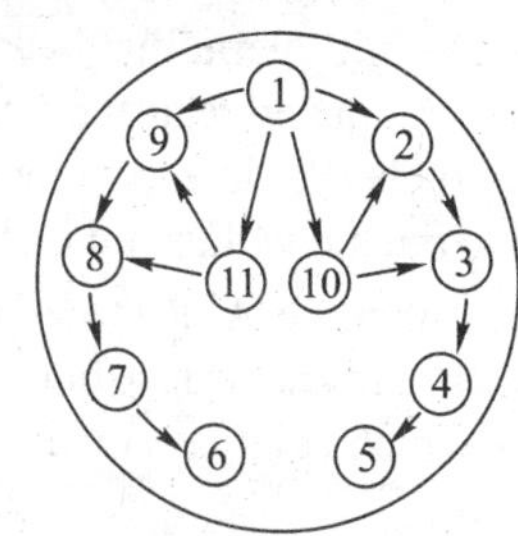

Fig. 16.6. Possible scheme for the transmission of a contractile impulse in flagellar fibrils according to localized contraction theory of Bradfield.

This theory of ciliary movement is abandoned, now, due to the lacking of adequate experimental evidences in the support of it and has been replaced by sliding mechanism theory which is most favoured one because the sliding of doublets during the bending of the cilium or flagellum has actually been observed and measured (see **De Robertis** *et al.*, 1975).

2. Sliding mechanism theory. According to this model, cilia and flagella move by sliding adjacent doublets past each other. It was first suggested by **Bjorn Afzelius** in 1959 and experimentally proved by **Peter Satir** and associates in 1960's. The displacement of the doublets during bending has been determined because the central microtubules extend to the very tip, whereas subfibres B terminate at a distance from the tip of 1 to 2 μm, and subfibres A terminate slightly beyond subfibres B. This microtubular arrangement has also made possible to demonstrate that the subfibres do not move relative to one another within the one another (**Slater**, 1968). **Sleigh** (1971) have shown that the amount of sliding displacement depends on the distance separating the tubules and on the bend angle (see Fig. 16.7).

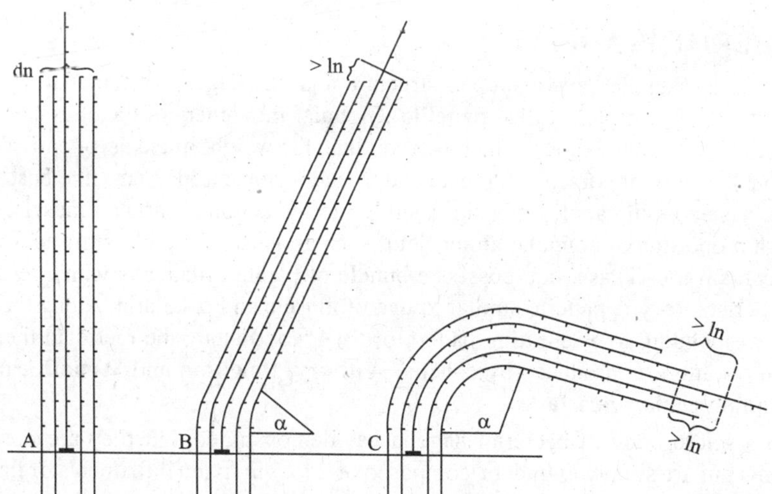

Fig. 16.7. Diagram of sliding model of the axoneme. The amount of sliding displacement (Δ ln) is a function of distance separating the microtubules (dn) and the bend angle (α). The central microtubules are represented by the longer lines (Sleigh, 1971).

Experimental work of **Summers** and **Gibbons** (1971) have demonstrated that the force needed to cause displacement between adjacent doublets and hence the bending of cilia and flagella is provided by hydrolysis of ATP (actually Mg^{2+}—ATP). This hydrolysis and conversion of chemical to mechanical energy is made possible by the dynein arms of subfibre A. The catalytic significance of dyne in in ciliary movement has been also confirmed very recently by **Afzelius** (1976, 1977). When a small group of male patients being examined because of sterility were found by **Afzelius** to have immotile sperm that lack dynein arms in their flagella. Most of these patients also suffer from chronic cough and recurrent lung infections due to poor ciliary action in the airways and consequent failure to clear efficiently mucous and inhaled particles from their lungs. The importance of dynein to the axoneme is thus quite clear.

Further, the ATP needed for ciliary movement is generated by mitochondria or by glycolysis in the cytoplasm and diffuse outward within the axoneme. Axoneme also contains the enzyme **adenylate kinase** which catalyzes the reaction 2 ADP $\rightarrow$ AMP + ATP.

16.5 FUNCTIONS OF THE CILIA AND FLAGELLA

1. The ciliary or flagellar movement provides the locomotion to the cell or organism.
2. The cilia create food currents in lower aquatic animals.
3. In the respiratory tract, the ciliary movements help in the elimination of the solid particles from it.
4. The eggs of amphibians and mammals are driven out from the oviduct by the aid of vibratile cilia of the latter.

Thus, the cilia and flagella serve many physiological processes of the cell, such as locomotion, alimentation, circulation, respiration, excretion and perception of sense.

16.6 DERIVATIVES OF CILIA

The cilia are modified into a variety of structures such as the rods and cones of the retina, crown cell of saccus vasculosus of third ventricle of fishes, primitive sensory cells of the pineal eye and cnidocil of the nematocysts of the coelenterates.

16.7 BACTERIAL FLAGELLA

The bacterial flagella have a simpler structure than the flagella of flagellates. Chemically it is composed of a single protein called **flagellin**. Globular monomers of flagellin have a molecular weight of 20,000 to 40,000 daltons, which is lower than the weight of eukaryotic tubulin (50,000 to 60,000 daltons). These monomers aggregate end to end to form a filament, like beads on a string. The flagellin has an amino acid composition similar to the action of striated muscle, especially in having a high proportion of nonpolar amino acids such as aspartic and glutamic acids. The flagella of bacteria contain no ATPase, but, possess a bundle of parallel filaments which remain arranged in the characteristic α-type pattern, similar to that of muscle and α-keratin. Along the axis there is a spacing corresponding to a repeating pattern of 5.1A°, and along the meridian there is a 9.8A° spacing. The α-pattern is produced by α-helix. **Astbury**, **Beighton** and **Weibull** called bacterial flagella '**monomolecular muscles**'.

Electron microscopy of bacterial flagella has demonstrated that they are not made up of 9 + 2 filaments but are simply cylinders, composed of 2 to 5 individual filaments of flagellin which are only 40–50A° wide but upto several μm long and are arranged in a hexagonal packing with a helical twist (Fig. 16.8). No membrane encloses the flagellum, except in spirochetes. Bacterial flagella grow at the tip, where as eukaryotic flagella grow at their basal end next to the centriole (basal body). The flagellum consists of three portions, a terminal **hook**, a main **shaft**, and a **basal region** which is attached to a granule embedded within the protoplast, but it bears no resmblance to a centriole or basal body (Fig. 16.9). According to **Lowy** and **Spencer**, bacterial flagella beat like whips and their motion is brought about by a rotating movement of the base. The rotating or oscillating movement of the base can possibly transmitt along the hollow axis by a progressive change in packing of the sub-units. ATP molecules are supposed to diffuse readily into the base of bacterial flagella.

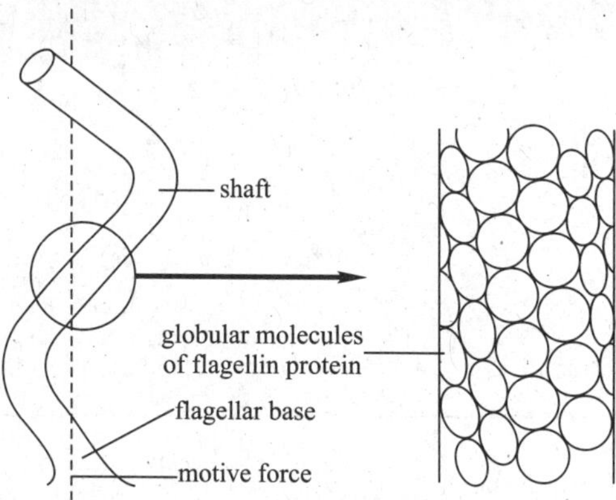

Fig. 16.8. Structure of bacterial flagella. The motive force is located at the base of the narrow shaft, which is composed of globular molecules, 40A° in diameter arranged in hexagonal packing with a helical twists (after Ambrose and Easty, 1970).

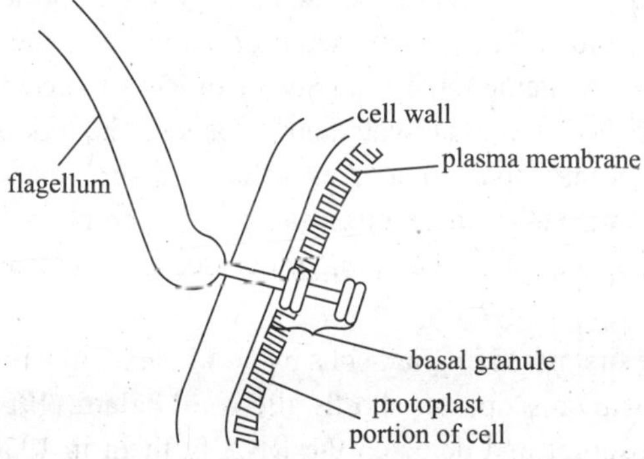

Fig. 16.9. Mode of insertion of basal region of a bacterial flagellum in a cell (after Avers, 1976).

REVISION QUESTIONS

1. Describe the structure of the axoneme. What features distinguish subfibre A from subfibre B?
2. Describe various theories of ciliary movement. Mention specifically the sliding microtubule model of axonemal movement.
3. Flagella and cilia, though identical in structure, commonly exhibit a quite different pattern of movement. Describe the two patterns and conditions under which one or the other would be more appropriate.
4. How do bacterial and eukaryotic flagella differ from each other in structure and movement?

17 Chapter

RIBOSOMES

The ribosomes are small, dense, rounded and granular particles of the ribonucleoprotein. They occur either freely in the matrix of mitochondria, chloroplasts and cytoplasm (*i.e.*, cytoplasmic matrix) or remain attached with the membranes of the endoplasmic reticulum and nucleus. The ribosomes have been found to be the universal components of all biological organisms. In other words, they occur in all prokaryotic and eukaryotic cells. They are used by the cell for protein synthesis the process by which amino acids are assembled in a definite sequence to produce the polypeptide chain. Protein synthesis requires the ordered interaction of three types of RNA molecules (*i.e.*, mRNA, tRNA and rRNA) of nuclear origin in addition to activated amino acids. Thus, ribosomes provide the surface on which protein synthesis takes place and they actively coordinate and catalytically assist the processes of **initiation**, **elongation** and **termination** of polypeptide molecules being synthesized. They are the activity centres for many interacting processes and molecule required for synthesis of every protein in the cell.

The ribosomes were first noted in plant cells by **Robinson** and **Brown** in 1953 when studying bean roots with the electron microscope and shortly afterward **Palade** (1955) observed them in animal cells. He isolated the ribosomes and detected the RNA in them in 1956. The present knowledge about the ribosomes have been gained by the cell fractionation, ultra-centrifugation, radioisotopy and electron microscopy.

17.1 OCCURRENCE AND DISTRIBUTION

The ribosomes occur in cells, both prokaryotic and eukaryotic cells. In prokaryotic cells the ribosomes often occur abundantly and freely in the cytoplasm. In eukaryotic cells the ribosomes either occur freely in the cytoplasm or remain attached to the outer surface of the membrane of endoplasmic reticulum. The yeast cells, reticulocytes or lymphocytes, meristamatic plant tissues, embryonic nerve cells and cancerous cells contain large number of ribosomes which often occur freely in the cytoplasmic matrix. The cells in which active protein synthesis takes place, the ribosomes remain attached with the membranes of the endoplasmic reticulum. Such cells are the pancreatic cells, plasma cells, hepatic parenchymal cells, Nissl bodies, osteoblasts, serous cells, or the submaxillary gland, Chief cells of the glandular stomach, thyroid cells and mammary gland cells. The cells which synthesize specific proteins for the intracellular utilization and storage often contain large number of free ribosomes. Such cells are the erythroblasts, developing muscle cells, skin and hair.

17.2 METHOD OF ISOLATION

The ribosomes are usually isolated from tne cell by the differential centrifugation method in which an analytical centrifuge is employed. The size of ribosomes and their subunits are usually given in **Svedberg units (S)**, a measure of particle size dependent on the speed with which particles sediment in the ultracentrifuge. One Svedberg unit is equal to 1×10^{-13} second, and larger the S value, the greater the size of the particle. On this basis a prokaryotic ribosome is a 70S particle and is composed of two major subunits: a 30S and a 50S subunit. Since sedimentation behaviour of particles and molecules is influenced by shape as well as size and molecular weight, the individual subunit values are higher than one might otherwise expect. The combined values for the two subunits are always higher than the S value of the monomer particle.

17.3 TYPES OF RIBOSOMES

Recently according to the size and the sedimentation coefficient (S) following types of ribosomes have been recognised:

1. 70S Ribosomes. The 70S ribosomes are comparatively smaller in size and have sedimentation cofficient 70S and the molecular weight 2.7×10^6 daltons. According to the data of electron microscopy the dimension of the dry particles of 70S ribosomes are 170 × 170 × 200A° (**Hall** and **Stayter**, 1959, **Huxley** and **Zubay**, 1960). They occur in the prokaryotic cells of the blue-green algae and bacteria and also in mitochondria and chloroplasts of many algae and higher plants.

2. 77S and 60S Ribosomes. The fungi generally possess mitochondrial ribosomes of an intermediate (77S) type, whereas animal mitochondrial ribosomes are small 60S structures (See **Goodenough** and **Levine**, 1974), The mitochondrial ribosomes of mammals however, have sedimentation coefficient 55S (See **De Robertis** *et al.*, 1975).

3. 80S Ribosomes. The 80S ribosomes have the sedimentaion coefficient of 80S and the molecular weight 40×10^6 daltons. The 80S ribosomes occur in eukaryotic cells of the plants and animals.

17.4 STRUCTURE OF RIBOSOMES

The ribosomes are oblate spheroid structures of 150 to 250 Å in diameter. Each ribosome is porous, hydrated and composed of two subunits. One ribosomal subunit is large in size and has a dome-like shape, while the other ribosomal subunit is smaller in size and occurring above the larger subunit and forming a cap-like structure.

The 70S ribosome consists of two subunits, *viz.*, 50S and 30S. The 50S ribosomal subunit is larger in size and has the size of 160 Å to 180 Å. The 30S ribosomal subunit is smaller in size and occurs above the 50S subunit like a cap. The 55S ribosomes of mammalian mitochondria contain a larger 35S subunit and a smaller 25S subunit. The 80S ribosome also consists of two subunits, *viz.*, 60S and 40S. The 60S ribosomal subunit is dome-shaped and larger in size. In the ribosomes which remain attached with the membranes of endoplasmic reticulum and nucleus, etc., the 60S subunit remains attached with the membranes. The 40S ribosomal subunit is smaller in size and occurs above the 60S subunit forming a cap-like structure. Both the subunits remain separated by a narrow cleft.

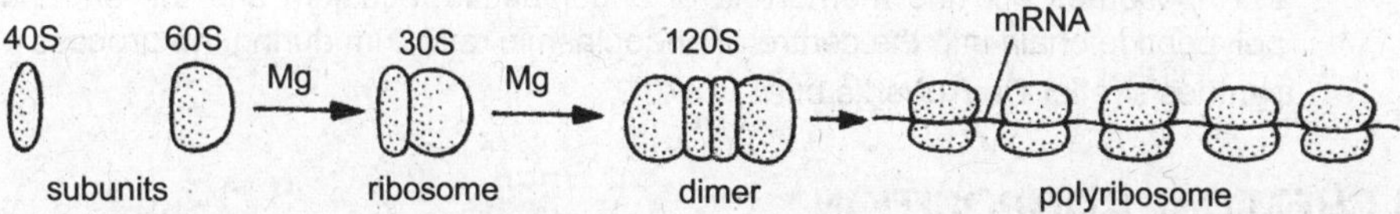

Fig. 17.1. Diagram of the subunit structure of the ribosome and the influence of Mg^{++} ions (after De Robertis *et al.*, 1970).

The two ribosomal subunits remain united with each other due to low concentration of the Mg^{++} (.001M) ions. When the concentration of Mg^{++} ions reduces in the matrix, both ribosomal subunits get separated. Actually in bacterial cells the two subunits are found to occur freely in the cytoplasm and they unite only during the process of protein synthesis. At high concentration of Mg^{++} ions (0.01 M) in the matrix, the two ribosomes combine to form a '**dimer**' with twice the molecular weight of the individual. Thus, Mg^{++} ions are required by ribosomes for their structural cohesion. Further, during protein synthesis many ribosomes are aggregated due to common messenger RNA and form the **polyribosomes** or **polysomes**.

17.5 ULTRASTRUCTURE

The fine structure of the ribosomes is still less worked out. However, **Nanninga** (1967) has observed that the 50S subunit of the 70S ribosome is pentagonal in shape and is a compact particle of 160 to 180A°. In the centre of this subunit occurs a round area of 40 to 60 A°. **Florendo** (1968) has observed a pore-like transparent area in the 50S subunit which does not allow the entrance of the proteolytic enzymes or ribonuclease enzyme.

In liver ribosomes (*i.e.*, 80S eukaryotic ribosomes) the 60S ribosomal subunit appears either round, with a diameter of 230 A° or triangular, with two convex sides and a third more flattened side that has a narrow depression or notch in the middle. The 40S ribosomal subunit is elongated and has a curved profile of about 230A° × 120A°, with a convex and a concave side. There is a line or partition that divides the 40S subunit into two unequal portions (**Florendo**, 1969). In the complete ribosome the smaller ribosomal subunit is attached by the concave side to the more flattened side of the large subunit and the partition in the small subunit is in coincidence with the notch of the 60S subunit, forming a kind of tunnel between the two. Some structural and biochemical studies support the view that the large subunit is traversed by a kind of channel or tunnel which contains the nascent polypeptide chain (Fig. 17.2).

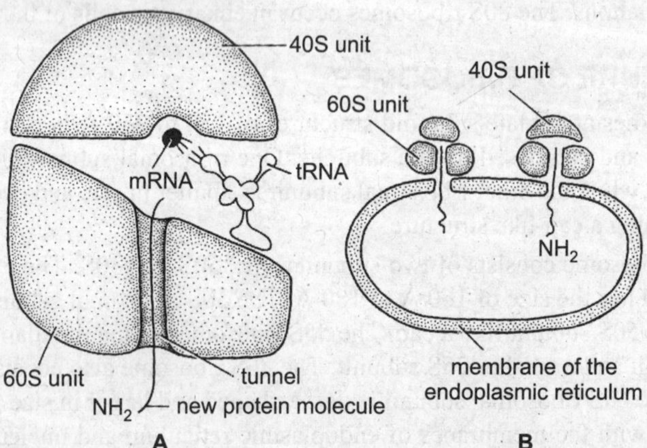

Fig. 17.2. Ultrastructure of the ribosome. A—Diagram of a ribosome showing the two subunits and the probable position of mRNA and tRNA; B—Diagram showing the relationship between the ribosomes and the membrane of endoplasmic reticulum and the entrance of the polypeptide chain into the centre of endoplasmic reticulum during the process of protein synthesis (afler De Robertis *et al.*, 1970).

17.6 CHEMICAL COMPOSITION

The ribosomes are chemically composed of RNA and proteins as their major constituents and little or no lipid molecules. In 70S and 80S ribosomes, the proteins and RNA present in approximately equal proportions. However, the 70S ribosomes contain more RNA (60 to 40%) than the proteins (36 to 37%), *e.g.*, the ribosomes of *E. coli* contain 63% rRNA and 37% protein. While the 80S ribosomes contain less RNA (40 to 44%) than the proteins (60 to 56%), *e.g.*, yeast ribosomes have 40 to 44% RNA and 60 to 56% proteins; ribosomes of pea seedling contain 40% RNA and 60% proteins and ribosomes of rat liver contain 40% RNA, 50 to 55% proteins and 5–10% lipids.

1. Ribosomal RNAs

The 70S ribosomes contain three types of rRNA, *viz.*, **23S rRNA, 16S rRNA and 5S rRNA**. The 23S and 5S rRNA occur in the larger 50S ribosomal subunit, while the 16S rRNA occurs in the smaller 30S ribosomal subunit. Assuming an average molecular weight for one nucleotide to be 330 daltons, one can calculate the total number of each type of rRNA. Thus, the 23S rRNA consists of 3300 nucleotides, 16S rRNA contains 1650 nucleotides and 5S rRNA includes 120 nucleotides in it (**Brownlee**, 1968; **Fellner**, 1972).

The 80S ribosomes contain four types of rRNA, *viz.*, **28S rRNA** (or **25-26 rRNA** in plants, fungi and protozoa), **18S rRNA, 5S rRNA** and **5.8S rRNA**. The 28S, 5S and 5.8S rRNAs occur in the larger 60S ribosomal subunit, while the 18S rRNA occurs in the smaller 40S ribosomal subunit. About 60 per cent of the rRNA is helical (*i.e.*, double stranded) and contains paired bases. These double stranded regions are due to hairpin loops between complimentary regions of the linear molecule.

The 28S rRNA has the molecular weight 1.6×10^6 daltons and its molecule is double stranded and having nitrogen bases in pairs. The 18S rRNA has the molecular weight 0.6×10^6 daltons and consists of 2100 nucleotides. The 18S and 28S ribosomal RNAs contain a characteristic number of methyl groups, mostly as 2′-O-methyl ribose. The molecule of 5S rRNA has a clover leaf shape and a length equal to 120 nucleotides (**Forget and Weissmann**, 1968). The 5.8S rRNA is intimately associated with the 28S rRNA molecule and has, therefore, been referred to as **28S-associated ribosomal RNA (28S-A rRNA) (Avers**, 1976).

The 55S ribosomes of mammalian mitochondria lack 5S rRNA but contain **21S** and **12S rRNAs**. The 21S rRNA occurs in larger or 35S ribosomal subunits, while 12S rRNA occur in smaller or 25S ribosomal subunit. The sedimentation coefficient of ribosomes, ribosomal subunits, rRNAs and number of ribosomal proteins of certain representative organisms have been tabulated in Table 17.1.

Table 17.1. Some characteristics of ribosomes of various organisms (Avers, 1976).

Source	Intact Ribosomes	Ribosome subunits	rRNA in subunit	Number of proteins in subunit
Prokaryotes	70S	30S	16S	21
		50S	23S, 5S	32–34
Eukaryotes	80S	40S		~30
		60S		~50
Animals		40S	18S	
		60S	28S, 5S, 5.8S	
Plants		40S	18S	
		60S	25–26S, 5S	
			5.8S	
Fungi		40S	18S	
		60S	25–26S, 5S	

Source	Intact Ribosomes	Ribosome subunits	rRNA in subunit	Number of proteins in subunit
Protozoa (some other protists)		40S 60S	5.8S 18S 25–26S, 5S 5.8S	

It is thought that each ribosomal subunit contains a highly folded ribonucleic acid filament to which the various proteins adhere (**Hart**, 1965). But as the ribosomes easily bind the basic dyes so it is concluded that RNA is exposed at the surface of the ribosomal subunits, and the protein is assumed to be in the interior in relation to non-helical part of the RNA.

2. Ribosomal Proteins

According to **Nomura** (1968, 1973) and **Garett** and **Wittmann** (1973) each 70S ribosome of *E. coli* is composed of about 55 **ribosomal proteins**. Out or these 55 proteins, about 21 different molecules have been isolated from the 30S ribosomal subunit, and some 32 to 34 proteins from the 50S ribosomal subunit. The primary structure of several of these proteins has been elucidated. Most of the recent knowledge about the structure of ribosomal proteins have been achieved by dissociation of ribosomal subunits into their component rRNA and protein molecules. When both 50S and 30S ribosomal subunits are dissociated by centrifuging both of them in a gradient of 5 M cesium chloride, then there are two inactive core particles (40S and 23S, respectively) which contain the RNA and some proteins called **core proteins (CP)** at the same time several other proteins—the so-called **split proteins (SP)**—are released from each particle (Fig. 17.3). There are SP50 and SP30 proteins which may reconstitute the functional ribosomal subunit when added to their corresponding core. Some of the split proteins are apparently specific for each ribosomal subunit. The split proteins have been further fractionated and divided into acidic (A) and basic (B) proteins. **Nomura** *et al*., (1968) fractionated at least six different groups of proteins in the ribosome (Fig. 17.3).

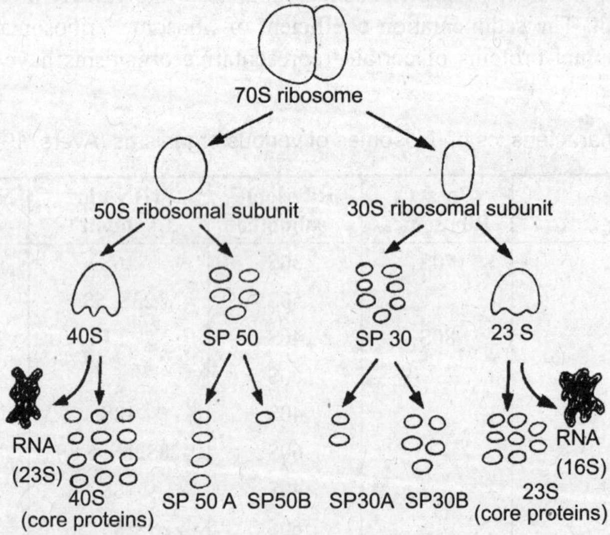

Fig. 17.3. The protein components of a 70S ribosome (after De Robertis *et al.*, 1975).

Further, it has been found that both the core and the split proteins are present in the ribosome with a different stoichiometry. The so-called **unit proteins** are present in one copy per ribosome; the **fractional proteins**, in 0.5 copy per ribosome; and the **marginal proteins**, in 0.7 to 0.8 copy per ribosome (**Kurland**, 1972). Therefore, all ribosomes of a cell are not identical. For example, one ribosomal protein called **S14 protein** is essential for ribosomal function, and at the same time is represented by only 0.5 copy per ribosome. The conclusion is that normally there are two types of ribosomes: S14 (+), that are active and, S14 (–) that should be inactive.

3. Ribosomal Enzymes and Protein Factors

Ribosomes have very significant participaticn in the process of protein synthesis, as during protein synthesis ribosomes mediate (1) the codon-anticodon recognition events happening between the tRNA and mRNA molecule; (2) formation of peptide bonds between amino acid and, (3) movement of mRNA so that codons are exposed to anticodons of tRNA in a sequential fashion. For these divergent activities such as initiation, elongation and termination of the polypeptide chain, for holding and moving mRNA and for the mobilization of tRNA, the ribosomes contain a wide array of protein factors and ribosomal enzymes, all of which have been tabulated in Table 17.2. The ribosomal enzymes and protein factors can be studied under following headings:

Table 17.2. Protein factors in protein synthesis (**Lipmann**, 1973).

	Phase	Factor	Source	Function
1.	Initiation	F_3 IF_1, IF_2, IF_3 } GTP	High salt 30S Ribosomal wash	Dissociation of ribosomal subunits. Binding of mRNA and initiator to tRNA 30S subunit.
2.	Elongation	Tu, Ts } T + GTP	Supernatant fraction	Binding of aminoacyl-tRNA Tu-GTP complex to ribosome.
		Peptidyl transferase	50S ribosomal subunit	Peptidyl transfer from peptidyl-tRNA to aminoacyl-tRNA.
		G + GTP	Supernatant fraction	Translocation of peptidyl-tRNA; release of free tRNA.
3.	Termination	R_1, R_2	Supernatant fraction	Release of protein at UAA, UAG or UGA codons.

A. Initiation factors. Three initiation factors (IF_1, IF_2 and IF_3) have been separated by washing ribosomes with NH_4Cl and submitting them to column chromatography in Ochoa's laboratory by a team of molecular biologists (**Stanley** *et al.*, 1966 ; **Iwasaki** *et al.*, 1968 and **Ochoa**, 1968). These initiation factors are proteins loosely associated with the 30S subunit. The **IF_1 factor** is a basic protein with a molecular weight of 9200 daltons and it is involved in the binding of F-met-tRNA. The **IF_2 factor** is also a protein having molecular weight of 80,000 daltons and contain essential—SH groups upon which its binding with GTP (guanosine triphosphate) depends. **Zasloff** and **Ochoa** (1972) have isolated a protein factor similar to IF_2 factor from eukaryotic ribosomes but that does not require GTP. The **IF_3 factor** is a basic protein which has a molecular weight of 30,000 daltons and is involved in the binding of the mRNA to the 30S subunit. IF_3 factor also may function as dissociation factor for 70S ribosomes. In *E. coli* certain protein factors called **interference factors (i factors)** have been reported. These i factors bind to factor IF_3, change its specificity and thus, regulate the translation of the genetic message at its initiation (**Le-Huang** and **Ochoa**, 1972, **Revel** *et al.*, 1973).

B. Elongation factors. In Lipmann's laboratory soluble protein fractions present in the post-ribosomal supernatant were found to be active in the elongation of the polypeptide chain (**Nishizuka** *et al.*, 1966; **Allende** *et al.*, 1967; **Ertel** *et al.*, 1968; and **Lucas-Lenard** and **Haenni**, 1968). At first, only the EFT and EFG factors were isolated, but later the **EFT factor** was found to comprise two proteins: **Tu**, which is temperature-unstable, and **Ts**, which is temperature stable. The EFTu factor + GTP form a complex with aminoacyl-tRNA prior to its binding to the acceptor site of ribosome and formation of this complex is catalyzed by factor Ts.

The **EFG factor**, also called **G factor** or **translocase**, is involved in the translocation of the mRNA. The isolated translocase from *E. coli* has a molecular weight of 72,000 daltons and appears to consist of a single polypeptide chain (**Ledar** *et al.*, 1969). According to **Laszlo** and **Lucas-lenard** (1973) EFT + GTP stimulates the binding of aminoacyl tRNA and EFG + GTP promotes the translocation of the newly elongated peptidyl-tRNA.

Further, 50S ribosomal subunit contains an enzyme called **peptidyl transferase**, or **peptide synthetase** which is involved in the formation of the peptide bond.

C. Termination factors. Two releasing factors, R_1 and R_2, of protein nature have been isolated from the supernatant of ribosomes (**Capecchi**, 1966, 1967).

17.7 RECONSTITUTION OR SELF-ASSEMBLY

To understand the three-dimensional organisation of ribosomal proteins in the ribosomes and also for the investigation of interactions between the molecules of rRNA and proteins, following kinds of approaches have been adopted in recent time:

1. One approach, developed in **M. Nomura's** laboratory, has been to take purified 30S ribosomal subunits, dissociate them by chemical means into their component RNAs and proteins and then allow them to reassociate under appropriate ionic conditions. Dissociation of 30S subunit may be achieved by treatment with four molar urea and two molar LiCl, which separate the proteins. If the 16S rRNAs previously extracted with phenol is placed in the presence of 20 different protein molecules of 30S ribosomal subunit, the reconstitution or self-assembly of 30S ribosomal subunit takes place in two steps:

$$\text{16S RNA} + \xrightarrow[\text{proteins}]{R_1} \text{RI particles} \xrightarrow{\text{heat}} \text{RI * particles} \xrightarrow{\text{+S proteins}} \text{30S ribosomal subunit}$$

In the first step, performed at a low temperature, the 16S RNA binds some of the 30S ribosomal proteins, forming an RI particle (*i.e.*, a reconstitution intermediate) that is inactive. In the second step, the RI particles are heated at 40°C in the presence of the other proteins that have remained in the supernatant (*i.e.*, S proteins) thereby forming an excited intermediate, RI*, within 20 minutes fully active 30S ribosomal subunits are formed. The self-assembly of 30S subunit is highly specific. It can be achieved with 16S RNA of other bacteria, but not with 16S RNA from yeast or the 23S RNA from *E. coli*.

In similar manner, reconstitution of 50S ribosomal subunit is achieved. Finally, a complete functional ribosome is reconstituted spontaneously. **Nomura** (1973) performed such reconstitution experiments on 40S ribosomal subunits. During all these investigations, it has been noted that some proteins become directly bounded to the 16S RNA with various binding affinities, while certain other proteins require the prior attachment of other proteins in order to be incorporated in a stepwise and cooperative manner. (Thus, the previous attachments of certain proteins facilitates the binding of others). Further, while certain ribosomal proteins play a structural role in the assembly of the ribosomes, others are definitely engaged in the specific ribosomal functions (See chapter of protein synthesis).

2. The *in vitro* reconstitution or self-assembly of ribosomal components into complete ribosomes has been observed *in vivo*. Several small precursor forms have been found in *E. coli* cells before final, mature subunits are formed, and mutant strains of *E. coli* have been selected by **C. Gutherie** and **M. Nomura** (1969) that are blocked at discrete stages in this self-assembly process and, therefore, accumulate the smaller precursor forms. Such mutations would ordinarily be lethal since only mature

ribosomal subunits can participate in protein synthesis and the strains must therefore be isolated as conditional lethal strains. The screening process for obtaining such *sad* (self-assembly-deficient) mutant strains begins by selecting cells that grow normally at 37°C but die at 20°C. Optimal rates of self-assembly occur in the cell at 37°C, and therefore if any ribosomal proteins or rRNAs carry mutations should be particularly debilitating in the cold. The study of the defects carried by *sad* strains also help in the understanding interactions between rRNAs and proteins.

3. For investigating out the molecular structure of ribosomes, one of the Nomura's elegant experiment made a use of antibiotics. A streptomycin-resistant strain of *E. coli* was found, by electrophoresis, to carry an alteration in a single ribosomal protein, denoted **P10**. To prove that the altered P10 protein is responsible for the altered response to streptomycin, P10 protein was isolated from a streptomycin sensitive strain and used to reconstitute 30S subunits in which all the proteins and RNA derived from resistant strain (Fig. 17.4). The reciprocal experiment was also performed by using P10 proteins from a streptomycin-resistant strain and other components from a sensitive strain. The results were clear: reconstituted subunits with the sensitive P10 protein were streptomycin-sensitive, even though all the other proteins and RNA come from resistant ribosomes. Conversely, the resistant P10 protein conferred resistance *in vitro*. Since the binding of streptomycin to ribosomes is known to interfere with the correct reading of the genetic code (*i.e.*, mRNA), the P10 protein is likely to be present at or near the ribosomal site at which the reading process occurs. It is in such a painstaking manner that the functions of the numerous proteins and the three rRNAs of the ribosome will be elucidated (see **Goodenough** and **Levine**, 1974).

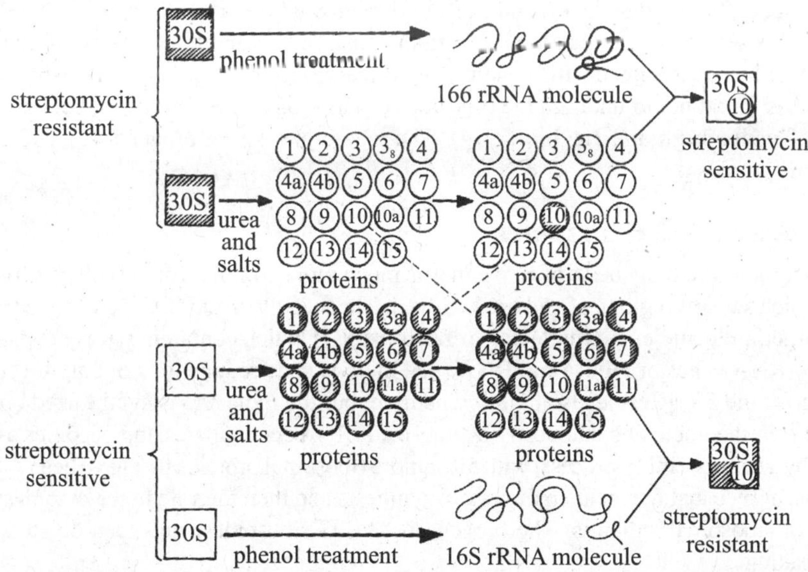

Fig. 17.4. Nomura's experiment showing that the P10 ribosomal protein of 30S subunit is responsible for a ribosome's senstivity or resistance to streptomycin (after Goodenough and Levine, 1974).

17.8 BIOGENESIS OF RIBOSOMES

The complete molecular organisation of the ribosomes with their three kinds of rRNA molecules and their 50 or more specific proteins, implies that more than 50 genes are involved in their formation. The biogenesis of bacterial 70S ribosomes differs markedly with that of eukaryotic 80S ribosomes.

1. Biogenesis of 70S Ribosomes

Smith *et al.*, (1968) have suggested that in bacteria the RNA genes coding for the 5S, 23S, and 16S ribosomal RNAs are tightly clustered in a region of the chromosome and are present in only few copies. In other words, the ribosomal genes are in a single operon which is transcribed as a unit to synthesize a large molecule of RNA containing the 16S, 23S and 5S rRNA sequences. About 0.4 per cent of an *E. coli* chromosome is devoted to carrying rRNA sequences. In contrast, about 80 per cent of the RNA in an *E. coli* cell is rRNA. This discrepancy in percentages can be explained as follows—First, rRNA is greatly stabilized and protected by ribosomal proteins, and thus any rRNA molecule that is synthesized is expected to have a far longer lifetime than other RNA species (*i.e.*, tRNA, mRNA). Second, in contrast to other genes that may be transcribed only a few times or perhaps not at all during the life of a cell, the rRNA genes are in a state of perpetual transcription. Indeed, after a polymerase enzyme has attached to an rRNA promoter site and moved along the gene a certain distance, a second polymerase attaches and begins to read, then a third, and so on. As a result at least 30 polymerase molecules are working in tandem on a given gene at anyone time, and strands of rRNA of progressively longer lengths are observed coming off the template. This process has been observed directly with the electron microscope by **Hamkalo** and **Miller** (1973).

Thus, in bacteria a single gene transcript containing the sequences of 16S, 23S and 5S rRNAs, is synthesized by a rRNA operon and this larger molecule, is thought to undergo both tailoring and chemical modifications before each rRNA molecule assumes its mature form. During tailoring of larger rRNA molecule, 16S rRNA sequence is first of all cleared off and is separated from the 23S and 5S sequences. The fragment containing 16S information is still larger than the mature 16S rRNA by at least 100 bases and is not methylated: both the methylation and the tailoring of this molecule takes place after it has associated with a number of proteins to form the percursor ribosomal subunits. The 5S rRNA is found not to undergo the processes of tailoring and methylation, before it becomes mature (see **Goodenough** and **Levine**, 1974). The whole process of biogensis of 70S ribosomes takes place in cytoplasm.

2. Biogenesis of 80S Ribosomes

In eukaryotes, the biogenesis of ribosomes is much more complex and involves a long-lasting process in which several regions of cell are involved. The 5.8S, 18S and 28S rRNAs are transcribed as a much larger molecule in the **nucleolar organizer (NO)** which containing many copies of 5.8S, 18S and 28S rRNA genes or **ribosomal DNA** (*i.e.*, there is gene redundancy or amplification). The DNA coding for the 5S rRNA is also highly repetitive, but the molecule is synthesized out side the nucleolus. It is in the nucleolus that newly synthesized rRNA accumulates and becomes associated, presumably by a self-assembly process, with 50 or more ribosomal proteins that have been synthesized in the cytoplasm by usual mechanism of protein synthesis and then migrate to the cytoplasm of cell, in the form of ribosomal subunits. The biogenesis of 80S ribosomes, thus, can be studied under following headings:

A. Nucleolar organizer and ribosomal DNA. In eukaryotes 5.8S, 18S and 28S rRNA gene sequences are clustered in a chromosomal region called the **nucleolar organizer (NO)**. By definition a NO lies in the heart of a nucleolus. Direct evidence that the nucleolus is responsible for the synthesis of rRNA was obtained in 1964, when it was discovered that an anucleolate mutant of amphibian *Xenopus laevis* was incapable of rRNA synthesis (**Brown** and **Gurdon**, 1964). Diploid cells of the wild type of *X. laevis* have two nucleoli; the heterozygous mutant contains only one nucleolus per diploid cell and the homozygous mutant is anucleolate (**O-nu** or **zero-nucleolus** mutant). Anucleolate condition is lethal and the embryo dies at the tail bud stage. Until then, homozygous mutants depend on maternal ribosomes for protein synthesis. By DNA-RNA hybridization technique, **Hall** and **Spiegelman** (1961) demonstrated that the DNA associated with nucleolus is responsible for coding rRNA. In *Xenopus laevis* the nucleolar organizer represent 0.2 per cent of the genome and carries 400 copies of each sequence (*viz.*, 5.8S, 18S and 28S rRNA). The heterozygous mutant of *X. laevis* contains half rDNA cistrons for 18S and 28S rRNA of the wild type (*i.e.*, it contains only 200 rDNA cistrons for each 5.8S, 18S and 28S rRNAs). The homozygous mutant is found to contain no rDNA cistron at all (**Wallace** and **Birnstiel**, 1966).

A similar type of experiment was performed with *Drosophila melanogaster* by **F. Ritossa** and **S. Spiegelman** (1965). In *D. melanogaster* the nucleolar organizer is contained in a heterochromatic region of the X or Y chromosome; therefore normal male (XY) and female (XX) flies will carry two **NO doses**. The NO can be deleted from the X, and male flies carrying the deleted X and normal Y can be bred; they carry one NO dose. A duplication for the NO region can also occur in the X chromosome; males carrying the duplication and a normal Y will have three NO doses, and females carrying two duplicated X chromosomes will have four NO doses. In the so-called "bobbed" mutant of *Drosophila*, the number of DNA cistrons may be be reduced, and it can be calculated that death will occur when fewer than 40 copies, of rDNA cistrons are present at the nucleolar organizer (**Ritossa**, 1968).

Ritossa and **Spiegelman** isolated DNA from the one-, two-, three-, and four- dose flies and compared the ability of each DNA preparation to hybridize with 18S and 28S rRNA. The dose of NO clearly correlates with the amount of DNA complementary to 18S and 28S rRNA. Again, 5S rRNA sequences are found to be absent from the NO. In fact, it has been established that the 5S sequences (*i.e.*, rDNA for 58 rRNA) are not even carried in the sex chromosomes in *D. melanogaster* but are instead clustered in one of the autosomes (**Pardue**, 1973). It has also been calculated that in *D. melanogaster* the NO constitutes 0.3 per cent of the genome and contains 130 copies each of the 18S and 28S sequences. At this stage if we compare rDNA of NO of *Xenopus laevis*, *Drosophila melanogaster* and *E. coli*, then it becomes evidently clear that as the size of the genome increases, the number of genes for rRNA also increases, but the relative proportion (0.2 to 0.4 per cent, remains, surprisingly, about the same for *E. coli*, *Drosophila* and *Xenopus*.

Molecular structure of nucleolar organizer. The molecular biology of nucleolar organizer reveals following two important aspects about it:

(*a*) Spacer DNA and satellite ribosomal DNA. The ribosomal DNA present in the nucleolar organizer has been isolated in its purified state in a number of species by virtue of the fact that it has a higher % GC content and, therefore, bands in a satellite position in cesium chloride (CsCl) gradient. In *X. laevis* this DNA has high buoyant density than rest of the DNA (*i.e.*, 1.723, as compared to 1.698) due to high GC contents (*viz.*, about 70%) and it represents only 0.15 to 0.20 per cent of the total DNA and is called **satellite ribosomal DNA** (see **De Robertis** *et al.*, 1975). When this satellite ribosomal DNA is hybridized against radioisotopically labelled 18S and 28S RNA, then it is found that large portion of nucleolar organizer DNA is not complementary to rRNA at all.

The extra DNA in the nucleolar organizer, when it was first detected, was given the name spacer DNA to indicate that it occupies the spaces between rRNA genes in the NO (see **Goodenough** and **Levine**, 1974). Electron microscopic investigations have shown that the spacer DNA is not transcribed in the NO region of Amphibia (**Miller** and **Beatty**, 1969). The exact significance of spacer DNA is still unknown.

(*b*) Amplification or Redundancy of the rDNA. While discussing the examples of *Drosophila* and *X. laeivs*, we have observed a considerable degree of amplification or redundancy of rDNA genes in total DNA. Such amplification of rDNA cistrons is particularly evident in many amphibian oocytes, in which the nucleus may reach a diameter of more than 0.5 mm and contain 1000 or more nucleoli. Such gene amplification may help these oocytes to accomplish an intense rRNA synthesis that may be 100,000 times greater per genome than in a liver cell. The percentage of total DNA involved in rRNA synthesis and the degree of amplification per haploid genome in various organisms, can be tabulated in the following Table 17.3.

Redundancy or amplification of rDNA genes is one way that the cell has to control the production of ribosomes, but apparently it is not the only way. Because, certain hybridization experiments of **Ritossa** *et al.*, (1966), with somatic chicken tissues (*i.e.*, kidney, liver, embryo, all with different rates of rRNA synthesis) have demonstrated the presence of a similar number of rDNA cistrons of about 100 per haploid genome. Even in sperm cells and erythrocytes in which the production of ribosomes has stopped there is the same level of DNA-RNA saturation. Likewise, in certain plants, the rDNA cistron amplification which varies from 1,600 to 13,000 per diploid nucleus, remain constant from embryo upto adult plant (**Ingle** and **Sinclair**, 1972). The exact significance of gene redundancy is still not clear.

Table 17.3. Amplification of rDNA genes in different organisms (**De Robertis** *et al.*, 1975).

Organism	% DNA	rDNA genes per haploid genome
E. coli	0.42–0.65	8–22
B. subtilis	0.38	9–10
HeLa cells	0.005–0.02	160–640
Drosophila (wild type)	0.27	130
Xenopus (wild type)	0.06–0.11	1200–3000

B. Biogenesis of 5S RNA. In contrast to prokaryotes, in eukaryotes the 5S rRNA is not related to me nucleolar organizer. In *X. laevis*, by use of the DNA—RNA hybridization technique, it was found that there are much more 5S genes (*i.e.*, about 27,000) than 18S and 28S rRNA genes and that they are not spatially related (**Brown** and **Weber**, 1968). Because of this fact, the presence of 5S rRNA was detected in the anucleolate mutant of *X. laevis* (**Brown**, 1966). HeLa cells are found to contain about 10,000 copies of 50S rRNA genes. In *Drosophila* the number of 5S rRNA genes is about the same as that of 18S and 28S genes (**Perry** *et al.*, 1970).

C. Processing of the ribosomal RNA in nucleolus. In eukaryotes original gene transcripts carrying 5.8S, 18S and 28S rRNA sequences undergo both tailoring and chemical modifications before they assume their mature forms. It is still not clear that how 5.8S rRNA is tormed from 45S rRNA molecule. However, processing of, 28S rRNA, and 188 rRNA includes following series of events:

(*i*) The original gene transcipt for 5.8S, 18S and 28S rRNA a single large RNA molecule with a sedimentation coefficient of 38 t 45S, depending on the species. The 45S rRNA molecule has a molecular weight of 4.5×10^6 daltons and a length of about 4.5 μm. It is transcribed from the rDNA of nucleolar organizer in about 2.2 minutes (in HeLa cells) and is present in the fibrillar region of the nucleolus. It is assumed that 20 RNA polymerases are transcribing simultaneously on the rDNA cistron.

(*ii*) During the transcription process certain regions of the 45S rRNA become methylated in the ribose moiety producing 2′—O-methyl ribose. The regions of the 45S RNA that are methylated correspond to the future 28S and 18S ribosomal RNAs.

(*iii*) The 45S rRNA has a life time of about 15 minutes and is followed by cleavage and degradation into smaller components (see **Perry**, 1972). Consequently, 45S rRNA molecule is cleaved into a 41S and 20S rRNA by the help of an enzyme called endonuclease.

(*iv*) The 20S rRNA is degraded in its non methylated region by an exonuclease enzyme and thus, producing the 18S rRNA, which is rapidly released to the cytoplasm (**Perry** and **Kelley**, 1972).

(*v*) The 41S rRNA undergoes a series of degradations by exo-nuclease enzymes which attack the non-methylated regions; by this process the 36S and 32S intermediates are produced.

(*vi*) The 32S rRNA molecule remains in tne granular part of the nucleolus for about 40 minutes and is then degraded to the 28S rRNA. The 28S rRNA remains in the nucleolus fot another 30 minutes before entering the cytoplasm. Consequently, during tailoring of 45S rRNA about half portion, which mainly composed of non-methylated regions and regions of high GC contents, is lost. The processing of the ribosomal RNA leads to an increase in methyl groups and to a decrease in GC.

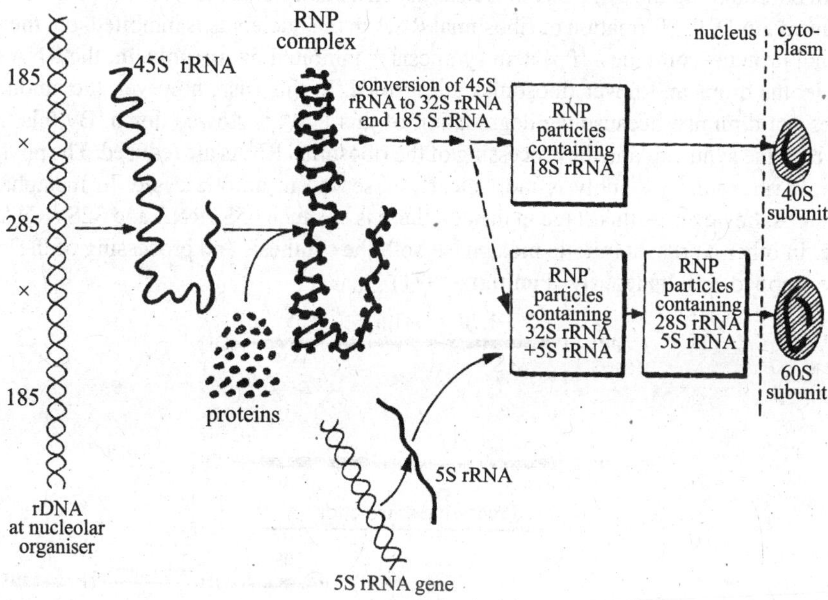

Fig. 17.5. Flow diagram showing the components and sequences of synthesis and packaging of eukaryotic ribosome subunits (after Avers, 1976).

D. Synthesis of ribosomal protein and ribosomal assembly. The process which involves the assembly of 50 or more ribosomal proteins and three rRNA molecules, is still little understood one. **Flamm** and **Birnstiel** (1964) and **Bimstiel** *et al.*, (1966) have demonstrated that the so-called structural core proteins are linked early to the nascent rRNA, and the other proteins are probably bound during a later phase. Thus, as soon as 45S rRNA precursor is transcribed from rDNA or NO, it becomes associated with certain ribosomal proteins to form a particle of about 80S (**Warner** and **Soeiro**, 1967). All the transitions between the 45S and the final 28S and 18S occur within ribonucleoprotein particles, and in this way both subunits are exported to the cytoplasm. **Perry** (1969) has suggested that during maturation of the ribosomal subunits there is a progressive conformational change that starts from extended strands and terminates in relatively compact particles. Further, during maturation of ribosomal subunits, in addition to progressive loss of rRNA, a loss of ribosomal proteins is also postulated (**Lian** and **Perry**, 1969). It is still not well understood that how the extranucleolar synthesis of the 5S rRNA is coordinated with that of the 455. However, the 58 rRNA is transcribed by the cistrons occurring out side the nucleolar organizer and before it leaves the nucleus for the cytoplasm, where it becomes incorporated with the ribonucleoprotein (RNP) particle or granule having 28S RNA. The 28S rRNP and 5S rRNA form the 60S ribosomal subunit in the cytoplasm. The 40S ribosomal subunits containing 18S rRNA, however, are the first to appear in the cytoplasm. In the cytoplasm, during protein synthesis the two ribosomal subunits unite to form a complete ribosome.

The transport of ribonucleoprotein particles into the cytoplasm is easily observed in dipterans and in amphibian oocytes, in which material of nucleolar origin may be seen passing through the pores of the nuclear envelope into the cytoplasm. These particles apparently go by way of the annuli in an elongate configuration in the salivary glands of the dipteran *Chironomus* (**Stevens** and **Swift**, 1967). **Stevens** (1967) made similar observations of migration of RNP granules through nucleopores of *Amoeba proteus*.

E. Regulation of ribosomal assembly. Certain recent evidences suggest that there is a mechanism coordinating the synthesis of ribosomal RNA and ribosomal proteins. If a cell is treated with **actinomycin D**, the formation of ribosomal RNA in the nucleolus is inhibited, but the synthesis of ribosomal proteins continues. If protein synthesis is inhibited by **puromycin**, the RNA synthesis in the nucleolus drops and fewer ribosomes are formed. In this case, however, the amount of 45S rRNA does not diminish because the degradation of this RNA is slowed down. By this treatment, therefore, both the synthesis and the processing of the ribosomal RNAs are reduced. The physiological regulation of ribosomal assembly is most clearly observed in mitotic cycle. In metaphase, RNA synthesis stops, however, at this stage in the cell there is as much 45S rRNA and 32S rRNA as in the interphase. In other words, at mitotic metaphase both the synthesis and processing of the ribosomal RNA have stopped simultaneously (**Penman**, 1971).

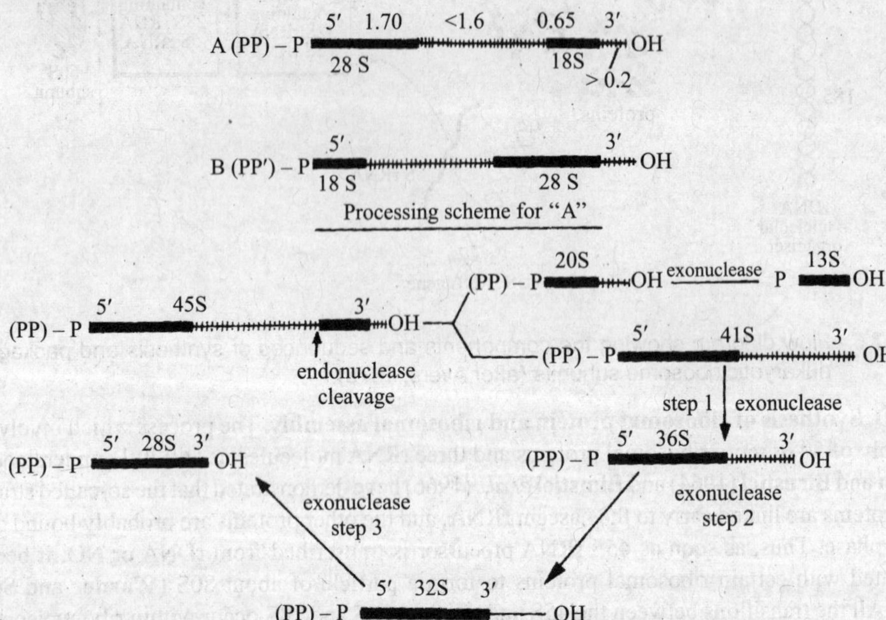

Fig. 17.6. Diagram showing possible arrangement of 28S and I8S rRNA sequences within the 45S rRNA molecule and possible processing mechanisms. The stepwise tailoring (cleavage and degradation) of 45S rRNA into 18S and 28S rRNA by exonuclease and endonuclease enzymes has also been shown in the diagram (after Perry and Kelley, 1972).

17.9 FUNCTIONS

Ribosomes play a very significant role during biosynthesis of proteins and that will be discussed in a separate chapter.

REVISION QUESTIONS

1. What are the ribosomes? What is meant by a 70S and 80S ribosome? Describe the structure of both types of ribosomes.
2. How many types of RNA and proteins are found in the 70S and 80S ribosomes?
3. Describe the process of biogenesis of ribosomes.
4. Describe the Nomura's experiment of ribosomal self-assembly.

18 Chapter NUCLEUS

The nucleus (L., *nux*-nut) is the heart of the cell. It is here that almost all of the cell's DNA is confined, replicated and transcribed. The nucleus, thus, controls different metabolic as well as hereditary activities of the cell. The nucleus is discovered by **Robert Brown** in 1831. Since its discovery the cytologists became interested in it more because of its extra-ordinary participation in the cellular metabolism and heredity mechanism.

18.1 OCCURRENCE AND POSITION

The nucleus is found in all the eukaryotic cells of the plants and animals. However, certain eukaryotic cells such as the mature sieve tubes of higher plants, cells of some areas of the lens of eye, and mammalian erythrocytes contain no nucleus. In such cells, nuclei are present during the early stages of development. The prokaryotic cells of the bacteria do not have true nucleus, *i.e.*, the single, circular and large DNA molecule remains in direct contacts with the cytoplasm. The position or location of the nucleus in a cell is usually the characteristic of the cell type and it is often variable. Usually the nucleus remains located in the centre. But its position may change from time to time according to the metabolic states of the cell. For example, in the embryonic cells the nucleus generally occupies the geometric centre of the cells but as the cells start to differentiate and the rate of the metabolic activities increases, the displacement in the position of the nucleus takes place. In certain cell such as the glandular cells the nucleus remains located in the basal portion of the cell.

18.2 MORPHOLOGY

Number

Usually the cells contain single nucleus but the number of the nucleus may very from cell to cell. According to the number of the nuclei following types of cells have been recognised:

1. **Mononucleate cells.** Most plant and animal cells contain single nucleus, such cells are known as **mononucleate cells.**
2. **Binucleate cells.** The cells which contain two nuclei are known as **binucleate cells**. Such cells occur in certain protozoans such as *Paramecium* and cells of cartilage and liver.
3. **Polynucleate cells.** The cells which contain many (from 3 to 100) nuclei are known as **polynucleate cells**. The polynucleate cells of the animals are termed as **syncytial cells**, while the polynucleate cells of the plants are known as **coenocytes**. The most common example of the syncytial cells are the osteoblasts (polykaryocytes of the bone marrow) which contain about 100 nuclei per cell and striated muscle fibres contain many hundred nuclei. The siphonal algae *Vaucheria* contains hundreds of nuclei and certain fungi are the best example of the coenocyte plant cells.

Shape

The shape of the nucleus normally remains related with the shape of the cell, but certain nuclei are almost irregular in shape. The spheroid, cuboid or polyhedral cells (isodiametrical cells) contain the **spheroid** nuclei. The nuclei of the cylindrical, prismatic or fusiform cells are **ellipsoid** in shape. The cells of the squamous epithelium contain the **discoidal** nuclei. The leukocytes, certain infusoria, glandular cells of some insects and spermatozoa contain the irregular shaped nuclei.

Size

The size of the nucleus of various cells is also variable. The size of the nucleus is directly proportional to that of the cytoplasm. **R. Hertwig** has given the following formula for the deduction of the size of the nucleus of a particular cell.

$$NP = \frac{V_n}{V_c - V_n}$$

where NP is the nucleoprotein index, V_n is the volume of the nucleus and V_c is the volume of the cell.

Moreover, the size of the nucleus is related with the number of the chromosomes or ploidy. The haploid cells contain small sized nuclei in comparison to the nuclei of the diploid cells. Likewise the polyploid cells contain larger nuclei than the diploid cells. Thus, the size of the nucleus of a cell depends on the volume of the cell, amount of the DNA and proteins and metabolic phase of the cell.

18.3 CYTOCHEMISTRY OF NUCLEUS

The chemical organization of the nucleus have been investigated by two main approaches. The first, which is essentially biochemical, consists of isolating a large enough number of nuclei to permit analysis by biochemical methods. The second approach, which is essentially cytologic, uses the cytophotometric land radio-autographic methods. Both the approaches are complimentary, therefore, following integrated discussion about cytochemistry of nucleus is desirable:

Miescher (1869) was probably the first cytochemist, who analyzed the chemical composition of pus cells, spermatozoa and haemolyzed nucleated red cells of birds and other organisms, and demonstrated that nucleic acids are one of the main components of the nucleus. Certain recent informations about the biochemical organization of nucleus has been provided from the use of HeLa cells (a tumor of human origin) and other cultured cells. To isolate the nuclei the cells are first swollen hypotonically and then gently homogenized. The nuclei are centrifuged and treated with some surface-active agents to free from adherent cytoplasm. This treatment strips off the outer nuclear envelope together with the few remaining ribosomes. A nucleolar fraction may be obtained by treating the nuclei with highly ionic solutions and digesting the chromatin with DNAse (**Penman** *et al.*, 1966). The number of nuclei can be measured easily in a chamber similar to that used for blood counts.

Various biochemical and cytochemical investigations have revealed that the nucleus chemically contains following molecules:

1. Nucleic acids (DNA and RNA),
2. Nuclear proteins,
3. Mineral salts, etc.

1. Nucleic Acids

Nuclei of eukaryotes contain large amount of DNA and RNA which often remain combined with nuclear proteins. The amount of DNA in an eukaryotic nucleus can be determined by microspectrophotometry, a technique that measures with precision the amount of Feulgen staining material each nucleus contains. By this and other procedures it is found that a typical eukaryotic nucleus will contain perhaps a thousands time more DNA than a bacterium and a hundred thousand times more than a virus (see Table 18.1).

Table 18.1. DNA content per nucleus of various organisms (McCarthy, 1969).

	Organism	Daltons	Nucleotide pairs
1.	**Viruses**		
	Bacterial		
	$\phi \times 174$	1.6×10^6	5500
	λ	30×10^6	45×10^3
	T_5	85×10^6	130×10^3
	T_2	130×10^6	200×10^3
	Animal		
	Shope papilloma	5×10^6	7.5×10^3
	Adenovirus 12	14×10^6	20×10^3
	Fowl pox	230×10^6	350×10^3
2.	**Bacteria (Haploid cells)**		
	Mycoplasma gallisepticum	0.2×10^1	0.3×10^6
	Hemophilus influenza	0.7×10^9	1×10^6
	Escherichia coli	2.6×10^9	4×10^6
	Bacillus subtilis	1.3×10^9	2×10^6
3.	**Fungi (Diploid cells)**		
	Saccharomyces cerevisiae	13×10^9	20×10^6
4.	**Plants (Diploid cells)**		
	Arabidopsis thaliana	2.6×10^{12}	4×10^9
	Zea mays	20×10^{12}	30×10^9
	Tradescantia paludosa	40×10^{12}	60×10^9
5.	**Invertebrates**		
	Tube sponge	0.05×10^{12}	9.1×10^9
	Jellyfish (Haploid)	0.2×10^{12}	0.3×10^9
	Sea urchin („)	0.5×10^{12}	0.8×10^9
	Nereid worm („)	1×10^{12}	1.4×10^9
	Snail, *Tectorius muricatus* (Haploid)	4×10^{12}	6.3×10^9
	Cliff crab	1×10^{12}	1.4×10^9
	Drosophila melanogaster	0.12×10^{12}	0.2×10^9
6.	**Vertebrates**		
	Lung fish	60×10^{12}	94×10^9

Organism	Daltons	Nucleotide pairs
Frog	28×10^{12}	45×10^{9}
Amphiuma (Salamander)	120×10^{12}	180×10^{9}
Carcharias obscurus (Shark)	3.4×10^{12}	5.2×10^{9}
Carp	2×10^{12}	3.3×10^{9}
Chicken	1.2×10^{12}	2.1×10^{9}
Mouse	3.0×10^{12}	4.7×10^{9}
Human	3.6×10^{12}	5.6×10^{9}

The data of Table 18.1 suggest that fungus such as yeast contains not much more DNA than *E. coli*, whereas the nuclei of salamanders and other tailed amphibia contain much more DNA than human nuclei. Among invertebrates, the lowest DNA values are found in the most primitive animals, such as sponges and coelenterates. In fishes, the DNA content per cell tends to remain constant within the different species of a family. In amphibians the DNA varies from 168 pg in *Amphiuma* to 7.33 pg in the toad. Diploid cells of various tissues of the fowl contain approximately 2.5 picograms (1 pg = 10^{-12} g) of DNA, whereas the haploid sperm has half that amount. In various species of mammals, variations in DNA content are small but characteristic for that species.

DNA contents and ploidy. DNA contents of a nucleus have a definite relation with the number of chromosome sets (n, ploidy) which is 2n is most somatic cells. In the liver there are large nuclei which contain two and four times as much DNA as the diploid nuclei (Table 18.2). This duplication or quadruplication of DNA content obviously correspond to polyploidy (**Pollister** *et al.*, 1951).

Table 18.2. DNA content and chromosome complement.

Cells	Mean DNA-Feulgen content	Presumed chromosome set
Spermatid	1.68	haploid (n)
Liver	3.16	diploid (2n)
Liver	6.30	tetraploid (4n)
Liver	12.80	octoploid (8n)

Spermatogenesis also presents an interesting example of correlation of DNA content with ploidy level (Table 18.3). Before meiosis occurs there are two classes of cells (spermatogonia) having different DNA contents (2n and 4n). The early primary spermatocyte is tetraploid (4n). After the first maturation division the secondary spermatocyte contain half the DNA content, corresponding to diploid (2n) condition. Finally, the second maturation division results in four spermatids; these cells have the DNA of only one chromosomal set (halploid cell). Similar results have been observed in oogenesis during maturation of oocytes.

Table 18.3. DNA content at different stages of spermatogenesis, (**Pollister** *et al.*, 1951).

Cell type	DNA–Feulgen Content
Premeiotic — class 2n	3.28 ± 0.07
Premeiotic — class 4n	5.96 ± 0.07
Primary spermatocyte	6.28 ± 0.07
Secondary spermatocyte	3.35 ± 0.04
Spermatid	1.68 ± 0.02

DNA content and length of the DNA molecules. Since DNA is a highly polymerized macromolecule (see chapter 5 and 21), it is interesting to compare the DNA content of a cell nucleus to the probable length of the molecule. Thus, mitochondrial DNA is a circle with a circumference of about five micrometres; in viruses it may be several micrometres long and bacterial DNA may reach a length of one millimetre. Considering that one picogram of DNA is equivalent to 31 cm of DNA, it is possible to calculate that there are about 174 cm of DNA in the human diploid cells (5.6 pg), and 37 metres in *Trillium* (120 pg), and 95 metres in polytenic chromosome of *Drosophila* (293 pg), (**DuPraw**, 1968). **Rudkin** in 1967 has estimated DNA contents of 46 human chromosomes by ultraviolet cytophotometry and he suggested that DNA content is proportional to the size of the chromosome. Thus, the largest human chromosome (1), which is 10 μm long, should accomodate about 7.2 cm of DNA in a tightly packed form.

Besides DNA, nuclei of eukaryotes also contain RNA. In liver nuclei it is shown that less than 5 per cent of the dry mass is RNA, whereas 85 to 90 per cent of the total RNA is in the cytoplasm. The nuclear RNA is distributed in the nucleolus, chromatin, and nuclear sap.

2. Nuclear Proteins

The protein part of the nucleus is complex and has several components. Of these, the best known are two strongly basic and simple proteins—the protamines and the histones. In addition to these there are several acidic proteins, the so-called non-histone proteins and nuclear enzymes, which may constitute the main component of the interphase nucleus.

A. Nucleoprotamines. Protamines are simple, basic proteins with a very low molecular weight (4000 daltons). They are very rich in the basic amino acid **arginine** and thus have pH value from 10 to 11. They are found in spermatozoa of some fishes and are tightly bound to DNA by salt linkages. In general, they consist of a 28 residue polypeptide, with a total length of 100 A°, and contain 19 arginines and 8 or 9 non-basic amino acids (**Callanan** *et al.*, 1957). In the nucleus of trout spermatozoon the DNA-protamine complex accounts for 91 per cent of the dry weight. **Feughelman** *et al.* (1955) have demonstrated by X-ray diffraction analysis that the protamines wraps helically around the DNA molecule. **Alfert** (1956) has shown cytochemically that during the development of the spermatozoon there is a progressive replacement of the histone by protamine. This may be due to higher affinity of protamines for DNA. Biochemically there are at least three classes of spermatozoa, depending on whether the DNA is in complex with protamine (salmon, herring, trout, rooster snail, squid), with histones (plants, carp, sea urchin) or with other types of proteins (most mammals) (**Vendrely** *et al.*, 1960).

B. Nucleohistones. Histones are also basic proteins, but they exhibit greater heterogeneity than protamines. Histones are basic proteins because of a high proportion of the amino acids **arginine** and **lysine**, both of which have positively charged amino groups ($-\overset{+}{N}H_4$) at neutral pH. They lack **tryptophan**, have molecular weight in the range of 11,000 to 21,000, and together comprise a mass that is always about equal to that of the DNA itself (*i.e.*, at a 1:1 ratio, see Table 18.4). In most eukaryotic nuclei there are only five principal histone types, called **H1**, **H2b**, **H2a**, **H3** and **H4** (an older system of nomenclature, still used, refers to them as **f1**, **f2b**, **f2a2**, **f3** and **f2a1**, respectively). In the order given, they vary in composition from "very lysine rich" (29% lysine, 2% arginine in calf thymus H1), to "argine rich" (11% lysine, 14% arginine). Avian erythrocytes, which retain a non-functioning nucleus in the mature cell, have an additional histone called **H5** or **f2C**. Except for **H1**, histones of the same class from different eukaryotes have very similar amino acid sequences. In particular, H4 has been rigidly conserved through evolution, varying by two amino acids out of 102 between calf thymus and pea seedlings. This strict conservation implies an important function, the interference with which is apt to be lethal (**Dyson**, 1978). **Histones** act as repressor or inhibitors of genes (*i.e.*, they prevent transcription of DNA into RN A molecules). However, they seem to regulate gene transcription in a non-selective way, since histones lack tissue specificity, and contain small degree of heterogeneity than acidic proteins.

Table 18.4. Chemical composition of chromatin of liver cells and pea embryonic cell.

Component	(Dry % weight)	Pea embryo (Dry % weight)
DNA	31	31
RNA	5	17.5
Histone	36	33
Acidic protein	28	18

C. Non-histone or acidic proteins. Interphase nuclei, as well as chromatin (Table 18.4), contain abundant non-histone proteins some of which may be linked to DNA (**Steele** and **Busch**, 1963). Among those not linked to DNA are the so-called **residual proteins**. Many acidic proteins because carry a net negative charge and so qualify as acidic proteins. Most prominent DNA linked acidic protein is a heterogeneous group of **phosphoproteins**—proteins carrying amino acids that have become phosphorylated (see **Goodenough** and **Levine**, 1974).

Phosphoproteins remain concentrated in the chromatin of metabolically active cells, whereas, they are relatively deficient in inactive cells (*e.g.*, spermatozoon). In neurons, the large nucleus contains 20 times more acidic proteins than the sperm head. Further, in contrast to histones, acidic proteins have a rapid turn over, are very heterogeneous, and show phylogenetic as well as tissue specificity (**Busch**, 1965; **Wang**, 1967). Acidic proteins show selective binding to DNA and have stimulatory effects on transcription (**Teng** and **Teng**, 1971). Certain hormones such as hydrocortisone and estradiol are found to influence selectively to certain acidic proteins.

Moreover, histone and acidic proteins have a difference in the time of their synthesis within the cell cycle. Whereas, histones are synthesized during the S period, the synthesis of acidic nuclear proteins goes on throughout the entire cell cycle (**Borun** and **Stein**, 1972). In both cases, the synthesis of chromosomal proteins takes place in the cytoplasm, and the proteins are then transported into the nucleus.

Recent studies indicate that acidic proteins may play a fundamental role in the control of genic expression by reactivating regions of genome that are masked by histones (see **Goodenough** and **Levine**, 1974; **DeRobertis** *et al.*, 1975).

D. Nuclear enzymes. Enzymes are also non-histone proteins. Of the nuclear enzymes the most important are those involved in the synthesis and repairing of nucleic acids *e.g.*, **DNA polymerase**, **RNA polymerase**, **endonuclease**, **exonuclease**, **ligase**, etc.). These enzymes will be discussed in detail in ensuing chapters. Some enzymes of nucleus which are related to nucleoside metabolism, are found in high concentration in the nucleus (*e.g.*, **adenosine diaminase**, **nucleoside phosphorylase** and **guanase**). Bound to DNA are **NAD synthetase**, **nucleoside triphosphatase**, and the **histone acetylases**.

Although the nucleus does not contain cytochrome oxidase or succinic dehydrogenase, it does contain the soluble enzymes of anaerobic glycolysis, including **aldolase**, **enolase**, 3—**phosphoglyceraldehyde dehydrogenase**, and **pyruvate kinase** (**McEven**, **Allfrey** and **Mirsky**, 1963). These findings suggest that the cell nucleus uses glycolysis as the main source of energy.

3. Mineral Salts and Other Nuclear Contents

Nuclei contain large amounts of cofactors, precursor molecules, and minerals, NAD, ATP, and acetyl-CoA are present, as are other nucleoside mono-and triphosphates, and the intermediates of glycolysis. Nuclei contain no lipid content (see **DeRobertis** *et al.*, 1975).

Distribution of minerals has been studied by microincineration. The **spodogram** (ash picture) shows that the ash of the nucleus is more concentrated than that of the cytoplasm. The nuclear ash is composed of **phosphorus**, **potassium**, **sodium**, **calcium** and **magnesium**. Apparently minerals are found in greater proportion in chromatin. Calcium plays a significant structural role when it is bound to DNA.

Phosphate occurs in large amount in the nucleolus, where the existence of a phosphate pool has been verified by electron microscopy and electron diffraction. **Tandler** and **Solari** (1968) have suggested that the phosphate pool may be involved in the cycle of chromatin condensation during mitosis.

18.4 ULTRASTRUCTURE

The nucleus is composed of following structures:

1. The nuclear membrane or karyotheca,
2. The nucleolus,
3. The nuclear sap or nucleoplasm, and
4. The chromatin fibres.

1 . Nuclear Membrane

The nuclear membrane or karyotheca forms an envelope-like structure called **nuclear envelope** around the nuclear contents. The nuclear envelope separates the nucleoplasm from the cytoplasm.

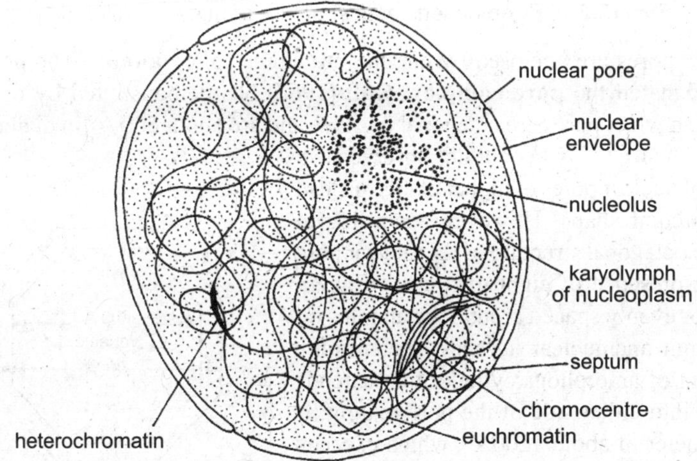

Fig. 18.1. Structure of a metaphase nucleus.

The electron microscopic studies of the nuclear envelope have shown that it is composed of two unit membranes, *viz.*, an outer membrane and an inner membrane. Each membrane is about 75 to 90 A° thick and lipoproteinous in nature. The outer and inner nuclear membranes remain separated by a space of 100 to 150A° (**DeRobertis** *et al.*, 1970, 1975), 100 to 300 A° (**Cohn**, 1970) or 400 to 700 A° (**Burke**, 1970). This inter-membranous space is known as **perinuclear space** or **cisterna**. The outer nuclear membrane often remains rough due to attached ribosomes with it. Sometimes it remains continuous with the membranes of the endoplasmic reticulum, Golgi complex, mitochondria, etc. The inner nuclear membrane contains no ribosomes and sometimes it also remains associated with the chromatin. Further, the nuclear membrane is followed by a supporting membrane of a uniform thickness known as **fibrous lamina** which is 300 A° in thickness.

Nuclear Pores

The nuclear membranes are not altogether continuous but at several places they are broken by the **nuclear openings** or **pores**. Around the margins of these nuclear pores both nuclear membranes are in continuity. At their nuclear side the pores are generally aligned with channels of nucleoplasm situated between more condensed lumps of chromatin.

The number of the pores for a particular nucleus is variable and often depends on the species and the type of the cell. For instance, the oocytes of the sea-urchin have 40 to 80 nuclear pores per square micron of the nucleus. However, the number of pores varies form 40 to 145 per square micrometre in nuclei of various plants and animals. **Watson** (1959) has calculated the nuclear pores of the mammalian cells as the 10 per cent of the total surface area of the nucleus. At their highest density the nuclear pores are packed in hexagonal array with centre-to-centre pore distance of about 1500 A°.

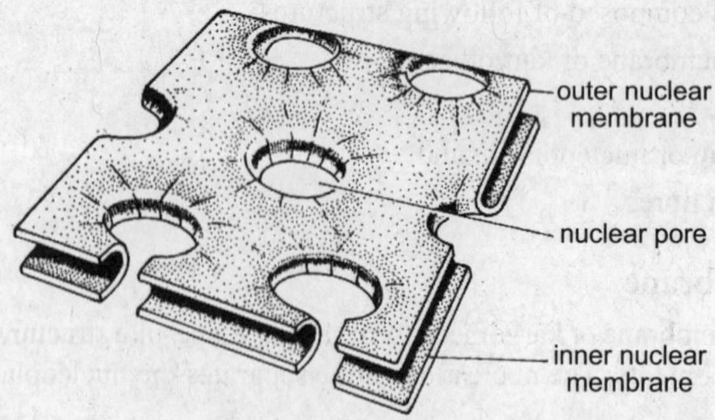

Fig. 18.2. Three dimensional structure of nuclear envelope.

The nuclear pores are enclosed by circular structures called **annuli**. The pores and annuli, together, are designated the **pore complex**. **Gall** (1967) has demonstrated by negative staining technique that the nuclear pores are octagonal in shape and are about 600 A° in diameter (Fig. 18.3). **Roberts** and **Northcote** (1970) could not observe such octagonal shape of nuclear pores of higher plants, instead they observed circular shape. However, according to **Frank** (1970) the octagonal structure of the nuclear pore is a result of the presence of eight **granules** of about 150A° in diameter evenly spaced around the annulus on both the cytoplasmic and nuclear surfaces. The **annular material** is a kind of amorphous cylinder that extends through the pore into either side of the pore margin. It has an outer diameter of about 1200A°, which exceeds that of the pore (Fig. 18.3 and 18.4). The central hole of the annulus varies from 300 to 500A°. This material is digested by trypsin and remains untouched when exposed to ribonuclease and deoxyribonuclease enzymes. These findings suggest that the annular material is protein in nature.

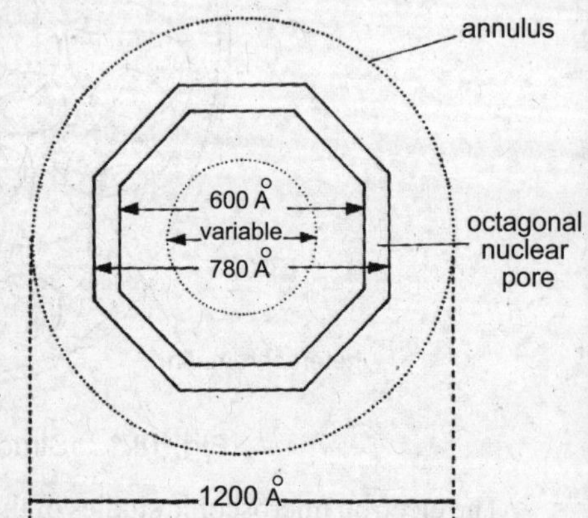

Fig. 18.3. Structure of a nuclear pore (Gall, 1967).

The pore complex is apparently a rather rigid structure present in a fixed number according to cell type. In certain physiological stages, however, they may change in number. For example, they are reduced in number in maturing erythroblasts and in spermatids.

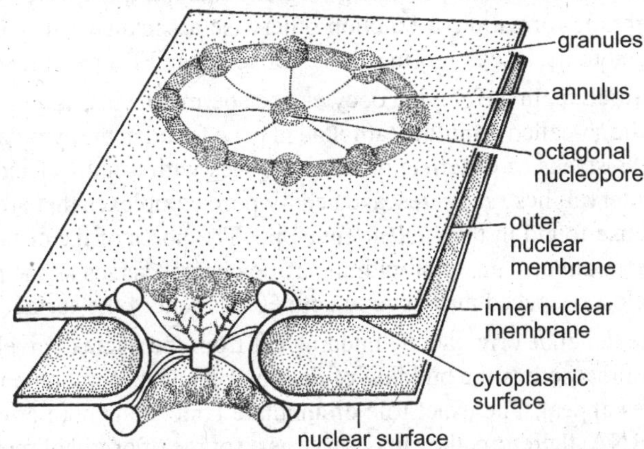

Fig. 18.4. Diagram of the pore complex (after Frank, 1970).

Origin of Nuclear Envelope

The nuclear envelope is the derivative of the membrane of the endoplasmic reticulum. In telophase of the mitosis, it has been observed that the cisternae of the endoplasmic reticulum collect around the chromosomes and by fusing together form the nuclear envelope.

Functions of Nuclear Membrane and Nuclear Pores

The nuclear membranes perform various important functions for the nucleus, such as, in certain cells (oocytes) the nuclear membranes allow free exchange of ions between the nucleus and the cytoplasm, while certain nuclear membranes as of the cells of the salivary glands of the *Drosophila* act as barrier for the diffusion of substance and even the ions of K^+, Na^+ and Cl^-. A Mg^{2+}—activated ATPase is associated with the nuclear membranes as well as with pore complexes. This enzyme could contribute to active transport of molecules and ions across the membrane (**Avers**, 1976).

Regardless of the selectivity conferred by the pore complex, there is considerable traffic through it. Nucleotides must be able to get in readily and transfer RNA, messenger RNA and immature ribosomes must get out. The use of radioactive tracers shows that histones and other nuclear proteins, including ribosomal proteins which are synthesized outside the nucleus, rapidly and efficiently collect in the nucleoplasm. The annuli regulate the exchange of the macromolecules through the pore complex according to their chemical nature and the size.

Relationship to the cytoskeleton. Microfilaments and microtubules are frequently seen in the vicinity of, and are sometimes attached to, the nuclear membranes. In simpler eukaryotic cells (*e.g.*, dinoflagellates; ciliated protozoans, *i.e.*, macronucleus of *Paramecium*; slime mold, *Polysphondylium*; etc.) Special areas of the nuclear membrane clearly serve as microtubule organizing centres to assemble the spindle apparatus needed for chromosome separation during cell division. The nuclear membrane thus serves in place of centrioles in these cells. In addition, microtubules can be assembled to the outer membrane of many nuclei and extend from there into the cytoplasm. They probably serve to direct cytoplasmic streaming of substances toward and awav from the nucleus and to anchor the nucleus in place (**Dyson**, 1978).

Nuclear blebbing. An irregular ruffling of the outer nuclear membrane is often observed and in some instances (*e.g.*, algae, *Botrydium granulatum*, cells of adrenal cortex of rat and lung cells of human foetus), blebbing has been seen. Pouches or blebs are finger-like extensions of the outer nuclear membrane that may be pinched off to form vesicles. Many workers believe that those regions of the outer nuclear membrane exhibiting blebbing (regions that are always free of ribosomes) represent sites of new membrane formation, a function otherwise associated with the ER itself and that the vesicles are destined to coalesce to form new lamellae of the ER or Golgi complex.

Annulate lamellae. In developing oocytes and spermatocytes, as well as in certain embryonic and tumour cells, the so-called **annulate lamellae** may be found in the cytoplasm. These membranous structures appear as stacks of cisternae or flattened sacs with a intra-saccular space 100 to 200A° wide. At regular interval these sacs are traversed by pore complexes that are similar in morphology and structure to those found in the nuclear envelope. The pores of the cisternae have an octagonal shape and contain an annular material with the same characteristics as the pore complexes (**Maul**, 1970). These are closely spaced may occupy upto 50 per cent of the surface of the membrane.

The annulate lamellae originate by budding off from the nuclear envelope. **Kessel** (1968) has demonstrated that first there is the budding of the outer nuclear membrane into flattened sacs; later the pore complexes appear. The exact role of annulate lamellae is not known, but, as they contain high contents of rRNA, therefore, they may serve as a source of origin of membrane of endoplasmic reticulum.

2. Nucleolus

The nucleus contains a large, eccentrically situated, spherical and acidophilic dense granule as **nucleolus**. It was first described by **Fontana** in 1781. It was well established in 19th century that the size of the nucleolus is related with the synthetic activity of the cell. Therefore, the cells with little or no synthetic activities, *e.g.*, sperm cells, blastomeres, muscle cells, etc., are found to contain smaller or no nucleoli, while the oocytes, neurons and secretory cells which synthesize the proteins or other substances contain comparatively large-sized nucleoli. The number of the nucleoli in the nucleus depends on species and the number of chromosomes. The number of the nucleoli in the cells may be one, two or four.

The light microscope generally reveals the nucleolus as structurally homogeneous, although small corpuscles or vacuoles are sometimes noted. The nucleolus is frequently attached to the nuclear membranes, and some of these vacuoles and material from the dense part of the nucleolus seem to pass into the cytoplasm.

Cytochemistry of nucleolus. Nucleoli have been isolated from oocytes of marine animals and from liver cells. They contained 3 to 5 per cent RNA. In nucleoli from pea embryos, the RNA content is 10 per cent, or 20 per cent of the total nuclear RNA. The nucleolar RNA resembles very closely with the ribosomal RNA in its base composition. The nucleolus contains large amount of the proteins, mainly phosphoproteins. There occur no histone. There is cytochemical evidence for the existence of a high concentration of orthophosphate, which may serve as precursor of the RNA phosphorus. The nucleolus also contains certain enzymes such as acid phosphatase, nucleoside phosphorylase, and NAD^+ synthesizing enzymes for the biosynthesis of some coenzymes, nucleotides and the ribosomal RNA. **RNA methylase**, an enzyme that transfers methyl groups to the RNA bases, has been localized in the nucleolus of certain cells (**Sirlin** *et al.*, 1963). Nucleolus contains no DNA, but it may be surrounded by a ring of heterochromatin.

Fine structure of nucleolus. In certain cells the nucleolus may exist in a fragmented or diffused form. But most nuclei contain compact nucleoli. The nucleolus is composed of the following four zones:

1. **Granular zone.** The granular zone occurs at the periphery of the nucleolus and composed of dense granules of 150 to 200A° diameter. The granular zone consists of ribonucleic proteins.
2. **Fibrillar zone.** The fibrillar zone is known as the **nucleolonema**. The nucleolonema is composed of many fibrils of 50 to 80A° long. Sometimes very long as 500A° fibrils have been reported in certain nucleoli. The fibrils are composed of ribonucleic proteins.

3. **Amorphous zone (pars amorpha).** The amorphous zone has low electron density and it is found only in certain nucleoli.
4. **Nucleolar-associated chromatin** is composed of fibres of 100A° thickness situated around the nucleolus and extending into it. These chromatin fibres may occupy special areas within the nucleolus or may be spread rather diffusely. They contain DNA.

Radioautographical and ultracentrifugal studies have made it clear that fibrillar portion of nucleolus is a precursor of the granular portion, and that both contain ribonucleoproteins which are precursors of the cytoplasmic ribosomes.

Further, the nucleolus possesses no limiting membrane and the calcium ions are supposed to maintain the intact organization of the nucleolus.

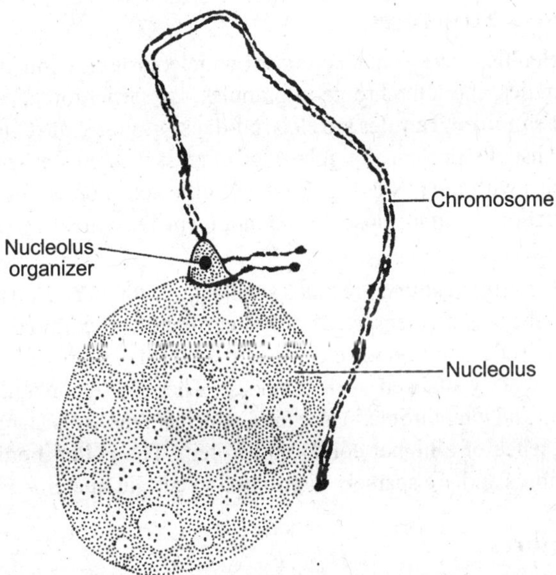

Fig. 18.5. Chromosome 6 in meiotic prophase in maize showing its nucleolus organizer in contact with the nucleolus (after King, 1965).

Nucleolar cycle. The nucleolus shows the cyclic changes in itself during the process of cell division. For instance, the nucleolus disappears at the prophase stage and reappears at the telophase.The nucleolar cycle remains associated with a region of the chromosome known as **nucleolar organizer region**. The nucleolus remains attached with this region and thus comes in direct contact with the rDNA which contains coded informations for the synthesis of the nucleolus and ribosomal RNA.

In the meristematic cells of *Allium cepa* it has been observed that the nucleolus contains a loop of chromatin (DNA) which extends from nucleolar chromosome. During late prophase this chromatin loop gradually retracts and coils inside the nucleolar zone of the corresponding chromosome. Simultaneously, there is a gradual dispersion of the fibrillar and granular components of the nucleolus into the nucleoplasm. During telophase, nucleolar reconstitution follows two steps: at early and middle telophase, the emerging nucleolus consists of a convoluted chromatin loop which uncoils from the nucleolar organizer and becomes surrounded by fibrillar and granular material; at late telophase, it exhibits all the characteristics of a mature interphase nucleolus (**Chouinard**, 1971).

Function of the nucleolus. The main function of nucleolus is the biogenesis of ribosomes. It stores all the proteins of ribosomes and also rRNA which is transcribed by rDNA. The tailoring of 45S rRNA which is transcribed by rDNA. The tailoring of 45S rRNA into 5.8S rRNA. 18S rRNA and 28S rRNA and their subsequent methylation occur in nucleolus. The final assembly of ribosomal proteins and rRNA molecules to form the ribosomal subunits also occur in nucleolus.

3. Nucleoplasm

The space between the nuclear envelope and the nucleolus is filled by a transparent, semi-solid, granular and slightly acidophilic ground substance or the matrix known as the **nuclear sap**, **nucleoplasm** or **karyolymph**. The nuclear components such as chromatin threads, nucleoprotein granules, nucleolus, etc., remain suspended in the nucleoplasm.

The nucleoplasm contains complex chemical organization and in fact, the cytochemistry of interphase nucleus represents the biochemistry of nucleoplasm.

Ribonucleoprotein Structures

Besides nucleolus, there occur certain ribonucleoprotein containing structures, such as the perichromatin granules, the interchromatin granules, the perichromatin fibres and so-called coiled bodies. The **perichromatin granules** are electron-dense granules of about 400 to 450A°, surrounded by a clear halo and usually present along the edge of masses of condensed chromatin. The number of these granules varies with the physiological state of the cell. For example, they increase in number with the administration of small doses of actinomycin D, which interferes with the synthesis of ribosomal RNA.

The **interchromatin granules** are much smaller (*i.e.*, 200 to 250A°) and more widely distributed, forming clusters in the less-condensed regions of chromatin (**Bernhard**, 1968). The **perichromatin fibres** are found at the edges of masses of chromatin. They may represent a fibrous RNA product of the chromosome that is readily attacked by ribonuclease. These RNA containing fibres may be precursors of the perichromatin and interchromatin granules, which are more resistant to ribonuclease—probably because of the presence of a higher content of protein. The **coiled bodies** are composed of rather coarse masses of fibres and are sparsely distributed in certain nuclei.

4. Chromatin Fibres

The nucleoplasm contains many thread-like, coiled and much elongated structures which take readily the basic stains such as the basic fuchsin. These thread-like structures are known as the **chromatin** (Gr., *chrome*-colour) **substance** or **chromatin fibres**. The fibres of chromatin are twisted, fine anastomose and uniformly distributed in the nucleoplasm. Such chromatin fibres are observed only in the interphase nucleus. During cell divisions (mitosis and meiosis) chromatin fibres become thick ribbon-like structures which are known as the **chromosomes**. The chromatin and chromosomes will be discussed in quite detail in next chapter.

REVISION QUESTIONS

1. Describe the nuclear envelope and the structure of its pores. What similarities occur between nuclear envelope and endoplasmic reticulum?
2. Describe the ultrastructure of nucleus.
3. Discuss the cytochemistry of nucleus.
4. What is meant by nuclear blebbing?
5. How many types of proteins and nucleic acids are found in the nucleus?
6. Describe the structure and function of the nucleolus. How is it formed?
7. Does amount of DNA has any correlation with the ploidy of the cell? What?

19
Chapter
CHROMOSOMES

The chromosomes are the nuclear components of special organization, individuality and function. They are capable of self-reproduction and play a vital role in heredity, mutation, variation and evolutionary development of the species.

19.1 HISTORICAL

W. Fleming (1879) first of all described the splitting of chomosomes and coined the term **chromatin** for stainable material of the nucleus. **W. Roux** (1883) suspected the involvement of the chromosomes in the mechanism of inheritance. **Benden** and **Bovery** (1887) reported that number of chromosomes for each species was constant. The present name **chromosome** (Gr., *chrom*-colour, *soma*-body) was coined by **W. Waldeyer** (1888) to darkly stained bodies of nucleus. **W.S. Sutton** and **T. Boveri** in 1902 suggested that chromosomes were the physical structures which acted as messengers of heredity. **Morgan** (1933) discovered the function of chromosomes in the transmission of heredity traits. **Heitz** (1935), **Kuwanda** (1939), **Geitter** (1940), and **Kaufmann** (1948) have described the morphology of chromosomes. The molecular organization of chromosomes have been recently worked out.

19.2 CHROMOSOME NUMBER

The number of the chromosomes is constant for a particular species. Therefore, these are of great importance in the determination of the phylogeny and taxonomy of the species. The organism with the lowest number of the chromosomes is the nematode, *Ascaris megalacephalus univalens* which has only two chromosomes in the somatic cells. The chromosome number of some animals and plants is tabulaled as follows:

Table 19.1. Chromosome number of some organisms.

Group	Common name	Scientific name	Diploid chromosome number
Animals:			
Protozoa	Paramecium	*Paramecium aurelia*	30–40
Cnidaria	Hydra	*Hydra vulgaris*	32
Nematoda	Round worm	*Ascaris lumbricoides*	24
Mollusca	Roman snail	*Helix pomatia*	54

Group	Common name	Scientific name	Diploid chromosome number
Arthropoda	Silkworm	*Bombyx mori*	56
	House fiy	*Musca domestica*	12
	Fruit fiy	*Drosophila melanogaster*	8
	Grasshoppers	—	24
	Honey bee	*Apis mellifica*	32, 16
	Mosquito	*Culex pipiens*	6
Pisces	Gold fish	*Carassius auratus*	100
Amphibia	Frog	*Rana pipiens*	26
	Toad	*Bufo americanus*	22
	Toad	*Xenopus laevis*	36
Aves	Chicken	*Gallus domesticus*	78
	Pigeon	*Columba livia*	80
	Duck	*Anas platyrhyncha*	80
Mammalia	Oppossum	*Didelphys virginiana*	22
	Mouse	*Mus musculus*	40
	Rabbit	*Oryctolagus cuniculus*	44
	Common rat	*Rattus rattus*	42
	Chinese hamster	*Cricetus griseus*	22
	Guinea pig	*Cavia cobaya*	64
	Dog	*Canis familiaris*	78
	Cat	*Felis domestica*	38
	Horse	*Equus caballus*	64
	Donkey	*Equus asinus*	62
	Pig	*Sus scrofa*	40
	Sheep	*Ovis aries*	54
	Goat	*Copra hircus*	60
	Cattle	*Bos taurus*	60
	Rhesus monkey	*Macaca mulatta*	42
	Gorilla	*Gorilla gorilla*	48
	Chimpanzee	*Pan troglodytes*	48
	Man	*Homo sapiens*	46
Plants:			
Algae	Chlamydomonas	*Chlamydomonas reinhardii*	10? 12? 16? (Haploid sets)
Fungi	Bread mold	*Mucor heimalis*	2
Gymnosperm	Yellow pine	*Pinus ponderosa*	24
Angiosperm	Cabbage	*Brassica oleracea*	18
	Radish	*Raphanus sativus*	18
	Papaya	*Carica papaya*	18
	Cotton	*Gossypium hirsutum*	52

Group	Common name	Scientific name	Diploid chromosome number
	Coffee	*Coffea arabica*	44
	Sunflower	*Helianthus annuus*	34
	Potato	*Solanum tuberosum*	48
	Tomato	*Lycopersicum solanum*	24
	Tobacco	*Nicotiana tabacum*	48
	Banana	*Musa paradisiaca*	22, 44, 55, 77, 88
	Garden pea	*Pisum sativum*	14
	Bean	*Phaseolus vulgaris*	22
	Orange	*Citrus sinensis*	18, 27, 36
	Apple	*Malus silvestris*	34, 51
	Indian corn	*Zea mays*	20
	Barley	*Hordeum vulgare*	14
	Bread wheat	*Triticum vulgare*	42
	Rice	*Oryza sativa*	24
	Bajra	*Sorghum vulgare*	10, 20, 40
	Sugarcane	*Saccharum officinarum*	80
	Field bean	*Vicia faba*	12
	Onion	*Allium cepa*	16
	Eucalyptus	*Eucalyptus sps.*	22

Haploid and diploid. The number and set of the chromosomes of the gametic cells such as sperms and ova is known as the gametic, reduced or **haploid** sets of chromosomes. The haploid set of the chromosomes is also known as the **genome**. The somatic or body cells of most organisms contain two haploid sets or genomes and are known as the **diploid cells**. The diploid cells achieve the diploid set of the chromosomes by the union of the haploid male and female gametes in the sexual reproduction.

19.3 MORPHOLOGY

Size

The size of the chromosomes varies from species to species and relatively remains constant for a particular species. The length of the chromosomes may vary from 0.2 to 50 μm. The diameter of the chromosomes may be from 0.2 to 20 μm. For instance, the human chromosomes are up to 6 μm in length. Moreover, the organisms with less number of chromosomes contain comparatively large-sized chromosomes than the chromosomes of the organisms having many chromosomes.

The monocotyledon plants contain large-sized chromosome than the dicotyledon plants. The plants in general have large-sized chromosomes in comparison to the animals. Further, the chromosomes in a cell are never alike in size, some may be exceptionally large and other may be too small. The largest chromosomes ar lampbrush chromosomes of certain vertebrate oocytes and polyten chromosomes of certain dipteran insects.

Shape

The shape of the chromosomes is changeable from phase to phase in the continuous process of the cell growth and cell division. In the resting phase or interphase stage of the cell, the chromosomes occur in the form of thin, coiled, elastic and contractile, thread-like stainable structures, the chromatin threads. In the metaphase and the anaphase, the chromosomes become thick and filamentous. Each chromosome contains a clear zone, known as **centromere** or **kinetochore**, along their length. The centromere divides the chromosomes into two parts, each part is called **chromosome arm**. The position of centromere vary from chromosome to chromosome and it provides different shapes to the latter which are following:

1. **Telocentric.** The rod-like chromosomes which have the centromere on the proximal end are known as the **telocentric chromosomes**.
2. **Acrocentric.** The acrocentric chromosomes are also rod-like in shape but these have the centromere at one end and thus giving a very short arm and an exceptionally long arm. The locusts (Acrididae) have the acrocentric chromosomes.
3. **Submetacentric.** The submetacentric chromosomes are J- or L-shaped. In these, the centromere occurs near the centre or a medium portion of the chromosome and thus forming two unequal arms.
4. **Metacentric.** The metacentric chromosomes are V-shaped and in these chromosomes the centromere occurs in the centre and forming two equal arms. The amphibians have metacentric chromosomes.

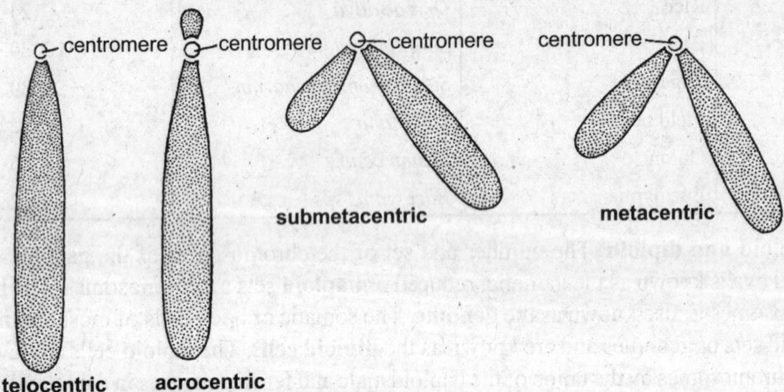

Fig. 19.1. The four morphological types of chromosomes according to the position of the centromere (after De Robertis *et al.*, 1970).

Karyotype and Idiogram

The characters by which a set of the chromosomes of a species is identified, are known as their **karyotypes**. When the karyotypes of a species are represented by a diagram then such diagram is called **idiogram**. (For technique of idiogram preparation, see chapter 3).

Kinds of Chromosomes

The eukaryotic chromosomes have been classified into **autosomes** and **sex choromosomes**. The autosomes have nothing to do with the determination of sex and exceed in number than sex chromosomes. The sex chromosomes which are also known as **accessory chromosomes**, **allosomes** or **hetero-chromosomes**, determine the sex of their bearer. They are usually two in number and are usually of two kinds: **X chromosomes** and **Y chromosomes**. One of the sexes has a pair of identical sex chromosomes (XX), the other may have a single sex chromosome, which may be unpaired (XO) or paired with a Y chromosome. The XY pair is also called heteromorphic because of the different morphology of the chromosomes.

19.4 STRUCTURE

According to classical cytology the chromosomes are composed of the chromonema and the centromeres.

Chromonema

In less compact chromosomes, under the optical microscope, a coiled filament is seen in the chromosome. The coiled filament was called **chromonema** by **Vejdovsky** in 1912.

The chromonema may be composed of two, four or more fibres according to the species. Further, the number of threads in the chromonema may depend on the different phases because at one phase the chromonema may contain one thread and at other phase it may contain three or four threads. The threads or fibrils of the chromonema remain coiled with each other. The coils may be of the following two types:

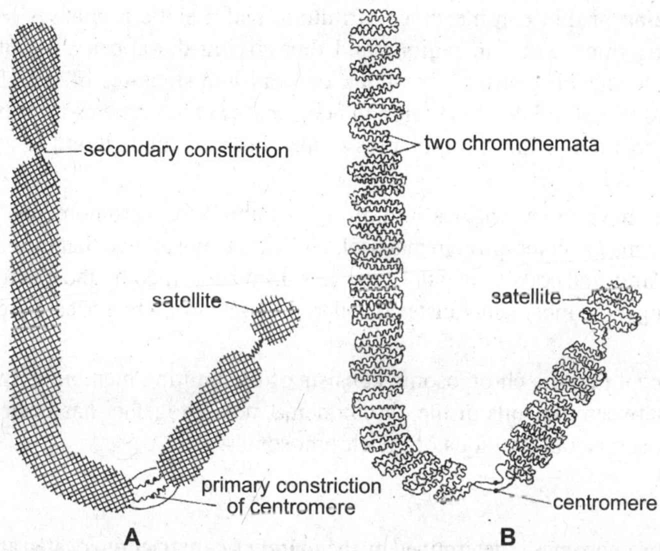

Fig. 19.2. Diagram of a metacentric chromosome. A—External structure; B—Internal structure (after De Robertis *et al.*, 1970).

***(i)* Paranemic coils.** When the subunits or the chromonemal fibrils or threads are easily separable from their coils then such coils are known as paranemic coils.

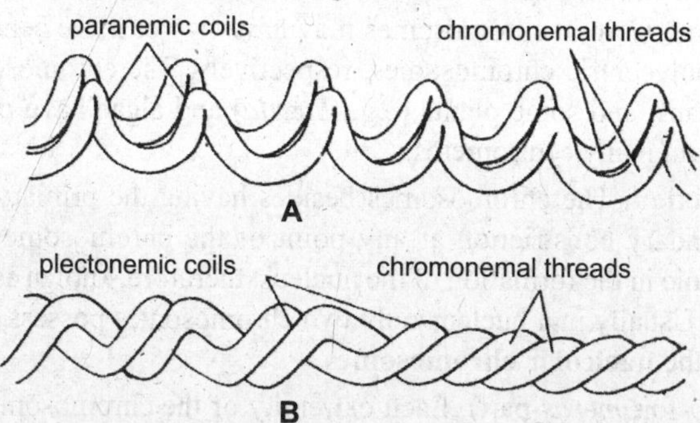

Fig. 19.3. Two types of coils of chromonemal threads. A—Paranemic coils; B—Plectonemic coils (after De Robertis *et al.*, 1970).

(ii) **Plectonemic coils.** When the chromosomal threads remain intertwined so intimately that they cannot be separated easily. This type of the coils are known as plectonemic coils.

The degree of the coiling in the chromonemal threads at mitosis and meiosis is variable and often depends on the length of the chromosomes. The chromosomes at the time of meiosis and mitosis contain three peculiar types of coils which are as follows:

1. **Major coils.** The major coils of the chromonema contain 10 to 30 gyres.
2. **Minor coils.** The minor coils of the chromonema lie perpendicularly to the major coils and contain many gyres in comparison to the major coils.
3. **Standard or somatic coils.** The chromonema of the mitosis has also been reported to contain helical structures which resemble with the major coils of the meiotic chromosomes. Such coils are known as standard or somatic coils.

Chromomeres

The chromonema of thin chromosomes of mitotic and meiotic prophases have been found to contain alternating thick and thin regions and thus giving the appearance of a necklace in which several beads occur on a string. The thick or bead-like stuctures of the chromonema are known as the **chromomeres** and the thin region in between the chromomeres is termed as the **inter-chromomeres**. The position of the chromomeres in the chromonema is found to be constant for a given chromosome.

The cytologists have given various interpretations about the chromomeres. Some consider chromomeres as condensed nucleo-protein material, while other postulated that the chromomeres are regions of the super-imposed coils. The latter view has been confirmed by the electron microscopic observations. For long-time most geneticists considered these chromomeres as **genes**, *i.e.*, the units of heredity.

The early concept that the chromosome consists of the limiting membrane (pellicle) and the amorphous matrix between the coils of the chromonema, now altogether has been rejected by the recent electron microscopic observations of the chromosomes.

Centromere

The shape of chromosomes is determined by the **primary constriction** located at the point where the arms of a chromosome meet (Fig. 19.2A). Within the constriction is a clear zone containing a small granule, or spherule. This clear region is the so called **centromere** or **kinetochore**. The centromere of the chromosome; of the *Trillium* has the diameter of 3 μm and the spherules have the diameter of 0.2 μm. The chromonema remains connected with the spherules of the centromere.

The chromosomes of most organisms contain only one centromere and are known as **monocentric** chromosomes. Certain chromosomes may have two or more centromeres and can be termed as dicentric and polycentric chromosomes, respectively. The chromosomes of the *Ascaris megalocephala*, hemipterans, and some plants (*e.g.*, *Luzula*) and algae have **diffused type of the centromere**, as they contain many centromeres.

Secondary constriction. The chromosomes besides having the primary constriction or the centromere possess secondary constriction at any point of the chromosome. Certain secondary constrictions play a vital role in the formation of the nucleus, therefore, known as the **nucleolar zone** or **nucleolar organizers**. Usually in a nucleus only two chromosomes possess such nucleolar zone and, therefore, known as the **nucleolar chromosomes**.

Telomere. (Gr., *telò*-for; *meras*-part). Each extremity of the chromosome has a polarity and therefore, it prevents other chromosomal segments to be fused with it. The chromosomal ends are known as the **telomeres**.

Satellite. Sometimes the chromosomes bear round elongated or knob-like appendages known as **satellites**. The satellite remains connected with the rest of the chromosome by a thin chromatin filament. The chromosomes with the satellite are designated as the **sat-chromosomes**. The shape and size of the satellite and the chromatin filament remain constant.

19.5 HETEROCHROMATIN AND EUCHROMATIN

The composing material of the chromosomes is the chromatin substance (DNA + nucleoproteins, etc.) which may occur in the form of euchromatin and heterochromatin. In 1928 **Heitz** defined **heterochromatin** as those regions of chromosome that remain condensed during interphase and early prophase and form the so called **chromocenters** or **false nucleoli**. The rest of the chromosome, which remains in a non-condensed state, was called **euchromatin**. There occur a mass of heterochromatin in close contact with the nucleolus, and correspond to the **nucleolar organizer**. During mitosis the heterochromatic regions appear localized at the centromeres, at the telomeres; or are intercalated in other parts of the chromosomes. Such regions may stain more strongly or weakly than the euchromatic regions, showing what is called a **positive** or a **negative heteropyknosis** (Gr., hetero- +pyknosis, different staining).

Heterochromatin and euchromatin are seen with the electron microscope to differ in their physical structure. Heterochromatin is composed of 250Å fibrils, whereas euchromatin contains mostly 30 to 80Å fibres. So, heterochromatin represents a condensed intercoiled state of chromatin, containing two to three times more DNA than euchromatin. However, it is genetically inert as it does not direct synthesis of RNA (*i.e.*, transcription) and protein and is often replicated at a different time from the rest of the DNA. **Brown** (1966) has recognized following two kinds of heterochromatin:

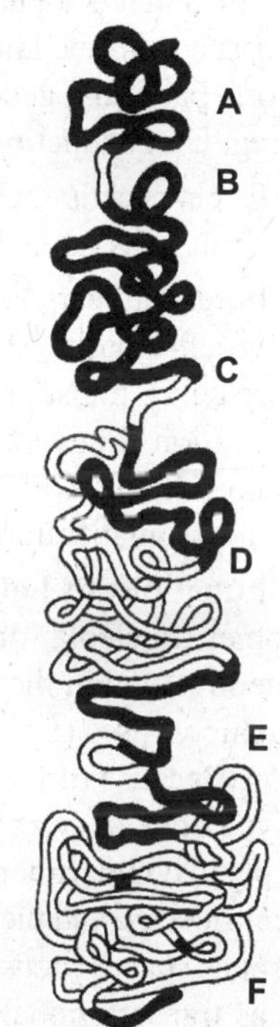

Fig. 19.4. Model of constitutive heterochromatin in a mammalian metaphase chromosome. A—Constitutive heterochromatin; B—Secondary constriction; I or nucleolar organizer; C—Primary constriction or centromere; D—Euchromatin; E—Secondary constriction II-possible site of 5S rRNA cistrons; F—Telomere (after De Robertis *et al.*, 1975).

1. Constitutive heterochromatin. It is a most common type of heterochromatin and is present at all times and in the nuclei of virtually, all the cells of an organism. It may be found in centromeric region, in the telomeres, or as bands in other parts of the chromosomes (Fig. 19.4). In *Drosophila*, for example, most pupal, larval and adult cells contain large blocks of constitutive heterochromatin that lie adjacent to the centromeres. These blocks of heterochromatin are found to be the sites in which highly repetitive satellite DNA is located. This DNA is **late replicating**: it fails to replicate until late in the S phase and is then replicated during a brief period just before the G_2.

For many years the regions of the chromosome which contain constitutive heterochromatin, were considered to be devoid of genetic activity. In recent times, however, important genes are recognized to be present in heterochromatin. For example, the polygenes that codify for the ribosomal RNA in the nucleolar organizer and those making the 5S and the transfer RNA are localized in heterochromatic regions.

2. Facultative heterochromatin. The facultative heterochromatin reflects the existence of a regulatory device designed to adjust the "dosages" of certain genes in the nucleus. It is originated during a process called **facultative heterochromatization**—a chromosome or a set of chromosomes becomes heterochromatic (turned off) in cells of one sex, while remaining set of chromosome becomes euchromatic (turned on) in the cells of opposite sex. The best known case is that of the X chromosomes in the mammalian female, one of which is active and remains euchromatic, whereas the other is inactive and forms the sex chromatin or Barr body, at interphase. This type of heterochromatin is acquired during embryogenesis; in the human, the sex chromatin appears in the embryo between the sixteenth and eighteenth days. Before that time, both X chromosomes are euchromatic. Thus, facultative heterochromatization remains indirectly related to sexual differentiation.

According to **Goodenough** and **Levine** (1974), there occur another kind of heterochromatin called **condensed heterochromatin**. This heterochromatin is deeply staining and tightly coiled chromatin and it is found in many interphase nuclei. This heterochromatin is distributed differentially from tissue to tissue and appears during the course of cell maturation via a process that appears to "turn off" particular genetic information in particular cells. The condensed heterochromatin has some gene regulatory function.

In plant cells there are constitutive heterochromatin and large amounts of repetitive DNA; however there is no facultative heterochromatin (**Britten** and **Kohne**, 1968).

In recent years, a specific role of histone H1 has been observed in determining the structure of heterochromatin. Histone H1 is absent or much reduced in chromatin that is uncoiled and actively being transcribed (*i.e.*, euchromatin), whereas the other histones are present in the usual concentration. Conversely, untranscribed heterochromatin has much H1. In chicken, accumulation of histone H5 in the mature erythrocyte is found to cause progressive inhibition of transcription due to heterochromatization of chromatin (**Dyson**, 1978).

Functions of heterochromatin. The heterochromatin has specific role in the biogenesis of ribosomes (nucleolar organizer and 5S rDNA) and tRNA molecules. Centromeric heterochromatin may be involved in the separation of chromosomes during cell division. It has been postulated that oncogenic viruses (*i.e.*, viruses capable of inducing cancer) may be inserted in the heterochromatic regions. Because of the repetitive nature, these regions could also be less susceptible to mutagens. This type of DNA (*viz.*, **repetitious** or **redundant** DNA) appears with evolution in the higher cells—probably to compartmentalize the genome into several functional parts, as for example, the nucleolus, the centromeres, and the multiple initiation points of DNA replication. Some of the repeated sequences are kept as spacers between genetically active regions. Within the euchromatin these sequences may serve as transcriptional stops, initiation points for RNA polymerase, or sites of attachment to the nuclear membrane. The sequences may also be used in pairing of homologous chromosomes and crossing over sites in meiosis (**Yunis** and **Yashmineh**, 1971).

Chromosome Banding

Beginning in 1969 new methods were developed to stain chromosome regions differentially. These methods produced distinctive bands of stained chromatin interspersed with unstained interband areas. Such chromosome banding studies have opened a completely new avenue to explore the structure and function of small-sized chromosomes of human and other organisms and their nucleoprotein components.

Two main categories of the chromosome banding patterns have been described:

1. Bands of presumptive heterochromatin distributed along the arms of the chromosomes have been revealed by staining with fluorescent dyes such as quinacrine mustards (**Q-bands**) or Giemsa and other non-fluorescent stains (**G-bands**). A reverse band (**R-band**) pattern occur when method is varied slightly, producing R-bands that are reciprocal of Q-bands and G-bands.

Q-banding is found to result from interaction between quinacrine and regions of DNA that are rich in adenine and thymine. Guanine and cytosine quench fluorescence, so regions rich in these bases would be present in the unstained interband.

2. **C-bands** that distinguish constitutive heterochromatin regions, particularly around the centromere, are visualized by Giemsa staining after special pretreatments that include HCl and NaOH denaturing steps.

C-banding is found to occur because a greater concentration of DNA remains in C-banded regions than in other regions of the chromosome after specific pretreatments.

Thus, banding patterns provide much greater resolution of heterochromatic regions along each chromosome than either the study of condensed interphase chromatin or autoradiographic study of replication time.

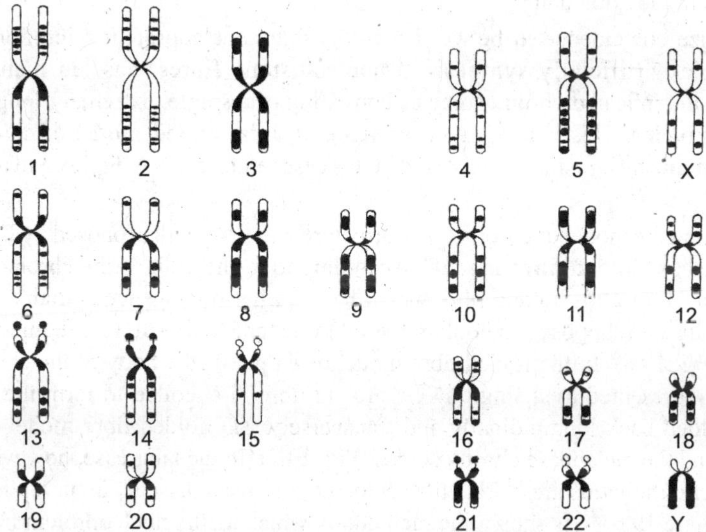

Fig. 19.5. Diagram showing the banding pattern of human chromosomes revealed with Giemsa stain. Since the banding is specific for each chromosome pair, this method, as well as, that involving fluorescent stains, is of great help in preparing a more refined analysis of normal and abnormal chromosomes (after De Robertis *et al.*, 1975).

Molecular Compounds of Chromosomes

Chemically the chromosomes of most prokaryotes and eukaryotes are composed of mainly DNA which may or may not be wrapped in histone and nonhistone proteins. The DNA of bacteria, viruses, and cellular organelles (*viz.*, mitochondria and chloroplasts) may have some protein associated with it—but this protein is not intimately associated with the nucleic acid, and "naked" fibres of DNA are readily visualized when bacterial, viral, or organelle chromosomes are examined with the electron microscope. In contrast, the chromosomal DNA of the eukaryotic nucleus associates with specific nuclear proteins—the histone and non-histone or acidic proteins, to form a stable nucleoprotein complex, the chromatin. Besides the proteins a number of enzymes (**DNA** and **RNA polymerases**, etc.) and various amounts of RNA and phospholipids are also intimately associated with chromatin.

Physical Organization of an Interphase Chromosome

Early light microscopical investigations have suggested the occurrence of **microfibrils**, ranging from 30Å to 170Å in chromatin. The finest microfibrils have been postulated to represent single nucleoprotein (*i.e.*, DNA + protein) molecules (De **Robertis**, 1964; **Sotelo** and **Wettstein**, 1965). Later on, electron microscopical observations of euchromatin confirmed the occurrence of microfibrils of 30Å thickness in it. Consequently, 30Å thick microfibrils of nucleoproteins (DNA + proteins) were considered as the basic structural units of eukaryotic chromosomes. This conclusion was further supported by an experiment in which a single nucleohistone fibre of 30Å diameter as synthesized artificially: when isolated DNA is allowed to interact with histones under laboratory conditions, nucleohistone fibre of 30Å diameter are formed. The histones presumably adopt a long flattened configuration in these fibres, for a DNA duplex is itself 20Å in diameter and histones would measure an additional 30Å if they were to assume a globular conformation (see **Goodenough** and **Levine**, 1974). As the DNA associates with the histone, a large portion of the DNA's PO_4^- groups are neutralized. The association of histone with DNA is found to confer on the DNA a number of distinct physical properties: for example, the DNA becomes stabilized against heat denaturation and protected from radiation damage.

The size coincidence in between the 30Å thick nucleoprotein microfibrils of euchromatin and 30Å thick artificially synthesized nucleohistone fibres, has led many investigators to envisage an unreplicated chromosome as consisting of a single, extremely long DNA duplex with associated proteins. This is termed an **unineine** or **unistranded model** of chromosome structure (Fig. 19.6); **neme** means strand and strand in this case refers to DNA duplex and not a polynucleotide chain.

The unineme model of chromosome structure was first of all proposed by **Dupraw** in 1965 and it was termed as "**folded fibre model**". According to it, the bulk of the chromosome is visualized to composed of a tightly folded fibre which has a rather homogeneous diameter of 200 to 300Å. This folded fibre is supposed to contain the DNA histone helix (of 30Å diameter) in a supercoiled condition (Fig. 19.6). In the folded fibre model of **Dupraw**, the body of the chromatid of classical cytology is represented by a single-DNA-protein fibre, first coiled to form the 250 to 300Å fibre, and then folded back longitudinally and transversely. The folded fibre model applies to both the interphase and the metaphase chromosomes (Fig. 19.7). In the later case, however, it is thought that the two sister chromatids are held at the centomere until anaphase by an unreplicatcd fibre segment of DNA. Figure 19.6A has shown the method, by which a 30Å nucleoprotein fibre (DNA duplex + proteins) folds back on itself or super coils around itself to produce a fibre, of 80Å diameter. Further intertwinings between two lengths of 80Å fibres in turn could produce the 250Å fibres found in stained heterochromatin.

The alternate models of chromosome structure called **multineme** or **multistranded models** visualize the chromosome quite differently. They propose that a replicated chromosome contains two (or several) enormous DNA duplexes with associated proteins, each of which contains identical genetic informations (Fig. 19.6 B). Thus, while the genes H, L, I, J, and K (in Fig. 19.6) appear once in a unineme chromosome, they would each appear twice in the multineme chromosome. In multineme chromosomes the 80 and 250Å fibres would, not necessarily represent the infoldings of a single 30Å fibre; more likely they would represent two or more independent fibres interacting with one another.

Present biochemical and cytological data suggest that genes can be present in the single copies and an eukaryotic chromosome is composed of a single highly folded DNA-protein fibre (see **Dupraw**, 1968; **Goodenough** and **Levine**, 1974; **De Robertis**' *et at.*, 1975). Further, some of the evidence for the folded fibre model with a single DNA molecule per chromosomes stems from the discovery of extremely long segments of DNA in the interphase nucleus. For example, in sea urchin sperm, molecules 50 to 90 μm were observed under the electron microscope (**Solari**, 1965), and continuous DNA molecules 1 to 22 mm long have been detected in various mammalian nuclei by radioautography (**Sasaki** and **Norman**, 1966).

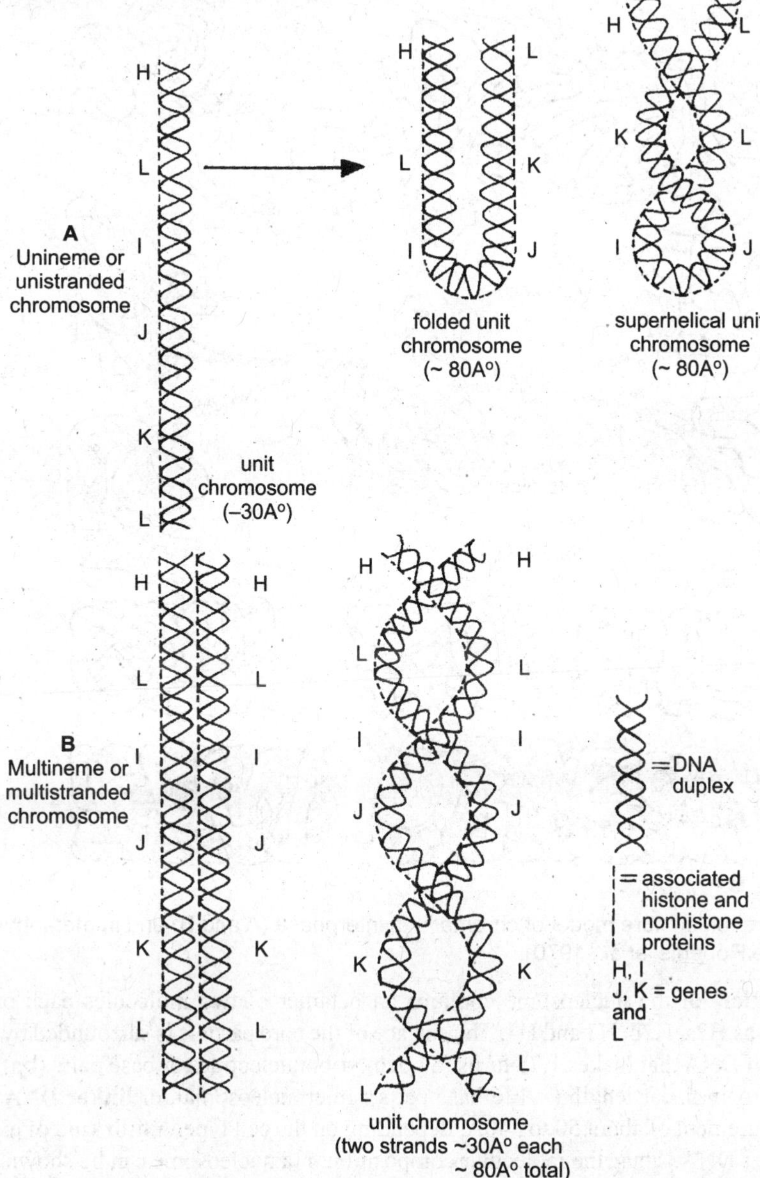

Fig. 19.6. Diagram contrasting A—Unineme and B—Multineme models of the unreplicated unit chromosome indicating how each model envisages the formation of 80Å fibres.

Nucleosomes

The DNA double helix, which runs the length of the eukaryotic chromosome, is coiled around into a bead structure called ν **(nu) bodies**, **PS particles**, or **nucleosomes**. The current popular name **nucleosome** was suggested by **Oudet** and colleagues in 1975. Both X-ray diffraction and neutron scatter studies of the nucleosomes have suggested that each nucleosome is a disc-shaped particle with approximate measurements of 110Å (diameter) by 55 to 57Å (height), containing tightly coiled DNA around it (see **Bradbury** *et al.*, 1981). Each nucleosome is found to consists of a core particle and linker DNA.

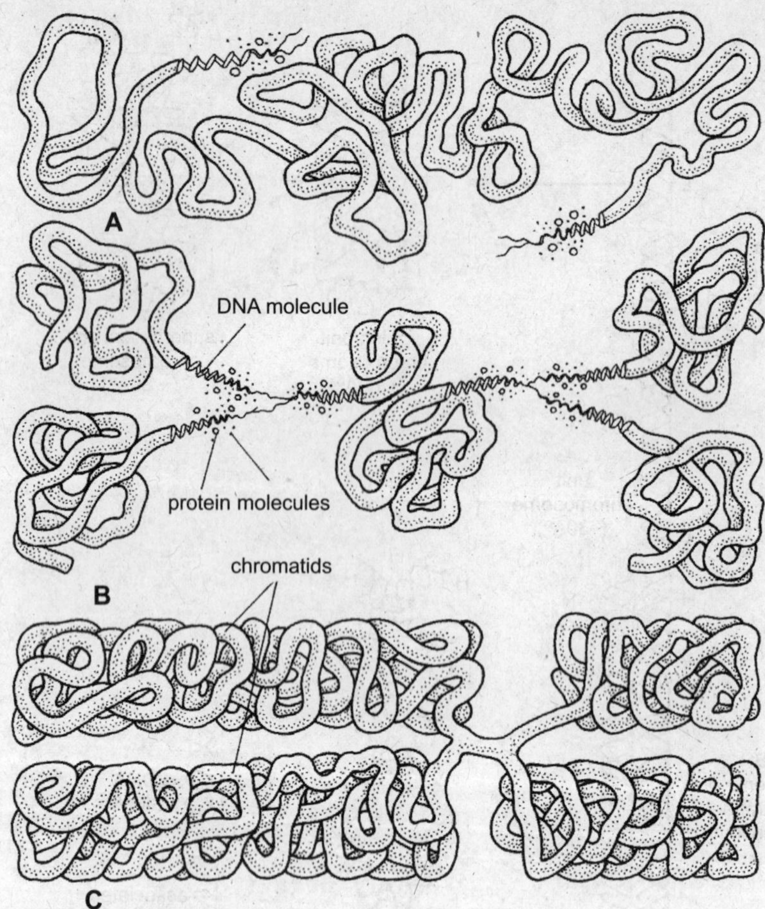

Fig. 19.7. Dupraw's folded fibre model of chromatin in interphase (A and B) and in metaphase (C) (after De Robertis' *et al.*, 1970).

The **core particle** of the nucleosome contains an octamer of two molecules each of four histones, designated as H2a, H2b, H3 and H4. The surface of the core particle is surrounded by a flat, superhelical strand of DNA that makes 1.75 turns (84 deoxyribonucleotides or base pairs (bp) each) and totals about 476Å in linear length (= 146 base pairs). Internucleosomal, or **linker DNA** has a variable linear measurement of about 50 to 340Å, depending on the cell type. A fifth kind of histone, H1, is bound to linker DNA. Thus, the molecular composition of a nucleosome can be shown in the form of the following equation (**Bradbury** *et al.*, 1981):

$$\text{Nucleosome} = \underbrace{\text{146 bp DNA} + 2\,(\text{H2a, H2b, H3, H4})}_{\text{Core particle}} + \text{Linker DNA} + \text{H1}$$

Recent investigations have suggested the occurrence of the follwoing DNA-histone arrangement in the nucleosome: two turns of DNA with 84 bp of DNA per turn and involves a histone core of the tetramer $(H3, H4)_2$ and the apolar regions of H2a and H2b. H1 is bound to the edge of the disc across the two turns of DNA and completes the 168 bp particle. The variable N-terminal regions of H2a and H2b and the variable N- and C-terminal regions of H1 are thought to act outside of this conserved structural unit. H1 is found to involve in higher order chromatin structures. H1 molecule seals off two turns of the DNA coil around the histone octamer of the conserved core particle structure (**Bradbury** *et al.*, 1981). H1 is reported to be phosphorylated just before mitotic and meitotic cell divisions to make possible the higher levels of coiling (see **Mays**, 1981).

The packaging of the eukaryotic DNA is based on the nucleosomes. During the cell cycle (G_1, S, G_2, M) nucleosomes are the smallest packaging units at all times. During the interphase (G_1, S, and G_2) gene expression may require association of nonhistone proteins with the genes, modifying and loosening the histone—DNA interactions of the nucleosomes. During mitosis or meiosis, the prophase is the stage during which the chromosomes become shorter and thicker due to multiple coiling as proposed by **Du Praw** and others. The hypothesis of a solenoidal structure, with coils of coils had renaissance since nucleosomal substructure has been discovered. Recall that nucleosomes already have two layers of coiling: (1) the double helix, and (2) the helical wrapping of the double helix: around the histone bead. A string of nucleosomes with each internucleosomal DNA bridge interacting maximally with its neighbouring histones, is thought to form a 100Å **unit fibre**. This fibre may then be coiled and that coil may be coiled again. Coiling proceeds for approximately seven levels, resulting in about a 500-fold shortening. The nucleosomes remain the basis of all this structure, it is not disrupted or distorted (**Mays**, 1981).

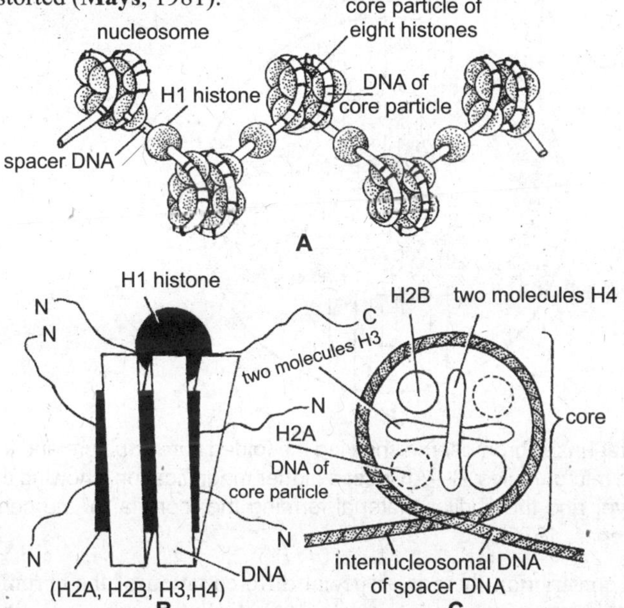

Fig. 19.8. A—A part of chromatin showing five nucleosomes; B—Ultrastructure of a nucleosome; C—Mode of arrangement of histone proteins in a nucleosome (after **Burns**, 1980).

During the process of prophase coiling, the chromatin attains a beaded appearance on a much larger scale than nucleosomes. These beads are visible through a light microscope. Since these beads stain very darkly, they were named **chromosomeres**.

A nucleosomal unit is not big enough to contain a gene. Since an average gene is around 1000 base pairs long, it should be packaged into five nucleosomes. During the transcription, the nucleosome structure is changed but not disrupted.

Ultrastructure of Primary Constriction and Centromeres

The primary constriction is a region in which there is a narrowing of chromosome, causing a division of the chromosomes into two arms. The primary constriction shows a faintly positive Feulgen reaction, indicating that there is DNA extending through it (**Kezer** and **MacGregor**, 1971).

The presence of DNA of the repititive type has been also demonstrated by hybridization experiments (see Chapter 21) constituting the so called **centromeric heterochromatin** (**MacGregor** and **Kezer**, 1971). Electron microscopy also demonstrated the passage of nucleoprotein fibres from one arm of the chromatid to the other. Five to seven fibres have been observed to pass through it (Fig. 19.9A) (**Dupraw**, 1968).

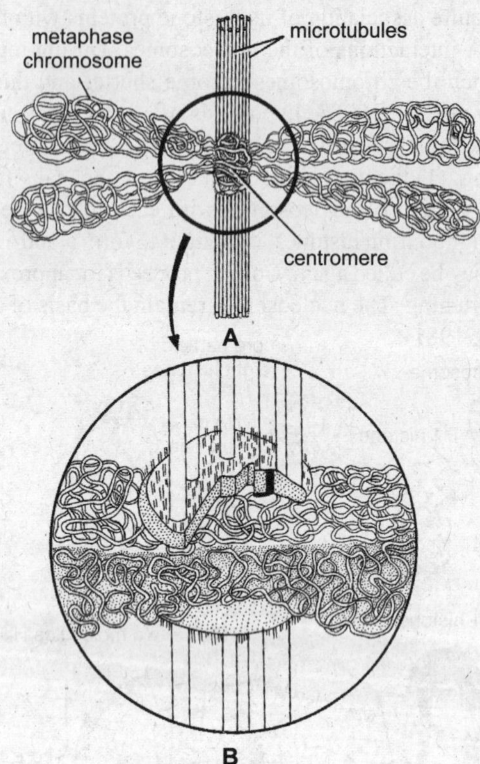

Fig. 19.9. A—A metaphase chromosome showing the folded fibre structure and the centromere with implanted microtubules; B—An inset a higher magnification, showing the convex electron dense layer and the fibrillar material forming the "corona" of the centromere (after De Robertis *et al.*, 1975).

In the primary constriction there is a special differentiation of the chromosome, called the centromere or kinetochore. The centromere is the site of implantation of the microtubules that constitute the chromosomal spindle fibres, for this reason it has been considered as functionally related to the chromosomal movements during mitosis. Usually two kinetochores, one in each chromatid, are observed. Under the electron microscope the centromere appears as a plate or cup-like disc, 0.20 to 0.25 μm in diameter, plastered upon the primary constriction. In cross-section it usually consists of an electrone dense layer 300 to 400Å thick and having a convex outer surface (Fig. 19.9B). Between this layer and the underlying chromatin fibres there is a less dense zone 150 to 300Å thick. On the convex side there is a fibrillar material which forms a kind of electrone dense "**corona**" (**Bajer**, 1968).

The exact chemical nature of the centromere is unknown, although it is thought. that it represents a non-chromatin material added to the surface of the primary constriction. **Luykx** (1970) has suggested that the kinetochore is a gene product and that it's activity is genetically controlled.

Functions of centromere. The main function of centromere related to attachment of the chromosomal microtubules. A related function may be to serve as nucleation centres for the polymerization of tubulin, the microtubular protein (**Dietz**, 1972).

19.6 THE FOLDED CHROMOSOME OF *E. COLI*

The 1300 μm-long circular DNA molecule is packed into a nucleoid region only 1 μm in diameter in *E. coli*. How is folding of chromosome accomplished? The answer to this question has been sought by **A. Worcel** and others (1974). The interaction that lead to folding must involve only DNA duplex itself since there is no nuclear membrane to provide additional packaging constraints in prokaryotic cells such as *E. coli*.

The chemical analysis of the isolated intact nucleoid shows that on a weight basis, there is about 30% RNA, about 1% protein (mainly RNA polymerase) and between 60 to 70% DNA. There are evidences which indicate that RNA is responsible for stabilizing the condensed state of DNA and continued RNA synthesis is required to maintain DNA in its folded configuration in the living cell.

These observations implies that the folding of *E. coli* DNA molecule must keep all genes exposed for transcription and not masked by tangles of DNA helix. **D. Pettijohn** and **R. Hecht** (1973) have proposed a model for the folded chromosome of *E. coli* that would lead to a structure about 30 μm in diameter after folding and 1–2 μm in diameter if the folded regions are super coiled (Fig. 19.10). Genes are accessible for transcription in this model and the calculated size of the molecule corresponds to known nucleoid diameter in the cell. Folding and supercoiling apparently occur by independent means because it is possible to relax supercoils without unfolding and to unfold molecules partially without changing the supercoils.

The exact chemical nature of RNA involved in folding of *E. coli* chromosome is not yet known. However, it is fairly clear that proteins do not serve as stabilizing agents for chromosome condensation in *E. coli* since RNA polymerase is virtually the only kind of protein isolated from nucleoids and it has no structural function. In this sense, prokaryotic DNA packaging is very different from packaging mechanisms in eukaryotic chromosomes in which histones complex with DNA to stabilize the structure and contribute its condensation (**Avers**, 1976).

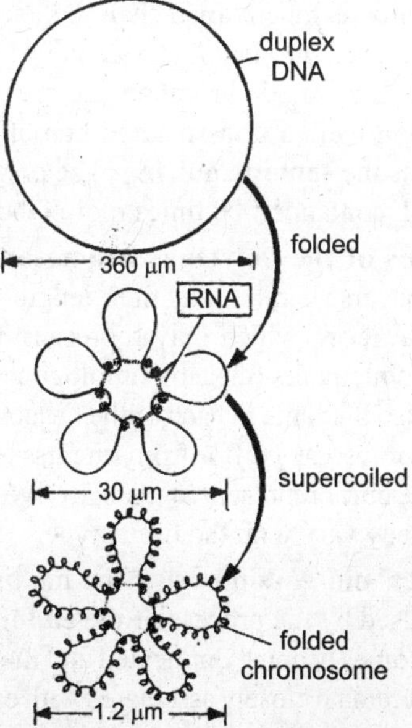

Fig. 19.10. Pettijohn and Hecht model of the folded chromosome of *E. coli*. The circular DNA is folded into a more compact arrangement that is stabilized by bound RNA molecules. Further compaction is achieved through supercoiling of the major DNA folded regions themselves (after Avers, 1976).

19.7 GIANT CHROMOSOMES

Some cells at certain particular stages contain large nuclei with giant or large-sized chromosomes. The giant chromosomes are the **polytene** and **lampbrush** chromosomes.

1. Polytene Chromosomes

The polytene chromosomes occur in the tissues of the salivary glands, gut, trachea, fat body cells and Malpighian tubules of many insects of the order Diptera. The polytene chromosomes were first of all reported by **E.G. Balbiani** in 1881 and the name **polytene** was suggested by **Kollar** due to occurrence of many chromonemae in them. Various cytologists such as **Carnoy**, **Alverdes**, **Costoff**, **Painter**, **Heitz**, **Baner** and **Bridges** have investigated the cytogenetical importance of the polytene chromosomes.

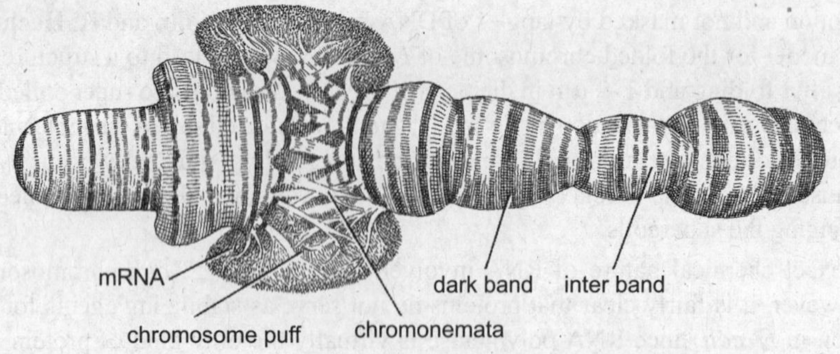

Fig. 19.11. Polytene chromosome of an insect.

The polytene chromosomes are larger in size in comparison to other somatic chromosomes. For instance, the four stranded polytene chromosomes of the *Drosophila melanogaster* have the total length about 200 μm which is much larger than the length 7.5 μm of a somatic chromosome. This enormous size of the polytene chromosome is achieved by the duplication of the chromonema for nine or ten times and the duplicated chromonemae are not separated. Moreover, the polytene chromosomes consist of closely coiled or associated homologous pairs of the chromosomes. This sort of association is known as the **somatic pairing**. The polytene chromosomes are the permanent prophase chromosomes which contain 1,000 times more DNA than the somatic chromosomes.

Bands and inter-bands of the polytene chromosomes. The polytene chromosomes bear alternating dark and light transverse bands along their length. There is a total of about 5,000 of these dark bands, called **chromosomeres**, which may represent individual genetic loci. The pattern of banding is identical in the two members of each homologous pair, but different from one pair to the next. The banding pattern is also the same in each of the tissues in which these polytene chromosomes are visible. However, the chromosomes differ from one tissue to the next in the pattern of localized uncoiling called **puffs**. Since, puffs represent areas of active gene transcription, so puffing pattern, but not the banding pattern, may vary with the tissue type.

Polytene chromosomes and endomitosis. The multistranded or polytenic structure of the polytene chromosomes is caused by the process of the **endomitosis** or **endoploidy**. In endomitosis chromonemae of the chromosomes become duplicated and the resulted chromonemae do not separate to form new chromosomes but remain closely associated with each other. In the process of endomitosis, the nuclear membrane does not rupture and no spindle formation takes place.

Puffs and Balbiani rings of the polytene chromosome. During certain developmental stages the polytene chromosomes of the larvae of certain dipterous insects develop swellings at a particular point of the dark band or the interband. Such chromosomal swellings are known as the **chromosome puffs** or **bulbs**. The process of puff formation is cyclic and is controlled by certain specific genes. The puffs are related with synthesis of RNA and proteins. **Edstrom** (1962) found that the chromosomal RNA differs from the nucleolar and cytoplasmic RNA and even the RNA of different puffs differ from each other in chemical composition. The process of puffing involves several processes such as the accumulation of acidic proteins, despiralization of DNA, synthesis of mRNA and storage of newly synthesized mRNA in the chromosomes.

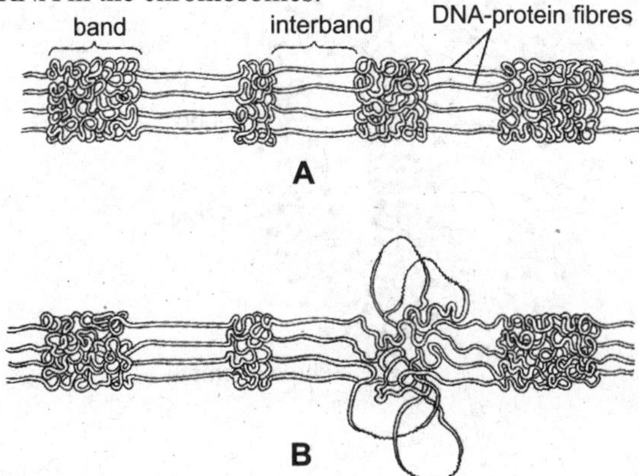

Fig. 19.12. A—Model of Dupraw and Rae showing band and interband structure in giant chromosome. B—The same model showing a possible method of "puffing" in one of the bands.

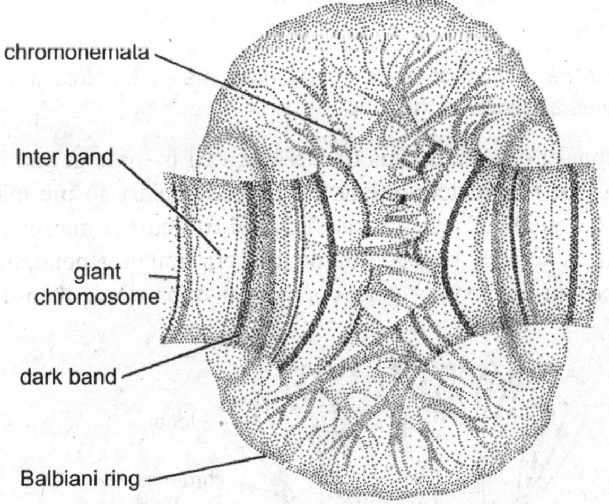

Fig. 19.13. Structure of a chromosome puff.

The chromonema of the polytene chromosomes gives out many series of the loops laterally. These rings are known as the **Balbiani ring** and they are rich in DNA and mRNA. The formation and function of the Balbiani rings are similar to the chromosomal puffs.

2. Lampbrush Chromosomes

In diplotene stage of the meiosis, the yolk rich oocytes of many vertebrates such as fishes, amphibians, reptiles and birds contain exceptionally large-sized chromosomes known as the **lampbrush chromosomes**. The lampbrush chromosomes were discovered by **Ruckert** in 1892.

The lampbrush chromosomes are much larger than the polytene chromosomes. The length of the lampbrush chromosomes of certain urodele oocytes may reach upto 5900 μm or three times longer than the polytene chromosomes. The lampbrush chromosomes are composed of the **main axis** and the **lateral loops**. The main axis is composed of four chromatids or two bivalent chromosomes. The chromonema of these chromatids gives out fine loops at the lateral sides giving the appearance of lampbrush or test tube brush. The chromosomes develop their lampbrush appearance when RNA synthesis is intense.

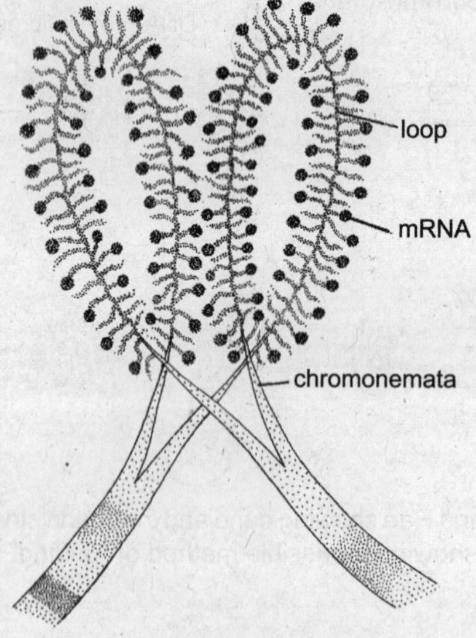

Fig. 19.14. Suggested form of the individual loops in chromosome puffs. Note the tiny fibrils with dense RNA granules attached to the loop.

Each loop appears to consist of a main axis of DNA coated by protein and RNA. Electron micrographs reveal fine fibrils of ribonucleoproteins set perpendiculary to the main loop. RNA synthesis seems to occur at the point of attachment of the fibril and the main axis of the loop. Presumably, **RNA polymerase** is actively engaged in the transcription of genetic, information into RNA. The fibril lengthens until all the gene or gene complex is transcribed; then it drops off into the cell fluids.

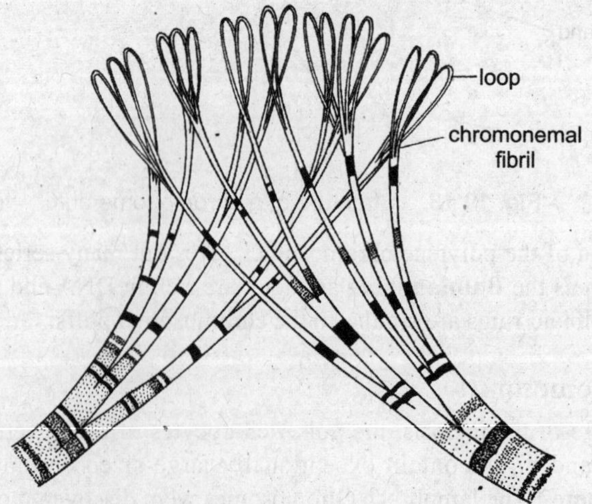

Fig. 19.15. A chromonemal loop of chromosome puff.

Further, there is evidence that the chromosome loop continuously spins out from the main chromosome axis at one of its ends, while it recoils into the chromosome at the other end. Thus a given gene would be available for transcription for only prescribed times before being incorporated into the rest of the chromosome structure. This intense period of transcription lasts for many days in some animals; then the RNA material is given off and loop collapses into the main body of the chromosome. Most of the RNA formed in the oocyte is used to form ribosomes (*i.e.*, it is rRNA). In addition, some mRNA is synthesized. This mRNA is stored in the cytoplasm and is used later in embryogenesis (*i.e.*, cleavage).

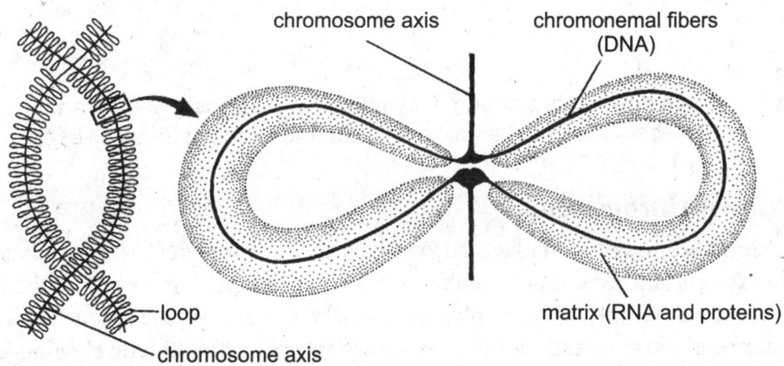

Fig. 19.16. Lampbrush chromosomes. A—At low magnification; B—Loop magnified.

3. B-chromosomes

Many plants (maize, etc.) and animals (such as insects and small mammals), besides having autosomes (A-chromosomes) and sex-chromosomes possess a special category of chromosomes called **B-chromosomes** without obvious genetic function. About 600 species of flowering plants and more than 100 animal species are now known to carry such B-chromosomes (**Jones**, 1975). These B-chromosomes (also called supernumerary chromosomes, accessory fragments, etc.) usually have a normal structure, are somewhat smaller than the autosomes and can be predominantly heterochromatic (many insects, maize, etc.) or predominantly euchromatic (rye). In maize, their number per cell can vary from 0 to 30 and they adversely affect development and fertility only when occur in large amount. In animals, the B-chromosomes disappear from the non-reproductive (somatic) tissue and are maintained only in the cell-lines that lead to the reproductive organs. B-chromosomes have negative consequences for the organism, as they have deleterious effect because of abnormal crossing over during the meiosis of animals and abnormal nuclear divisions of the gametophyte plants. In animals, B-chromosomes occur more frequently in females and the basis is non-disjunction. The non-disjunction of B-chromosomes of rye plant is found to be caused due to the presence of a heterochromatic knob at the end of long arm of B-chromosome.

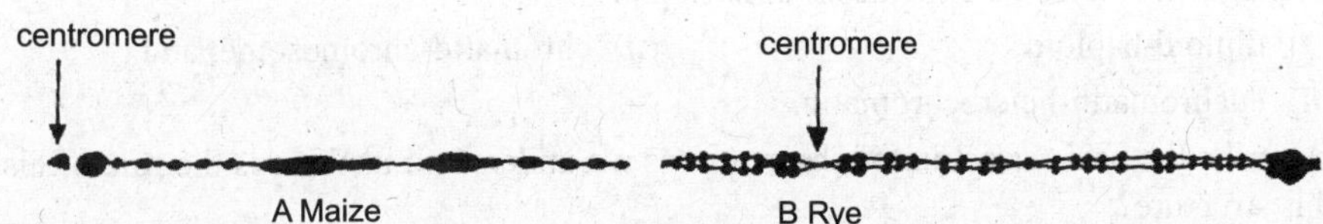

Fig. 19.17. B-chromosomes of maize (A) and rye (B) at pachytene (after Sybenga, 1972).

The origin of the B-chromosomes is uncertain. In some animals they may be derivatives of sex chromosomes, but this is not the rule. They generally do not show any pairing affinity with the

A-chromosomes. **Gibson** and **Hewitt** (1970) found the base composition of the DNA of B-chromosomes of the grasshopper *Myrmeleotettix* to be different from that of the A-chromosomes. According to **Sybenga** (1972) B-chromosomes are stabilized remanants of interspecific hybridization with a non-disjunction system restricted to critical stages whose accumulation instead of elimination results.

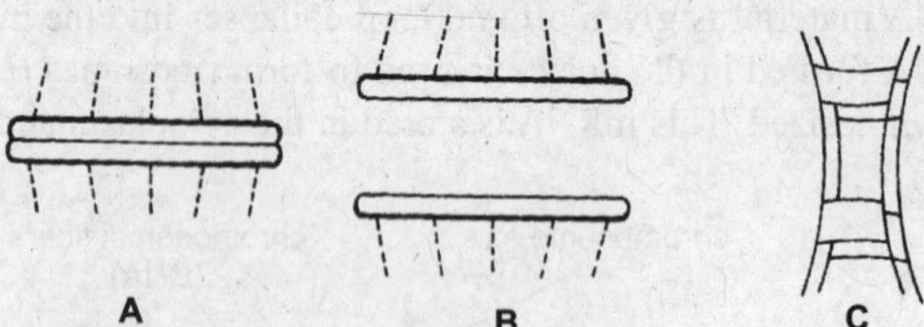

Fig. 19.18. A—Holokinetic chromosome at mitotic metaphase; B—At anaphase; C—Meiotic metaphase I bivalent of a holokinetic chromosome pair (after Sybenga, 1972).

4. Holokinetic Chromosomes

The chromosomes of most plants and animals have centromeres that are situated at one specific position in each chromosomes. In a number of animals, especially in insects of the order Hemiptera and a few, mostly monocotyledonous plants (*Juncales*, *Cyperales*), the kinetic activity is distributed over the entire chromosome and such chromosomes are called **holokinetic chromosomes (Sybenga,** 1972). The term diffuse centromere has been used as an alternative but is not quite logical. In 1966 **Flach** observed this type of centromere in some primitive dicotyledons (Ranales: *Myristica*). *Ascaris* and pseudoscorpion *Tityus* also possess such polycentric chromosomes.

In mitotic metaphase, the chromatids of a holokinetic chromosome orient parallel in the equator: one chromatid towards one pole the other towards the other pole (Fig. 19.18A). This is also the way they separate in anaphase (Fig. 19.18B) and they maintain this orientation until they arrive at the poles. Probably kinetic activity starts at one point and proceed from there on, orienting each unit to the preceding one.

19.8 CYTOGENETICAL FUNCTIONS OF CHROMOSOMES

The chromosomes are the most significant components of the cell. They control most of the cell biological and genetical activities of a species. They contain the genetical material, the DNA which ultimately influences all the biological phenomena at molecular, physiological and gross morphological levels. In the forthcoming chapters an attempt shall be made to describe the cytological, molecular biological and genetical role of chromosomes.

REVISION QUESTIONS

1. Give an account of the morphology, ultrastructure and chemistry of the chromosomes.
2. Distinguish between the members of each pair:
   (*i*) diploid-haploid; (*ii*) chromatid-chromosome; and
   (*iii*) euchromatin-heterochromatin.
3. Describe the basic structure of chromatin as we understand it. What is the role of histones in this structure?
4. Describe the structure of the prokaryotic chromosome.
5. Write short notes on the following: Chromosomal proteins; nucleosome; B-chromosomes; polytene chromosome; and lampbrush chromosomes.
6. Why the study of the chromosome. has become very significant in the field of biology?

20 Chapter CHROMOSOMAL VARIATIONS

The chromosomes of each species has a characteristic morphology (structure) and number. But, sometimes due to certain accidents or irregularities at the time of cell division, crossing over or fertilization some alterations in the morphology and number of chromosomes is manifested phenotypically and is of great genetical interest. We can study both types of variations separately under the following headings:

A. Variation in chromosome number,

B. Variation in chromosome morphology.

20.1 VARIATION IN CHROMOSOME NUMBER

Each species has a characteristic number of chromosomes in the nuclei of its gametes and somatic cells. The gametic chromosome number constitutes a basic set of chromosome called **genome**. A gamete cell contains single genome and is called **haploid**. When haploid gametes of both sexes (male and female) unite in the process of fertilization a **diploid** zygote with two genomes is formed. The diploid zygote undergoes embryological development and forms an adult animal which upon attaining sexual maturity produce haploid gametes. And this alteration of generation continues between haploidic and diploidic generation in most species. But sometimes the size of haploidic or diploidic genome or number of chromosome in a haploid or diploid cell does not remain constant (same) but alters variously. Variation in number of sets of chromosomes (*ploidy*) is commonly encountered in nature and may be of the following two types:

1. Euploidy,
2. Aneuploidy.

1. Euploidy

The term **euploidy** (Gr., *eu* = even or true; *ploid* = unit) designates genomes containing whole sets of chromosomes. The euploids are those organisms which contain balanced set or sets of chromosomes in any number. The euploids may be of the following types:

(i) Monoploid. The monoploid organisms have one set of chromosomes or one genome (n) in the nuclei of their body cells. The monoploid plants are often weak and sterile, *e.g.*, some algae, fungi, bryophytes, *Sorghum, Triticum, Hordeum, Datura* and hymenopteran insects such as wasps and bees.

Cytology of monoploids. In a monoploid or haploid set, the chromosomes are non-homologous and lack any homologue to pairwith, therefore, they are found as univalents at metaphase I of meiosis. During anaphase I, these univalents distribute at random. For instance, a haploid in maize (2n = 20) will have 10 chromosomes and the number of chromosomes in a gamete can range from 0 — 10. Consequently, considerable sterility will be found in a monoploid maize. Further, some gametes will contain complete haploid set of chromosomes, and thus, will act in a normal fashion.

(ii) Triploid. The triploid organisms have three sets of chromosomes or genomes (3n) in the nuclei of their body cells. A triploid may originate by the union of a monoploid gamete (n) with a diploid gamete (2n). The extra set of chromosomes of the triploid is distributed in various combinations to the germ cells resulting in the genetically unbalanced gametes. Triploids are usually sterile, *e.g.*, some cells of birds, reptiles, man and other vertebrates (**Ohno**, 1963, **Pennock**, 1965).

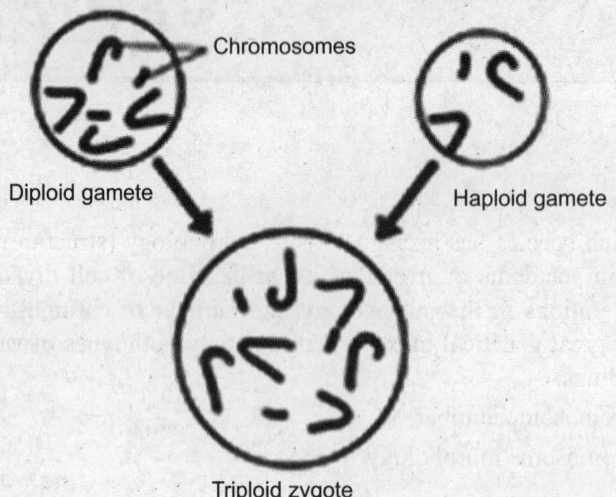

Fig. 20.1. Diagram showing the origin of a triploid (after SRB, Owen and Edger, 1965)

(iii) Tetraploid. The organisms with four genomes (4n) in the nuclei of their somatic cells are called tetraploids. The tetraploidy is arised by somatic doubling of the chromosome number. Doubling is accomplished either spontaneously or it can be included in high frequency by exposure to chemicals such as *cochicine*, *acenaphthene* and **veratrine** and also by exposure to heat or cold. *e.g.*, wheat, *Chrysanthemum*, Solanum, man (**Carr**, 1967), salamander, etc.

(iv) Polyploid. Any organism with more than two genomes (2n) is called a polyploid. Ploidy levels higher than tetraploid are not commonly encountered in natural populations, but our most important crops and ornamental flowers are polyploids, *e.g.*, wheat (hexaploid, 6n), strawberries (octaploid, 8n), many commercial fruits and ornamental plants, liver cells of man, etc.

Types of polyploids. The polyploids may be of the following two types:

(a) Autopolyploid. The autopolyploids are those polyploids, which consist of same basic set of chromosomes multiplied. For example, if a diploid species has two similar sets of chromosomes or genomes (AA), an autotriploid will have three similar genomes (AAA), and an autotetraploid will have four such genomes (AAAA). Since an autotriploid remains sterile and cannot produce seeds, therefore, it (autopolyploidy) has great commercial value in producing seedless varieties of economic plants. For example, in Japan, **H. Kihara** produced seedless watermelons, which were autotriploids; common 'doob' grass of U.P. and Bihar is an autotriploid. Other seedless autopolyploids are grapes, sugarbeet, banana, etc. Whenever autopolyploids, originate in nature, these would be eliminated due to natural selection. In *O. lamarckiana*, the giant mutant described by **de Vries** was later discovered as an autotetraploid.

Induced autopolyploidy. The autopolyploidy have been induced in many plant and animal cells by artificial means such as chemical (*e.g.*, chloral hydrate, colchicine, sulfanil amide, mercury chloride, hexachlorcyclohexane, etc.), radioactive substances, (*e.g.*, radium and X-ray) and temperature shocks. These inducers usually disturb the mitotic or meiotic spindle and cause non-segregation of already duplicated chromosomes, during cell divisions.

(b) Allopolyploids. When the polyploidy results due the doubling of chromosome number in a F_1 hybrid which is derived from two distinctly different species, then, it is called **allopolyploidy** and the resultant species is called an allopolyploid. Let A represent a set of chromosomes (genome) in species X, and let B represent another genome in a species Y. The F_1 hybrids of these species then would have one A genome and another B genome. The doubling of chromosomes in the F_1 hybrids will give rise to allotetraploids with two A and two B genomes (see Fig. 20.2)

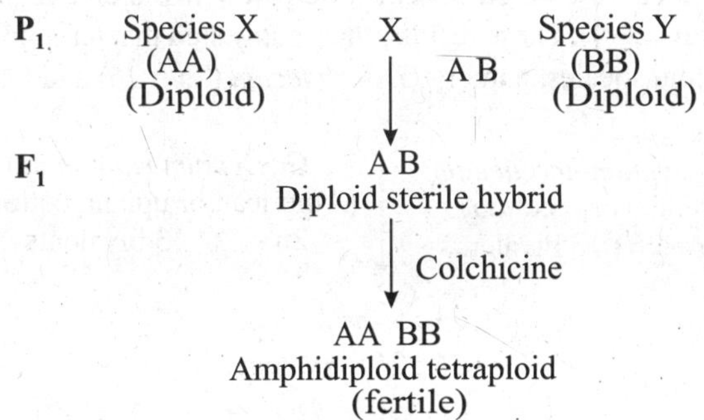

Fig. 20.2. Formation of allotetraploid.

Raphanobrassica is a classical example of allopolyploidy or amphipolyploidy. In 1927, a Russian geneticist, **G.D. Karpechenko** performed a cross between radish (*Raphanus sativum*, 2n = 18) and cabbage (*Brassica oleracea*, 2n = 18) and in F_1 got sterile (diploid) hybrids. Among these sterile F_1 hybrids, he found certain fertile plants which were found to contain 36 chromosomes. These fertile tetraploids were called *Raphanobrassica*.

Synthesized Allopolyploids

To find out the origin of naturally occurring allopolyploids some cytogeneticists produced certain allopolyploids in laboratory by employing artificial means. Common hexaploid wheat and tetraploid cotton furnish two such examples.

(i) *Triticum spelta*, is a hexaploid, wheat which was artificially synthesized in 1946 by **E. S. McFadden** and **E. R. Sears** and also by **H. Kihara**. They crossed an emmer wheat, *Triticum dicoccoides*, (tetraploid: 2n = 28) with goat grass, *Aegilops squarrosa* (diploid: 2n = 14) and doubled the chromosome number in the F_1 hybrids (Fig. 20.3). This artificially synthesized hexaploid wheat

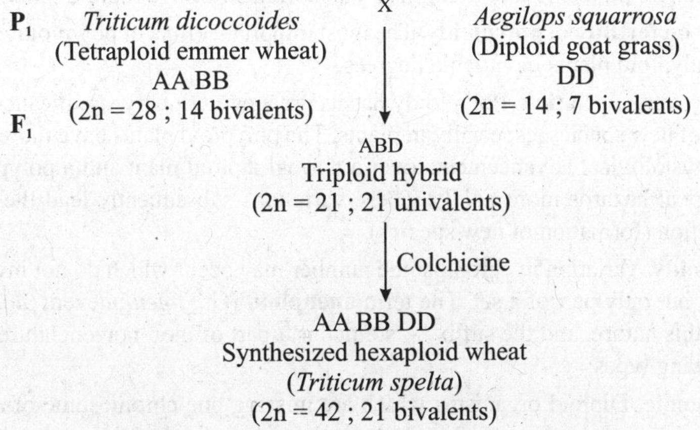

Fig. 20.3. Artificial synthesis of hexaploid wheat.

was found to be similar to the primitive wheat *T. spelta.* When the synthesized hexaploid wheat was crossed with naturally occurring *T. spelta*, the F_1 hybrid was completly fertile. This suggested that hexaploid wheat must have originated in the past due to natural hybridization between tetraploid wheat and goat grass followed by subsequent chromosome doubling.

(ii) *Gossypium hirsutum* the new world cotton plant, is another interesting example of allopolyploidy. Old world cotton *Gassypium herbaceum*, has 13 pairs of chromosomes, while, American or "upland cotton" also contains 13 pairs of chromosomes. *J.O. Beasley* crossed the Old world and American cottons and doubled, the chromosome number in the F_1 hybrids. The allopolyploids thus produced, resembled the cultivated New world cotton and when crossed with it gave fertile F_1 hybrids (Fig. 20.4). These results, thus, suggested that tetraploid *Gossypium hirsutum* originated from two diploid species, namely *G. herbaceum* (2n = 26) and G. *raimondii* (2n = 26).

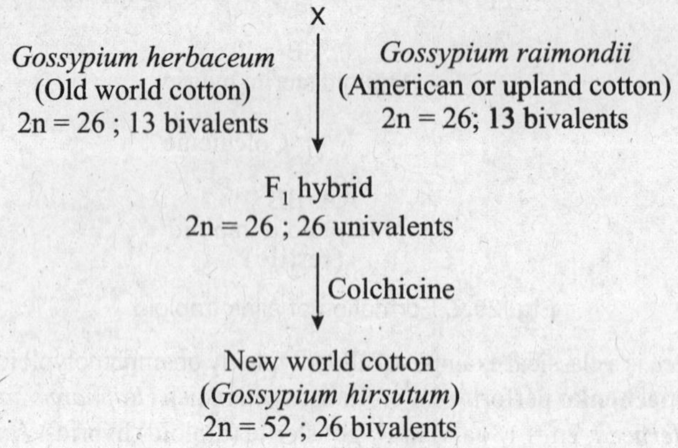

Fig. 20.4. Artificial synthesis of New world cotton.

Phenotypic Consequences of Polyploidy

The increase in the genome's size beyond the diploid level is often caused following detectable phenotypic characteristics in a polyploid organism:

(i) Morphological effect of polyploidy. The polyploidy is invariably related with **gigantism**. The polyploid plants have been found to contain large-sized pollen grains, cells, leaves, stomata, xylem, etc. The polyploid plants are more vigorous than diploids.

(ii) Physiological effect of polyploidy. The ascorbic acid content has been reported to be higher in tetraploid cabbages and tomatoes than in corresponding diploids. Likewise corn meal of a tetraploid maize seed contain 40 per cent more vitamin A than cornmeal from a diploid plant.

(iii) Effect on fertility of polyploidy. The most important effect of polyploidy is that it reduces the fertility of polyploid plants in variable degrees.

Polyploidy and speciation. Polyploidy has its great evolutionary significance, because it is a means of origin of new species, especially in plants. The polyploid plants have more morphological, genetical and physiological advancements over a normal diploid plant and a polyploid plant often faces the ecological hazards more boldly. These variations subsequently lead the polyploid plant toward specification (formation of new species).

2. Aneuploidy. Variation in chromosome number may occur which do not involve whole sets of chromosome, but only part of a set. The term **aneuploid** (Gr., *aneu*-uneven; *ploid*-unit) is given to variations of this nature, and the suffix "– somic" is a part of their nomenclature. The aneuploid may be of following types:

(*i*) Monosomic. Diploid organisms which are missing one chromosome of a single pair are monosomic with the genomic formula 2n – 1. A monosomic individual forms gametes of two types,

(n) and (2n – 1). The n – 1 gametes do not survive in plants, but, in animals that may cause genetic imbalance, which is manifested by high mortality or reduced fertility of resulted organism.

(ii) Nullisomic. An organism which has lost a chromosome pair is nullosomic. The nullosomic organism has the genomic formula (2n – 2). A nullisomic diploid often does not survive, however, a nullisonmic polyploid (*e.g.*, hexaploid wheat, 6X – 2) may survive but exhibit reduced vigour and fertility.

(iii) Trisomic. Diploids which have one extra chromosome are represented by the chromosomal formula 2n + 1. One of the pairs of chromosome has an extra number, so that a trivalent structure may be formed during meiotic prophase. If two chromosomes of the trivalent go to one pole and the third goes to the opposite pole, then gametes will be (n + 1) and (n), respectively. Trisomy can produce different phenotypes, depending upon which chromosome of the complement is present in the triplicate. In man, trisomy has very deleterious effect resulting in **Down's syndrome**, formerly called **mongolism**. A mongole person is mentally retarded, short in structure, exhibits characteristic abnormalities of palm prints and certain other malformations, especially of heart, ear, hands and feet. In them sexual maturity are rarely attained.

(iv) Double trisomic. In a diploid organism when two different chromosomes are represented in triplicate, the double trisomic is resulted. The double trisomic causes great genetic imbalance and has the genomic formula 2n + 1 + 1.

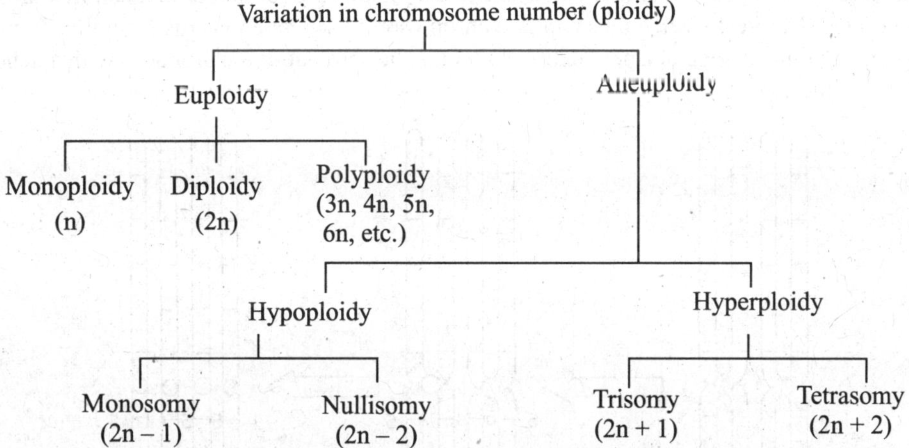

(v) Tetrasomic. The diploid organisms having two extra chromosomes are known as tetrasomic. They have the genomic formula 2n + 2. All the 21 possible tetrasomic are available in wheat.

Different types of ploidies have been summarized in the chart above.

20.2 VARIATION IN CHROMOSOME MORPHOLOGY OR CHROMOSOMAL ABERRATIONS

Chromosomes are structures with definite organization. They carry genes which remain arranged in them in linear order. In ordinary conditions, though the chromosomes remain unchangeable but under certain natural or artificial conditions some structural changes may occur in them. These structural changes are collectively called **chromosomal aberrations.**

Most chromosomal aberrations are caused due to accidental, natural, or induced breakage of chromosomes. The induced chromosome breakage may be caused by radiation, and chemicals such as Lysergic acid diethylamide LSD, etc. The chromosomal aberrations may remain confined to a single chromosome, or may extend to both of the member of a pair or may involve two or more pairs of chromosomes. The chromosomal aberrations, may be of following two kinds:

1. Intrachromosomal aberrations,

2. Interchromosomal aberrations.

1. Intrachromosomal Aberrations. The intrachromosomal or homosomal aberrations occur in one and the same chromosome and are of following kinds:

(i) Deficiency or deletion. When a chromosome lacks in a **intercalary** or **terminal** segment, the deficiency or deletion occurs. The lost chromosomal segment, if lacks in a centromere, lag in anaphasic movement and is lost from reorganizing nuclei. A loss of any considerable portion of chromosome is usually lethal to a diploid organism because of genetic imbalance, *e.g.*, maize, *Drosophila*, man, etc.

(ii) Duplication. Duplication occurs when a segment of the chromosome is represented two or more times in the chromosomes. The extra segment may be attached to the chromosome whose loci are repeated or to a different linkage group, or even be present as a separate fragment. The duplications of chromosomes are not deleterious to the organism like the deficiency and they usually protect the organism from the effect of a deleterious recessive gene or from otherwise lethal deletions. Moreover, the duplication is useful in the evolution of new genetic material and in altering the phenotype due to reallocation of chromosomal material (position effect), *e.g., Drosophila,* etc.

(iii) Inversion. An inversion is a chromosomal aberration in which a segment is inverted at 110 degree. Inversions are called **pericentric** when the segment includes the centromere and **paracentric** if the centromere is located outside the segment. When a crossing over occurs within inverted segment of a paracentric inversion, dicentric and acentric chromatids are formed. The dicentric chromatids form a bridge that breaks when the anaphase chromosomes separate towards the poles. If crossing over occurs within the loop of a pericentric inversion, the chromatids are produced with a deficiency and a duplication.

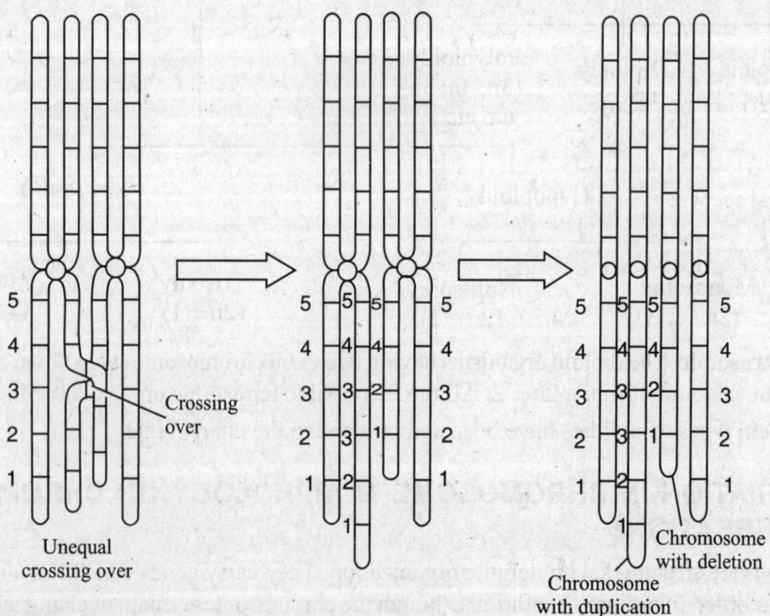

Fig. 20.5. Production of deletion and duplication in chromosomes due to unequal crossing over (after Sutton, 1965)

Isochromosomes. An isochromosome is a chromosome in which both arms are identical. It is thought to arise when a centromere divides in the wrong plane, yielding two daughter chromosomes, each of which carries the information of one arm only but present twice.

2. Interchromosomal Aberrations. When breaks occur in non-homologous chromosomes and resulting fragments are interchanged by both of the non-homologous chromosomes, the interchromosomal aberration occurs. The inter-chromosomal aberrations include following one type:

Translocation. Translocation involves the shifting of a part of one chromosome to another non-homologous chromosome. If two non-homologous chromosomes exchange parts, which need not be of same size, the result is a **reciprocal translocation**. The reciprocal translocation may be of following types.

(i) Homozygotic translocation. In homozygotic translocation normal meiosis occurs and that cannot be detected cytologically. Genetically they are marked by altered linkage groups and by the fact that a gene with "new neighbours" may produce a somewhat different effect in its new location.

(ii) Hetrozygotic translocation. In hetrozygotic translocation a considerable degree of meiotic irregularity occurs. Typically a cross-shaped formation is seen in prophase I; this often opens out into a ring as chiasmata terminalize. The heterozygous translocation produces semisterile organism because between half and two third of gametes (in animals) or meiospores (in plants) fail to receive the full complements of genes required for normal development of sex. The heterozygotic translocation is common in maize plant.

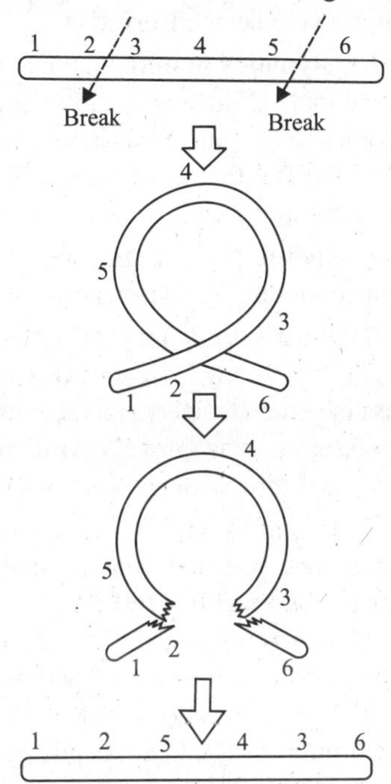

Fig. 20.6. Origin of an inversion in a chromosome (after Stansfield, 1969)

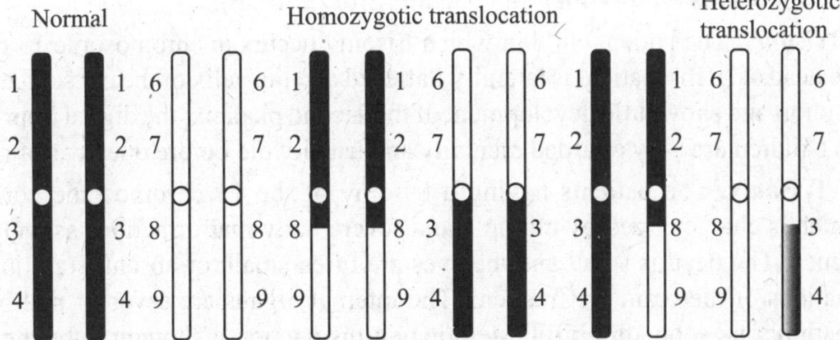

Fig. 20.7. Schematic representation of homozygotic and heterozygotic reciprocal translocation compared with the normal arrangement (after De Rebertis *et al.*, 1970).

20.3 HUMAN CYTOGENETICS : ABNORMAL HUMAN KARYOTYPES

The normal chromosome number of man is 46, but various types of chromosomal abnormalities either in their number or morphology have been observed. These chromosomal abnormalities are expressed in a defective phenotype *i.e.*, various defects occur in the morphology and physiology of an organism all of which cause different symptoms of a particular disease and called a *syndrome*. The chromosomal abnormalities can be studied under the following headings:

A. Autosomal Abnormalities

Following types of autosomal abnormalities have been recorded in man:

(a) Numerical autosomal aberrations. In man following kinds of autosomal numerical variations have been observed:

1. Polyploidy in man. In man some type of polyploidy are commonly encountered. A severely defective male child was found to be **triploid** with total of 69 chromosomes (66 autosomes + two X-chromosomes +one Y chromosome). Further, an extensive survey of human cytogenetics have revealed the fact that most human individuals are **mosaics**, have both diploid and triploid cells in skin and tetraploid cells in liver.

2. Aneuploidy in man. In man several kinds of autosomal aneuploidies have been reported. Certain commonly known trisomic and monosomic aneuploidies of man are following:

(i) Down's syndrome (21-Trisomy). One of the most familiar human aneuploidy is trisomy 21. Originally studied by **Langdon Down** in 1866, it had been termed **mongoloid idiocy** or **mongolism** because of certain facial characteristics that suggested resemblance to oriental features. The condition is now referred to as **Down's syndrome** which diplomatically removes the nuances of associating mental retardation with any particular group of people (*i.e.*, Mongols) (see **Pai,** 1974).

Down's syndrome is a congenital syndrome, usually recognizable at birth by an experienced physician, and one that is associated with multiple malformations (characteristic facial features, palmprint abnormalities, etc.; severe mental retardation and markedly defective development of the central nervous system. The face of such a patient has a special moon-like aspect, with oblique palpebral fissures, increased separation between the eyes, and a skin fold (epicanthus) at the inner part of the eyes. The nose is flattened, the ears are malformed; the mouth is constantly open; and the tounge protrudes. The heart, hands and feet too remain defective in a mongoloid.

The riddle of Down's syndrome was essentially solved when **J. Lejeune** and **R. Turpin** showed in 1959 that it is associated with an extra chromosome 21. Thus mongoloids have 47 chromosomes instead of 46, with three copies of chromosome 21 instead of the usual two (hence, Down's sydrome is also called trisomy 21). This chromosomal aberration originates from non-disjunction of pair 21 during meiosis (for details see **Bodmer** and **Cavalli-Sforza,** 1976).

(ii) 18-Trisomy. The patient child in which trisomy occurs in chromosome 18 remains small and weak. The head of such a patient is laterally flattened and the helix of the ear scarcely developed. The hands are short and show little development of the second phalanx; the digital imprints are rather simple. These children are very retarded mentally and usually **die before** one year of age.

(iii) 13-Trisomy. The patients having a trisomy of the **13 chromosome** contain **Patau's syndrome** which is characterized by multiple and severe body malformations as well as profound mental deficiency. The head is small and the eyes are often small, or absent. Harelip, cleft palate, and malformations of the brain are frequent. The internal organs are severely malformed, and in most cases death occurs soon after birth. Meiotic non-disjunction is thought to be the cause of this chromosomal aberration.

(iv) 21-Monosomy. When one chromosome of the pair of chromosome 21 become completely deleted 21-monosomy occurs and it remains lethal to the patient. But when large part of one 21 chromosome is lacking, children exhibit morphological characteristics, just opposite to mongolism or Down's syndrome. In 21-monosomics, the nose remains prominent, the distance between eyes is shorter than normal, the ears are large and the muscles are contracted.

(v) 18-Monosomy. This is the opposite syndrome in which a partial deletion of one chromosome of the pair occurs (**Grouchy** *et. al.,* 1966). The ears are voluminous, the fingers long, and the digital imprints are complex and convoluted.

(b) Structural autosomal aberrations. Cases carrying all kinds of structural aberrations have been reported in man. Translocations of several types, deletions, duplications, ring chromosomes, inversions, and isochromosomes have frequently been associated with congenital diseases. These chromosomal abnormalities appear sporadically in the general population, and they usually lead to characteristic phenotypic changes.

One of the most remarkable phenotypes associated with partial deletion of the short arm of chromosomes 5 is the condition called **catcry syndrome (Lejeune**, 1963) or **cri du chat syndrome (Lejune** *et al*., 1965). The affected baby has a strange mewing cry, multiple malformations and mental retardation. Another type of patient showing facial alternation, skeletal and ophthalmologic abnormalities, along with profound mental retardation is the carrier of a deletion of the long arm of chromosome 18.

B. Sex-Chromosomal Abnormalities

In man different kinds of sex-chromosomal numerical aberrations have been detected. Most of them are caused either by mitotic non-disjunctions or meiotic non-disjunctions. They are expressed phenotypically in the following different kinds of syndromes.

(1) Klinefelter syndrome. Persons with klinefelter syndrome or seminiferous tubule dysgenesis have been found to contain a positive sex chromatin and 47 chromosomes: 44 autosomes, two X-chromosomes and one Y-chromosome (44 autosomes+XXY). The patients with klinefelter syndrome in their puberty have male phenotype; small soft testes with excessive fibrous tissues; only Sertoli cells in the lining epithelium of seminiferous tubules; no spermatogenesis; high urinary excretion of pituitary follicle stimulating hormone (FSH) and low excretion of 17-ketosteroids. The patients of this syndrome also have **gynecomastia** (a tendency for formation of female-like enlarged breast), tendancy of tallness, obesity, long limbs, under developed genetalia, and sparse body hairs and idiocy.

(2) Turner's syndrome. The persons with the karyotype of 45 chromosomes (44 autosomes and one X-chromosome) have the symptoms of disease called female gonadal dysgenesis **Turner's syndrome**. Such persons have female phenotype, but with rudimentary gonads and without menstruation cycle during puberty. Further, a patient of Turner's syndrome is characterized by short stature, congenital malformations, shield chest, pronounced webbing of the neck, short fourth metacarpel, hypoblastic nails (nails are small, narrow and deep set in nail pit or square with increased lateral curvature), recessive X-linked conditions such as colour blindness and diabetes and usually impaired intelligence.

REVISION QUESTIONS

1. What is polyploidy? Describe different kinds of polyploidies and discuss their phenotypic effects.
2. Describe different types of euploidy and aneuploidy.
3. What is chromosomal aberration? Describe various types of chromosomal aberrations.
4. Write an essay on 'abnormal human karyotypes and their phenotypic effects.'
5. Write short notes on the following:

(*i*) Polyploidy; (*ii*) Down's syndrome;
(*iii*) Cat-cry syndrome; (*iv*) Turner's syndrome.

21 Chapter DEOXYRIBONUCLEIC ACID (DNA)

The deoxyribonucleic acid or DNA is the most important chemical compound of the living beings which carries hereditary informations from generation to generation of the cell or the entire organism as a whole. The DNA has attracted the attention of the modern biologists like the atom did for the chemists and physicists in the last century. Because DNA has been found associated with almost all biological activities, therefore, enormous investigations have been done and still are in process to understand more and more about the DNA. The DNA has occupied a central place in the cytology, genetics, molecular biology, microbiology, developmental biology, biochemistry and evolution.

21.1 HISTORICAL

The DNA molecule was first of all isolated by **F. Miescher** in 1869 from the pus cell, spermatozoa and from the nucleus of the red blood cells of the birds. But he could not recognize its exact chemical nature and named it as **'nuclein'. Fischer** in 1880's identified the pyrimidine and purines in the nucleic acids. **Kossel** demonstrated two pyrimidines (cytosine and thymine) and two purines (adenine and guanine) in it and got Nobel prize in 1910 for this discovery. **Levene,** a Russian born biochemist, recognized the 5 carbon ribose sugar in 1910 and later also discovered deoxyribose in nucleic acids. He also suggested the presence of phosphoric acid in the nucleic acid. **Robert Feulgen** in 1914 demonstrated a colour test known as **Feulgen reaction** for the DNA. **Avery, Macleod** and **Mc Carthy** in 1944 first of all demonstrated that DNA is directly involved in inheritance. The chemical study of DNA was made by **Chargaff** in 1947. He showed that DNA consists of equal proportions of the large purine bases and smaller pyrimidine and that adenine and thymine are present in equimolecular proportion and so are cytosine and guanine. In 1950 **Wilkins** and his co-workers by X-ray diffraction method found that in DNA molecule the purines and pyrimidines bases were placed at a distance of 3.4 A°. They also found that another regularity in structure occurred at repeating distance of 34 A° (*i.e.,* every 10 nucleotide units) and suggested that molecule was not linear but twisted into a helix, one complete turn occurring every 34 A°. **Pauling** and **Corey** in 1951 worked out α-helicle structure of fibrous proteins and later extended these ideas to the DNA molecule. In 1952 **A.D. Hershey** and **M. Chase** demonstrated that only the DNA of T_4 bacteriophage enters the host, the bacterium *Escherichia coli,* whereas the protein (*i.e.,* capsid) remains behind. They thus confirmed that DNA is the genetic material of most living organisms. In 1953 **Watson** and **Crick** constructed the double helix (duplex) model for the DNA molecule which could successfully demonstrate the various activities of the DNA molecule. **Kornberg** (1957) has proved the DNA double helix model of Watson and Crick by synthesizing the DNA molecule in the cell free system. In 1967 **Kornberg** synthesized a DNA molecule from the 6,000 nucleotides.

21.2 OCCURRENCE

Except a few viruses all the living organisms possess DNA. In the cell the greatest amount of DNA remains concentrated in the nucleus especially in the chromosomes. The DNA molecules also occur in the mitochondria, plastids and centrioles. In certain cases *e.g., Paramecium, Tetrahymena, Amoeba proteus,* amphibians and ferns, the DNA molecules occur in the cytoplasmic matrix.

21.3 DNA CONTENTS OF NUCLEUS

The amount of DNA is usually measured by the microunit of the weight known as the picogram. One picogram (1 Pg) is equal to 10^{-12} grams. The amount of DNA has been found to be constant from cell to cell and species (see Table 18.1). For instance, the DNA amount of various diploid cells of fowl has been measured as 2.5 picograms. Their sperms contain just half (approximately 1.25 pg) of the DNA amount of the diploid cell (see Table 18.3).

The DNA amount of a cell is also related to the ploidy or number of chromosomes of that cell. For instance, the tetraploid liver cell has been found to contain double amount of DNA than the other diploid cells (see Table 18.2). Among the invertebrates, the sponges and coelenterates contain the lowest amount of DNA. The amount of the DNA in general varies from species to species. Such variations may be less in the case of mammalian species or may be great in case of different species of the fishes, amphibians and birds. Among the amphibians, the DNA contents of the nucleus may vary from 1.68 pg in *Amphiuma* to 7.73 pg in the toad (for details see chapter 18).

21.4 MORPHOLOGY

Shape

The DNA molecule of the eukaryotic cells is thread-like, straight and unbranched in shape, while the DNA molecule of the prokaryotic cells, mitochondria and plastids has the circular shape.

Size

The size of DNA molecule varies from species to species. The DNA molecule of the mitochondria has been measured as 5 μm.

The viruses contain several microns long DNA molecule. The single DNA molecule of the bacteria has been measured as 1.4 mm long.

Because the eukaryotic cells contain comparatively large amount of the DNA so in them one straight DNA molecule cannot exist like the prokaryotic cells (viruses, bacteria, etc.) and the mitochondria, plastids, etc. Thus in these cells the DNA molecule is subdivided into several separate subunits each of which forms the chromosome of the classical cytology.

In eukaryotic cells, various sizes of the DNA molecule have been reported by different investigators. The DNA molecule of 50 to 60 μm long (**Solari**, 1965), 500 μm long (**Cairus**, 1966) and 1.6 to 1.8 mm long (**Huberman** and **Riggs,** 1966) have been measured in various eukaryotic cells.

Because one picogram of DNA has the molecule of 31 cm long, so by taking the weight of DNA amount in the nucleus the size of the DNA molecule can be calculated easily. By employing this method **Dupraw** and **Bahr** (1968) have calculated that the human diploid cells with the 5.6 pg DNA amount contain 174 cm long DNA molecule. Likewise they measured that the *Trillium* cells with 120 pg DNA contain 37 metres long DNA molecule and the polytenic chromosomes of the *Drosophila* with 293 pg DNA contents having 97 metres long DNA molecule.

21.5 CHEMICAL COMPOSITION OF DNA

The DNA is a complex macromolecular chemical compound which is composed of three kinds of molecules which are as follows:

1. A pentose sugar known as **deoxyribose**.
2. **A phosphoric acid**.
3. **Nitrogen bases**. The nitrogen containing organic compounds of the DNA are of two basic types, *viz.*, (*i*) **pyrimidines** and (*ii*) **purines**.

(*i*) **Pyrimidines**. The pyrimidines contain single ring of atoms in their molecules. The DNA contains only two pyrimidines, *e.g.*, **cytosine** and **thymine**. The chemical formulae of both have been shown in Fig. 21.2 and Fig. 21.3.

(*ii*) **Purines**. The purines are the organic compounds which contain two rings of atoms in their molecules. The DNA contains two purines, *e.g.*, **adenine** and **guanine** (Fig. 21.4 and 21.5).

Fig. 21.1. Chemical formula of deoxyribose.

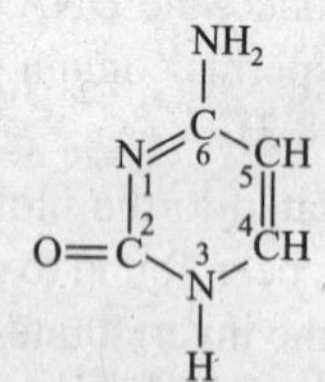

Fig. 21.2. Chemical formula of cytosine (2-hydroxy-6-aminopyrimidine, MW = 111.10 daltons).

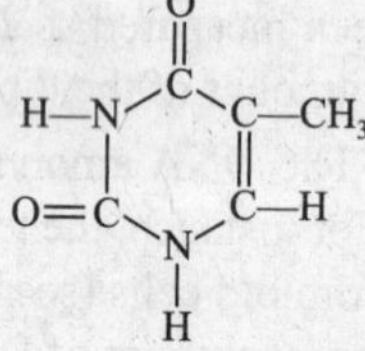

Fig. 21.3. Chemical formula of thymine (2.6-dihydroxy-5-methylpyrimidine, MW = 126.12 daltons).

Fig. 21.4. Chemical formula of adenine (6-aminopurine MW = 135.13 daltons).

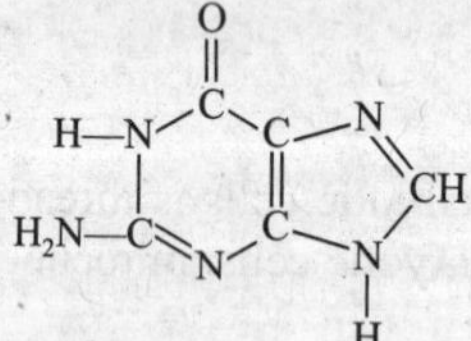

Fig. 21.5. Chemical formula of guanine (2-amino-6-hydroxypurine, MW = 151.13 daltons).

21.6 MOLECULAR STRUCTURE OF DNA

Purines (*i.e.*, adenine and guanine) and pyrimidines (*i.e.*, cytosine and thymine) can form chemical linkages with the pentose (5-carbon) sugar, the deoxyribose. The carbon atoms on the sugar are designated 1′, 2′, 3′, 4′ and 5′ and it is the 1′ carbon of the sugar that becomes bonded to the nitrogen atom in position 1 of pyrimidine or the nitrogen atom in position 9 of a purine. Such molecules are known as **nucleosides** or **deoxyribonucleosides** and they can serve as elementary precursors for DNA synthesis. But, before a nucleoside can become part of a DNA molecule it must become complexed with a phosphate group to form a **nucleotide** or **deoxyribonucleotide**. The four kinds of deoxyribonucleosides and deoxyribonucleotides have been tabulated in Table 21.1.

Nucleotides with a single phosphate group are known as nucleoside monophosphates, an example being adenine deoxyribonucleoside monophosphate or dAMP (Fig. 21.6). Nucleotides can also possess two or three phosphate groups (*i.e.*, ADP or ATP). It is the nucleoside triphosphates that serve directly as precursors for DNA synthesis. The triphosphates of four deoxyribonucleotides namely, deoxyadenosine triphosphate (dATP), deoxyguanosine triphosphate (dGTP), deoxycytidine triphosphate (dCTP) and thymidine triphosphate (TTP) are energy rich compounds which occur freely in nucleoplasm and cytoplasm. The significance of occurrence of deoxyribonucleotides in triphosphate forms lies in the fact that during DNA replication, the DNA polymerase enzyme can act only on triphosphates of deoxyribonucleotides.

DNA is simply a long polymer of nucleotides called **polynucleotides**. Only one phosphate group of each precursor nucleotide triphosphate is included in the polymer. This phosphate group, which is bonded to the 5′-carbon of the sugar (Fig. 21.6), becomes chemically bound to the 3′-carbon in the sugar of a second nucleotide, and so on, so that a long series of 5′—3′ **linkages** is found along the length of the polymer. The phosphate bonds are known as covalent ester bonds and are extremely strong. The phosphate residues (PO^-) along the chain are acidic.

Further, once a sugar-phosphate 'backbone' has been formed, the position of the purine and pyrimidine bases is quite rigidly fixed. Each base will be staked on top of the next, like a stack of pennies, with one base 3.4 A° away from its neighbour. Since purines and pyrimidines are essentially flat, two-dimensional structures, there is no stereochemical interference between the bases in a stack. Indeed, weak bonds form between the staked bases and add to the stability of the molecule.

Single-stranded polynucleotide chain of DNA has been adopted as the genetic material in certain viruses, but most prokaryotes and eukaryotes have made use of a double-stranded DNA molecule in their chromosomes. The detailed structure of double-stranded DNA has been worked out in the following way:

Table 21.1. Four nitrogen bases, nucleosides and nucleotides of DNA molecule.

Nitrogen base	**Base + deoxyribose = deoxyribonucleoside***	**Deoxyribonucleoside + phosphoric acid = deoxyribonucleotide**	**Abbreviation for nucleotide**
1. Adenine (A)	Deoxyadenosine	Deoxyadenylic acid (Deoxyadenosine monophosphate)	dAMP
2. Guanine (G)	Deoxyguanosine	Deoxyguanylic acid (Deoxyguanosine monophosphate)	dGMP
3. Cytosine (C)	Deoxycytidine	Deoxycytidylic acid (Deoxycytidine monophosphate)	dCMP
4. Thymine (T)	Thymidine	Thymidylic acid (Thymidine monophosphate)	TMP

* Note that the names for the pyrimidine nucleosides end with "— dine", whereas the purine nucleosides end with "— sine".

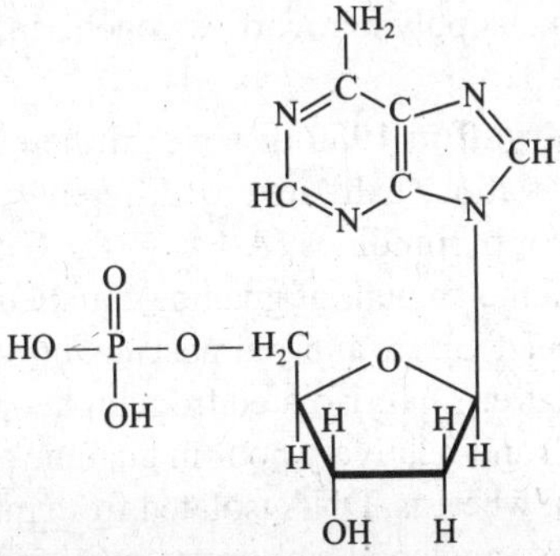

Fig. 21.6. A deoxynucleotide, deoxyadenosine 5′-monophosphate (deoxyadenylic acid; dAMP).

Molar Ratios of Nitrogen Bases in DNA Molecule

When many samples of DNA were isolated, purified and analysed by various techniques, such as paper chromatography, etc., it was found by **Hotchkiss** and **Chargaff** in 1948 that contrary to *Levene's* (1920's) *tetranucleotide theory* which considered DNA as a monotonous polymer having four DNA bases in approximately equal molar proportions, the four nucleotide bases are not necessarily present in DNA in exactly equal proportions. **Chargaff** reported that the DNA extracted from calf-thymus nuclei contains the four bases in the following molar proportions: 28% adenine, 24% guanine, 20%

cytosine and 28% thymine. When he analysed the DNA samples of varied animals, he found that the exact base composition of DNA differs according to its biological source. The relative amounts of purines and pyrimidines in samples of DNA of different living organisms have been tabulated in Table 21.2.

Table 21.2. Relative amounts of nitrogen bases in different samples of DNA (Chargaff and Davidson, 1955).

S.N.	Source	Adenine	Guanine	Cytosine	Thymine	$\frac{A+T}{G+C}$
1.	Beef sperm	28.7	22.2	22.0	72.2	1.26
2.	Human thymus	30.9	19.9	19.8	29.4	1.52
3.	Human liver	30.3	19.5	19.9	30.3	1.53
4.	Human sperm	30.7	19.3	18.8	31.2	1.62
5.	Hen red cells	28.8	20.5	21.5	29.2	1.38
6.	Rat bone marrow	28.6	21.4	21.5	28.4	1.33
7.	Herring sperm	27.8	22.2	22.6	27.5	1.23
8.	*Paracentrotus lividus* (sea urchin) sperm	32.8	17.7	18.4	32.1	1.85
9.	Salmon	29.7	20.8	20.4	29.1	1.43
10.	Wheat germ	26.5	23.5	23.0	27.0	1.19
11.	Yeast	31.3	18.7	17.1	32.9	1.79
12.	*Diplococcus pneumoniae*	29.8	20.5	18.0	31.6	1.59
13.	*K-12 Escherichia coli*	26.0	24.9	25.2	23.9	1.00
14.	*Mycobacterium tuberculosis*	15	34.9	35.4	14.6	0.42
15.	Bacteriophage T_2	32.5	18.2	16.7	32.6	1.86

These different values of A, G, C, and T in different samples of DNA are suggesting that DNA rather than being a monotonous polymer, carries genetic information in the form of specific nucleotide base sequences.

The equivalence rule. Chargaff in 1950 discovered the equivalence rule which suggested that despite wide compositional variations exhibited by different types of DNA, the total amount of purines equalled the total amount of pyrimidines (A + G = T + C); the amount of adenine equalled the amount of thymine (A = T) and the amount of guanine equalled the amount of cytosine (G = C). **Chargaff's** equivalence rule has been found to apply almost universally in different organisms (viruses, bacteria, plants and animals). However, DNA isolated from higher plants and animals was in general rich in adenine and thymine (A : T) and relatively poor in guanine and cytosine (G : C) (*e.g.*, AT/GC ratio of DNA of man was 1.40 : 1); whereas, DNA isolated from micro-organisms (viruses, bacteria and lower plants and animals) was in general rich in guanine and cytosine and relatively poor in adenine and thymine (*e.g.*, AT/GC ratio of DNA of *Mycobacterium tuberculosis* was 0.60 : 1). These differences in AT/GC ratios of micro-organisms and higher organisms undoubtedly reflect difference in genetic information carried by these hereditary molecules and also phylogenetic, evolutionary and taxonomical significance of them.

Geometrical Organization of DNA

The first person to give any thought to the three dimensional structure of DNA was **W. T. Astbury** who by his X-ray crystallographic studies of DNA molecule concluded in 1940's that because DNA has high density, so, its polynucleotide was a stack of flat nucleotides, each of which was oriented perpendicularly to the long axis of the molecule and was situated every 3.4 A° along the stack. The X-ray crystallographic studies of Astbury were continued by **Wilkins** and his associates who managed to prepare highly oriented DNA fibres that allowed them to obtain an X-ray diffraction photograph. One of his female associates **Rosalind Franklin** obtained a superior X-ray diffraction photograph of DNA which confirmed Astbury's earlier inference of 3.4 internucleotide distance and suggested helical configuration for DNA molecule. **Watson** and **Crick** who were already engaged in constructing some suitable model for DNA structure, when observed Franklin's picture of DNA molecule, they immediately utilized that information in constructing a molecular model for DNA. In April 1953, **Watson** and **Crick** published their conclusions about the structure of the DNA in the same issue of '**Nature**' in which **Wilkins** and his colleagues presented the X-ray evidence for that structure.

Considerations of Watson and Crick in the construction of double helical structure of DNA molecule. **Watson** and **Crick** concluded directly from the X-ray diffraction photograph of DNA taken by *Franklin* that (1) the DNA polynucleotide chain has the form of a regular helix, (2) the helix has a diameter of about 20 A° and, (3) the helix makes one complete turn every 34 A° along its length, and hence, since the internucleotide distance is 3.4 A°, consists a stack of ten nucleotides per turn. Considering the known density of the DNA molecule, **Watson** and **Crick** next concluded that the DNA helix is double-helical or *duplex* containing two polynucleotide chains, or two stacks of ten nucleotides each per turn, since the density of a cylinder 20 A° in diameter and 34 A° long would be too low if it contained but a single stack of ten, and too high if it contained three or more stacks of ten nucleotides each. Before trying to arrange these two polynucleotide chains into a regular helix of the required dimensions, however, **Watson** and **Crick** placed a further restriction on their model. A restriction that derived from their knowledge that DNA is, after all, the genetic material. If DNA is to contain hereditary information so they reasoned, and if that information is inscribed as a specific sequence of the four bases along the polynucleotide chain, then the molecular structure of DNA must be able to accommodate any arbitrary sequence of bases along its polynucleotide chains. Otherwise the capacity of DNA as an information carrier would be too severely limited. Hence, they felt the need of construction of such a regular helix that though, it is composed of two polynucleotide chains containing an arbitrary sequence of nucleotide bases every 3.4 A° along their length, as would nevertheless, as a constant diameter of 20 A°. Since the dimension of the purine ring is greater than that of the pyrimidine ring **Watson** and **Crick** hit upon the idea that the two-chain helix could have a constant diameter if there existed a complementary relation between the two nucleotide stacks, so that at every level one stack harbours a purine base and the other a pyrimidine base. Finally, to endow the helix with thermodynamic stability, the structure would have ample opportunities for the formation of hydrogen bonds between amino or hydroxyl-hydrogens and keto-oxygens or immino-nitrogens of the purines and pyrimidine bases. These considerations led them to construct a double helix model for the molecular structure of DNA molecule.

Watson and Crick's Structural Model of DNA

In DNA molecule the adjacent deoxyribonucleotides are joined in a chain by 3′5′ phospho-diester bridges or bonds which link the 5′ carbon of the deoxyribose of one mono-nucleotide unit with the 3′ carbon of the deoxyribose of the next mononucleotide unit. According to **Watson** and **Crick** DNA molecule consists of two such polynucleotide chains wrapped helically around each other, with the sugar-phosphate chain on the outside (forming ribbon-like back bone of double helix) and purines and pyrimidines on the inside of the helix (projecting between two sugar phosphate backbones as transverse bars). The two polynucleotide strands are held together by hydrogen bonds between specific pairs of purines and pyrimidines.

The hydrogen bonds between purines and pyrimidines are such that adenine can bond only to thymine by two hydrogen bonds, and guanine can bond only to cytosine by three hydrogen bonds and no other alternative is possible between them. The specificity of the kind of hydrogen bonds that can be formed assures that for every adenine in one chain there will be a thymine in the other. For every guanine in first chain there will be a cytosine in the other and so on. Thus, the two chains are complementary to each other; that is, the sequence of nucleotides in one chain dictates the sequence of nucleotides in the other. The two strands run anti-parallely—that is, have opposite directions. One strand has phosphodiester linkage in 3′ → 5′ direction while other strand has phosphodiester linkage in just reverse or 5′ → 3′ direction. Further the adenine-thymine and guanine-cytosine base pairs are of precisely the same size and shape, therefore, DNA duplex has a constant diameter of 20 A° along its entire length and most importantly, any sequence of base pairs is possible within a two-stranded molecule. The coiling of double helix is right handed and a complete turn occurs every 34 A°. Since each nucleotide occupies 3.4 A° distance along the length of a polynucleotide strand, ten mononucleotides occur per complete turn.

The double helical molecule is a remarkably stable conformation as a result of two sets of forces: (1) hydrogen bonding between all the bases along the length of the chain pair, and (2) hydrophobic interaction between stacked bases in the vertical sequence of the individual chains (see **Avers**, 1976).

Fig. 21.7. Watson-Crick model of double helical DNA molecule.

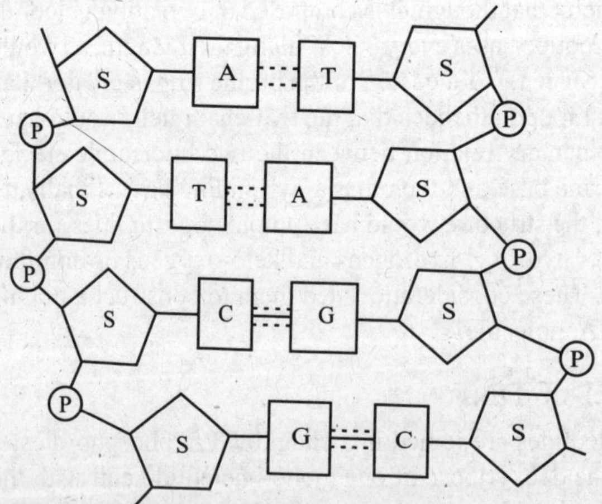

Fig. 21.8. A segment of DNA molecule showing arrangements of different components (S = deoxyribose, P = phosphate, A = adenine. T = thymine; G = guanine and C = cytosine) (after, De Robertis *et. al.*, 1970.)

Denaturation and Renaturation of DNA

In a DNA duplex, the two polynucleotide strands remain held together by weak hydrogen bonds. If a solution containing DNA molecules is heated, its hydrogen bonds become increasingly unstable with rising temperature, and eventually the two strands of the DNA helices can be caused to separate. This is melted or **denatured** DNA. Denaturation can also be effected by treating the DNA with a strong alkali which interferes with the hydrogen bond formed between the bases. If the solution is now cooled, or slowly neutralized the formation of new base pairs again becomes thermally or chemically probable and eventually new double-stranded molecules are formed. This process is termed **renaturation** or **reannealing**. This experimental technique of denaturation and renaturation of DNA first developed by **J. Marmur** and associates in 1963.

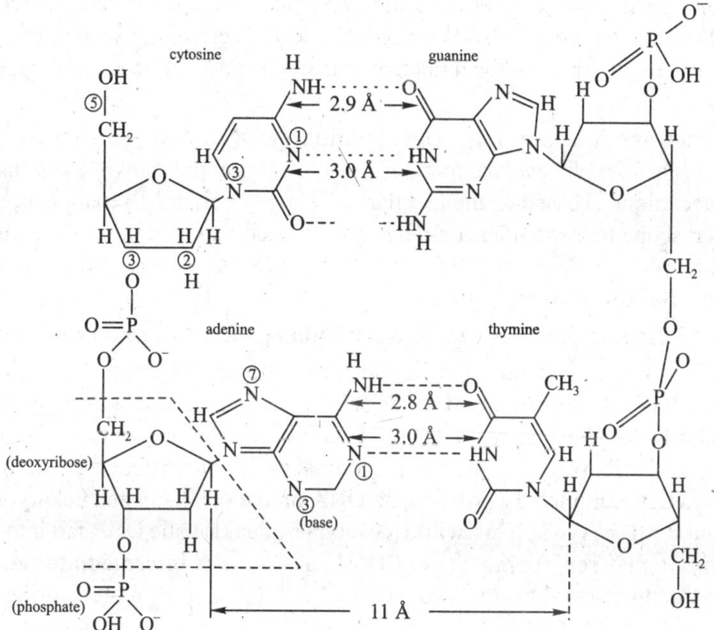

Fig. 21.9. Segment of a DNA molecule (after Levine, 1969)

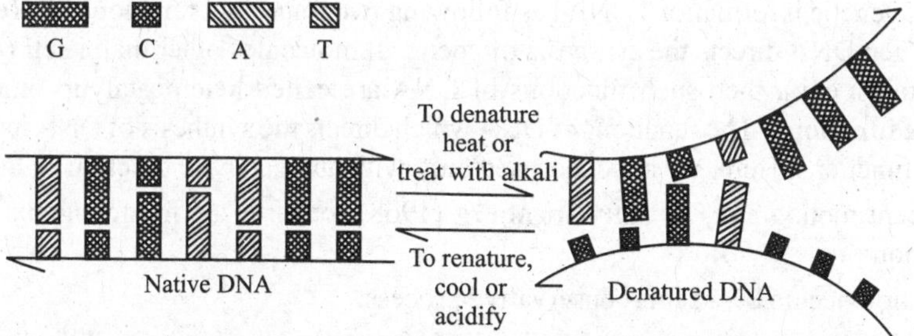

Fig. 21.10. Denaturation and renaturation of duplex DNA.

From this experiment it should be evident that if two strands of DNA that have quite different nucleotide sequences come together, stable hydrogen bonding cannot occur: the Chargaff's rule of A—T and G—C pairs specificity and the structure of the double helix dictate that stable renaturation can occur only if the two strands that lie in register are exactly, or almost exactly, complementary to one another.

Nucleic acid hybridization. Renaturation of DNA is a very useful tool in molecular biology. For example, hybrid molecules can be formed between DNAs of different species and the amount of **hybridization** will indicate the degree of genetic similarity. This technique has been developed by **M. Pardue** and **J. Gall** (1970). By this experimental technique, the single strands of DNA also form hybrids with RNA by complementary base pairing.

In a hybridization experiment, DNA duplexes are heated so that they denature into their component single strands. At this point, the denatured DNA is presented with single-strand fragments of DNA or RNA that derive from another source (*i.e.,* another animal or another species). The mixture is then allowed to cool slowly so that duplex formation can occur. If the fragments and the denatured DNA carry homologous base sequences, "hybrid" DNA—DNA or DNA—RNA duplexes will form, where no homology exists no hybridization will occur.

This property of renaturation has been used to recognize which part of DNA has been used as a template for a given RNA species. Renaturation studies have led to the discovery of **repeated sequences** of DNA in eukaryotic cells. When certain sequences are repeated many times (upto 10^6 copies), the rate of renaturation will be much faster than for those sequence (*i.e.,* genes) represented only once.

Partial denaturation mapping. Denaturation of DNA done under carefully controlled conditions may be used for physical mapping of DNA in a technique known as **partial denaturation mapping**. This technique is based on the fact that the regions rich in AT separate more easily. Under the electron microscope those regions are detected as single-stranded loops. The distance between the loops and the end of the DNA molecule can be measured; this distance is a characteristic of the DNA species (see **De Robertis** *et al.,* 1975).

Molecular Comparisons between Nuclear Eukaryotic and Prokaryotic DNA.

At this point we can cite three characteristic properties of eukaryotic DNA that distinguish it from prokaryotic: there is much more of it per cell; it has a more stable average GC content; and it is typically non-homogeneous, for it exhibits satellite DNA fragments in CsCl gradients (for details see chapter 17 : ribosomes). The fourth and final molecular difference relates to the different **renaturation kinetics** exhibited by prokaryotic DNA on the one hand and eukaryotic DNA on the other (**Kohne** and **Britten,** 1968). Thus while most types of eukaryotic DNA fall into following three general categories: a **fast-renaturing** class of DNA, a class with **intermediate renaturation** rates and a **slow-renaturing** class, almost all prokaryotic DNA falls into slow-renaturing class.

21.7 REPLICATION OF DNA

As a carrier of genetic informations DNA has following two important functions: **1. Heterocatalytic function**—When DNA directs the synthesis of chemical molecules other than itself (*e.g.,* synthesis of RNA, proteins, etc.), then such functions of DNA are called heterocatalytic functions; and **2. Autocatalytic function**—The functions of DNA which directs the synthesis of DNA itself, and called autocatalytic functions. Here, we are concerned only with autocatalytic function of DNA.

In a recent monograph, **Arthur Kornberg** (1968) set forth the following six basic rules of DNA replication:

1. Replication occurs by a semi-conservative process.
2. Replication proceeds in one or both directions from a given point, usually in both directions.
3. Replication starts at a unique point, or origin, and there may be one or more origins in a DNA molecule.
4. Both strands replicate by addition of nucleotide monomers in the 5′ to 3′ direction.
5. Replication occurs in short, discontinuous pulses, which produce short fragments that later are joined to the main body of the molecule.
6. A short segment of RNA primer is required to initiate DNA polymerase action in lengthening the polynucleotide chain.

Each of these rules of replication has been supported by the following experimental evidences:

1. The semi-conservative model of DNA replication. Continuity of life requires conservation of genetic information from generation to generation. The explanation lies in the mechanism by which new DNA (set of genes) is manufactured so that identical replicate molecules are synthesized accurately in every cycle. One compelling feature of the Watson-Crick model for DNA was that it could from the basis of a model of replication which would be guided by the property of complementary base pairing inherent in the structure of molecule itself. Watson and Crick suggested that the two strands of the duplex out of which each could serve as a template for synthesis of a new complementary partner, thus producing two identical molecules from the original duplex. Since only one strand of the old duplex is conserved in each new duplex, this mode of replication has been called **semi-conservative**; the two other theoretically possible mechanisms are the **dispersive** and the **conservative** modes (Fig. 21.11).

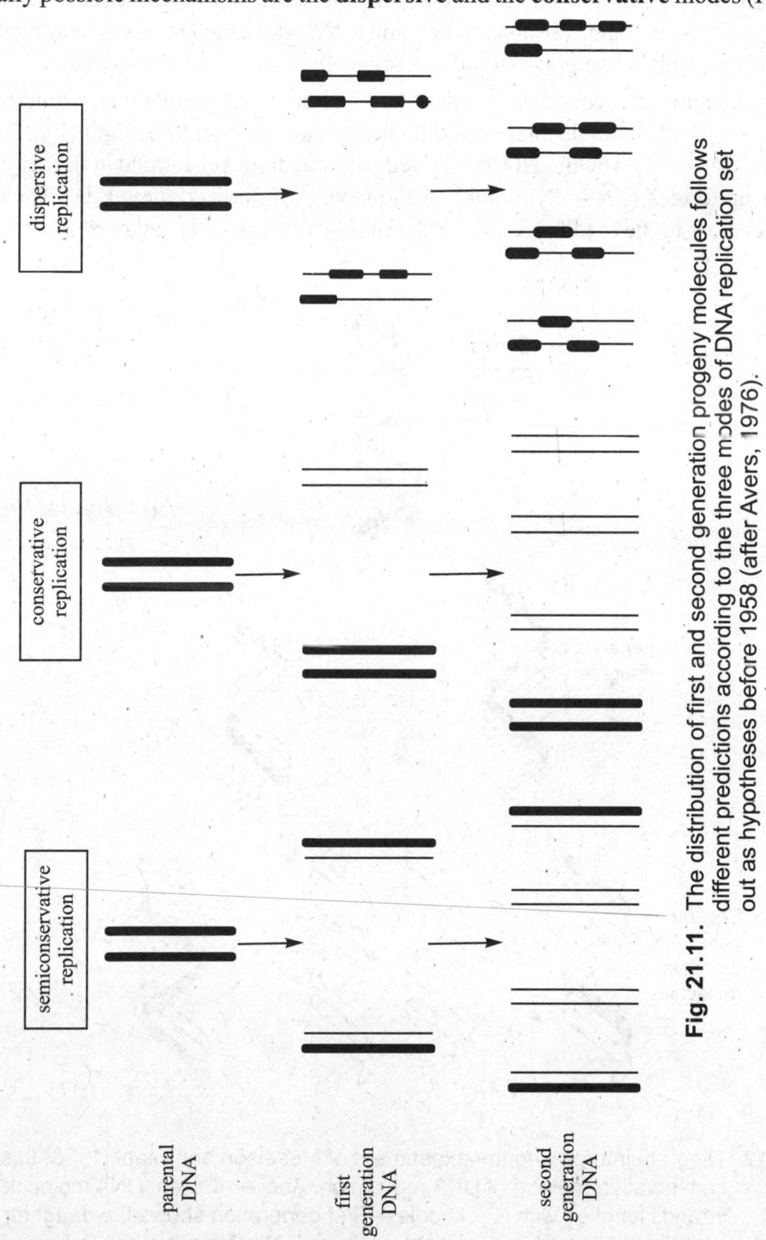

Fig. 21.11. The distribution of first and second generation progeny molecules follows different predictions according to the three modes of DNA replication set out as hypotheses before 1958 (after Avers, 1976).

Matthew Meselson and **Franklin Stahl** (1958) provided strong evidence which supported the semiconservative mode of DNA replication and worked against the other two possibilities. Using the method of equilibrium density gradient centrifugation to separate DNA is cesium chloride (CsCl) gradients, **Meselson and Stahl** designed their experiments to obtain data that could support only one of the theoretical possibilities and simultaneously exclude the other two. The utilized the fact that if *E. coli* cells are grown in a medium containing the heavy nitrogen isotope ^{15}N, their DNA will become heavier than ordinary DNA and this density difference can be distinguished by centrifugation in a CsCl gradient.

In Meselson-Stahl experiment, the *E. coli* cultures to be analysed has previously grown in media containing the heavy nitrogen isotope ^{15}N, so that the parent DNA was uniformly labelled at time—zero. These ^{15}N-labelled cells were transferred afterwards to media containing the ordinary ^{14}N isotope. In the first generation after cell and DNA doubling, DNA was extracted and centrifuged to identify the kinds of isotope-marked molecules that had been synthesized.

If replication was conservative, then two distinct DNA populations would be identified after centrifugation: half the molecules would be heavy and half would be light (Fig. 21.12). The heavy molecules (^{15}N—^{15}N) would be the conserved parental duplexes formed in the original ^{15}N-medium. The light molecules (^{14}N—^{14}N) would be the newly synthesized duplex DNA manufactured from ^{14}N—precursors in the medium in which the first generation cells had been produced.

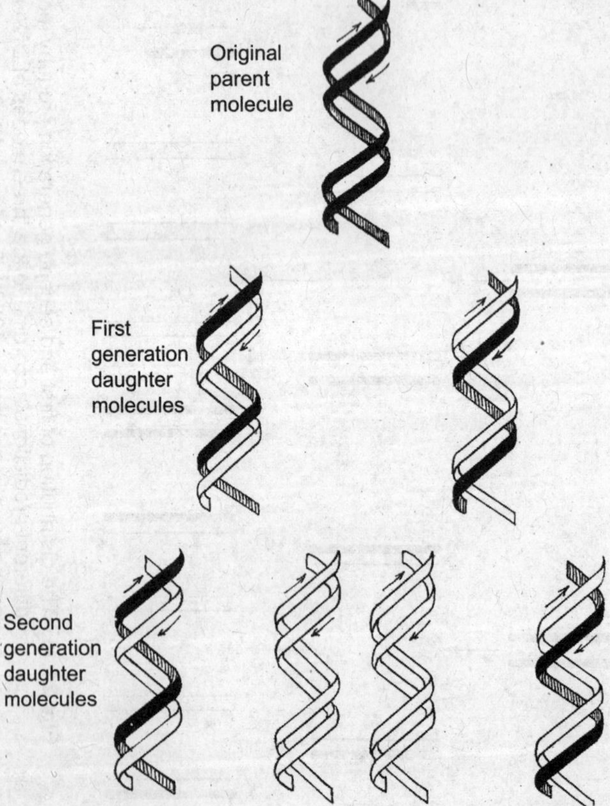

Fig. 21.12. Diagram interpreting the experiment of Meselson and Stahl (1958) to show the semi-conservative method of DNA replication. Above—Parent DNA molecule with both strands labelled with N^{15}; Middle—First generation shows the daughter molecules (in white) synthesized in a medium containing N^{15} (Note that the DNA molecules are hybrids of N^{15}— and N^{14} DNA strands); Below—At the second generation two molecules are hybrids and two are not (after De Robertis et al., 1970).

If replication was semi-conservative, it was predicted that all first-generation DNA molecules would be hybrid $^{15}N—^{14}N$, that is, all would be half heavy. If replication was dispersive, the population of DNA molecules would contain varying amounts of ^{15}N— and ^{14}N—DNA, depending on which original ^{15}N-pieces and how much of the original had been incorporated into the new molecules along with new ^{14}N-labelled sequences.

Sedimentation of extracted and purified DNA was carried out using high-speed centrifugation and a CsCl density gradient. At equilibrium the DNA molecules would settle in a specific region of the density gradient that corresponded to the buoyant density of DNA in CsCl. The $^{15}N—^{15}N$, $^{15}N—^{14}N$, and $^{14}N—^{14}N$ duplexes each settle in a distinct region that does not overlap with the others. The contents of the centrifuge tubes were photographed and interpreted. All DNA molecules from first generation cells were half-heavy ^{15}N-^{14}N, an observation which supported the semi-conservative mode of replication of DNA in *E. coli.*

Since 1958, the mode of DNA synthesis by semi-conservative replication has been verified many times by independent experiments. Experiments of the Meselson-Stahl design have also been conducted in the studies of DNA replication in cellular organelles. In 1967, **K. S. Chiang** and **S. Sueoka** showed that chloroplast DNA in unicellular *Chlamydomonas reinhardii* replicated semiconservatively.

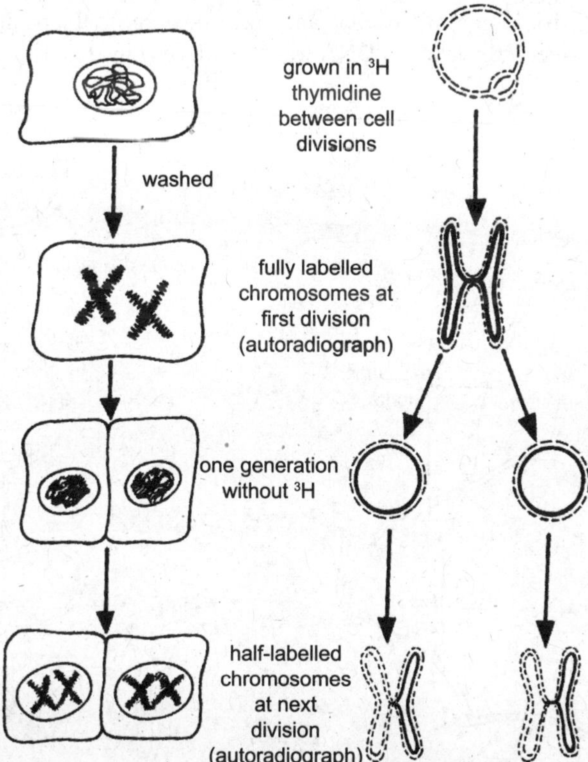

Fig. 21.13. Taylor's autoradiographic evidence showing semi-conservative replication of DNA of eukaryotic chromosomes (after Dyson, 1978).

A variation on the Meselson-Stahl experimental design was exploited by **J. Herbert Taylor** (1958) to examine the mode of replication in whole eukaryotic chromosomes. **Taylor** incubated the root cells of a plant (*Bellavalia romana*) in medium containing thymidine which was labelled with the radioactive isotope **tritium** (^{3}H) between cell divisions and found that when the chromatin formed visible chromosomes, the two sister chromatids were equally labelled. When cells treated in this way were allowed to proceed through a second division cycle, this time without radioactivity (*i.e.,* unlabelled or ^{1}H-thymidine), the chromosomes appeared with one labelled chromatid and one chromatid free of label (Fig. 21.13). Thus, DNA of eukaryotic chromosomes is also replicated by semiconservative method.

2. Direction of DNA replication. The first experimental evidence showing that replication proceeded in a specific direction was provided in 1963 by **John Cairns. Cairns** used autoradiography to capture *E. coli* chromosomes in the process of replication. In this experiment, *E. coli* cultures were grown in ^{3}H-thymidine for one 30-minute generation to label the DNA entirely. Afterward they were allowed to grow in the same medium for varying intervals during the second 30-minute cycle before they were removed for autoradiography.

The replicating regions of the large molecule would thus have twice the label density as regions that had not yet been replicated. Next, the cells were placed in a cellulose casing and disrupted with detergent. When the solution was removed from the casing, some DNA molecules were left behind, absorbed to the surface of the container. The casing was then transferred to a microscope slide and coated with a fine-grain photographic emulsion. As the tritium atoms decayed, the released electrons (*i.e.,* β-rays) caused the conversion of the silver halide in the emulsion to silver grains, in much the same way as photons of light would do. After several months, the emulsion was developed to reveal a trail of silver grains visible in a microscope and corresponding to the positions of the decaying molecules. Thus the shape of the labelled DNA was visualized (Fig. 21.14).

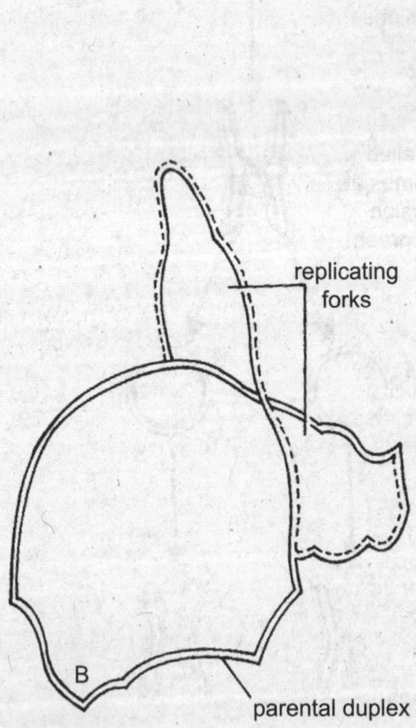

Fig. 21.14. Replicating DNA of E. coli K_{12}, as diagrammed from a autoradiograph visualized by Cairns (1963). Replicating DNA is divided into three sections (A, B, and C) that arise at the two replication forks (X and Y), (after Goodenough and Levine, 1974).

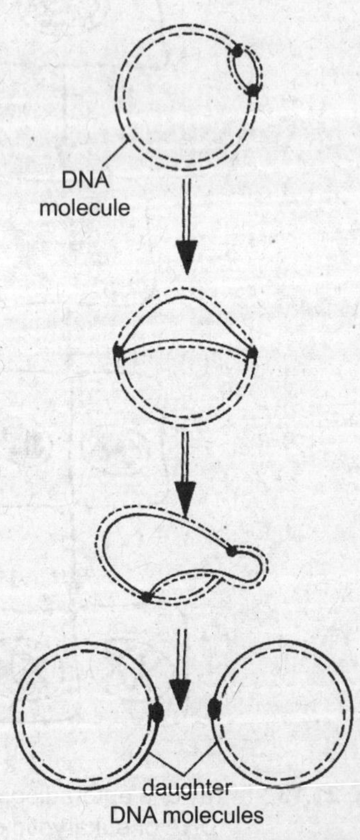

Fig. 21.15. The replication scheme suggested by autoradiography. Here, the addition of tritium is synchronized with the beginning of replication (after Dyson, 1978).

Autoradiography allowed Cairns to see the shape of the complete chromosome. It turned out to be a closed circle having a circumference of 1100-1400 μm even during replication. It appears as if new molecules are separated from the original in the same way that a closed zipper with its two ends sewed together would yield two circles when unzipped. There is a point on the molecule, called the **origin**, from which replication starts. Cairns suggested that a **replication fork** took off from this point in one direction, *i.e.,* DNA replication was **unidirectional**. However, **M. Masters** and **P. Broda** (1971) have shown that the replication of *E. coli* DNA is **bidirectional**, *i.e.,* a replication fork takes off from the point of origin in each direction. When the two replication forks meet on the other side of the circle, replication is completed and two daughter chromosomes, each containing one new and one old strand, are formed.

Bidirectional pattern of DNA replication has also been observed to occur in most viruses, prokaryotes and eukaryotes.

Further, molecules of eukaryotic chromosomal DNA show multiple origins, in the form of "eyes" or loops along the molecule while most viral and bacterial DNA contain only one origin point. Replication may begin at the same fixed origin in prokaryotes and viruses while an earlier round is still in progress.

3. Addition of nucleotide monomers. If the same enzymatic mechanisms are responsible for synthesis of both new strands, then chain growth cannot be simultaneous and synchronous for the two strands at the growing fork. It was predicted that (1) newly added monomers for both strands would occur only at the 3′ end of the replicating chains, and (2) asymmetric single-strand would be found in the duplex in the region where the opposite strand was being replicated. Chemical and enzymatic analysis verified the first prediction, and electron microscopy verified the second. The first prediction, is also found to be commonly occurred one in most virus, prokaryotes and eukaryotes.

In phage lambda (λ) DNA, the size of an asymmetric single-strand unit was measured to be upto 0.4 μm, which is equivalent to about 1000 base-pairs. Such asymmetric single-strand regions have also been identified in replicating mitochondrial DNA from animal cells (**D. R. Wolstenholme**, 1973) from centrifugation and electron microscopic studies, In the 5 μm long circles of animal mitochondrial DNA, there is a novel replication pattern in which replication begins along the light or L-strand of the duplex, causing the heavy or H-strand to be displaced. In the displaced or **D-loop** molecules it is possible to isolate the newly formed L-strand component, if the hydrogen bonds that bind segment to the replicating DNA are broken. The identity of the isolated fragments can be confirmed by centrifugation analysis and by hybridizing the newly synthesized L-strands with complementary L-strands from duplex DNA. Replication of the parental H-strand is initiated later. The process, therefore, takes place by a staggered copying: the L-strand is copied first and the H-strand is copied later, with each proceeding unidirectionally from the 5′ to the 3′ end of their respective chains (Fig. 21.16)

4. Synthesis of short pieces. R. Okazaki (1968, 1971) first showed that the most recently synthesized DNA occurred in short pieces that were later incorporated into the high-molecular-weight DNA chains. When growing cultures of *E. coli* were provided with labelled precursor in brief pulses at low temperature almost all the precursor label could be found in DNA fragments, called **replication fragments** or **Okazaki fragments.** Mutants which lacked enzymes necessary to extend the DNA chain or to join the short fragments were particularly useful because all their newly synthesized DNA occurred as short pieces. This finding suggested that synthesized proceeded along both chains of the duplex in brief, discontinuous pulses.

These replication or Okazaki fragments were employed to verify that nucleotide monomers were added in the 5′ $\rightarrow$ 3′ direction along both chains. The most recently added monomers regularly were found at the 3′ end of fragments for both antiparallel chains of the double helix.

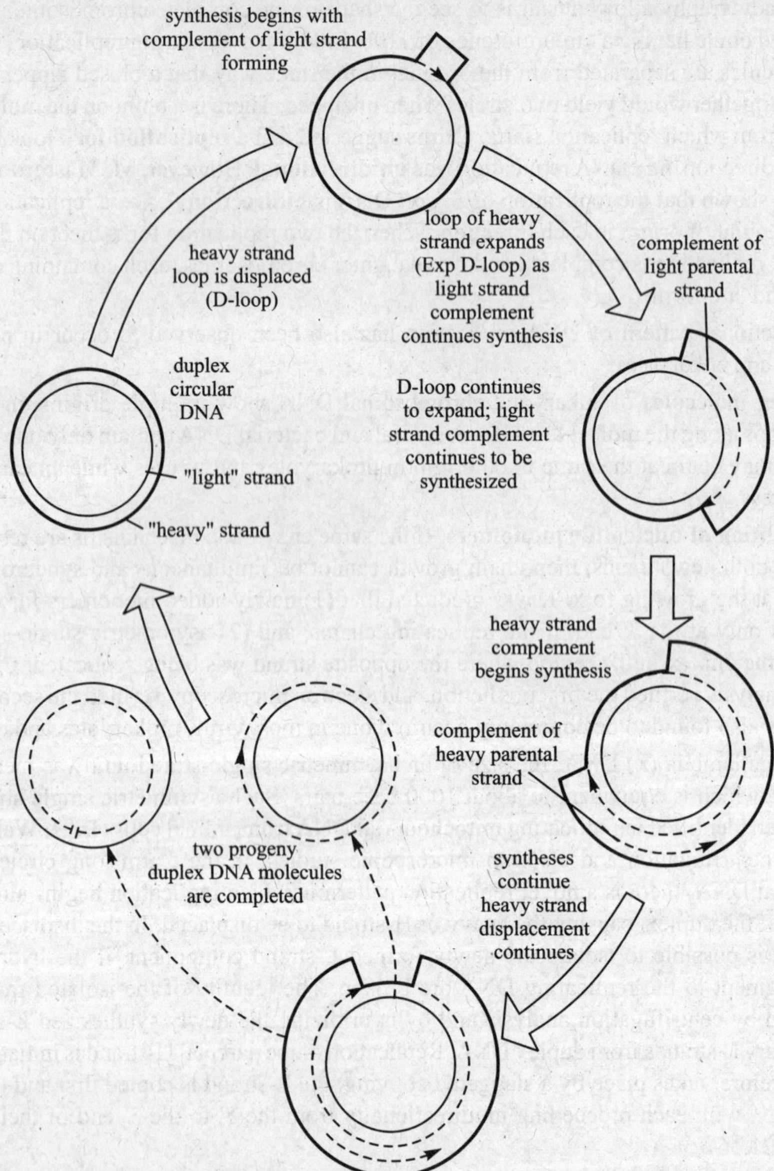

Fig. 21.16. Replication of mitochondrial DNA. Diagram illustrating the staggered copying of the parental DNA strands during D-loop synthesis of mouse mitochondrial DNA. Heavy strands are shown thicker than light complementary strands, and new strands are shown by dashed lines (after Avers, 1976).

5. Linking of short pieces. A DNA ligase is found to be the enzyme responsible for joining the replication fragments to the main DNA chain.

6. Initiation of replication by RNA primer. In 1970, **A. Kornberg, R. Okazaki,** and colleagues have reported the requirement of **RNA primer** in DNA synthesis. It had been known for a long time that no known DNA polymerase could start a new DNA chain, although the polymerases could catalyse chain growth. Initiation of DNA chain synthesis occurs as a brief transcriptional event catalysed by a **DNA-directed RNA polymerase.** The priming pieces of RNA must later be excized from the chain by some nuclease enzyme that specifically recognizes the region where the 3′ primer terminus is covalently bonded to the 5′ deoxyribonucleotide position. After the RNA primer is excised, the gap must be filled in with deoxyribonucleotides by DNA polymerase action, thus reconstituting the continuous DNA chain that continues to grow in this way along both strands in the 5′ → 3′ direction.

The event of chain initiation by a RNA primer was first supported by experimental studies of **A. Kornberg** on the replication of bacteriophage M13 DNA system. Later, RNA involvement in DNA chain initiation was found to be widespread feature in prokaryotic and eukaryotic species (see **Avers**, 1976; **Dyson**, 1978). In all cases, the size of RNA primer was found to be 10 per cent of the length of a replication fragment.

7. Unwinding the double helix. It had been postulated for a long time that some proteins must be present to facilitate unwinding of the duplex DNA in advance of the replicating fork. The first **unwinding protein** to be isolated and characterized was the protein product of gene 32 in *E. coli* phage T_4, reported in 1970 by **B. Alberts** and **L. Frey** other unwinding proteins have since been recognized in eukaryotic species.

The protein product of gene 32 converts a duplex DNA to single strands at temperatures 40° below the Tm (= midpoint melting temperature, *i.e.,* at temperature the midpoint of transition of a preparation of duplex DNA molecules to single strands during melting) for this DNA because tight binding occurs between the protein and single-stranded DNA and little binding with duplex DNA or RNA takes place. The unwinding protein binds to A—T rich lowmelting regions of DNA first, and the energy of this binding drives the melting to completion. The unwinding protein binds to the sugar-phosphate backbone so that no sequence specificity, other than for lowmelting regions rich in A—T pairs is involved. The elongated shape of the protein molecule permits it to bind tightly to about 10-nucleotide-long stretches. Because protein-protein interactions are highly favoured, and protein molecules bind cooperatively thus line up adjacent to one another rather than at isolated sites on DNA (Fig. 21.17).

Unwinding proteins not only melt duplex DNA by preferential binding to single-stranded sugarphosphate backbone, but they also facilitate base-pair alignment between single strands during DNA replication and recombination. Phage T_4 has an absolute requirement for gene 32 protein product for its DNA replication.

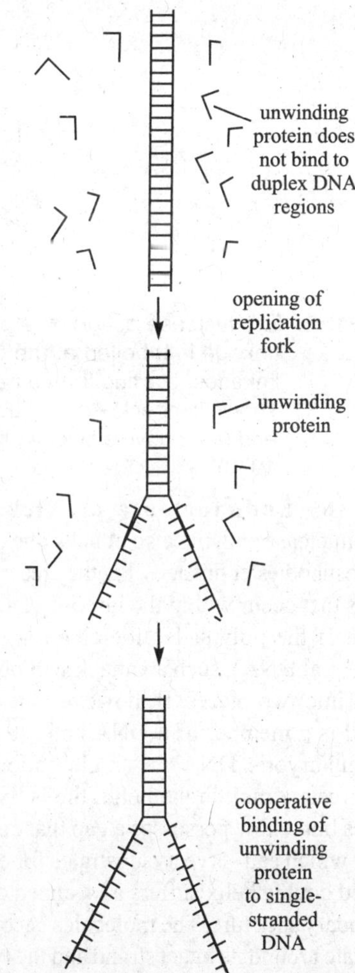

Fig. 21.17. Diagram showing the mode of action and effect of unwinding protein at the replication fork of duplex DNA (after Avers, 1976)

Enzymes Involved in DNA Replication

DNA replication in *E. coli* and other prokaryotic cells is found to be catalysed by following nuclear enzymes:

(i) Nuclease Enzyme

The nuclease enzymes act to hydrolyse or break down a polynucleotide chain into its component nucleotides. A polynucleotide is held together by 3′, 5′ phosphodiester bonds and a nuclease enzyme will attack either the 3′ or the 5′ end of this linkage. The nuclease enzymes may be of following two kinds:

(a) Exonuclease enzymes. A nuclease enzyme which begins its attack from a free end of a polynucleotide is called **exonuclease.** Therefore, depending on the specificity of the enzyme, an exonuclease will either being at a free 3′—OH end of a polynucleotide and progressively cleave the bonds on the 3′—OH side of the phosphodiester backbone or it will begin at a free 5′—P end and digest the polynucleotide in 5′ → 3′ direction. In both cases the enzyme travels along the chain in a stepwise manner, liberating single nucleoside monophosphate molecules and eventually digesting the entire polymer.

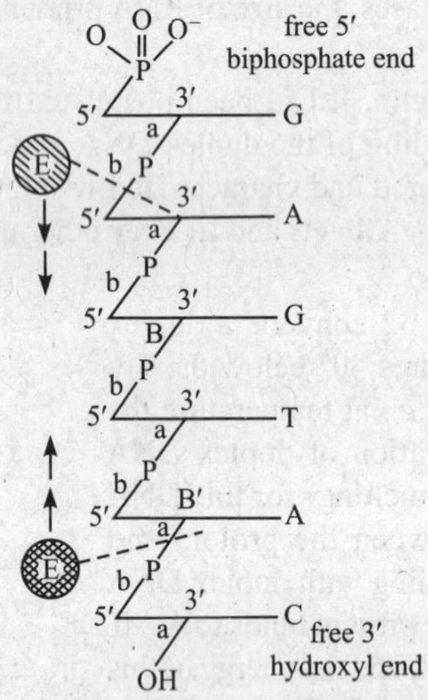

Fig. 21.18. Exonuclease action on a polynucleotide chain. The 3′ side of each phosphodiester linkage is labelled a, the 5′ side is labelled *b*. An exonuclease (E) that cleaves *a* linkages, starting from a free 3′—OH end (*e.g.,* snake venom phosphodiesterase) is shown in check. An exonuclease (E) that cleaves b linkages, starting from a free 5′—P end (*e.g.,* bovine spleen phosphodiesterase is shown in line shade (from Lehninger, 1970).

(b) Endonuclease or **Nickase enzyme**. Endonuclease enzyme also attacks one of the two sides of phosphodiester linkages, but they react only with those bonds that occur within the interior of a polynucleotide chain. If the polynucleotide chain is single-stranded (*e.g.,* viral DNA), such an attack will obviously cut the chain into two pieces. If, however, the polynucleotide strand is a member of a DNA helix (*e.g.,* prokaryotic and eukaryotic DNA), a single endonucleolytic cut will create a **nick** in the helix; the helix remain in one pieces but it now possesses a gap that contains two free ends, which can serve as substrates for exonucleases. A nicked double helix suffers a localized disruption of its secondary structure. The molecules become free to bend or rotate around its intact strand and the two broken ends are free to dangle. The increased molecular motion in the region of the nick will very likely interrupt hydrogen bonding between bases in the vicinity of the nick, thus effecting a limited "unraveling" of the helix.

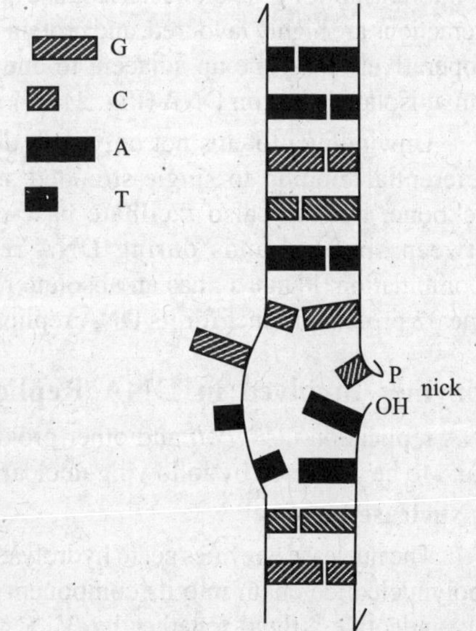

Fig. 21.19. A nicked duplex DNA molecule such as is formed by an endonuclease enzyme (after Goodenough and Levine, 1974)

(ii) Polymerase or Replicase Enzymes

A polymerase enzyme catalyses the formation of a polymer and cellular polymerase enzymes of genetic interest are those that bring about the synthesis of one polynucleotide chain that is a copy of another. A polymerase enzyme is called **replicase enzyme** when the copy of polynucleotide chain so produced are inherited by daughter cells or viruses, that is, when the enzyme brings about chromosome replication (see **Goodenough** and **Levine**, 1974).

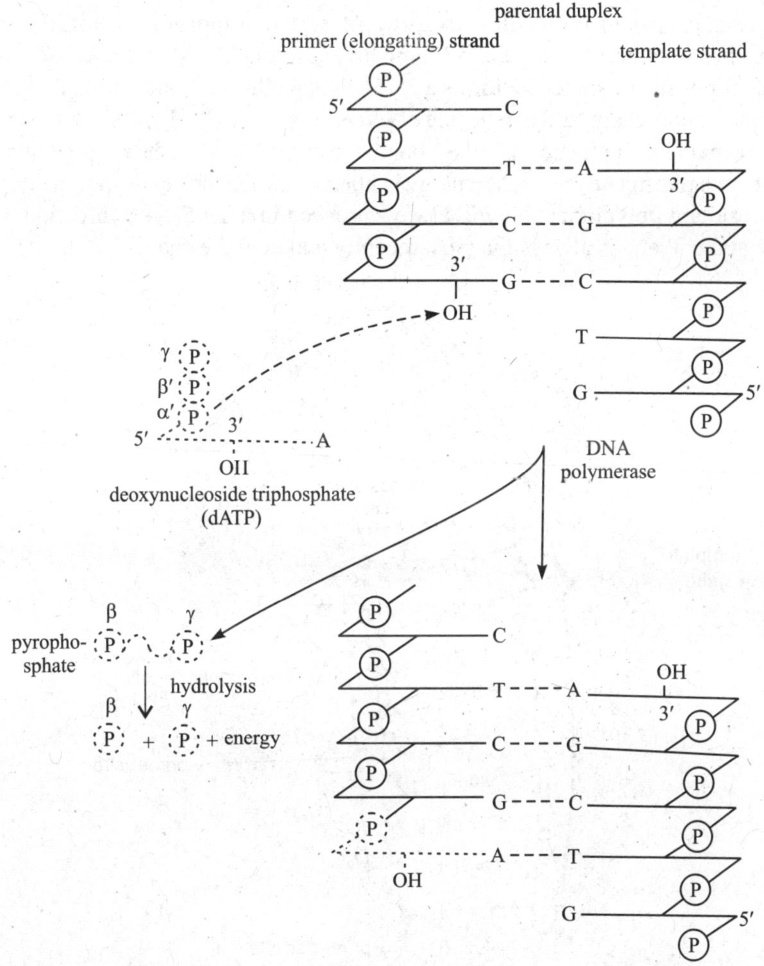

Fig. 21.20. DNA polymerization, A dATP molecule is shown being added to a parental DNA duplex or helix at its 3′—OH end. As DNA polymerase catalyses the formation of the phosphodiester bond pyrophosphate (P ~ P) is hydrolysed into two phosphate molecules (after Goodenough and Levine, 1974).

In vitro DNA polymerization. To understand the mechanism of DNA-replication inside the living cell (*in vivo*), molecular biologists tried *in vitro* polymerization of DNA and found that in addition to DNA polymerase enzyme, three classes of organic molecules are essential for *in vitro* reaction. The first are **deoxynucleoside triphosphates**. These are the familiar deoxynucleotide monophosphates (*i.e.*, d AMP, d CMP, d GMP, and d TMP) with two additional phosphate groups attached to the initial or α-phosphate group (*e.g.*, dATP, dCTP, dGTP, and dTTP). The second class of essential molecules for many DNA polymerase enzymes are polynucleotide chains with free 3′—OH ends, many DNA strands (often called **primer strands**), meaning that they cannot initiate the *de novo* synthesis of a new strand. The third class of essential molecules for DNA polymerase enzymes are **template strands**. All biologically important DNA polmerases possess a critical property: they will add nucleotides to a primer strand only in response to the base sequence found on a second template strand. Just as **Watson** and **Crick** suggested in their original model of DNA replication, the polymerase enzymes observe the rules of complementary base pairing. Thus, if a free 3′—OH group on a primer strand lies opposite a thymine on a template strand (see Fig. 21.20), a polymerase enzyme will add only an adenine group to the primer, even when dCTP, dTTP and dGTP are also present in the reaction mixture.

Once the appropriate molecules are present and the appropriate ionic conditions are maintained, *in vitro* polymerization reaction summarized in Fig. 21.20 will occur. The α-phosphate of a nucleoside triphosphate molecule forms a 3′, 5′ phosphodiester bond with a free 3′—OH in the growing polynucleotide chain, and a molecule of **pyrophosphate** (P ~ P), is simultaneously released Pyrophosphate contains a "high-energy" or "~" bond, meaning that when the released pyrophosphate is hydrolysed into two phosphate molecules energy is liberated which drives the polymerization process forward. The resultant polymerization will always proceed in a net 5′ → 3 direction, meaning that the nucleotide at the 3′ end is always the most recently added to the chain.

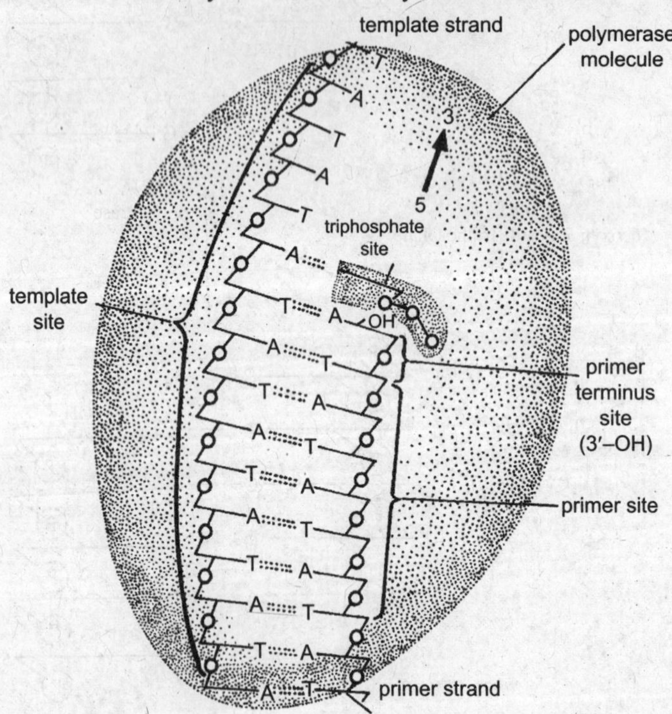

Fig. 21.21. Diagram of the centre of the DNA polymerase I of *E. coli* (after Goodenough and Levine, 1974).

The Kornberg enzyme. A. Kornberg (1969) first of all used **DNA polymerase I** of *E. coli* which later on named as **Kornberg enzyme** or **Kornberg polymerase** after its discoverer, in *in vitro* polymerization of DNA. His early experiments which indicated that the polymerase enzyme makes faithful complementary copies of DNA molecules, made use of artificially synthesized template strands with alternating A and T [poly d(AT)]. When such template strands were incubated with Kornberg polymerase and with the four nucleoside triphosphates carrying radioactive label, radioactive DNA that contained only alternating A and T was synthesized. In other words, even though a great deal of dGTP and dCTP was present in the solution, none was ever incorporated into DNA in response to poly d(AT) strand. When more complex biological DNAs with heterogeneous base sequence were used, then by a molecular biological technique called **nearest neighbour analysis,** it was found that the Kornberg polymerase catalyses the synthesis of complementary copies of template DNA.

Chemically the Kornberg enzyme is presently known to be a single polypeptide chain with a molecular weight of 109,000 – one of the largest single-chain globular protein known (Fig. 21.21). Only one site on the enzyme appears capable of interacting with free nucleoside triphosphates. It is supposed, therefore, that once the polymerase enzyme encounters to a given base in the template it can catalyse phosphodiester bond formation in the daughter strand only when the correct complementary triphosphate comes to occupy this triphosphate site. Presumably only the complementary base will have the correct geometry to align properly with the elongating daughter strand and so be in the correct position to form an ester bond; if, for instance, a pyrimidine is called for, a purine might "bulge out" too far. Once an ester bond is formed, the Kornberg enzyme is presumably free to move along to the next base in the template, where a new complementary triphosphate enters the site, another bond is formed and so on, until the entire template is faithfully copied. The Kornberg enzyme, therefore, like most DNA polymerases, stimulates 5′ → 3′ synthesis of DNA by adding complementary nucleoside triphosphates to the 3′—OH end of a DNA strand. The Kornberg enzyme also possesses two exonuclease activities: 1. An exonuclease activity that degrades a strand from its exposed 3′ end (*i.e.*, 3′ → 5′ exonuclease activity); and 2. A 5′ → 3′ exonuclease activity. (**Dyson,** 1978)

DNA polymerase II and DNA polymerase III. The first known *E. coli* polymerase, DNA polymerase I was not generally accepted as the primary replicating enzyme because its behaviour had a number of peculiar aspects *in vitro*. For example, branched DNA chains were synthesized in the presence of DNA polymerase I *in vitro*, whereas unbranched DNA is the only form synthesized *in vivo*. In 1969 a polymerase I-deficient mutant was isolated by **P. Delucia** and **J. Cairns**. This *pol A⁻* mutant synthesized DNA at normal rate despite very low (virtually undetectable) amounts of polymerase I, and a search was initiated for other polymerizing enzymes, using this mutant strain as an experimental system.

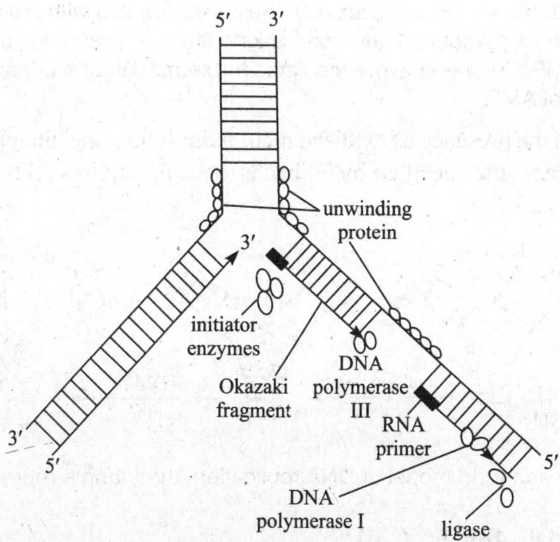

Fig. 21.22. Summary diagram of requirements and events relative to replication of duplex DNA molecules (after Avers 1976).

Polymerase I activity is so high in wild type cells that it masks activities of other enzymes involved in nucleotide incorporation, but in *pol A⁻* mutants, **DNA polymerase II** and then **DNA**

polymerase III were found. Another polymerase β mutant *bol B*⁻ was found to lack DNA polymerase II, but it still synthesized DNA at normal rates. DNA polymerase II did not seem to be the primary replicate either. Mutants deficient in DNA polymerase III, *pol C*⁻ strains have suggested the DNA polymerase III to be the main replicate of *E. coli*. Without it, cells cannot reproduce.

According to Kornberg (1974) and others, DNA polymerase I fills in the gaps between Okazaki fragments and removes segments of RNA primer at the 5′ end of each newly synthesized fragment (see **Dyson** 1978).

(iii) DNA Ligases

DNA ligase enzymes are capable of catalysing phosphodiester bond formation between free 3′—OH and free 5′—P groups of a nick of DNA which is created by endonuclease enzyme, thereby restoring an intact DNA duplex. Many DNA ligases have already been discovered. The ligase enzyme

1. E (mammalian or phage induced) + ATP ⇌ E-AMP + PP
   E (E. coli) + NAD ⇌ E-AMP + NMN (Nicotinamide mononucleotide)
2. E-AMP + 3′ — OH — P — 3′ → 3′ — OH — P — 3′ ; P --- A
3. 3′ — OH — P — 3′ ; P --- A →(E) + AMP

G C A T

Fig. 21.23. Postulated mechanism of DNA ligase reaction. (1) The enzyme (E) forms an enzyme-adenylate (E—AMP) complex. (2) The E-AMP reacts with a nicked DNA chain, generating a pyrophosphate bond linking the 5′—P terminus of the DNA to the P group of the AMP. (3) The enzyme mediates the formation of a phosphodiester bond with the release of AMP.

from *E. coli* requires the presence of oxidized nicotinamide adenine dinucleotide (NAD+) a cofactor, whereas, the ligase enzyme specified by T_4 bacteriophage requires ATP to bring about the joining reaction (See Fig. 21.23).

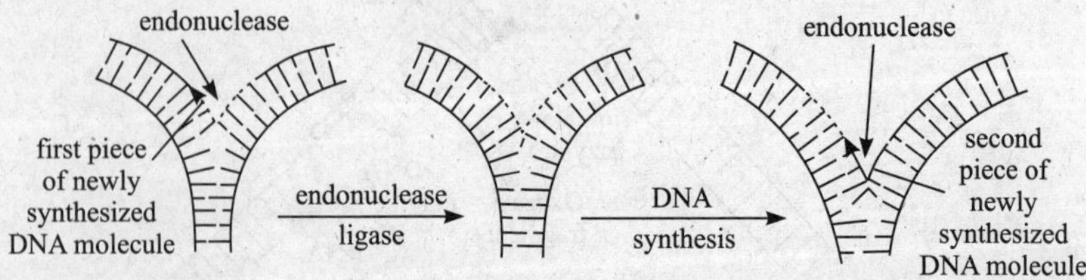

Fig. 21.24. "Knife and fork" model of DNA replication, the triangle represents an endonuclease.

Replication Models for E. Coli

The following three models have been proposed by molecular biologists to explain DNA replication in *E.coli.*

(i) Knife and fork model for DNA replication. According to the knife and fork model which proposed by **R. Barzilai** and **C. Thomas** (1970), a single DNA polymerase first copies one strand, then jumps across the replicating fork and, continuing to elongate the same DNA molecule, copies the other strand in the opposite direction until it encounters the barrier of already replicated DNA. Two events now occur: ligase joins the free ends of the second daughter strand as before and an endonuclease (the "knife") cut the newly synthesized strand in the forked region, thus creating two DNA molecules. A second polymerase now enters the fork, elongate one chain, jumps to the other side of the fork, and so on.

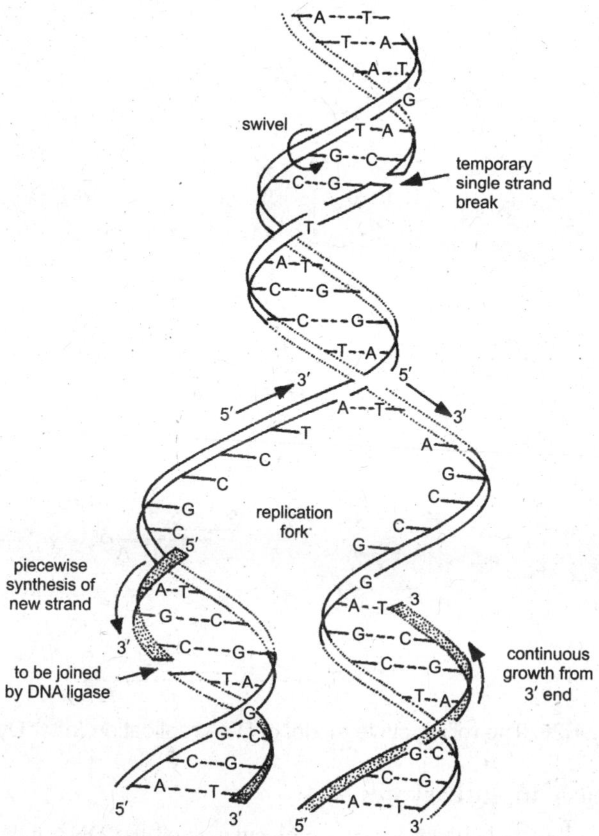

Fig. 21.25. This discontinuous synthesis of DNA (after Dyson, 1978)

***(ii)* Discontinuous model for DNA replication.** This model is most widely accepted and supported one. According to this model, the parent helix undergoes a localized unwinding or denaturation so that its internal bases are exposed for replication. An enzyme called endonuclease creates a transient break (a "nick") in one strand safely ahead of the replication fork (Fig. 21.25). The nick permits swiveling about the P—O—P bonds in the intact chain without the necessity for twisting the whole molecule. The unwinding proteins stabilize the denatured configuration at the growing point (Fig. 21.22).

Now in the presence of DNA polymerase III, one new strand grows more or less continuously from its 3′ end at a replication fork (*i.e.,* in the 5′ → 3′ direction). The other new strand is being put together from small pieces, called Okazaki fragments, each synthesized in the 5′ → 3′ direction by a replicate (DNA Polymerase III) and then laced together by DNA polymerase I and ligase to provide an overall direction of growth that is 3′ → 5′ (Fig. 21.25). Such a discontinuous synthesis of DNA strand is also called **backfilling**.

(iii) Rolling circle model. This scheme of DNA replication is also dependent on backfilling or discontinuous DNA synthesis and is probably used during transfer of DNA from one bacterium to another during mating and also during gene amplification in nucleoli of eukaryotic cells (**Dyson,** 1978). In it, the 5′ end at a nick is peeled off the circle and a complementary strand laid down on it by piecewise backfilling. Meanwhile, the circle retains its double-stranded structure by growth from the free 3′ end (Fig. 21.26).

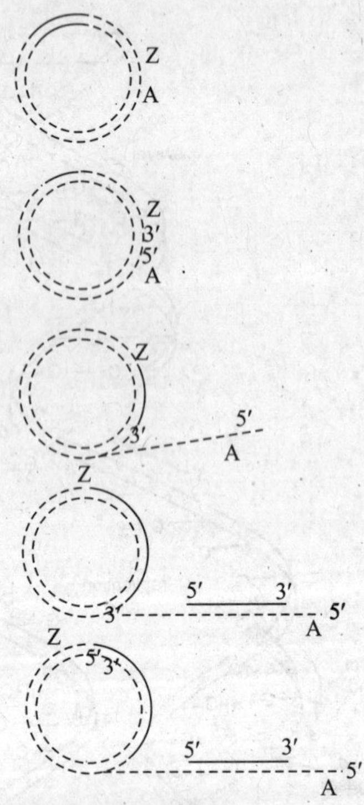

Fig. 21.26. The rolling circle model of DNA replication (after Dyson, 1978)

DNA Replication in Eukaryotes

Most molecular biologists believe that at a molecular level the DNA in a nuclear chromosome is replicated by the same kinds of enzymes (*e.g.,* exonucleases, endonucleases, polymerases, and ligases) and by the same sorts of steps as DNA replication in bacterial chromosomes. In most eukaryotes the molecular study of DNA replication remains difficult due to the fact that their DNA exists as heterogeneous chromatin and the chromatin is aggregated in a variable jungle of twisted fibres whose fundamental pattern of organization is unknown. However, some information about DNA replication in eukaryotes has been received from dipteran polytene chromosomes, lampbrush chromosomes of amphibian oocytes, and chromosomes of some eukaryotes.

Time of DNA replication in eukaryotes. In rapidly growing bacteria DNA synthesis occurs from the time a cell originates at division to the time it gives rise to daughter cells by division. A similar pattern is observed in simple eukaryotes such as yeast, in which DNA synthesis takes place throughout the interphase and ceases only during the brief period of nuclear and cell division. In higher plants and animals, however, DNA replication occurs only during a discrete interval of interphase known as **synthesis** or S period. Since histones are also synthesized during this time, the S period can be considered a time of chromosomal as well as DNA replications. The length of a S phase is a constant property of any one cell type.

Replication units. For studying DNA replication in eukaryotes, in one of the experiment, diploid cells are grown in a tissue culture medium containing H^3-thymidine for brief periods of time; large DNA fragments are spread onto a surface and subjected to auto-radiography. **J. Huberman** and **A. Riggs** (1968) measured the lengths of individual radioactive chromosomal segments in preparations derived from a human cell line known as **HeL** a (Hela cells were originally derived from the cervical cancer of one *Henrietta Lacks*), and calculated that the DNA is replicated at about 1 μm/min (in contrast to 30 μm/min for *E coli*), or about 60 μm/hr. When we consider that an average chromosome contains about 30,000 μm of DNA, it becomes clear that if replication was to initiate at one end and proceed sequentially to the other end, it would take 500 hours. Instead, replication typically occurs within six to eight hours. This and a number of other considerations have led to the conclusion that during a typical S phase each chromosome is "worked on" by replication enzymes at many different places at once. In other words, each chromosome contains a number of **different replication units.** Autoradiographical studies have shown that each replication unit functions independently of one another.

Further, all the DNA in a cell must be replicated in advance of mitosis, or meiosis if daughter cells are to receive complete sets of genetic information. Since individual replication units behave independently, some generalized kind of mechanism must exist which takes cognizance of the fact that DNA replication has been completed throughout the genome and which then triggers the onset of the G_2 (Gap period of interphase which follows S phase and includes growth and metabolic activity) and M (mitosis) phases of the cell cycle. The nature of this mechanism is totally unknown.

Eukaryotic DNA Replication at a Molecular Level

The detailed mechanism of eukaryotic DNA replication is no better understood than that of prokaryotic DNA. According to well accepted **bidirectional model** of eukaryotic DNA replication, DNA synthesis

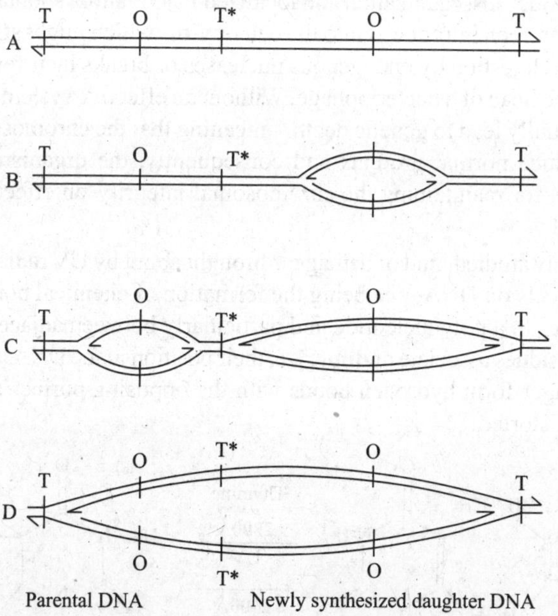

Fig. 21.27. Bidirectional model for mammalian chromosomal DNA replication. Origins are indicated by O and termini by T. (A) DNA prior to replication; (B) replication started in right-hand replication unit; (C) replication started in left-hand replication unit completed at termini of right-hand unit; (D) replication completed, sister duplexes joined at common terminus T (after De Robertis *et al.*, 1975).

within a given replication unit is initiated some where at or near the midpoint of the unit at a site termed the **origin** (O). Two replicating forks are then believed to travel in opposite directions until they reach either end of that unit, the two end points being called **termini** (T). A given replication unit may or may not undergo bidirectional synthesis in synchrony with contiguous units. In either case the newly replicated strands in adjacent units will eventually meet. These strands are then linked, perhaps by a DNA ligase to form long, continuous daughter DNA strands.

The model shown in Fig. 21.27 describes DNA replication in eukaryotes as being semiconservative, and extensive evidence supports this assumption. Specifically, a number of investigators have performed experiments similar to those of **Meselson** and **Stahl** (1958) and have found that heavy DNA from eukaryotes becomes hybrid in density after one round of replication in light medium.

21.8 MUTATION AND DNA REPAIR SYNTHESIS

Though the gene is generally stable, it may change by a process called **mutation**. The capacity to mutate is a property of the genetic material that is as important as stability. Mutation takes place in all living organisms and is the origin of hereditary variations. A genetic mutation, which may originate either spontaneously or due to some mutagenic agent, becomes incorporated in the population and is transmitted by sexual reproduction. A mutation may correspond to the change of a single nucleotide, of a long polynucleotide chain, or even of an entire chromosome arm. When the locus is restricted, the resume called a **gene mutation**, when it is extended, involving the chromosomes structure, it is considered as a **chromosomal mutation or aberration** (see chapter 20).

Further it is known that the DNA in the chromosomes may be come mutated or damaged by a variety of chemicals, such as nitrogen mustard or mitomycin C or by the radiation produced by ^{32}P decay, X-rays, or ultraviolet (UV) light. In addition, chromosomes probably undergo a continuous process of "spontaneous" disorganization and localized inactivation; spontaneous in the sense that no known toxic agent has been introduced into the cell or virus which might stimulate the damage. Such events might include digestion by endogenous nucleases or breaks incurred during the packaging of chromosomes into the head of a bacteriophage. Without an effective system of repair, these mutations and damages will usually lead to genetic death—meaning that the chromosome cannot be replicated, genes will not produce normal proteins and consequently, the organism cannot generate viable offspring. Therefore, for maintaining the chromosomal integrity, an effective repairing mechanism is essentially needed.

The most widely studied kind of damage is brought about by UV radiation. Ultraviolet radiation produces several effects on DNA, one being the formation of chemical bonds between two adjacent pyrimidine molecules in a polynucleotide and particularly between adjacent thymine residues (Fig. 21.28). As the two residues associate or **dimerize**, their position in the DNA helix becomes so displaced that they can no longer form hydrogen bonds with the opposing purines and thus the regularity of the helix becomes distorted.

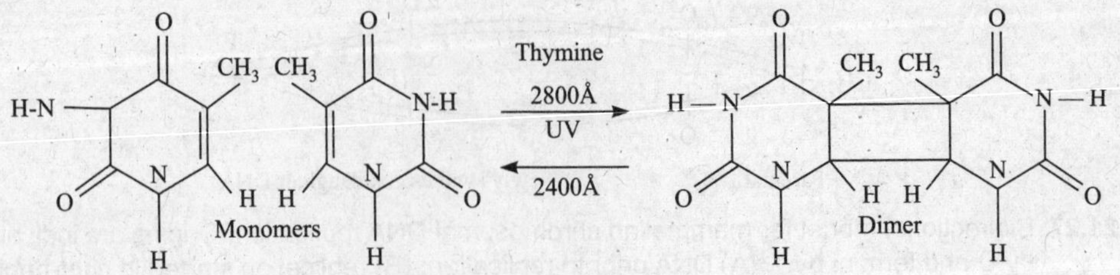

Monomers — Thymine 2800Å UV → ; ← 2400Å — Dimer

Fig. 21.28. Formation of dimer of thymine

Thymine dimers are removed from a chromosome in at least three ways—by **photoreactivation**, by **excision repair**, and by **post-replication repair**. The last mechanism involves both DNA replication and recombination and falls into the category of genetics, therefore, cannot be discussed here.

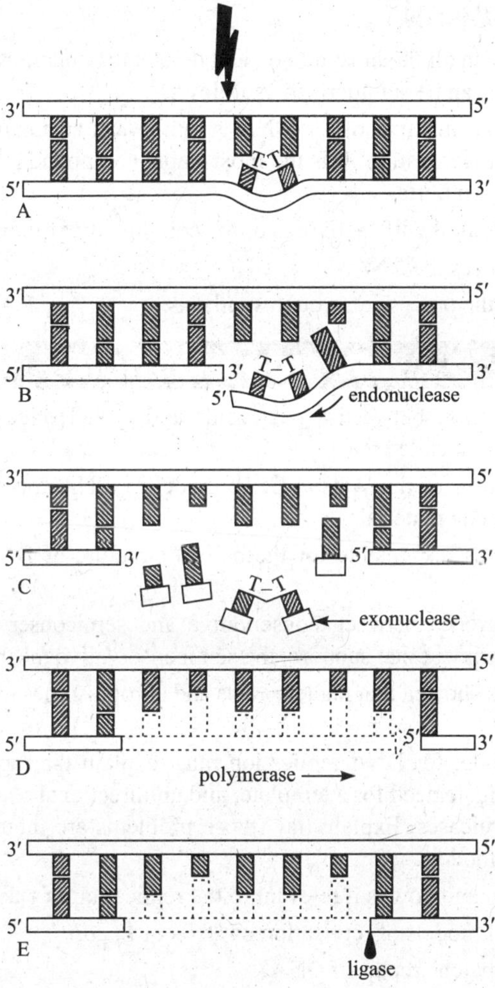

Fig. 21.29. Diagram showing the effect of ultraviolet light (UV) on DNA molecule and the mechanism of DNA repair (after De Rebertis *et al.*, 1975)

Photoreactivation is a process that requires a specific and interesting enzyme, the product of which is able to cleave the bond that has formed between thymine dimers and thereby convert them to monomers. This photoreactivating enzyme can associate with a dimer in the dark, but it must absorb a photon of visible light before it can bring about monomerization.

Excision repair can occur in dark and involves more enzymes than photoreactivation (Fig. 21.29 A) (1) the recognition and incision of the affected DNA strand by an endonuclease (Fig. 21.29 B), (2) excision and broadening of the gap by an exonuclease (*e.g.,* DNA polymerase) (Fig. 21.29 C), (3) filling of the gap by repair replication by DNA polymerase (Fig. 21.29 D), and (4) covalent joining of the polynucleotide by the ligase (Fig. 21.29 E) (**Howard**, 1968). In this mechanism, step 1 is very important, because, it involves nuclease enzymes. Nucleases are specific enzymes that can recognize sequence of nucleotides (primary structure) as well as secondary and tertiary structures in the DNA molecule (for example, the existence of loops). Further, the production of pyrimidine dimers in special regions of the DNA (*i.e.*, the promoter) may have important consequences, since it will impair both DNA duplication and transcription (**Radman** *et al.*, 1970).

21.9 FUNCTIONS OF DNA

The DNA has a key role in all the biosynthetic and hereditary functions of the living organisms. Its few important functions can be summarized as follows:

1. The most important function of the DNA is that it acts as a carrier of genetic informations from generation to generation. It is the most stable compound of the biological world which can be considered immortal.
2. The DNA controls all the life activities of the cell directly or indirectly.
3. The DNA synthesizes the RNA.
4. The DNA guides the process of protein synthesis.

REVISION QUESTIONS

1. What is the difference between a nucleoside and a nucleotide? What is a phosphodiester linkage, and why is it called that?
2. Describe the features of the Watson-Crick model of DNA and state why these features are needed by the genetic material.
3. What are the forces responsible for the helical structure of DNA? For its double-stranded structure?
4. What is the difference between conservative and semiconservative replication of DNA? Describe the experiment that supports the semiconservative mechanism.
5. What experiments showed that nucleic acids and chromosomes replicated in the same general manner?
6. A satisfactory model for DNA replication must explain the rapid unwinding of the parent molecule, the obligate need for a template, and unidirectional $5' \rightarrow 3'$ chain growth catalysed by the known replicases. Explain how those problems are thought to be solved by current DNA replication models.
7. What is a replicon and how is it relevant to the replication of eukaryotic DNA?
8. Describe different models of replication of DNA of *E. coli.*
9. What is "cut and patch" repair of DNA?
10. The melting temperature (Tm) of DNA increases in a quite predictable way with the ratio [(G + C) / (A + T)]. Why?
11. A typical human cell contains about 4×10^{12} daltons (6×10^{-12} g) of DNA. If that amount of DNA were in a single double stranded helix how long would it be? (The average mass of a nucleotide in DNA is about 300 daltons)
    (**Ans.** about 7 feet).

22 Chapter GENETIC CODE

As DNA is a genetic material, it carries genetic informations from cell to cell and from generation to generation. At this stage, an attempt will be made to determine that in what manner the genetic informations are existed in DNA molecule? Are they written in articulated or coded language on DNA molecule? If in the language of codes what is the nature of genetic code?

A DNA molecule is composed of three kinds of moieties: (i) phosphoric acid, (ii) deoxyribose sugar, and (iii) nitrogen bases. The genetic informations may be written in anyone of the three moieties of DNA. But the poly-sugar-phosphate backbone is always the same, and it is, therefore, unlikely that these moieties of DNA molecule carry the genetic informations. The nitrogen bases, however, vary from one segment of DNA to another so the informations might well depend on their sequences. The sequences of nitrogen base of a given segment of DNA molecule, actually has been found to be identical to linear sequence of amino acids in a protein molecule. The proof of such a **colinearity** between DNA nitrogen base sequence and amino acid sequence in protein molecules has first obtained from an analysis of mutants of head protein of bacteriophage T_4 (**Sarabhai** *et al.*, 1964) and the A protein of tryptophan synthetase of *Escherichia coli* (**Yanofski** *et al.*, 1964). The colinearity of protein molecules and DNA polynucleotides has given the clue that the specific arrangement of four nitrogen bases (*e.g.*, A, T, C and G) in DNA polynucleotide chains somehow, determines the sequence of amino acids in protein molecules. Therefore, these four DNA bases can be considered as four alphabets of DNA molecule. All the genetic informations, therefore, should be written by these four alphabets of DNA. Now the question arises that whether the genetic informations are written in articulated language or coded language? If genetic informations might have occurred in an articulated language, the DNA molecule might require various alphabets, a complex system of grammar and ample amount of space on it. All of which might be practically impossible and troublesome too for the DNA. Therefore, it was safe to conclude for molecular biologists that genetic informations were existed in DNA molecule in the form of certain special language of code words which might utilize the four nitrogen bases of DNA for its symbols. Any coded message is commonly called **cryptogram**.

22.1 BASIS OF CRYPTOANALYSIS

The basic problem of such a genetic code is to indicate how information written in a four letter language (four nucleotides or nitrogen bases of DNA) can be translated into a twenty letter language (twenty amino acids of proteins). The group of nucleotides that specifies one amino acid is a **code word** or **codon**. By the **genetic code** one means the collection of base sequences (codons) that correspond to each amino acid and to translation signals. We can consider here the classical but logical reasoning done by **George Gamov** (1954) about the possible size of a codon. The simplest possible code is a **singlet code** (a code of single letter) in which one nucleotide codes for one amino acid could be specified. A **doublet code** (a code of two letters) is also inadequate, because it could specify only sixteen (4 × 4) amino acids, whereas a **triplet code** (a code of three letters) could specify sixty four (4 × 4 × 4) amino acids. Therefore, it is likely that there may be 64 triplet codes for 20 amino acids. The possible singlet, doublet and triplet codes, which are customarily represented in terms of "**mRNA language**" [mRNA is a complementary molecule which copies the genetic informations (cryptogram of DNA) during its transcription], have been illustrated in Table 22.1.

Table 22.1. Possible singlet, doublet and triplet codes of mRNA.

Note : The genetic code is usually described in terms of the codons in messenger RNA transcripts rather than directly in DNA codewords. This convention arose from the fact that almost all experimental studies have employed RNA transcripts involved in protein translation, because it is easier than working with the DNA.

Single code (4 words)	Doublet code (16 words)				Triplet code (64 words)			
					AAA	AAG	AAC	AAU
					AGA	AGG	AGC	AGU
					ACA	ACG	ACC	ACU
					AUA	AUG	AUC	AUU
					GAA	GAG	GAC	GAU
					GGA	GGG	GGC	GGU
A	AA	AG	AC	AU	GCA	GCG	GCC	GCU
G	GA	GG	GC	GU	GUA	GUG	GUC	GUU
C	CA	CG	CC	CU	CAA	CAG	CAC	CAU
U	UA	UG	UC	UU	CGA	CGG	CGC	CGU
					CCA	CCG	CCC	CCU
					CUA	CUG	CUC	CUU
					UAA	UAG	UAC	UAU
					UGA	UGG	UGC	UGU
					UCA	UCG	UCC	UCU
					UUA	UUG	UUC	UUU

The first experimental evidence in support to the concept of triplet code is provided by **Crick** and coworkers in 1961. During their experiments, when they added or deleted single or double base pairs in a particular region of DNA of T_4 bacteriophages of *E.coli*, they found that such bacteriophages ceased to perform their normal functions. However, bacteriophages with addition or deletion of three base pairs in DNA molecule, had performed normal functions. From this experiment, they concluded that a genetic code is in **triplet** form, because the addition of one or two nucleotides has put the reading of the code out of order, while the addition of third nucleotide resulted in a return to the proper reading of the message.

22.2 METHODS OF CRYPTOANALYSIS OF GENETIC CODE OR METHODS OF CRACKING OF GENETIC CODE

The genetic code has been cracked or deciphered by the following kinds of approaches:

1. The *in vitro* Codon Assignment

Marshall Nirenberg in 1961 first of all, provided the means for a much more rapid decipherment of the genetic code. He made *in vitro* studies on the incorporation of radioactive amino acids in cell free protein synthetic systems containing artificial (synthetic) ribopolynucleotides or mRNA. A cell free system for protein synthesis includes ribosomes, enzymes, tRNA, etc. To produce such a cell free protein synthetic system, the protein synthesizing components of broken cell (usually *E. coli*) were separated from the remainder by gentle centrifugation. During these manipulations natural mRNA is subjected to mechanical and enzymatic break down. Artificial messenger RNAs were then introduced. The artificial mRNA was prepared for each nitrogen base with the aid of a **polynucleotide phosphorylase enzyme** obtained from *Azobacter vinelandii* or *Micrococcus lysodeikticus*. The enzyme differed from RNA polymerase enzyme in not requiring the presence of DNA as a primer or template for the synthesis of RNA. Thus **Nirenberg** prepared a **polyuridylic acid** (UUUU...), **polycytidylic acid** (CCCCC...), **polyadenylic acid** (AAAAA...) and **polyguanylic acid** (GGGGG...) from uracil, cytosine, adenine and guanine respectively. When he introduced these artificial homopolymeric polyribonucleotides or mRNA (*e.g.*, poly U, poly C, poly A and poly G acids) in different cell free protein synthetic systems of *E. coli* containing radioactive amino acids, he found that each artificial mRNA stimulated the synthesis of polypeptides of single kind of amino acids. For example, poly U acid stimulates the *in vitro* synthesis of monotonous polypeptide-namely polyphenylalanine whose amino acid residues were phenylalanine. Therefore, he concluded that a sequence of UUU coded for phenylalanine. Likewise because polycytidylic acid was found to direct synthesis of polyproline hence, the sequence of CCC codes designates proline and because, polyadenylic acid directs synthesis of polylysine, so the sequence of AAA designates lysine. Later on the sequence of GGG was found to specify glycine.

In this way four of 64 codes or codons were easily accounted for. In order to gain some insight into the meaning of the remaining 60 codons containing more than one kind of nucleotide, **Nirenberg** continued these experiments by using artificially synthesized random ribopolynucleotides containing two, three or four different nucleotide constituents. By suing artificial mRNAs, *viz.*, poly UA, poly UC, and poly UG, he cracked the codes for arginine, alanine, serine, proline, tyrosine, isoleucine, valine, leucine, cysteine, tryptophan, glycine, methionine and glutamic acid.

After learning of Nirenberg's first success with poly U, **Ochoa** and his collaborators carried out entirely analogous sets of decoding experiments in which they used artificial random ribopolynucleotides. Through the parallel efforts of these two research groups the empirical formula of many amino acid codes or codon became known within a year or so. But this work could not establish the actual sequence of the nucleotides within any codon, except for UUU, CCC, AAA and GGG.

In order to ascertain that which structural isomer of a codon of a given empirical formula designates which amino acid, artificial mRNAs of known sequence were employed. In 1965, **H. G. Khorana** first of all, succeeded in synthesizing polyribonucleotides or mRNA of known sequences and he synthesized an alternating copolymer such as—UGUGUG—UGU—. Use of the particular alternating polynucleotide as a mRNA in the *in vitro* protein-synthesizing system give rise to the formation of the alternating polypeptide (*e.g.*, valine-cysteine-valine-cysteine) evidently directed by the codon sequence—UGU-GUG-UGU-GUG. This result established that the UUG (lucine) codon is not UGU, and that neither the UUG (tryptophan) nor the UGG (glycine) codon is GUG, but UUG (valine) is UGU, and GUG is a cysteine synonym, or that UUG (cysteine) is UGU and GUG is a valine synonym. Thus, **Khorana** determined the exact sequence of nucleotides in various genetic codons which discovered either by Nirenberg or by himself.

In 1964, while **Khorana** was just completing the difficult synthesis of the first artificial ribopolynucleotides of defined sequence, **Nirenberg** made a second discovery that made possible a rapid culmination of the code-breaking efforts. He found that addition of simple **trinucleotides** of known base sequences to ribosomes would cause these ribosomes to bind that, and only that, aminoacy-tRNA which carries the anticodon complementary to the trinucleotide added to the reaction mixture. For example, the trinucleotide GCC was found to be active in promoting the binding of alanyl-tRNA*ala* but not of any other aminoacyl-tRNA and it was, therefore, concluded that GCC is a codon for alanine. These studies enabled the preparation of the complete genetic code dictionary.

2. The *in vivo* Codon Assignment

The cell free protein synthetic systems, though have proved of great significance in decipheriment of the genetic code, but they could note tell us whether the genetic code so deciphered is used in the living systems of all organisms also. Three kinds of techniques are used by different molecular biologists to determine whether the same code is also used *in vivo* (*a*) amino acid replacement studies (*e.g.*, tryptophan synthetase synthesis in *E. coli* (**Yanofsky** *et al* 1963) and haemoglobin synthesis in humans), (*b*) frame shift mutations (*e.g.*, investigations of **Terzaghi** *et al* 1966, on lysozyme enzyme of T_4 bacteriophages, and (*c*) comparison of a DNA or mRNA polynucleotide cryptogram with its corresponding polypeptide clear text (*e.g.*, comparison of amino acid sequence of the R_{17} bacteriophage coat protein with the nucleotide sequence of the R_{17} mRNA in the region of the molecule that dictates coat-protein synthesis by **S. Cory** *et al* 1970).

Thus, *in vitro* and *in vivo* studies, so far described, gave the way to formulate a code table for twenty amino acids as follows:

Table 22.2. The genetic dictionary. The trinucleotide codons are written in the 5′ → 3′ direction.

First base	Second base				Third base
	U	C	A	G	
U	UUU } Phe UUC UUA } Leu UUG	UCU } Ser UCC UCA UCG	UAU } Tyr UAC UAA } Non-sense codon UAG	UGU } Cys UGC UGA } Nonsense codon UGG } Try	U C A G
C	CUU } Leu CUC CUA CUG	CCU } Pro CCC CCA CCG	CAU } His CAC CAA } Gin CAG	CGU } Arg CGC CGA CGG	U C A G
A	AUU } Ileu AUC AUA AUG*Met	ACU } Thr ACC ACA ACG	AAU } Asn AAC AAA } Lys AAG	AGU } Ser AGC AGA } Arg AGG	U C A G
G	GUU } Val GUC GUA GUG	GCU } Ala GCC GCA GCG	GAU } Asp GAC GAA } Glu GAG	GGU } Gly GGC GGA GGG	U C A G

* AUG—Met chain initiation codon;

The codon assignments given in Table 22.2 have been verified in the most direct way possible. In 1972, **W. Fiers** and his associates announced the complete nucleotide sequence of the gene coding for the coat protein of the small RNA phage MS2. Since the sequence of 129 amino acids in the protein was already known, a direct comparison between amino acid and nucleotide sequences was possible.

Patterns to the genetic code. A notable pattern emerged when the genetic code of above discussed table was studied. First, aminoacids with similar structural properties tend to have related codons. Thus the aspartic acid codons (GAU and GAC) are similar to glutamic acid codons (GAA and GAG); similarly, the codons for the aromatic amino acids phenylalanine (UUU, UUC), tyrosine (UAU, UAC) and tryptophan (UGG) all begins with uracil. This feature of the code is thought to have evolved to minimize the consequences of mistakes made during translation or of mutagenic base substitutions. If an amino acid in a protein is erroneously replaced by one with similar properties, the protein may still be functional.

22.3 CHARACTERISTICS OF TRIPLET CODON

The genetic dictionary of mRNA codons reveals following important features of triplet codons:

1. Degeneracy. The code contains many synonyms, in that almost all amino acids are represented by more than one codon. For example, the three amino acids—arginine, serine and leucine— each have six synonymous codons. However, for many of the synonym codons specifying the same amino acid the first two bases of the triplet are constant, whereas the third can vary; for example, all codons starting with CC specify proline (CCU, CCC, CCA and CCG) and all codons starting with AC specify threonine. This flexibility in the third nucleotide of a codon may well help to minimize the consequences of errors.

Wobble hypothesis. Examination of genetic code reveals an interesting pattern of degeneracy. In many cases the terminal (3′) nucleotide in a codon can be either of the two pyrimidines, U or C, and still specify the same amino acid. In other cases, the third codon may be either of the two purines, A or G, without changing the specificity. This observation led to the **wobble hypothesis** of **Crick,** in which the greatest importance is assigned to the first two bases, leaving a certain amount of freedom in the third. The result is almost a "2½" base code. The reason for the wobble lies with the geometry of the ribosome and with the properties of the tRNA molecules (**Dyson,** 1978).

2. Non-overlapping. The code is non-overlapping, meaning that no single base can take part in the formation of more than one codon.

3. Ambiguity. The genetic code is ambiguous, that is, same codon may specifies more than one amino acid. For example, UUU codon usually code for phenylalanine but in the presence of streptomycin, may also code for isoleucine, leucine or serine.

4. Commaless. The genetic code is commaless, which means that no codon is reserved for punctuations.

5. Starting codons. AUG codon is called starting or chain initiation codon, because, it initiates the synthesis of polypeptide chain.

6. Non-sense codon. The UAA (also called **ochre,**), UAG (also called **amber** because an investigator who studied the properties of this codon belonged to the Bernstein family, and Bernstein means "amber" in German) and UGA (also called **opal**) codons do not specify any amino-acid, so, are called nonsense codons. They are also called **termination codons,** because, these codons are used by the cell to signal the natural end of translation of a particular polypeptide. However, their inclusion in any mRNA results in the abrupt termination of the message at the point of their location even though the polypeptide chain has not been completed.

7. Universality. The genetic code has been found to be universal, because, same code applies in all kinds of living systems.

REVISION QUESTIONS

1. What is a codon ? How is it related to a cistron ? What is meant by the genetic code ?
2. List the main features of the genetic code.
3. Describe how the genetic code was deciphered.
4. One of the more popular early proposals for the genetic code had three bases per codon, but with each codon overlapping the next by one base. How do the results obtained with alternating RNA copolymers (*e.g.*, UGUGUG......) eliminate that scheme ? What does protein sequencing have to tell us about it ?
5. What observations indicate that the genetic code is identical in probably all forms of life ?
6. What is the basis for the "Wobble Hypothesis" ?

23 Chapter RIBONUCLEIC ACID (RNA)

Most prokaryotic and eukaryotic cells contain another important nucleic acid, the ribonucleic acid (RNA) besides DNA. Some viruses, however, contain no **DNA** but only RNA and in them, RNA being the sole genetic molecule, carries the responsibilities of DNA. Such RNA is called genetic **RNA**. Further in those cells in which the genetic substance is **DNA**, there occur another kind of RNA molecules which are called **non-genetic RNAs** and which have a **DNA dependent synthesis (transcription)** and which ultimately **translate** into the linear sequence of amino acids in a polypeptide chain (protein synthesis). Both kinds of RNAs, *i.e.*, genetic and non-genetic RNAs can be considered under following separate headings:

23.1 GENETIC RNA

Some plant viruses (*e.g.*, TMV, turnip yellow mosaic viruses, wound tumour viruses, etc.,), animal viruses (*e.g.*, influenza viruses, foot and mouth viruses; rous sarcoma viruses, poliomyelitis viruses, reoviruses, etc.) and bacteriophages (*e.g.*, MS_2, etc.) contain ribonucleic acid (RNA) as their genetic material. Like DNA, RNA is polymeric nucleic acid of four monomeric **ribotids** or **ribonucleotids**.

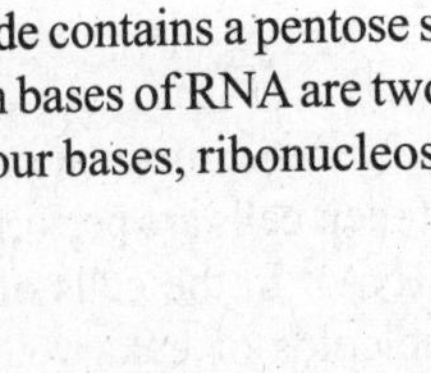

HOCH$_2$ O H H H H OH OH OH

Fig. 23.1. Chemical formula of D-ribose.

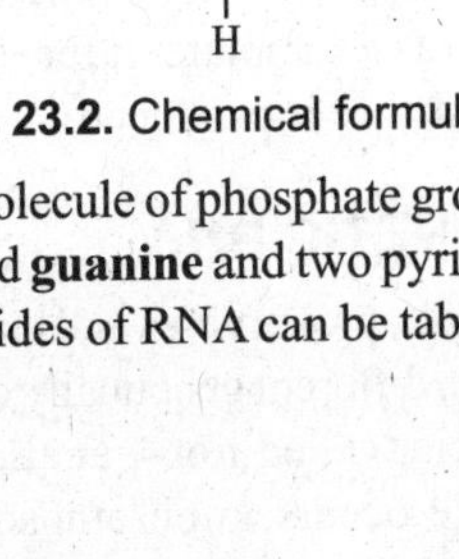

O C H—N C—H O=C C—H N H

Fig. 23.2. Chemical formula of Uracil.

Each ribonucleotide contains a pentose sugar (**D-ribose**); a molecule of phosphate group and a nitrogen base. The nitrogen bases of RNA are two purines, **adenine** and **guanine** and two pyrimidines, **cytosine** and **uracil**. The four bases, ribonucleosides and ribonucleotides of RNA can be tabulated as follows:

Table 23.1. Four nitrogen bases, ribonucleosides and ribonucleotides of RNA

Base	Ribonucleoside	Ribonucleotide	Abbreviation for ribonucleotide
1. Adenine (A)	Adenosine	Adenylic acid (Adenosine monophosphate)	AMP
2. Guanine (G)	Guanosine	Guanylic acid (Guanosine monophosphate)	GMP
3. Cytosine (C)	Cytidine	Cytidylic acid (Cytidine monophosphate)	CMP
4. Uracil (U)	Uridine	Uridylic acid (Uridine monophosphate)	UPM

The four ribonucleotides also occur freely in nucleoplasm but in the form of triphosphates of ribonucleosides such as adenosine triphosphate (ATP), guanosine triphosphate (GTP), cytidine triphosphate (CTP), and uridine triphosphate (UTP).

Molecular Structure of RNA

RNA molecule may be either single-stranded or double stranded but not helical like DNA molecule. **Single stranded** RNA occurs as genetic material in plant viruses (*e.g.*, TMV, TYM), animal viruses *e.g.*, influenza viruses, foot and mouth viruses, rous sarcoma viruses, poliomyelitis viruses and bacteriophages (*e.g.*, MS_2). The double stranded but non-helical RNA occurs as the genetic material in some plant viruses (*e.g.*, reoviruses). Each strand of RNA is polynucleotidic, that is, made up of many ribonucleotides. In the polynucleotide strand of RNA, the ribose and phosphoric acids of nucleotides remain linked by phosphodiester bonds.

Replication of Genetic RNA

The genetic RNA of viruses is self-replicating, that is, it can produce its own replica by itself. So its, mode of replication is called **RNA-dependent RNA synthesis**. The genetical research on genetic RNA has revealed following facts about it:

1. The viral RNA functions directly as a messenger RNA which, in association with the ribosomal apparatus of the host, directs the synthesis of both the **RNA polymerase enzyme** (require for RNA replication) and the proteins of the viral coat.
2. With the mediation of RNA polymerase and on the standard base-pairing principles, the viral RNA serves as a template in the synthesis of a complementary RNA chain and thus a double stranded structure is produced.

23.2 NON-GENETIC RNA

In the organisms (*viz.*, prokaryotes and eukaryotes), where coded genetic informations are contained in the DNA molecule, different genetically controlled functions of their cells are performed by a different kind of nucleic acid, called **non-genetic ribonucleic acid** (RNA). In the cells of such organisms, the DNA molecule occurs in chromosome of nucleus or nucleoids of eukaryotes or prokaryotes respectively and process of protein synthesis occurs in the cytoplasm. It is investigated that a DNA molecule does not leave the nucleus to participate directly in the process of protein synthesis, but employs different types of non-genetic ribonucleic acid molecules for carrying its genetic informations from the nucleus to the site of protein synthesis, *i.e.*, ribosomes. Thus, the DNA molecule acts as a template for the synthesis of different non-genetic RNA molecules which copy down the coded genetic informations of DNA molecule during their DNA dependent synthesis (*i.e.*, **transcription**).

Chemical Composition of Non-Genetic Ribonucleic Acid (RNA)

Chemically the non-genetic RNA is closely related with DNA. However, the non-genetic RNA is a single strand polymer of ribonucleotide units and is composed of phosphoric acid, ribose (pentose sugar) and nitrogen bases, which are purines (adenine and guanine) and pyrimidines (cytosine and uracil). The molecular weights of the various RNA molecules vary from about 25,000 to over one million. Its base composition does not follow the base composition of DNA although, in general, the proportion of A + C roughly equals G + U, as shown in the Table 23.2.

Table 23.2. Base ratios of RNA from various sources (as molar percentages) (From Hall et al 1974)

Source	Adenine	Guanine	Cytosine	Uracil
1. *Allium cepa* (onion seed)	24.9	29.8	24.7	20.6
2. *Phaseolus vulgaris* (bean seed)	24.9	31.4	24.1	19.6
3. *Cucurbita pepo* (pumpkin seed)	25.2	30.6	24.8	19.4
4. Ox liver	17.1	27.3	33.9	21.7
5. Yeast	25.4	24.6	22.6	27.4
6. *E. coli*	25.3	28.8	24.7	21.2

Further, some RNA molecules contain significant proportions of some methylated bases and an unusual nucleoside known as pseudouridine (ψU), in which the glycosidic bond is associated with position 5 of uracil rather than position z.

Comparison between DNA Replication and Transcription

The replication and transcription are two chief activities of DNA and they should be compared at the outset in the following manner:

1. In DNA replication an enzyme (or enzyme complex) matches up complementary deoxyribonucleoside triphosphates with a DNA template according to Watson-Crick pairing rules and the bases are polymerized to form a daughter DNA molecule. In DNA transcription a different enzyme, called **DNA-dependent RNA polymerase** mediates a similar process, except that complementary ribonucleoside triphosphates are matched with the DNA template and RNA polymers are formed. The base uracil (U) replaces thymine in RNA but, otherwise the DNA strand is faithfully copied. The RNA copy has the opposite polarity from the template so that for example the sequence $\xrightarrow{\text{TACAAC}}$ in DNA is transcribed as $\xleftarrow{\text{AUGUUG}}$ in RNA.
2. The RNA transcripts do not ordinarily remain hydrogen-bonded with their DNA templates as DNA daughter strands do. Instead, they "peel off" the template as they are formed, thus becoming available to participate in protein synthesis.
3. DNA of prokaryotes (*E. coli*) and eukaryotes has one or few initiation points for DNA replication, so that, at least large portions of genome are copied into enormous daughter DNA molecules. In contrast, the synthesis of RNA molecules is initiated at close intervals along the DNA and thus relatively short RNA copies are produced.

4. Lastly, replication and transcription have to serve two different functions. The purpose of replication is to conserve the entire genome for next generation, whereas the purpose of transcription is to make RNA copies of individual genes that the cell can use in the biochemistry. The copies are themselves not endowed with the same kind of permanence as the genetic material; instead, they are typically degraded by cellular nucleases once their functional usefulness has been spent.

23.3 RNA POLYMERASE ENZYMES

DNA-dependent RNA polymerase enzymes are remarkable enzymes. The recognize individual bases in DNA, select the appropriate complementary ribonucleotides, catalyze phosphodiester bond formation between ribonucleotides, pick the correct DNA strand to be transcribed, and initiate transcription at appropriate promoter sites along the chromosome. RNA polymerases of prokaryotes and eukaryotes have following characteristics:

(a) RNA Polymerases from Prokaryotes and Organelles

The isolated polymerase enzyme from *E. coli*, is one of the largest soluble proteins yet studied. It measures about 100 Å in diameter and has a molecular weight of about 490,000 daltons. RNA polymerase of *E. coli* is **holoenzyme** and is composed of two main subunits, a smaller subunit called **sigma factor** (σ) and a large unit called **core polymerase** which is composed of two **alpha**

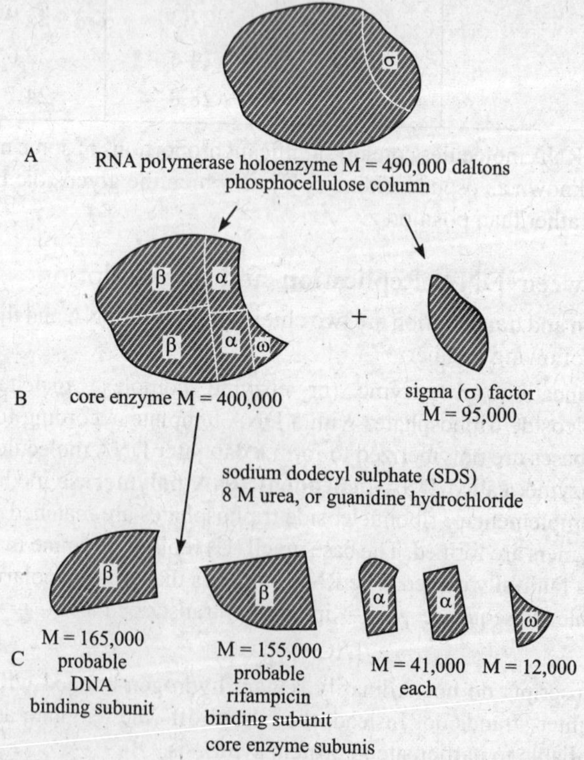

Fig. 23.3. The *E. coli* DNA-dependent RNA polymerase. All subunits are highly schematic: (A) Intact molecule or holoenzyme (B) The separated core enzyme and sigma units, (C) Subunits of the core enzyme. (after Goodenough and Levine, 1974)

(α) **units**, two **beta** (β) **units** and a **omega** (ω) **unit** (*i.e.*, core enzyme can be represented by formulae $\beta\beta'.\alpha_2\omega$). The core enzyme alone is capable of making a RNA copy of DNA, but it begins transcription at random along the template and copies both DNA strands. When sigma factor is added back to core enzyme, transcription begins at the true promoter sites and on the correct strand. A sigma factor is thought to initiate the transcription process by (1) recognizing a promoter region, possibly by its base sequence or possibly by its tertiary structure, and (2) mediating the binding of a core enzyme to the promoter. After a core enzyme is bound and begins to transcribe the continuous sequence into RNA the sigma is thought to be released so that it can associate with another core enzyme.

Out of 5 subunits of core enzyme, only β' subunit is directly involved in the binding of RNA polymerase to DNA. The others are thought to play still undefined roles in transcription, perhaps in its regulation. Lastly, the RNA polymerase of *E. coli* and of certain chloroplasts and mitochondria is sensitive to the antibiotic **rifampicin** which probably combines with the β subunit of the *E. coli* enzyme. However, RNA polymerases from higher plant chloroplasts and T, bacteriophages are found to be rifampicin-resistant.

(b) RNA Polymerases from Eukaryotes

In prokaryotes, while single RNA polymerase seems to handle all transcription, eukaryotic cells use a family of RNA polymerases consisting of at least three distinctly different enzymes, namely **Class A-, Class B-** and **Class C- RNA polymerases.** The purpose is presumably to subdivide the task and to provide flexible controls.

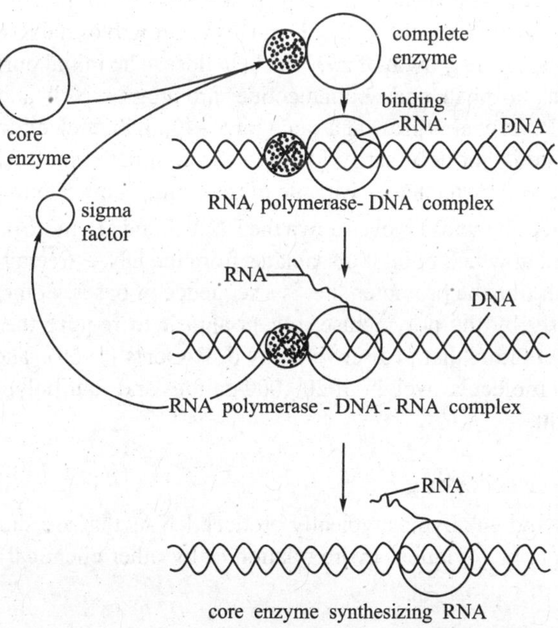

Fig. 23.4. Role of sigma factor and core enzyme of RNA polymerase of *E. coli* during transcription (after Lewin).

Class A-RNA polymerases are believed to be localized exclusively in the nucleolus and involved in the synthesis of ribosomal RNAs: Class B- and Class C-RNA polymerases are found outside the nucleolus and carry out the rest of the nuclear transcription: Class B-RNA polymerases produce mRNA and Class C-RNA polymerases produce tRNAs. All three enzymes have molecular weight greater than 500,000 and are presumed to be composed of subunits, but their molecular structures are not known like the prokaryotic enzymes.

RNA Synthesis and Chain Termination

One strand or two ? For transcription process entire chromosome (DNA) does not unwind and rewind but instead a local denaturation of the DNA helix takes place so that only those bases are exposed that constitute the gene to be transcribed. Further, no one strand of DNA has a monopoly on transcription. Rather, some of the genes are transcribed from one strand while others are transcribed from the alternate strand. In other words, the same gene is not ordinarily transcribed in both strands, an event that would lead to two messages bearing the same information in different (but complimentary) languages.

Start and stop signals. The role of the prokaryotic σ factor of RNA polymerase is to recognize start signals within the DNA molecule. These regions are called **promoter sites.** The promoter sites are not identical to each other, even though all attract the same RNA polymerase. The difference from one site to another gives some of them a competitive advantage, resulting in more frequent transcription of the associated DNA. Since not all genetic information need not to be turned into protein at the same rate, this difference in promoters presumably serves a useful function.

The recognition (promoter) site for RNA polymerase is not transcribed. Rather, as the polymerase begins to move down the gene it skips the first six or seven bases. Actual RNA initiation takes place. Once RNA synthesis is initiated, the first nucleoside triphosphate to be incorporated into the RNA chain is usually either ATP or GTP. This means (since the first base in the transcript is purine) that the first base of a gene will be a pyrimidine, either T or C in DNA. Growth of the RNA chain then proceeds in a $5' \rightarrow 3'$ direction, just as the growth of a DNA chain does. The initial purine is, therefore, found as a ribonucleoside 5′-triphosphate and ribonucleotides are progressively added to free 3′-hydroxyl groups. Once initiated, RNA chains grow at a rapid rate—40 to 50 nucleotides per second in *E. coli* at 37°C. The triphosphate is not necessarily found in the completed molecule, because completed RNAs are regularly attacked by nucleases capable of removing some 5′ nucleotides.

Once started, RNA polymerase moves down the DNA strand at a more or less constant rate until it comes to a **stop signal**, at which point it dissociates from the DNA, freeing the newly synthesized RNA strand. Stop signal, like the promoter site, is a sequence of bases. Some of these signals, seem to be recognized directly by the polymerase, others appear to require the help of an additional protein called a **rho** (ρ) **factor**, that is discovered by **J. Roberts** (1969). The rho terminator factor is a protein which has a molecular weight of 200,000 daltons and four polypeptide chain of 50,000 daltons molecular weight.

Post-transcriptional Processing

Both prokaryotes and eukaryotes typically produce RNAs that are shortened and chemically modified by deamination, methylation, hydroxylation or by other chemical change after synthesis and before use.

Time of Transcription

In most eukaryotes most transcription occurs only during interphase, a time when the chromosomes are in their highly diffuse state. However, in case of dipteran polytene chromosomes and lampbrush chromosomes of amphibian oocytes, condensed chromosomes are transcribed but, in them transcription occurs only in that portion of chromosome which becomes diffuse due to puff formation in polytene chromosomes or loop formations in lampbrush chromosomes.

23.4 TYPES OF NON-GENETIC RNA

According to their specific functions during the process of protein synthesis, following kinds of non-genetic RNA molecules have been recognized in prokaryotic cells:

(1) Ribosomal RNA (rRNA)

Ribosomal RNA (rRNA or **insoluble RNA** constitutes the largest part (up to 80%) of the total cellular RNA. It is found primarily in the ribosomes although, since it is synthesized in the nucleus it is also detected in that organelle. It contains the four major RNA bases with a slight degree of methylation, and shows differences in the relative proportions of the bases between species. Its molecules appear to be single polynucleotide strands which are unbranched and flexible. At low ionic strength, rRNA behaves as a random coil, but with increasing ionic strength, rRNA behaves as a random coil, but with increasing ionic strength the molecule shows helical regions produced by base pairing between adenine and uracil and guanine and cytosine.

Types and synthesis of rRNA. The eukaryotic cells have four kinds of rRNA molecules, namely **28S rRNA** (the sedimentation constant varies between 25S and 30S depending on the species), **18S rRNA, 5.8S** and **5S rRNA**. The 28S rRNA 5.8S and 5S rRNA occur in 60S ribosomal subunit, while 18S rRNA occurs in 40S ribosomal subunit of 80S ribosomes of eukaryotes. The prokaryotic cells contain three kinds of rRNA molecules, namely **23S rRNA, 16S rRNA** and **5S rRNA**. The 23S rRNA and 5S rRNA occur in 50S ribosomal subunit, while 16S rRNA occur in 30S ribosomal subunit of 70S ribosomes of prokaryotes. In eukaryotic cells of plants and animals the 18S and 28S rRNA molecules are transcribed by rDNA or nucleolar organizer (NO) region of chromosomes and nucleolus acts as a site of synthesis and maturation of these rRNA molecules. 5S rRNA is transcribed by rDNA which occur outside the nucleolar organizer region (For details see the chapter of ribosomes.)

The functions of rRNA molecules are still little understood. However, they are supposed to have some definite role in protein synthetic process, besides being the major constituent molecules of ribosomes.

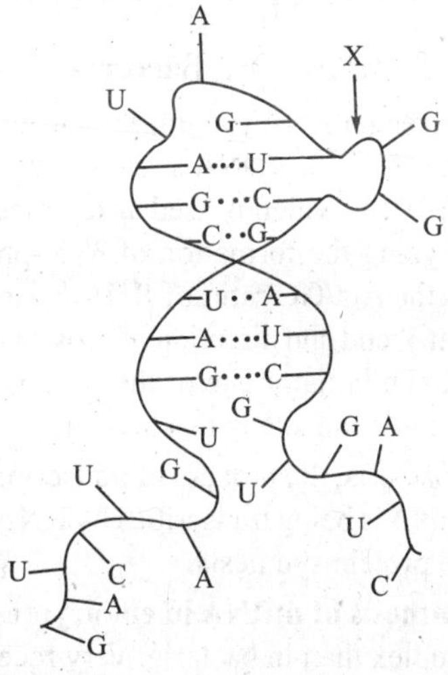

Fig. 23.5. The molecular (*i.e.*, secondary) structure of rRNA showing a helical region with complimentary base pairing and a looped outer region of the helix at X (Davidson, 1972).

(2) Messenger RNA (mRNA)

The RNA molecules which are transcribed from large number of genes of the total genome (*i.e.*, 99 per cent genes of the total genome of *E. coli*), and have base sequence complementary to DNA, carry DNA's genetic information for the assembly of amino acids into the polypeptide chains (protein molecules) to the cytoplasmic sites of protein synthesis, the ribosomes, to which they become associated to participate in codon anticodon interactions with tRNA, are called **informational** or **messenger RNAs (mRNA)**. The name messenger RNA has been proposed by **Jacob** and **Monod** (1961). The molecule of a mRNA is single-stranded like the rRNA molecule and it is DNA-like in its base composition so that GC contents of mRNA correspond to the GC contents of the genome's total DNA.

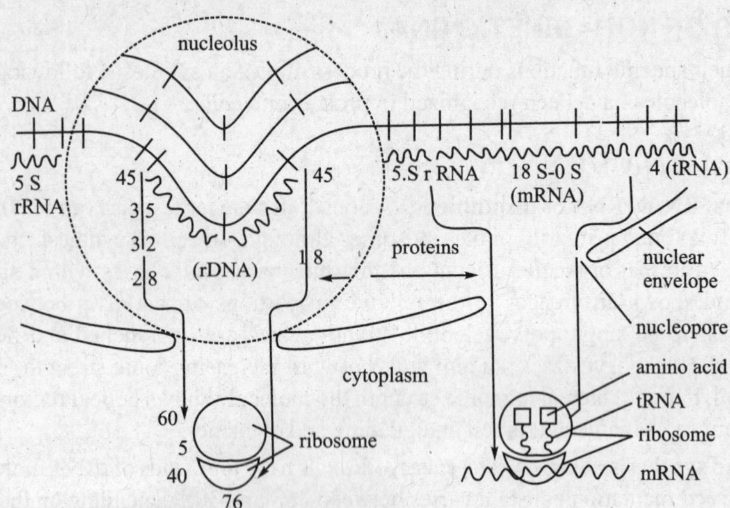

Fig. 23.6. Diagram of the transcription and transport of nuclear RNAs in a eukaryotic cell and participation of tRNA and mRNA in protein synthesis (after De Robertis *et al* 1970).

mRNA Synthesis in Bacteria

Messenger RNA is **complementary** to chromosomal DNA; it forms RNA-DNA hybrids after separation of the two DNA strands. Synthesis of mRNA is accomplished with only one of the two strands of DNA, which is used as template. The enzyme RNA polymerase joins the ribonucleotides, thus catalyzing the formation of 3′-5′-phosphodiester bonds that form the RNA backbone. In this synthesis the AU/GC ratio of RNA is similar to the AT/GC ratio of DNA. The mRNA synthesis is initiated at 5′ end and direction of growth is from the 5′ end to 3′ end. In bacteria, the RNA polymerase attaches to an initiator site of the structural gene, in the promoter and it catalyzes mRNA synthesis until a termination site is reached.

In bacteria, the process of transcription of mRNA is simultaneous with translation, *i.e.,* as soon as the mRNA is being transcribed by RNA polymerases the ribosomes become attached to the mRNA to initiate protein synthesis.

Synthesis of mRNA in eukaryotes. The origin and fate of mRNA in eukaryotic cells is much more complex than in bacteria. Very recently, it has been found that the formation of a functionally active mRNA molecule is the consequence of a complex series of steps that comprise: (1) the actual transcription of DNA into mRNA precursors, (2) the intranuclear processing (tailoring) of these precursors, and (3) the transport of the mRNAs into the cytoplasm and their association with ribosomes to initiate the process of translation of protein synthesis. Consequently synthesis of mRNA molecules includes following events:

1. Heterogeneous nuclear RNA. It has been suggested that mRNA is synthesized in the nucleus as the part of a heterogeneous population of large RNA molecules which constitute the so called **heterogeneous nuclear RNA (het-RNA** or **Hn-RNA)**. The Hn-RNA is also called high molecular weight RNA (**HMW-RNA**) or **DNA-like RNA (dRNA)**. The molecules of Hn-RNA range in size from 5×10^5 to 10^7 daltons and are degraded for the most part within the nucleus at a relatively rapid rate (**Darnell**, 1968). Only about 20 per cent of the Hn-RNA in terms of total nucleotide, is not degraded and has been postulated to convert into mRNA molecules.

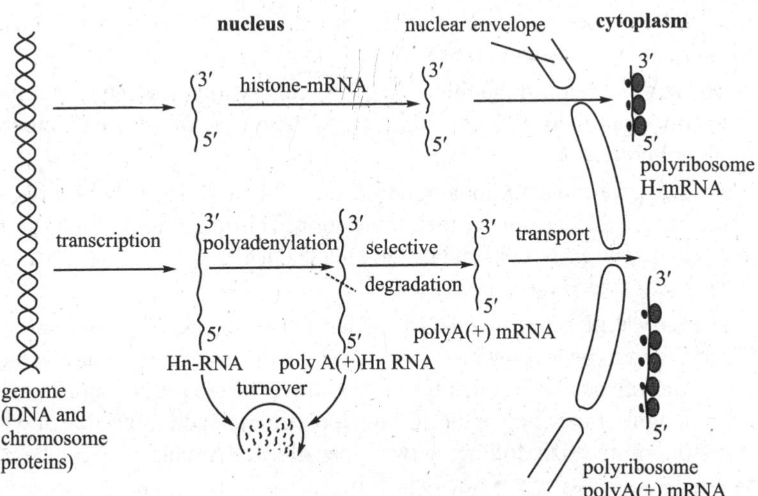

Fig. 23.7. Synthesis and processing of heterogeneous nuclear RNA (Hn-RNA), poly-A (+) messenger RNA (Poly-A (+) (mRNA) and histone-messenger RNA (histone mRNA). The steps of transcription, polyadenylation, selective degradation and transport of mRNA into cytoplasm are indicated (after De Robertis *et al* 1975).

Hn RNA molecules occur in nucleoplasm outside the nucleolus and they contain DNA-like base composition and readily hybridizes with DNA.

Before leaving the nucleus, eukaryotic mRNAs undergo three kinds of modifications: the addition of polyadenylate (Poly A) at the 3′ end; the addition of "caps" of special nucleotides at the 5′ end; and methylation of nucleotides at a few interval sites. The finished product is typically translated into a single polypeptide chain.

2. Polyadenylation. Recently it has been discovered that Hn-RNA contains a sequence of polyadenylic acid (poly A), approximately 200 nucleotides long at their 3′ end (**Kates**, 1970; **Lim** and **Canellakis**, 1970; **Edmons** *et al.*, 1971, and, **Darnell** *et al* 1971). This poly-A sequence is added to the Hn-RNA after the transcription is completed (**Darnell** *et al* 1971), and is attached to the 3′ — end of the RNA molecule (**Perry** *et al.*, 1973). **De Robertis** *et al* 1975) have suggested that once the Hn-RNA molecule is transcribed from DNA, the poly A sequence is added, in a stepwise fashion by the action of a **poly-A synthetase**. Simultaneous with or after polyadenylation and starting from the 5′ end a selective degradation of the Hn-RNA molecules takes place by the action of nucleases. The final product is **poly (+) mRNA**, which will finally reach the cytoplasm. Most of the eukaryotic mRNA molecules contain a 3′ terminal poly-A chain. The post-transcriptional attachment of poly-A may be a special step in the processing of mRNA and may be related either to its transport to the cytoplasm or to its greater longevity, since in some experimental systems survival time of the mRNA is very much shortened in the absence of a poly-A tail (**Dyson.** 1978).

Recently, it is also discovered that the mRNAs for the histones (called **histone mRNAs**) are directly transcribed from repetitive sequences in the DNA without the need for a giant precursor molecule (Hn-RNA) or polyadenylation. It has been demonstrated that the histone mRNAs enter the cytoplasm without delay, whereas the poly-A (+) mRNAs have a 15 minute delay before appearing attached to the polyribosomes. The long period has been attributed to the processing steps that poly-A (+) mRNAs undergo before passing into the cytoplasm.

3. 5′ capping. At the other end of the eukaryotic message, one usually finds a **5′ cap**. The cap consists of a methylated guanylate (*i.e.*, 7-methylguanosine triphosphate) stuck onto the chain "backward" (5′ to 5′) from the rest of the nucleotides. This configuration is abbreviated M^7 G (5′) pp′ (5′) X, where X is the normal 5′ terminus. In addition to 7-methylguanosine, cap structures include methylation of the first and sometimes second "normal" nucleotides at their 2′ OH. The presence of a cap seems to facilitate translation (see **Dyson,** 1978).

4. Methylation. The third modification of the eukaryotic message is **methylation** of internal adenylate nucleotides at their N-6 position (*i.e.*, at the amine of adenine's number 6 carbon). Its function is still unknown.

Besides these post-transcriptional modifications, eukaryotic mRNAs differ from prokaryotic mRNAs in leaving the nucleus prior to their translation. This migration is found to involve nucleolus. Current view is that new mRNAs associate with nucleolar-derived ribosomal precursors to facilitate exit from the nucleus (see **Dyson,** 1978).

Heterogeneity and types of mRNA. When the total mRNA population of an organism is considered, it is found to be heterogeneous in size, showing a wide range of S values of 6 to 30. This property of mRNA reflects the fact that the size or length of the mRNA molecule is directly related with the size or length of the codons for different protein molecules, the size of which may be quite variable. According to the size, following two types of mRNA molecules can be recognized:

(a) Monocistronic mRNA. Mostly the mRNA carries the codons of single cistron, (*i.e.*, codes for one complete protein molecule) of the DNA. Such mRNA molecule is called **monocistronic mRNA**. For example, for the synthesis of a polypeptide chain of 300 to 500 amino acid residues, a monocistronic mRNA of *E. coli* contains 900 to 1500 nucleotides in its molecule.

(b) Polygenic or **polycistronic mRNA**. Sometimes a mRNA molecule carries the codes from several adjacent DNA cistrons and become much longer in size. This type of mRNA is called **polygenic** or **polycistronic mRNA.** For example, for the metabolism of the histidine protein the cell synthesizes about 10 specific enzymatic proteins and a mRNA in this case may carry codons for all the 10 enzymes.

Life-span of mRNA. In most prokaryotic and eukaryotic cells, mRNA has short life-time. For example, the average life of mRNA of *E. coli* is about 2 minutes because it is attacked by the cytoplasmic ribonuclease enzyme. So that, at most times, mRNA makes up only 5% of the total cellular RNA. Likewise, in most eukaryotes the average life span of mRNA is one to four hours. However, in both bacteria and eukaryotes mRNAs are known that are metabolically stable and are apparently resistant to nucleases and survive for long period of time. For example, mRNA with life time of six hours has been detected in the bacterium *Bacillus cerus* at a time when the cells are induced to become long lived spores. Likewise, in differentiating eukaryotic cells mRNAs with a life time of days have been detected. For example, in the immature red blood cells (reticulocytes) of the mammals the mRNA is synthesized originally by the nucleus in early stages and expelled to the cytoplasm. In later stages the nuclei of maturing reticulocytes degenerate but the mRNA exists up to 2 days for prolong utilization in the synthesis of globin protein of haemoglobin. Further, in extreme cases, such as in the state of dormancy adopted by many animal eggs and plant seeds, mRNA is maintained in a stable form for the months or even years.

Informosomes. In the eukaryotic cells, the stability to the mRNA is provided by certain proteins. Several investigators, *e.g.,* **Spirin, Beltisina** and **Lerman** (1965), **Perry** and **Kelley** (1968) and **Henshaw** (1968) have reported that in certain eukaryotic cells the mRNA does not enter in the cytoplasm as a naked RNA strand but often remains ensheathed by certain proteins. **Spirin** (1965) has coined a new term **informosomes** to this mRNA and protein complex. The informosome is used by the cell when there is a delay in the translation. For instance, in the embryo the genetic expression is manifested late during organogenesis. In such cases mRNA occurs in the form of informosomes. The proteins of informosomes protect the mRNA from the degrading actions of the enzyme, ribonuclease. These proteins may also control the synthesis at the level of the translation and thus may regulate or modulate the protein synthetic process.

(3) Transfer RNA (tRNA)

The RNA which possesses the capacity to combine specifically with only one amino acid in a reaction mediated by a set of amino acid—specific enzymes called **aminoacyl-tRNA synthetases;** transfers that amino acid from the "amino acid pool" to the site of protein synthesis and recognises the codons of the mRNA is known as the **soluble RNA** (sRNA) or **transfer RNA (tRNA)**. Thus tRNA molecule acts as an interpreter of genetic code and has to perform several highly complex functions during protein synthesis—it interacts with a specific synthetase enzyme, possesses a site for binding an amino acid, possesses a second site for interacting with a ribosome, and contains an anticodon that must be expected to the codons of mRNA.

Structure and maturation of tRNA. Th tRNA molecules that perform all these functions account for 10 to 50 per cent of the total RNA in *E. coli.* Each tRNA has a sedimentation coefficient of 4S and contains 75 to 85 nucleotides. The sequence of alanine tRNA was first of all elucidated by **R. W. Holley** and collaborators in 1965. The primary structure of some 30 tRNA, from *E. coli* to mammalian liver cells to higher plant cells, is already known (**Smith,** 1973). Like the rRNA and mRNA molecules, the molecules of tRNA are found to be matured or tailored in the nucleus prior to their movement to the cytoplasm. For example, in *E. coli* the precursors of tRNA molecules have been isolated, each of which has about 40 extranucleotides, principally at 5′ end but also at the 3′ end. These extra nucleotides are subsequently cleaved off by still unidentified enzymes to yield a molecule of the final 70 to 80 nucleotide size.

Following such large scale tailoring each tRNA molecule is more delicately modified before it becomes fully active. Three bases, 5′-CCA-3′ are added to the 3′ end of every tRNA molecule, regardless of its amino-acid affinity, by an enzyme called **tRNA phosphorylase**. In addition, specific nucleotides in a given tRNA are transformed into what are called **minor** or **unusual bases** by specific chemical modifications: for example, methyl groups are added at certain positions to yield 3-methyl-cytosine or 1-methyl-guanosine; certain uracils are reduced to dihydrouracil or rearranged into a form, known as pseudoracil; and adenine is deaminated to yield inosine.

The significance of these unusual bases of tRNA was understood well by molecular biologists during the construction of two dimentional model from the primary-sequences of nucleotides of known tRNA. Thus, it was realized that most bases of tRNA pair according to Watson-Crick's pairing rule, but, unusual bases fail to do so because they carry substitutions or alternations in those positions that usually participate in hydrogen bonding. Consequently, the presence of these bases forces the model builder to construct several non-base-paired loops in the tRNA molecule. By working on these **lines, R. Holley** (1968) first of all proposed a **clover leaf model** for yeast tRNA*ala*. The clover leaf model of tRNA because accommodated several of the known functions of tRNA, so it gained general acceptance. A typical clover-leaf model of tRNA (Fig. 23.8) depicts following structural peculiarities:

(*i*) All tRNA molecules contain the same terminal sequence of 5′-CCA-3′ bases at 3′-end of the polynucleotide chain. The last residue, adenylic acid (A), is the **aminoacid attachment site**.

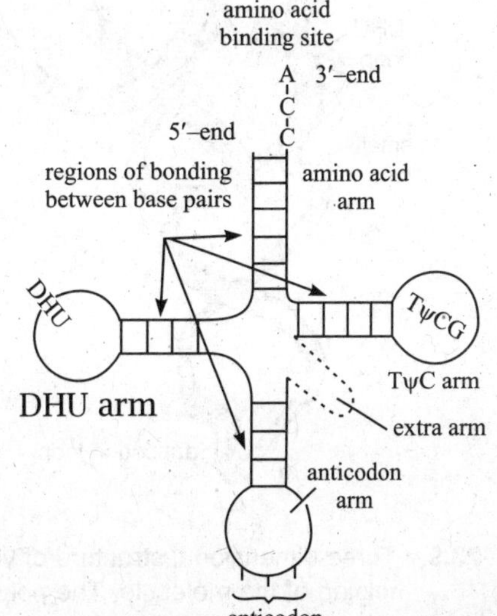

Fig. 23.8. Diagrammatic representation of clover leaf model of yeast alanine tRNA. (ψ–pseydouridine; DHU–dihydrouridine) (after Hall *et al.*, 1974).)

(*ii*) All tRNAs have a loop called TψC arm of seven unpaired bases including pseuouridine. The TψC arm is involved in the binding of tRNA molecules to the ribosomes.

(*iii*) All tRNA molecules contain a site for the recognition of the amino acid activating synthetase enzymes. This is the function of **dihydrouridine loop** or **DHU arm** which is made up of 8 to 12 unpaired bases.

(*iv*) There is one nucleotide triplet in the tRNA molecule which is different in all tRNAs examined. This is the codon **recognition site** or **anticodon** and it is complementary to the corresponding friplet codon of mRNA.

Here, the significance of wobble hypothesis can be observed for according to that concept the third position in the codon is less reliably matched than the others: In particular, either of the two pyrimidines, U or C, might be paired with an anticodon G; and either of the two purines, A or G, might be paired with an anticodon U. (on the other hand, an anticodon C or A in the third position is thought to be rather specific for G or U, respectively in the mRNA). Still more flexibility is derived from the appearance of inosine in the third position of the anticodon, for this base hydrogen bonds to U, A and to C.

(*v*) Some tRNA with long chains may form a short, **extra arm**.

As the clover leaf model is in two-dimensions, whereas the tRNA-synthetase enzyme interaction occurs between molecules that are three dimensional. Very recently, by X-ray diffraction analysis **S. H. Kim** and coworkers (1972, 1973) have proposed a three-dimenstional L-shaped configuration (Fig. 23.9) for a phenylalanine tRNA molecule of yeast cells. According to this model, the two major portions of the L consist of base-paired double helices that are joined by the unpaired segments of the molecule, whereas the anticodon is in one extremity of the L and the amino acid acceptor is in the other. This acceptor end sticks out from the rest of the molecule and may be capable of some degree of movement (**Kim** *et al* 1972).

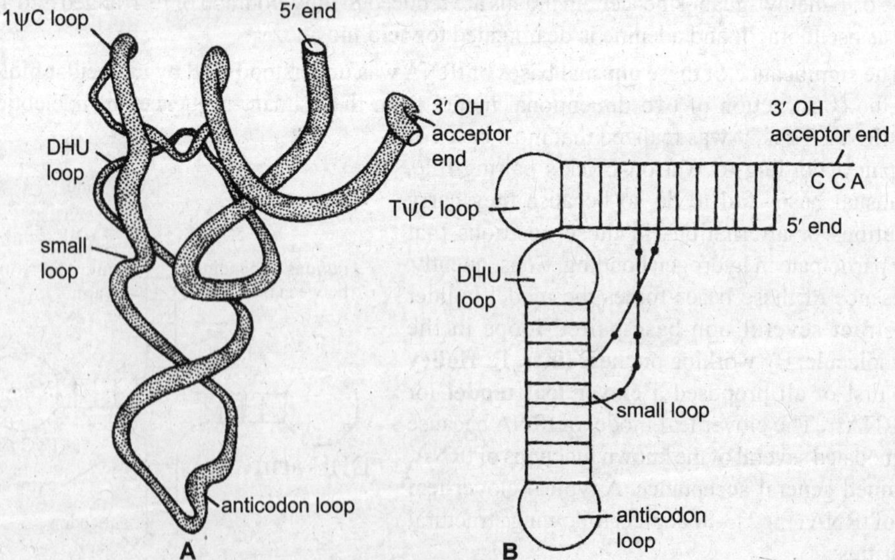

Fig. 23.9. Three dimensional structure of yeast phenylalanine tRNA. A – Actual appearance of the folding of the molecule. The polynucleotide chain is represented as a continuous coiled tube; B – The way that the cloverleaf representation must be transformed in order to show the physical connections between various parts of the molecule. Two double-stranded helical regions are seen, each oriented at the right angles to the other produce an L-shaped structure (after Goodenough and Levine, 1974).

Genes for tRNA. There are probably at least 30 to 40 different tRNA genes and tRNA molecules in *E. coli*. Higher organisms are found to contain 60 tRNA molecules and 60 tRNA genes. Since the cell uses only 20 amino acids in protein synthesis (and probably only 20 synthetase enzymes), it follows that several tRNAs will often have an affinity for the same amino acid. For example, *E. coli* cells contain five species of tRNA for leucine amino acid.

All the tRNA genes constitute for less than 1% of the total genome in both *E. coli* and eukaryotic cells, yet some 10 to 15% of between the number of tRNA genes and gene transcripts, occurs because of following facts— (1) The tRNA molecules are relatively stable compared with many kinds of RNA. (2) The tRNA molecules are transcribed continuously and more quickly by tRNA genes than other RNAs because they are needed in plentiful amounts.

Classification of Genes According to their Transcription in RNA molecules

All the RNA species are transcribed from the corresponding locus in the DNA molecule. Those regions of the genome transcribing the messenger RNAs are called the **structural genes.** The other regions, coding for the different ribosomal RNAs and transfer RNAs are generally called the **determinants for RNA.**

REVISION QUESTIONS

1. How do RNA molecules differ from DNA molecules ?
2. Describe the transcription, processing, and functioning of each of the three main classes of RNA in eukaryotes (that is, mRNA, rRNA and tRNA).
3. Describe the reaction catalyzed by RNA polymerase. What experiment first indicated that only one DNA strand in a gene region is transcribed ?
4. Contrast the prokaryotic and eukaryotic messengers with respect to gene content, relative precursor size, and 5′ and 3′ modifications.
5. Distinguish between each pair of terms listed: codon—anticodon, hnRNA—mRNA and monocistronic mRNA–polycistronic mRNA.

24
Chapter
BIOSYNTHESIS OF PROTEINS

The proteins have significant role in the structural and functional organization of the cell. The structural proteins constitute various cellular components and some extracellular parts such as cuticle and fibres, etc. The functional (*e.g.*, enzymatic and hormonal) proteins control almost all metabolic, biosynthetic, bioenergetic, growth regulating, sensory and reproductive activities of the cell. All the proteins which are required by the cell for its different purposes are synthesized by the cell itself intracellularly.

A cell, however, cannot synthesize all the required proteins of multicellular individual, therefore, different kinds of proteins are synthesized by different types of cell. Thus, the liver cells are specialized for the synthesis of liver and plasma proteins, the β-cells of pancreatic islets are specialized for synthesis of proteins of insulin hormone and cells of pituitary are specialised for synthesis of protein component of pituitary hormone and so on.

24.1 CENTRAL DOGMA AND CENTRAL DOGMA REVERSE

The process of synthesis of protein involves one of the central dogma of molecular biology (Fig. 24.1), which postulates that genetic information flows from nucleic acids to protein. (It was first forwarded by **Crick** in 1958). The first step of this central dogma is known as transcription and does not involve a change of code since DNA and mRNA are complementary. The second step involves a change of code from nucleotide sequences to amino acid sequences and is called translation. It can be illustrated as follows:

$$\text{DNA} \xrightarrow{\text{replication}} \text{DNA} \xrightarrow{\text{transcription}} \text{RNA} \xrightarrow{\text{translation}} \text{Proteins}$$

Thus, according to this central dogma, the flow of information is one way, *i.e.*, from DNA the information is transferred to RNA (mRNA) and from RNA to proteins. In 1968, **Barry Commoner** suggested a circular flow of information, *i.e.*, DNA transcribes RNA, translates into proteins, synthesize RNA and RNA synthesizes DNA, as has been illustrated in following figure:

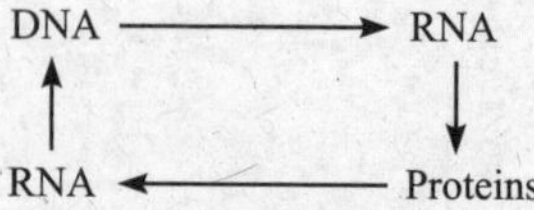

Very recently, **Baltimore** (1970) and **Mizushima** and **Temin** (1970) have reported the existence of an enzyme **"RNA dependent DNA polymerase" (inverse transcriptase)** in certain RNA containing oncogenic viruses and this enzyme could synthesize DNA from a single-stranded RNA template. This tumour viron contains the reverse transcriptase by which a RNA/DNA hybrid molecule can be produced (**Spiegelman *et al.***, 1970). In this way RNA viral genes can be integrated in the genome of the host cell. The viron also contains a DNA polymerase which can replicate the double-stranded

DNA. this exciting finding in molecular biology gave rise to the concept of **"central dogma reverse"** suggesting that the sequence of information flow is not necessrily from DNA to RNA to protein but can also take place from RNA to DNA. The central dogma reverse can be illustrated as follows :

$$\text{DNA} \underset{\text{reverse transcription}}{\overset{\text{transcription}}{\rightleftarrows}} \text{RNA} \xrightarrow{\text{translation}} \text{Proteins}$$

24.2 COMPONENTS OF PROTEIN SYNTHETIC MACHINERY

The process of protein synthesis is complicated and it employs following molecules and cellular organelles:

1. Amino acids,
2. DNA,
3. Non-genetic ribonucleic acids (RNAs),
4. Ribosomes and enzymes.

1. Amino Acids

Because, the proteins are the polymers of amino acids therefore, protein synthetic process requires the amino acids as the raw material. As we have already discussed in the chapter of cytoplasmic matrix, all the naturally occurring proteins of living organisms fundamentally are the polymers of about 20 amino acids. These amino acids occur in the matrix forming an **"amino acid pool"** and are readily available for the process of protein synthesis.

2. DNA

The chromosomal DNA is the master macromolecule of the cell. Its immediate function is the determination of the kind of the protein which a cell has to manufacture. In other words, the process of protein synthesis is initiated, guided, regulated, and controlled by the DNA molecule.

3. Non-Genetic Ribonucleic Acids (RNAs)

In the previous chapter three kinds of non-genetic RNAs, (*i.e.,* rRNA, mRNA and tRNA) have been described. All these three kinds of RNAs take an active part in protein synthesis. Thus, mRNA carries coded informations for protein synthesis—from DNA to the site of protein synthesis, the ribosomes; tRNAs transport activated amino acids from 'amino acid pool' to the site of protein synthesis; where they recognize the triplet codons of mRNA and get attached with that and lastly, rRNA though having no specific function at its disposal like mRNA and tRNA, but there are ample evidences which suggest that rRNA has a general function to perform.

4. Ribosomes and Enzymes

Ribosomes are macromolecular structures which guide the multiple interactions involved in the synthesis of proteins. To direct these interactions ribosomes contain required enzymatic protein factors and ions (for details see Chapter 17, ribosomes), and they function in groups called **polyribosomes** or **polysomes**. The number of ribosomes in a polysome is related to the length of the protein to be synthesized. For example, for the polypeptides of haemoglobin, a pentamer (*i.e.,* five ribosomes) is used. Each ribosome carries a nascent polypeptide chain. In the case of haemoglobin, therefore, five chains are formed at the same time along the mRNA.

Evidence for ribosomes as sites of protein synthesis. The first direct evidence relating ribosomes and protein synthesis was described by **Zamecnik** and coworkers in a series of investigations from 1952 onwards. Radioactive amino acids were injected into rats and at various time intervals after the injection the liver was removed, homogenized and centrifuged to separate the various cell organelles, which were studied for evidence of incorporation of amino acids into proteins. If examined shortly after injection, only the microsomal (ER) fraction contained labelled protein, whereas at later times labelled protein, whereas at later times labelled protein was found in all cell fractions. These results suggested that proteins were first synthesized in the microsomes and then transferred to other parts of the cell. It was later found that isolated microsomal fractions, which were supplemented with ATP, catalysed the incorporation of amino acids into proteins in the presence of the unsedimentable, soluble fraction which provided essential co-factors. Since this pioneer work, cell free systems capable of catalysing amino acid incorporation into protein have been isolated from a variety of species and have been shown to require the following components: ribosomes, the twenty common amino acids, tRNAs, mRNA and ATP generating system, GTP, Mg^{++} and K^+ ions and a supernatant enzyme fraction.

Other Functions of Ribosomes

The functions and other activities of the ribosomes and their subunits are given as follows:

1. Association and dissociation of the ribosomal subunits. When ribosomes are not involved in translation, they exist mostly as their free units. In free polysomes of bacteria and eukaryotes a **ribosome—polysome cycle** has been demonstrated in *E. coli* and in yeast cells by **Kaempfer** (1968, 1969); in reticulocytes by **Colombo** *et al*., (1968) and in liver cells by **Farber** (1969). The two ribosomal subunits exchange at the site of initiation and dissociate at the terminator end (see Fig 24.1). Thus subunits are exchanged and there is a pool of free ribosomal subunits. A dissociation factor (IF_3) of protein nature is involved in the separation of the two ribosomal subunits of *E. coli* at the end of the translation (**Subramanian,** *et al* 1969; **Algranati,** *et al* 1969).

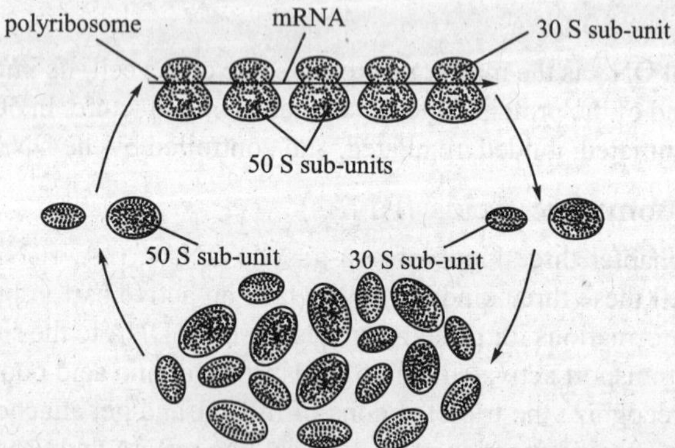

Fig. 24.1. Ribosome-polysome cycle during protein synthesis of *E. coli* (after De Robertis *et al* 1970).

Moreover, experiments on the dynamics of the assembly suggest that the 60S ribosomal subunit binds directly to the membrane of endoplasmic reticulum and then the 40S subunit, forming a complex with the mRNA, joins the 60S (**Baglioni** *et al* 1971). By *in vitro* experiments, **Borghese** *et al* (1973) have demonstrated that the small (40S) subunit of the membrane bound ribosome is capable of being exchanged with small subunits of free ribosomes. However, the large subunits are not exchanged, as they form a stable complex with the membrane of endoplasmic reticulum.

2. Function of 30S subunit. The 30S subunit provides the site for the binding of the mRNA to it. The mRNA binds with the 30S subunit and later on, N-formylmethionyl-tRNA get attached with AUG codon of mRNA in the presence of GTP and three non-ribosomal proteins called **initiation factors,** namely **IF_1**, **IF_2** and **IF_3**. These factors occur in 30S ribosomal subunit. Initiation factor IF_3 has two functions: (1) it stimulates binding of 30S subunit and appropriate recognition sites on mRNA; and (2) it assists in dissociation of 70S ribosome into 30S and 50S subunits. This second function also contributes to initiation because it leads to a pool of available 30S subunits. Initiation factor IF_2 promotes binding of N-fmet-tRNA to the 30S subunit-mRNA complex that formed first. The IF_2 protein has GTPase activity. The role of initiation factor IF_1 is uncertain at present, except that the factor somehow assists both IF_2 and IF_3 in their activities during initiation. When initiation is complete, the 50S subunit binds to the 30S-mRNA N-fmet-tRNA initiation complex and all the three initiation factors are then released from the 70S ribosome (**Avers**, 1976).

3. Function of 50S subunit. The formation of polypeptide chain occurs in the 50S ribosomal subunit. The 50S subunit is supposed to contain two binding sites, *viz.*, **aminoacyl-tRNA** or **acceptor side** ('A' site) and **peptidyl tRNA** or **donor site** ('P' or 'D' site) for the tRNA. The tRNAs which carry activated amino acids along them enter in the 50S subunit from one side and attach with the amino acyl tRNA site. After leaving the amino acids to peptidyl tRNA site, the tRNAs exit from other side. The peptidyl tRNA site contains the tRNA along with growing polypeptide chain. **W. D. Stansfield** (1969) has presumed three sites in the ribosome (*i*) a **decoding site** which binds the loaded tRNA with the mRNA by base pairing, (*ii*) a **condensing site** which joins the amino acid to the growing polypeptide chain and (*iii*) an **exit site ('E'**site) at which the tRNA detaches from the polypeptide, mRNA and ribosome.

According to **Avers** (1976), 70S ribosomes have the following four active sites or centres (Fig. 24.2): 1. **D site** situated largely on the 30S subunit; 2. The **A site** located largely on 50S subunit; 3. A **peptidyl transferase (synthetase)** centre exclusively on the 50S subunit (this enzyme is used in the formation of peptide bonds between amino acids); and 4. A **GTPase site** situated on the 50S subunit (This site also has **elongation factors T** and **G**, the latter is also called **translocase**) (Fig. 24.2).

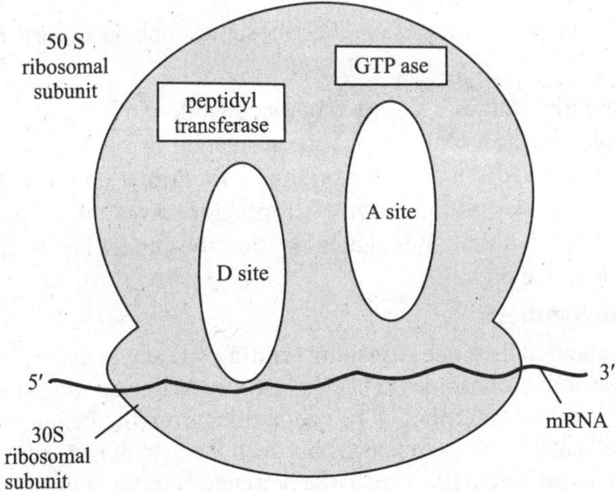

Fig. 24.2. Probable location of four active sites of the ribosome that are concerned with protein synthesis (after Avers, 1976)

4. Formation of polysomes or **polyribosomes.** During the process of protein synthesis because the codes of mRNA are read by many ribosomes, therefore, as soon as a ribosome has translated perhaps 25 codons of mRNA, the 5′ end of the mRNA becomes free to form a second initiation complex and a second ribosome begins moving along the messenger, mediating the synthesis of a second polypeptide chain. A third ribosome follows, and so on. The resulting structure, called a **polysome** or **polyribosome**, consists of a mRNA molecule which is being simultaneously translated by ribosomes into several polypeptide chains.

In a polysome each ribosome lies at a distance of 340 Å from each other. The number of the ribosome in a polysome depends on the length of the mRNA. For instance, a polysome with the mRNA of 900 nucleotides contains 8 to 12 ribosomes in it and synthesizes a protein molecule of

35,000 molecular weight. The polysomes of *E. coli* and cells of chick embryos composed of 50 unit ribosomes (**Rich**, 1967). The polysomes may occur freely in the cytoplasm or may remain attached with the endoplasmic reticulum or other membranes.

5. Function of 60S subunit. It has been reported by **Halliman, Murty** and **Grant** (1968) that the ribosome which remain attached with the endoplasmic reticulum synthesize proteins more efficiently than the free ribosomes.

In the 80S ribosome of eukaryotic cells, the large subunit 60S often remains attached with the membrane of the endoplasmic reticulum. The 60S ribosomal subunit remains separated from the 40S by a groove. The 60S ribosomal subunit contains a central channel or space by which this groove remains connected with the canal of endoplasmic reticulum. The protein synthesis occurs in the groove between the two subunits and the newly formed polypeptide chains are transported to endoplasmic reticulum via the channel or tunnel of 60S subunit where these proteins remain well protected from the enzymatic actions of proteolytic enzymes of the cytoplasm.

24.3 MECHANISM OF PROTEIN SYNTHESIS

The mechanism of protein synthesis has been investigated most thoroughly in bacteria usually (*E. coli*), therefore, the process of protein synthesis of *E. coli* which contains 70S ribosomes will be described in more detail and then this will be discussed in relation to our present knowledge of protein synthesis on 80S ribosomes of plants and animals.

A. Protein Synthesis on 70S Ribosomes

The mechanism of protein synthesis on 70S ribosomes includes following stages:

1. Transcription

The process of protein synthesis is started by the uncoiling of strands of DNA molecule. One strand of DNA molecule acts as a template for the formation of mRNA. In the presence of RNA polymerase enzyme the mRNA is formed according to the triplet codes of DNA by the copying or transcription process. As soon as the mRNA is formed it leaves the nucleus and reaches in the cytoplasm where it attaches with the 30S subunit of the ribosomes. The mRNA carries the triplet codons for the synthesis of the protein.

2. Initiation of Protein Synthesis

Every mRNA contains at least one **ribosome binding site** at which inactive ribosomal subunits assemble to establish an active ribosome. In bacterial systems, this binding site usually contains the base sequence AGGA at a location roughly 10 nucleotides from the beginning (*i.e.*, 5′ end) of the actual message. The 30S subunit binds first, possibly with the help of base pairing between the 3′ tail of its 16S RNA and the ribosome binding site, in the presence of initiation factors IF_3 and possibly IF_1.

Initiation begins when N-formylmethionyl-tRNA is accepted by the 30S-mRNA at the AUG codon which begins the message. This step is promoted by IF_2 and GTP and possibly IF_1. The 50S subunit is added last to the 30S-mRNA fmet-tRNA initiation complex and this step results in the hydrolysis of bound GTP (to GDP) and release of initiation factors from 70S ribosome.

N-formylmethionyl-tRNA (fmet-tRNA) is a methionine—charged tRNA that has been formylated at the free amino group of methionine. Although there are two methionine transfer RNAs, only one will permit the formylase enzyme—catalyzed formylation of its amino acid. The discovery of fmet-RNA in 1964 by **K. Marker** and **F. Sangar** immediately sparked a great deal of interest, for the previous year **J. P. Waller** had pointed out the surprising fact that nearly 45% of all proteins in *E. coli* have methionine at their amino ends even though methionine constitutes only about 2.5% of all amino acids in these same proteins. It was immediately suggested that fmet—tRNA might initiate polypeptide chain synthesis, for the amino end is the only position that formyl-methionine could occupy, since its own amino group is blocked.

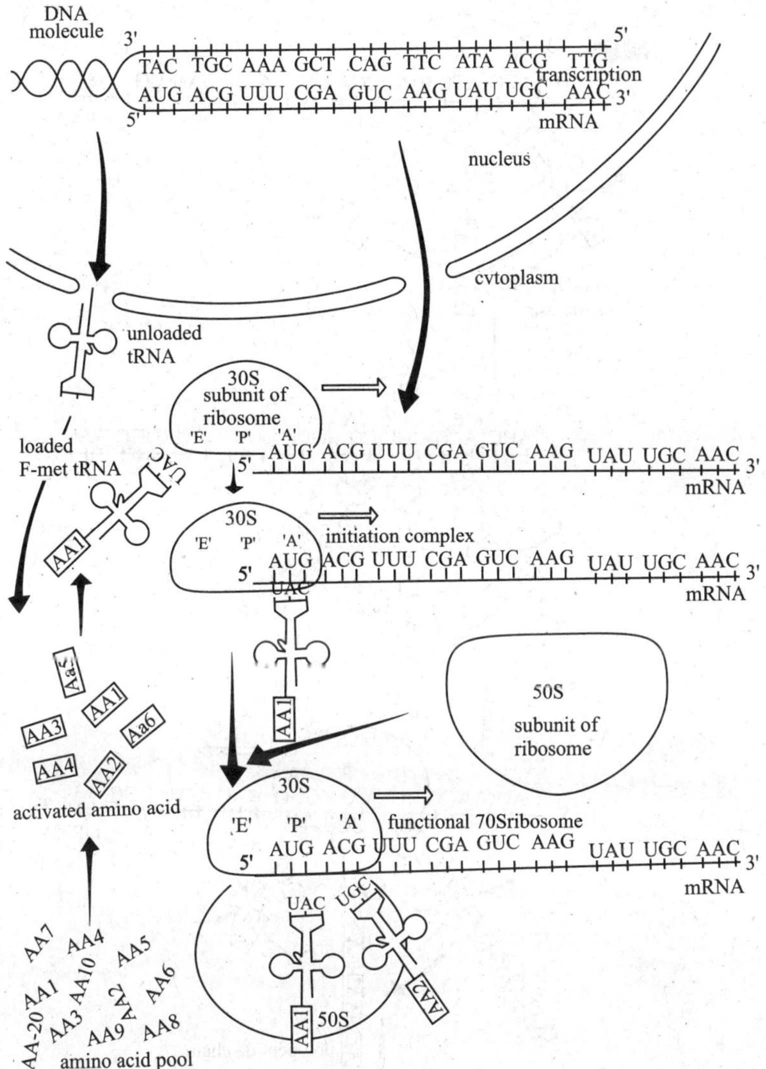

Fig. 24.3. Diagrammatic representation of the some early steps of the process of protein synthesis of *E. coli*. 'A' = aminoacyl site or decoding site, 'P' = peptidyl site or condensing site, 'E' = exit site, AA_1 = N- formyl methionine, AA_2 = threonine (cont. in Fig. 24.4).

Further, formylmethionyl-tRNA binds specifically to the normal methionine codon, AUG. It will also bind less efficiently to GUG, a valine codon. Although AUG seems to be the preferred start signal *in vivo*, proteins have been identified whose message begins instead with GUG. Thus, the same two codons that specify ordinary methionine and valine when they occur in the interior of a polypeptide are also responsible for chain initiation.

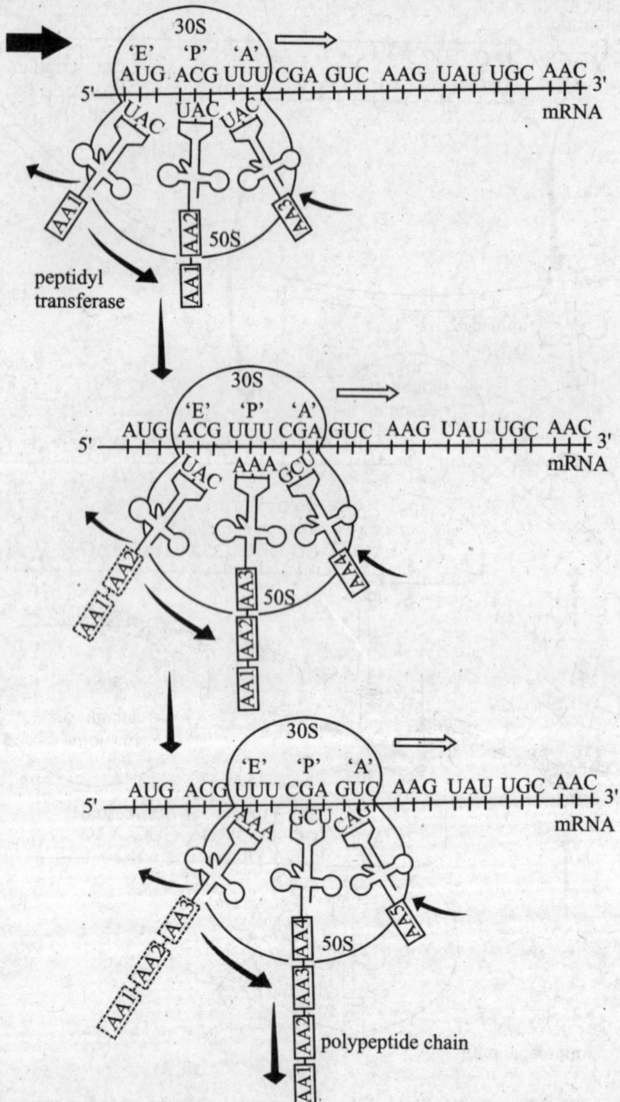

Fig. 24.4. Diagrammatic representation of some later stages of process of protein synthesis of *E. coli*. AA_3 = phenylalanine, AA_4 = arginine, AA_5 = valine, AA_6 = lysine (for rest of the abbreviations consult Fig. 24.3).

3. Transfer of Amino Acids to the Site of Protein Synthesis

The amino acids are transferred from the intra-cellular cytoplasmic 'amino acid pool' to the active ribosome by the transfer RNA molecules. Before an amino acid can be incorporated into a growing polypeptide chain at the active ribosome, it must first be esterified to a suitable transfer RNA. That event is catalyzed by an enzyme, called an **aminoacyl-tRNA synthetase**, which is specific for the amino acid in question and drives the reaction by coupling it to the hydrolysis of ATP to AMP. During the first reaction, the enzyme attaches the amino acid to AMP to form amino acid-adenylate (or AA-AMP) by using a high energy anhydride bond between the carboxylate of the amino acid and the phosphate of AMP and releasing pyrophosphate (PP). The amino acid-adenylate complex is bound to the enzyme until a second reaction replaces the anhydride bond with a lower energy ester linkage to the 3′ terminal hydroxyl of the ribose of the adenosine at CCA end of tRNA (Fig. 24.5):

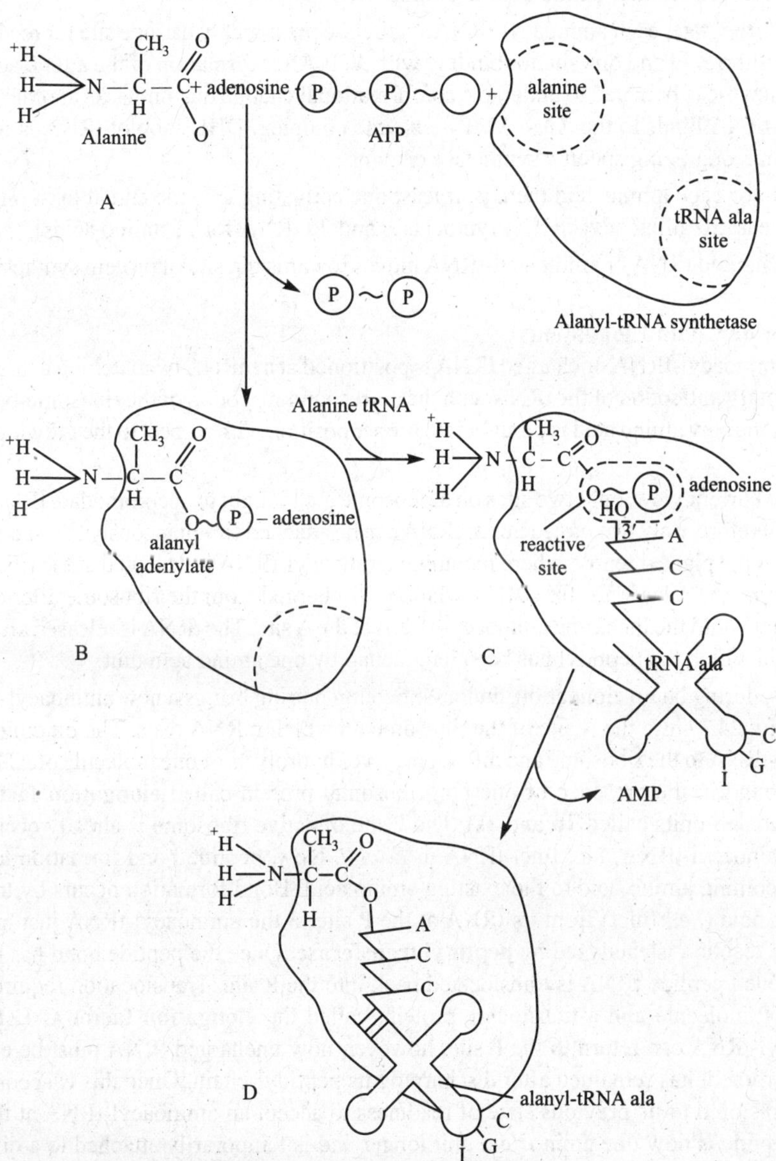

Fig. 24.5. A schematic view of the joining of an amino-acid (alanine) to its tRNA molecule as mediated by its synthetase enzyme.

Amino-acid + ATP + Enzyme → Amino-acid ≃ adenylate – Enzyme + Pyrophosphate

or AA + ATP + E → (AA ≃ AMP – E) + PP (24.1)

(AA ≃ AMP – E) + t RNA → AA – t RNA + E + AMP

Aminoacyl – tRNA or charged tRNA (24.2)

Free pyrophosphate gets hydrolyzed to P_i by the enzyme pyrophosphatase, thus helping to drive the reaction to the right. AMP is released into the medium and the freed enzyme can recycle to activate and attach another amino-acid to another tRNA.

In the free state, each aminoacyl-tRNA synthetase presumably has one site for recognition of its particular amino acid and one site for binding with ATP. After formation of the amino acid-adenylate bond, the enzyme is believed to undergo a conformational change that unmasks another site at which the correct tRNA binds to the AA – AMP – enzyme complex. DHU loop of tRNA is found to have some role in recognizing specific synthetase enzyme.

Thus, for each amino acid there is at least one activating enzyme and at least one tRNA (*i.e.*, cell has at least 20 aminoacyl-tRNA) synthetases and 20 tRNA for 20 amino acids).

The charged tRNA or aminoacyl-tRNA moves towards the site of protein synthesis, *i.e.*, active ribosomes.

4. Polypeptide Chain Elongation

An aminoacyl-tRNA or charged tRNA is positioned at a mRNA by matching a three-nucleotide complementary anticodon of the tRNA with the corresponding codon of the ribosome-bound mRNA. In this way, the new amino acid is brought into proper position with respect to the growing polypeptide chain.

In the current view, only two sites on a ribosome are thought to accommodate tRNAs at any one time and, therefore, only two molecules of tRNA can be attached simultaneously to an active ribosome. The **A site** is the place of entry, where incoming aminoacyl-tRNA is accepted at the ribosome. The **P site** is the place of release for free tRNA which is discharged from the ribosome after depositing its peptidyl chain onto the incoming aminoacyl-tRNA at the A site. The tRNA is released after a sequence of actions in which the peptidyl has been lengthened by one amino acid unit.

Thus, during chain elongation, codon-anticodon pairing brings a new aminoacyl-tRNA (AA_2–tRNA in Fig. 24.3) into the A site of the ribosome on which mRNA rests. The binding of incoming aminoacyl-tRNA to the ribosome and mRNA involves hydrolysis of one molecule of ATP-like energy rich compound in the presence of one non-ribosomal protein called **elongation factor T (EF-T,** actually two sub-units called **Tu** and **Ts**). The P site of active ribosome is already occupied by first coming aminoacyl-tRNA, *i.e.*, fmet-tRNA in *E. coli*. Now, peptide bond formation takes place to link the incoming amino acid to the existing amino acid. Bond formation occurs by transfer of the first amino acid (*i.e.*, fmet) from its tRNA at the P site to the aminoacyl-tRNA just brought to the A site. The reaction is catalyzed by **peptidyl transferase**. Once the peptide bond has been formed, the lengthened peptide tRNA is translocated back into the P site. Translocation requires hydrolysis of one GTP molecule and a translocase protein; called the **elongation factor G (EF-G)**. Before the peptidyl-tRNA can return to the P site, however, now uncharged tRNA must be expelled from the place where it has remained after discharging its peptidyl-chain. Once this is accomplished, the ribosome restored to its previous state of readiness to accept an aminoacyl-tRNA at the A site, but the polypeptide is now one amino acid unit longer and is temporarily attached to a different tRNA than it was at the beginning of the episode.

The ribosome moves to the next triplet codon after every cycle of peptide bond formation, from the 5′ toward the 3′ end of the mRNA strand attached to the 30S subunit. **H. M. Dintzis** (1961) has provided experimental evidence that amino acids are added sequentially and not through random insertions during chain elongation in reticulocytes.

There exists a great ambiguity about relative movement of ribosome and mRNA. According to one suggestion GTP hydrolysis during translocation event would provide the energy to drive a pulsating ribosome contraction after the formation of the peptide bond. This contraction would move the ribosome along the mRNA and change the status of the two bound tRNAs in one concerted movement (**Avers,** 1976). However, **Dyson'** (1978) held that mRNA is moved past the ribosome three nucleotides at a time, so that a tRNA and a mRNA codon occupy each of two ribosomal positions in turn.

The whole process of chain elongation occurs very rapidly, with growth rates up to 40 amino acids per second in *E. coli* and perhaps much faster in some eukaryotic cells (*e.g.*, 600 amino acids per minute in reticulocytes during haemoglobin synthesis). The cellular rate of protein synthesis is enhanced even further by the presence of multiple ribosomes on the same mRNA, forming **polysome**.

At this stage, sequence of events that takes place at the active ribosome during polypeptide chain elongation can be summarized as follows: 1. Incoming aminoacyl-tRNA enters the A site on the ribosome, recognizing the mRNA codon by its anticodon and binding with it in the presence of one GTP and one elongation factor T. Peptidyl-tRNA carrying the nascent polypeptide chain occupies the P site. 2. Peptide bond synthesis takes place by transfer of the polypeptide chain attached to the tRNA at the P site to the aminoacyl-tRNA at the A site. 3. Formation of the peptide bond is completed, catalyzed by enzyme peptidyl transferase. The A site is now occupied by a peptidyl-tRNA, while the freed tRNA at the P site is released to recycle. 4. The peptidyl-tRNA is translocated to the P site, a process that requires GTP and elongation factor G. The A site is again free to accept the next aminoacyl-tRNA, the ribosome is one codon farther along the message (moving toward 3′ end of the mRNA) and the polypeptide chain is one amino acid longer after each such cycle.

5. Termination and Release of Polypeptide Chain

The termination of polypeptide chain growth, like its initiation, takes place at specific codon—in this case UAA, UAG and UGA. Thesc arc "nonsense" codons that prematurely terminate translation when they appear by mutation. Once a terminator codon is encountered, no further polypeptide chain synthesis occurs.

Recognition of the terminator codon comes not from tRNA, but from proteins called **release factors (Capecchi,** 1966, 1967). At least two of these exist in *E. coli*, one of which (*i.e.*, $\mathbf{R_1}$) is involved in termination at UAA and UAG, the other (*i.e.*, $\mathbf{R_2}$) at UAA and UGA. When a ribosome encounters these codons in the presence of the appropriate release factor, the growing polypeptide chain is freed from its tRNA, a reaction that requires GTP. Hydrolysis of GTP thus powers each ribosome-associated step in translation.

The ribosome itself dissociates into its inactive subunits, an event that is mediated by IF_3 initiation faction. The dissociated ribosomal subunits and freed tRNA are now free to participate in another round of polypeptide synthesis.

6. Modification of Released Polypeptide

The released polypeptide chain contains the formylated methionine at its one end. An enzyme **deformylase** removes the formyl group of methionine. The **exopeptidase** enzyme may remove some amino acids from N-terminal end or the **C-terminal** end of polypeptide chain. At this stage the polypeptide (protein) possesses its primary and probably its secondary structures. The linear sequence of amino acids forms the primary structure; at least some portion of many proteins have a secondary structure in the form of an alpha-helix. The protein chain may then fold back upon itself, forming internal bonds (including strong disulphide bonds) which stabilize its tertiary structure into a precisely and often intricately folded pattern. Two or more tertiary structures may unite into a functional quarternary structure. For example, haemoglobin consists of four polypeptide chains, two identical α-chains and two identical β-chains. A protein does not become an active enzyme until it has assumed its tertiary or quarternary pattern.

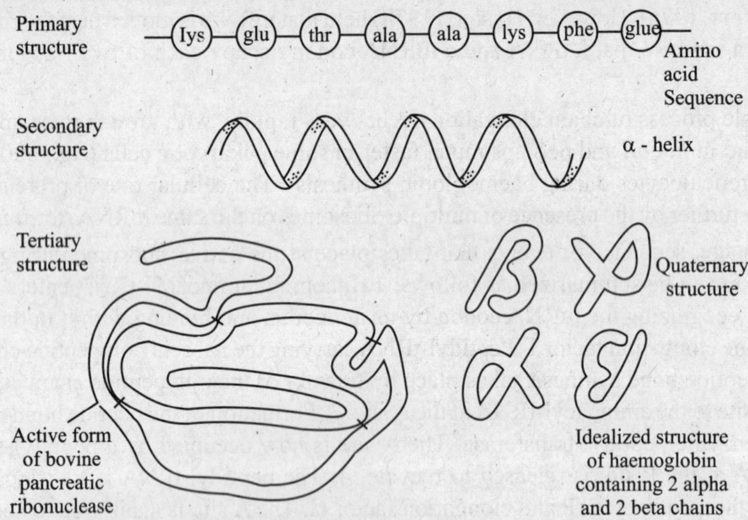

Fig. 24.6. Stages in the development of a functional protein (after Stansfield, 1969).

B. Protein Synthesis on 80S Ribosomes

The process of protein synthesis of eukaryotes is found to be similar to the mechanism of protein synthesis on 70S ribosomes of prokaryotes (see **Allende,** 1969; **Boulter, Ellis** and **Yarwood,** 1972; **Hall** *et al.* 1974 for full details of protein synthesis on 80S ribosome). However, the process of initiation of polypeptide of 80S ribosomes of eukaryotes, differs with that of prokaryotes, in following aspect:

In eukaryote systems met-tRNA (methionyl-tRNA) is not formylated. There are two different met-tRNA entities, however: **met-tRNA**$_f$ which can be enzymatically formylated *in vitro* and **met-tRNA**$_m$ which cannot be formylated. Even though this compound has the capacity to be formylated, a formylase enzyme does not seem to be present in eukaryotic cytoplasm. Because of these absence of a formylase, the usual initiator is met-tRNA$_f$. It is interesting to note that protein synthesis in mitochondria and chloroplasts of eukaryotes utilizes fmet-tRNA as the initiating aminoacyl-tRNA like the prokaryotic systems. A formylase enzyme is present in these organelles, even when it is absent in the cytoplasm of the very same cells of eukaryotes (**Avers,** 1976).

Further, the elongation factor T (EF-T) and elongation factor G (EF-G) of eukaryotes are called **EF-1** and **EF-2,** respectively.

Relating Genes to Proteins

If often becomes useful in genetic analyses to be able to determine by quick, rule of thumb estimates how much DNA corresponds to a gene, how many triplets are needed to specify a protein of a certain molecular weight and so on. In following table (after Goodenough and Levine, 1974) we have summarized some figures for maping such estimates:

Table 24.1. Method of relating genes with proteins

1. Average nucleotide = 600 daltons molecular weight.
2. Typical gene = 1000 nucleotides $\simeq$ 0.7 × 10^6 daltons of single-strand DNA.
3. 1 μm duplex DNA $\simeq$ 2 × 10^6 daltons of DNA $\simeq$ 1 × 10^6 daltons singlestrand DNA.
4. Typical mRNA = 1000 nucleotides = 300 triplet codons → polypeptide with 333 amino acids and a molecular weight of about 40,000 daltons.

A Genetic Perspective of Protein Synthesis

Our account of the mechanisms of protein synthesis in prokaryotes and eukaryotes has conveyed that translation of a mRNA sequence into a polypeptide requires exquisitely elaborate interactions between a host of nucleic acids and proteins. If we include the 50 odd ribosomal protein and the rRNAs, the tRNAs and aminoacyl tRNA synthetase, the GTP molecules and the various protein factors that promote initiation, elongation and termination events, the tally comes to well over 100 different kinds of macromolecules involve. Clearly, a substantial proportion of a cell's genetic information must be devoted to the synthesis and regulation of its protein, synthesizing apparatus along. Moreover this apparatus must be carefully designed to maximize the accurate translation of mRNA into protein: for example, the initiation of protein synthesis requires the interaction of two ribosomal subunits, two nucleic acids, three protein factors, and GTP and these multiple components presumably fit together in a productive manner only in a specific way, one then results in the correct alignment of the mRNA with respect to the aminoacyl and peptidyl sites and ribosome.

Action of Antibiotics in Protein Synthesis

During molecular biological studies of protein synthetic process molecular biologists have employed a variety of antibiotics to inhibit the protein synthesis at different desired steps, therefore, the mode of action of certain antibiotics will be quite useful for our understanding.

Aurintricarboxylic acid inhibits initiation by preventing association of ribosome subunit with mRNA both in prokaryotes and eukaryotes. **Streptomycin** inhibits initiation and chain elongation stages in prokaryotes: it releases bound fmet-tRNA from initiation complex; inhibits binding of aminoacyl-tRNA to ribosome and inhibits translocation on the ribosome. **Cycloheximide** prevents formation of initiation complex *in vitro* and also prevents chain elongation only in eukaryotic protein synthetic systems and has no effect in prokaryotic systems. It is found to inhibit tRNA movement on eukaryotic ribosomes. **Chloramphenicol** inhibits protein synthesis in bacteria, chloroplasts and mitochondria but remain uneffective in 80S ribosomes. It effects chain elongation by stopping amino acid incorporation into polypeptides by inhibiting peptidyl transferase. **Tetracycline** preferentially inhibits the binding of AA—tRNA at the "aminoacyl" site, whereas **puromycin** attacks the bound AA—tRNA at the "peptidyl" site. The latter acts as a kind of terminator by substituting for tRNA and forming a polypeptide—puromycin chain which is released. Puromycin may interrupt protein synthesis even a 0°C and tends to dissociate polysomes, thus leading to an accumulation of ribosomal subunits. Further, the antibiotic **fusidic acid** blocks the translocation which is induced by the G factor.

Actinomycin is an antibiotic which alters the structure and function of DNA. **Rifampicin** inhibits specifically bacterial RNA—polymerases. A toxic peptide, α-**amanitin** is used to differentiate between the RNA polymerase of the nucleolus and that of the nucleoplasm in eukaryotes (**Kersten**, 1971). Various other drugs inhibit termination stage of protein synthesis both in prokaryotes and eukaryotes by inhibiting releasing factors and by inhibiting ribosome release from mRNA.

REVISION QUESTIONS

1. Trace the flow of genetic information from a structural gene's DNA to mRNA to protein, according to current theory ?
2. For what is reverse transcription responsible ?

3. Differentiate between transcription and translation.
4. How do the functions of rRNA, mRNA, and tRNA differ ?
5. At which steps in translation is GTP involved ?
6. What are the functions of the A and P ribosomal sites ?
7. Summarize the events of initiation and termination during protein synthesis.
8. Describe in brief the complete process of protein synthesis.
9. Distinguish between each pair of terms listed: A site-P site; codon-anticodon; initiation-elongation; peptide bond-hydrogen bond; promoter-termination codon; ribosome-polysome; and wobble-degeneracy.

25 Chapter

REGULATION OF GENE ACTION OR GENETIC CONTROL OF GENE ACTION

DNA molecule has genetic informations for almost all the proteins which may be required by an organism, in specific amounts at certain definite times of the life cycle. But all the genes (cistrons) of DNA molecule cannot make polypeptide all the time because, if all of them were operative at the same time, the cell would become filled become filled with unnecessary proteins. There are many evidences which show that many proteins which play an important role in an adult animal are not synthesized during embryonic development and certain other proteins may be synthesized primarily during embryonic development but not during adulthood. Therefore, the flow of information from DNA (gene) to protein is regulated in some manner. Regulation, a fundamental property of living matter, is related to adaptation to the changing environment and to the phenomena of growth and differentiation. The mechanism of regulation of gene action has been extensively studied in certain micro-organisms such as *Escherichia coli* and in certain higher organisms. In both the mechanisms of gene regulation is somewhat different, therefore should, be discussed separately.

25.1 REGULATION OF GENE ACTION IN PROKARYOTES

The mechanism of gene action in prokaryotes or micro-organisms has been best studied in the bacteria *Escherichia coli. E. coli* is especially appropriate for this type of analysis since its circular chromosome contains the information to code for a total of only 3000 proteins. The DNA is transcribed in discrete segments that cover one two twenty genes at the same time and whose initiation and termination points are fixed. Among micro-organisms especially in *E.coli* following types of regulatory mechanisms of gene action have been reported:

A. Enzyme Regulation of Gene Action

The enzyme regulation of gene action can be well understood by knowing enzyme system and their mode of synthesis in *E. coli*. The synthesis of enzymes system in *E.coli* may be of following two types:

1. Unregulated enzyme production. Certain enzymes are produced continuously by an organism regardless of the presence or absence of its substrate in the environment. Such enzymes are called **constitutive enzymes** and they require no regulation. The constitutive enzymes are generally those that are needed at all times. Thus the enzymes involved in glucose metabolism—enzymes of glycolysis and the hexose monophosphate pathway—are constitutive, and one can imagine that the metabolism of glucose is sufficiently central to the physiology of *E. coli* and these pathways should be continuously functional.

2. Regulated enzyme production. The regulated enzymes are those enzymes which are synthesized in certain specific conditions and require one or other type of gene regulation. For example, the metabolism of less common sugars such as lactose, arabinose, and galactose, is effected by **regulated enzymes,** and it is clearly economical to elaborate such enzymes only on those occasions when their substrates are present. Regulated genes also specify enzymes of most biosynthetic pathways—pathways for the synthesis of amino acids, purines, pyrimidines, and so on—and these enzymes are synthesized according to the demand for their biosynthetic products. The regulated enzymes are of following two kinds:

(*i*) **Inducible enzyme.** An inducible enzyme is produced only when its substrate (inducer) is present in the environment. The phenomenon involved in the production of new enzymes due to a substrate or inducer is called **enzyme adaptation** or **induction**. This adaptation can be a reversible change, since in the absence of the **inducer** (substrate) the enzyme content may decrease (**deadaptation**).

Example

Lactose utilization in *Escherichia coli.* *E. coli* requires two enzymes, *viz.*, β-**galactoside permease** and β-**galactosidase** for lactose metabolism. The enzyme β-galactoside permease is responsible for transport of lactose into the cell and its concentration there, while the enzyme β-galactosidase catalyzes the hydrolysis of lactose to galactose and glucose. One strain of *E. coli* produces both enzymes whether lactose is present or not; this is a **constitutive strain**. Another strain produces these enzymes only in the presence of lactose; this is an **inductive** strain. Thus the lactose **induces** the synthesis of an enzyme in the inductive mutant strain. Lactose, the substrate, is acting here as an enzyme **inducer** or **effector** (**Monod**, 1956).

However, it has been demonstrated that an inducer of an enzyme and the substrate on which it acts may or may not be identical. In fact, not all inducers are substrates and not all substrates are inducers. For example, methyl-β-D-thiogalactoside is an inducer but not substrate and phenyl-β-D-galactoside is a substrate but not an inducer.

(*ii*) **Repressible enzymes.** Some enzymes are normally present in the cell but cease to be synthesized when high concentrations of their end product are present. Such enzymes are called **repressible enzymes;** while the end product is called **corepressor**. A gene called **regulator gene** produces a substance called **aporepressor** which units with corepressor to form a functional **repressor** molecule. This repressor molecule or substance inhibits synthesis of mRNA by all genes specifying enzymes in the synthetic pathway. Hormones may exert their phenotypic effects by derepressing genes previously repressed.

Example

In *E. coli*, when the amino acid, histidine occurs in high concentration in the medium, that start to act as corepressor. As a corepressor, this amino acid terminates the synthesis of 10 enzymes which are required in pathway to histidine. This kind of repression is called **coordinate repression.**

(*iii*) Feedback inhibition (End product inhibition). Feedback inhibition is a regulatory mechanism which does not effect enzyme synthesis, but rather inhibits enzyme activity. The end product of a biosynthetic pathway may combine loosely (if in high concentration) with the first enzyme in the pathway. This union does not occur at the catalytic site, but it does modify the tertiary structure of an enzyme and hence inactivates the catalytic site. This **allosteric transition** of protein molecule blocks its enzymatic activity and prevents overproduction of end products and their intermediate metabolities.

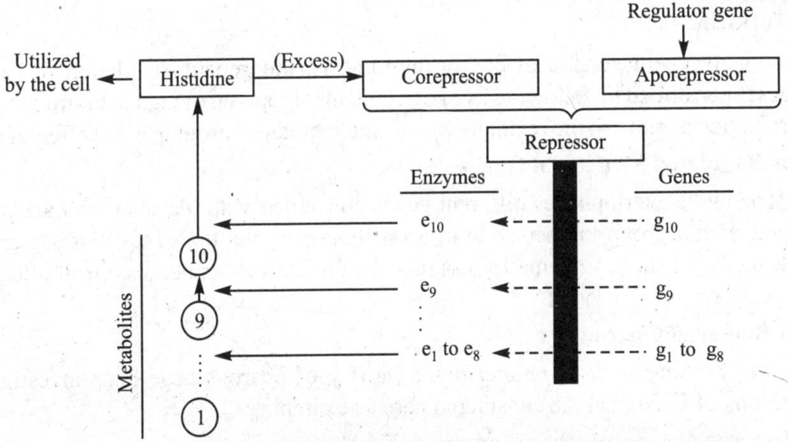

Fig. 25.1. Coordinate repression in *E. coli* (after Stansfield, 1969).

Example

The studies on isoleucine synthesis in *E. coli* (**Umbarger**, 1961) demonstrated that addition of isoleucine (the end product of a five step conversion of threonine) to a culture of the bacteria resulted in immediate blocking of the threonine → isoleucine pathway. In the presence of added isoleucine, the cells preferentially use this **exogenous** end produce (*i.e.*, isoleucine) and their own isoleucine synthesis become ceased. Moreover, the production of each of the five enzymes is not interfered with, but action of an enzyme responsible for deamination of threonine to α-ketobutyrate is inhibited by the end product, isoleucine.

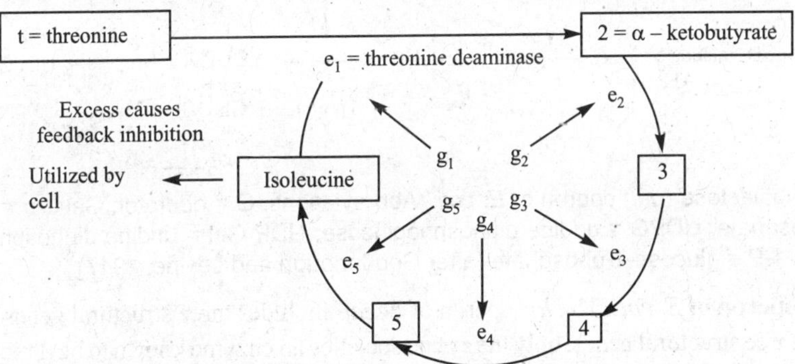

Fig. 25.2. Feedback inhibition in *E. coli* (after Stansfield, 1969).

B. Gene Regulation of Gene Action (Regulatory Genes)

Studies in bacterial genetics indicate that not all genes act by determining the structure of a given enzyme. Some are able to "regulate" the action of other genes and these have been called **regulatory genes.** The concept of gene regulation has come from the studies on *lac operon* of *E. coli* by **Jacob** and **Monod** (1961). Their studies and other later investigations have established that in prokaryotes the genes are regulated at a transcriptional level. To explain the regulating mechanisms of expression or action of regulated genes at transcriptional level, **Jacob** and **Monod** forwarded a hypothesis called **operon Hypothesis.**

Operon Hypothesis

According to recent version of operon hypothesis, the genetic regulation in bacteria and bacteriophages is performed by following five key elements: 1. operon or regulated structural genes; 2. the promoter; 3. the operator; 4. the regulatory gene and regulatory protein, 5. the effector or inducer.

1. Operon or Regulated Structural Genes

In bacteria and bacteriophages different genes concerned with the same trait are often found clustered together in a group known as an **operon**. For example, the genes in a bacterial operon determine structure of those enzymatic proteins which control sequential metabolic steps of a biochemical reaction.

Examples of Bacterial Operons

In *E. coli* and *Salmonella typhimurium*, a variety of operons have been investigated. Few important operons of *E. coli* can be considered here as examples:

(*i*) *Gal* **operon of** *E. coli*. In the *gal* operon of *E. coli*, the sequence of genes (*e.g.*, gal E, gal T and gal k) in the operon directly mirrors the sequence followed by the gene products (*e.g.*, galactokinase, galactose-1-phosphate uridyl transferase, and uridinediphospho-galactose-4-epimerase) as they carry out the degradation of galactose into glucose-1-phosphate and UDP-glucose.

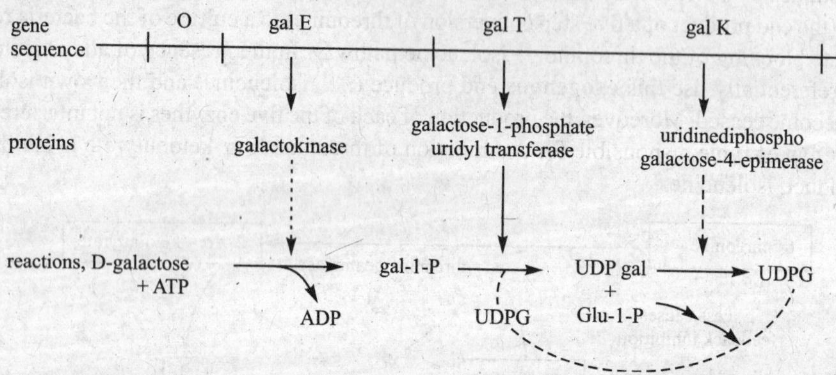

Fig. 25.3. The galactose (*gal*) operon of *E. coli*. Abbreviations: O = operator, Gal-1-p = glactose-1-phosphate, UDPG = uridine diphosphoglucose; UDP Gal = uridine diphosphogalactose; Glu-1-P = glucose-1-phosphate (after Goodenough and Levine, 1947)

(*ii*) *Lac* **operon of** *E. coli*. The *lac* operon of *E. coli* includes three structural genes (*z*, *y*, and *a*) and among its three structural genes, only the *z* gene specifies an enzyme known to be directly involved in the metabolic pathway for lactose utilization. The *z* gene product is a single long polypeptide chain (134,000 daltons); this combines with three other like chains to form the tetrameric enzyme **β-galactosidase** which catalyzes the hydrolysis of lactose (or other β-galactosides) into galactose and glucose. The *v* gene product, on the other hand, does not specify a catabolic enzyme at all but rather a molecule known as **M protein** or **galactoside permease** which is located in the bacterial cell membrane and acts to facilitate the specific uptake of lactose (and similar molecules) from the external medium. The last gene in the operon, gene *a*, specifies the enzyme **thiogalactoside transacetylase** which can, *in vitro*, transfer the acetyl group from acetyl coenzyme A to isopropyl-D-thiogalactoside (**IPTG**) a synthetic galactoside derivative. The function of this enzyme *in vivo* is unknown, but since bacterial strains carrying deletions of the *a* gene behave normally in all respects the gene appears not to specify an enzyme essential for lactose utilization.

Genetic Properties of Bacterial Operons

A bacterial operon always consists of two or more distinct genes. They are "ordinary" genes in the sense that a missense mutation in one gene is usually without effect on the expression of other genes in the operon. The operon genes are unlike ordinary genes in that they are all transcribed into *a single mRNA molecule,* often called a **polygenic** or **polycistronic messenger**, starting from a single promoter site. This has been shown most clearly by examining the mRNA produced by individual operons. The mRNA from the *lac* operon, for example has a molecular weight of 1.7×10^6 daltons, far greater than that needed to encode the sequence of β-galactosidase alone. This polygenic messenger contains several distinct translation "start" signals, each presumably heralded by an AUG. At a given time, therefore, one ribosome attached to such a messenger may be involved in the synthesis of β-galactosidase and the next in the synthesis of M protein.

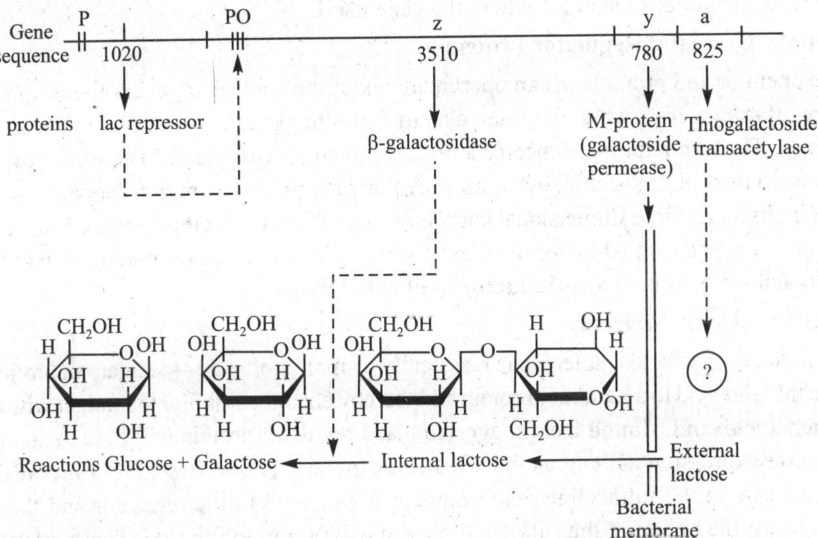

Fig. 25.4. The lactose (*lac*) operon of *E. coli.* Numbers represent the estimated number of base pairs of each gene. Abbreviations: P = promoter; O = operator; I = regulatory gene (after Goodenough and Levine, 1974)

Thus, bacterial operons possess following genetic features:

1. The component genes of an operon are clustered in the genetic map and specify different proteins concerned with the same trait.
2. The genes of an operon are independent in complementation tests but are co-transcribed into a single mRNA.
3. Nonsense mutation in promoter-proximal portions of the operon typically exert polar effects on the translation of distal genes.
4. The phenotypic expression of component genes of an operon is regulated by promoter, operator and regulator genes.

2. Promoter Gene

The promoter gene represents a sequence of bases that are recognized by a DNA-dependent RNA polymerase enzyme and promotor-polymerase binding **initiates transcription** of the neighbouring structural genes of an operon. The promoter is a key regulatory element, since it controls the rate of mRNA synthesis of a given operon. The initiation properties of a promoter gene can be modified by temporary changes in the environment. Specifically, certain promoters are regulated by certain specific proteins known as **regulator proteins** or **repressors**, which are specified by genes called **regulatory genes**. In the presence of a regulator protein, initiation of transcription by a regulated promoter is blocked. When other regulated promoters interact with other regulator molecules, initiation is stimulated.

3. Operator Gene

An operator gene also represents a sequence of bases that interacts with a repressor protein. The protein is also called a regulator molecule, and operator-regulator interaction will either prevent or promote transcription of the regulated gene, depending on which operator is being considered. The major distinction between an operator and a promoter is that *the operator is not normally the site of attachment of an RNA polymerase*. Instead, it ordinarily lies between the promoter and the beginning of a regulated gene of an operon and thus it comes to influence whether a polymerase is able to progress from its attachment site to the gene itself.

4. Regulatory Gene and Regulator Protein

The operator and promoter of an operon are under the control or yet another segment of DNA called a **regulatory gene,** which is situated apart from the operator, promoter and structural genes of an operon. The regulator gene specify a protein called a **repressor** or **regulator protein** which has the potential to bind specifically to an operator or a promoter region, apparently because of some specificity in its three-dimensional configuration. Obviously, if this binding is to regulate gene transcription, some additional factor must exist which governs whether binding in fact takes place. This additional factor is known as **inductor** or **effector molecule**.

5. Inducer or **Effector Molecule**

An inducer or effector molecule is classically a small molecule—a sugar, an amino acid, or a nucleotide that can bind to a regulator protein and thereby change its ability to interact with an operator or promoter. **Jacob** and **Monod** have suggested that a regulator protein will bind to an operator and inhibit operon expression as long as the effector or inducer is not present, but that if the effector molecule appears in the intracellular environment it will bind to the regulator and thereby "pull" the regulator off the operator, thus allowing operon expression to proceed. These relationships are diagrammed in figure 25.5. The inducer binds to a repressor and destroys its capacity to recognize the sequence of nucleotides defining the operator, presumably through a conformational change in the repressor protein (see **Dyson**, 1978).

Regulation of the Lac Operon of *E. coli*

As described in a preceding section, lactose utilization in *E. coli* involves the products of the three structural genes that constitute the ***lac*** operon: **β-galactosidase,** a lactose-splitting enzyme specified by gene *z*, **M protein**, a molecule necessary for lactose uptake and specified by gene *y*, and **transacetylase**, a poorly understood enzyme specified by gene *a*. The molecular basis for regulation of the *lac* operon is well understood. Briefly stated, the operon possesses a promoter locus (*p*) that is under **positive control**, meaning that when it interacts with its regulator protein operon transcription is stimulated. The operon also possesses on operator locus (*o*) that is under **negative control**, meaning that when it interacts with its regulator protein operon transcription is repressed. The regulator protein for the *lac* operon locus is commonly referred to as the **lac repressor**, and it is specified by the *i* gene that maps just outside the operon.

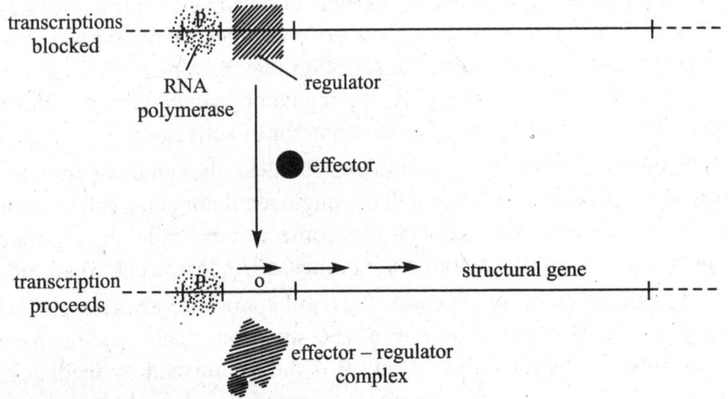

Fig. 25.5. Relationships between promoter (p), operator (o), and regulated structural gene (operon), showing RNA polymerase attachment to promoter, a regulator protein binding to the operator, and in the presence of inducer or effector, the effector-regulator binding which removes the regulator from the operon. This diagram presents the essence of the 1961 Jacob-Monod model for *lac* operon regulation (after Goodenough and Levine, 1974).

Experiments have demonstrated that the repressor binds to the operator in an uninduced cell and that it comes to leave the operator when lactose is introduced, thereby leaving the operon open to transcription. In other words, the molecular details of *lac* regulation conform to the pattern suggested by the Jacob-Monod model of gene regulation (Fig. 25.4 and 25.5). The further molecular details of *lac* regulation were worked out with a number of mutant strains of *E. coli* whose genetics have been extensively analyzed.

Molecular Biology of *lac* Operon

All available genetic and biochemical evidences in the mid-1960s indicated that an effector molecule such as **IPTG** (isopropylthiogalactose) interacted with a *lac* repressor protein to relieve some block in the transcription of the *lac* operon. **W. Gilbert** and **B. Muller-Hill** (1967) have isolated the *lac* repressor protein and a purified repressor protein proved to be a tetramer with a molecular weight of 160,000 daltons. The four subunits of the protein have since been shown to be identical, each having a molecular weight of 40,000 daltons, and each can bind a molecule of **IPTG**, meaning that the tetramer is capable of binding four **IPTGs**.

A. Riggs and **S. Bourgeosis** (1970) have suggested that the repressor is able to find specifically to the *lac* operator by recognizing the edges of the bases expose in the large and/or small grooves of the DNA helix. They note that the shape of the edge of an AT pair will be quite different from the shape of a GC pair and, since the repressor will presumably bind to the DNA with a fixed orientation that the grooves can potentially contain four types of edges: the A edge of an AT pair, the T edge of an AT pair, the G edge of a GC pair and the C edge of a GC pair. Assuming that a protein of the repressor can fit into the grooves and can establish specific hydrogen bonds only with the particular sequence of nucleotide edges found in the *lac* operator region, the specific repressor-operator binding can be explained, whether or not the model is correct for the *lac* operon it will undoubtedly prove important to give greater consideration to the information that a double-stranded DNA might carry within its grooves (**Goodenough** and **Levine,** 1974).

Further, the *lac* operator consists of apparently 21 nucleotides, including the start codon for operon transcription. The binding site for RNA polymerase (the promoter) overlaps the operator site slightly and is on the side away from the structural gene. Thus, the presence of a repressor physically blocks a portion of the promoter and prevents the binding of RNA polymerase. (**Dyson** 1978).

Thus, the operon is a set of adjacent genes whose coordinate expression is under the control of a repressor or regulator protein, itself the product of a regulator gene. When the regulator protein attaches to the operator site of the operon; transcription may be either inhibited (negative control) or made possible (positive control). The ability of a regulator protein to bind to the operator may be influenced by small molecules acting as either corepressor or activators.

Regulon. The operon concept is now firmly established, though there are many variations. In recent years, it has been investigated in *E. coli* that a single regulator gene, called **regulon** can control several operons at scattered sites around the chromosome. For example, the arginine pathway of *E. coli,* involves structural genes located at four distinct sites, all under the control of the same repressor.

Autogeneous regulation. In certain cases, the regulator protein does not produced by distantly located regulator gene, but it is made by one of the structural genes within the operon itself, a situation known as **autogenous** regulation. Control is the established by feedback, modulated by small molecules.

Another example of transcriptional control through modification of a polymerase—promoter interaction is the phenomenon of catabolic repression.

C. Catabolite Repression

B. Magasainc (1957) and others have shown that the presence of glucose inhibits the synthesis of enzymes involved with the utilization of such sugars as lactose, arabinose or galactose. This phenomenon is variously known as **catabolite repression** or the **glucose effect** and occurs in most micro-organisms including *E. coli* and yeast. For example, when a culture of *E. coli* cells is maintained on lactose and the growth medium is then supplemented with glucose, it was found that the synthesis of β-galactosidase become permanently repressed as long as glucose remains in the medium. This inhibitory effect of glucose remained poorly understood until it was noted that the presence of glucose leads to a marked drop in intracellular levels of **cyclic AMP** (3′, 5′-cyclic adenylic acid), the small nucleotide. This discovery was followed by studies made by **G. Zubay** and **J. Beckwith** (1970) who used the isolated *lac* operon DNA of *E. coli* and hypothesized that glucose by depressing cyclic AMP levels, effectively suppresses the transcription of the *lac* operon.

Cyclic AMP (cAMP) has a regulatory role in bacteria in activating and deactivating the inducible operons at the level of the promoter. In *E. coli* a cyclic **AMP receptor protein (CRP)** which is also known as **CAP** or **catabolite activator protein** (**Eron** *et al* 1971) has been reported. CRP is able to bind cyclic AMP with high affinity and is a soluble protein with two subunits (*i.e.*, a dimer) of 45,000 daltons molecular weight. After the CRP—cAMP complex is formed, it binds to the promoter and favours the recognition of this site by RNA polymerase, thus enhancing the transcription of the inducible operon. In the case of the *lac* operon, in addition to the negative control by the repressor, there is a positive control by the CRP—cAMP complex. In spite of its general role in regulation, cAMP is not essential for the life of the bacterium. Thus, mutants of *E. coli* that cannot synthesize cAMP can grow on a glucose substrate (**Brickman** *et al* 1973)

D. Stringent Control

In addition to the finely tuned regulation that bacterial cells have developed for individual genes and operons, a number of more generalized regulatory systems exist that affect many aspects of cellular metabolism. For instance, the **stringent control** is designed to conserve the resources of a cell in the "hard times" incurred during amino acid starvation. Such hard times exist, for example, when an auxotrophic bacterium is deprived of a required amino acid. They also exist in a *shift down* experiment prototrophic bacteria are first grown on a medium rich in amino acids to inhibit transcription of all repressible genes concerned with amino acid biosynthesis; they are then shifted to a medium free of amino acids so that they are forced to synthesize essential biosynthetic enzymes in the absence of a pool of exogenous amino acids.

Bacterial cells respond stringently to meet such emergencies: they greatly curtail their rates of synthesis of RNA, particularly rRNA and tRNA, and modify their rates of nucleotide biosynthesis phosphorylation, protein turnover, and many other processes, presumably to conserve their resources and thus maximize their chances of survival. **Ryan** and **Borek** (1971) have reported that *rel* (relaxed) gene of *E. coli* exerts a critical control over the stringent response and **guanosine tetraphosphate** or ppGpp molecules accumulated in response to amino acid starvation of rel^+ strain of *E. coli.* ppGpp, appears to bind directly to RNA polymerase, decreasing its ability to bind to rRNA promoters but not necessarily to other promoter sites.

25.2 CONTROL OF GENE EXPRESSION IN EUKARYOTES

In eukaryotes following two kinds of controls or regulations of gene expression occur: 1. **Short-term** or **reversible regulation** corresponds to the kind of regulation we studied in bacteria and it represents a cell's response to fluctuations in the environment specifically, it involves changes in activities or concentrations of enzymes as particular substrates and or hormone levels rise and fall. The changes a cell experiences during a cell cycle, particularly the fluctuations in rates of DNA, RNA, and protein synthesis that regularly occur with respect to the time of mitosis can also be placed in this category **2. Long-term** or **irreversible regulation** includes the phenomena associated with **determination, differentiation,** or more generally **development** it is involved in the numerous steps by which a fertilized egg becomes an organism of perhaps trillions of cells with diverse and ultimately quite permanent roles to play in the maintenance of the whole. Short-term regulations also occur in developing and differentiating eukaryotic cells side by side of long-term regulation. Therefore, for proper understanding of gene regulation in eukaryotes a brief discussion of cell differentiation and of nucleocytoplasmic interrelationship will be quite fruitful.

25.3 CELL DIFFERENTIATION

In multicellular organisms, most cells are adapted to specialized functions, and the morphology of the cell is modified accordingly. For example, nerve cells assume a shape and structure adapted to the functions of **irritability** and **conductivity** and these modifications enable them to react to stimuli and to transmit signals from one part of the organism to another. The progressive specialization in structure, biochemistry and functions constitutes in a restricted sense, **cytodifferentiation (Berrill** 1971) or **cell differentiation (De Robertis** *et al* 1975) Cell differentiation is thus a developmental process whereby cells achieve their distinctive, biochemical and functional characteristics. It may also be defined as the process by which stable differences arise between cells of an individual (**Gurdon**, 1973). One of the general principles of cell differentiation in animal tissues is that once a cell has specialized it becomes a **stable type**, which cannot revert back to the undifferentiated state. For example, a cultured cell from the skin epithelium remains epithelium and does not change into a muscle or another cell type.

Cell differentiation is a persistent change very different from the changes in enzyme induction or repression in bacteria. It occurs throughout the life of the organism. However, during the embryonic period it reaches a maximum and becomes one of the most important processes. Most organisms develop from a single cell—the **fertilized ovum**— that gives rise to all tissues and organs. This cell divides actively (*i.e.,* undergoes cleavage) to form the embryonic structure known as the **blastula**, in which tissues are not yet defined. In many species up to this time, this process is mainly **quantitative** and involves only an increase in the number of cells, but after the blastula is formed the process becomes **qualitative**, as well. The cells of blastula begin to rearrange themselves by a process called **gastrulation**, at which time the three germ layers (*viz.*, ectoderm, mesoderm and endoderm) are formed and the future organs are determined. Cell differentiation begins during gastrulation and continues through the process of tissue formation (**histogenesis**), which is followed by the formation of organ (**organogenesis**) (For details see **Verma, Agarwal** and **Tyagi**, 1980).

Determination. In many cases, before it is possible to recognize that a cell has differentiated, there is a period during which the cell is already committed to the change. In this state, called **determination**, the cell has already stabilized or fixed its capacity to follow a certain pattern of differentiation. Imaginal discs of *Drosophila* provide a classical example of determination. In the larva such discs contain cells that are apparently undifferentiated, but which, with time, give rise to legs, wings, antennae, and other body parts. Experiments in which an imaginal disc is transplanted into another larva or is serially grafted demonstrate that this capacity is already determined. These cells do not lose their determination and are still able to produce the corresponding part in the adult.

Instead of classical, purely morphologic approach, the phenomenon of cell differentiation has been recently analysed at cellular and molecular levels. In molecular terms cell differentiation implies the preferential synthesis of some specific proteins, *e.g.,* haemoglobin in erythrocytes, gamma globlulin in plasmocytes, actin and myosin in muscle, and crystalline protein of lens cells. To induce such synthesis, certain genes must be activated at a definite time in particular cells.

Nucleocytoplasmic Interrelation and Cell Differentiation

The nucleus and the cytoplasm are interdependent; one cannot survive without the other. The cytoplasm provides most of the energy for the cell through oxidative phosphorylation (in mitochondria) and anaerobic glycolysis, and the cytoplasmic ribosomes contain most of the "machinery" for protein synthesis. On the other hand, the nucleus provides templates for specific synthesis (mRNA) and also supplies the other important RNA molecules (rRNA and tRNA). The discussion of nucleocytoplasmic interrelation, therefore includes—(1) the mechanism by which the genes contained in the chromosomes exert their control on the metabolic processes of the cytoplasm and (2) the mechanisms by which the cytoplasm influence gene activity. Further, the interdependence and interactions between the nucleus and cytoplasm of eukaryotic cells have been exemplified by following experiments.

A. Nucleocytoplasmic interaction in Protozoa. Nuclear control of the cytoplasm was first considered during the last century by **Balbiani** in the so-called **merotomy** experiments, in which Protozoa were enucleated and studied. Such enucleated fragments are able to sustain most cellular activities, *e.g.,* they can form a cellulose membrane and carry on photosynthesis (plant cells), react to stimuli and ingest food (amoebae), activate cilia (ciliated cells), undergo cytoplasmic streaming, and so forth. However, these enucleated cells generally survive only a short-time and are incapable of growth and reproduction. Within 5 to 10 minutes after being enucleated by micromanipulation (*e.g.,* removal of cell nucleus by a hooked needle or a micropipette or centrifugation of a cell until it breaks into two pieces, one with and one without a nucleus), an amoeba (*Amoeba proteus*) loses its surface tension, becomes spheroid and develops numerous blunt pseudopodia. Its movement is slowed down and it can no longer digest foods. Further, it is intersting to note that an enucleate half of an amoeba will maintain a contractile vacuole included in the enucleated half but will not initiate a new one if the cut is made so as to remove both nucleus and contractile vacuole (**Flickinger** and **Coss**, 1970). In this state (*viz.,* **enucleated state**) it may survive for about 20 days. However, if a nucleus is successfully implanted within three days, the amoeba becomes extended, starts to move normally and digests food. Finally, it may divide and eventually produce a culture mass (**Fronbrune**, 1949). When a nucleus is transferred from one amoeba to another of same species (**homotransfer**) activation of cytoplasm, division and mass culture may occur readily. When a nucleus of another species is implanted (**heterotransfer**), the cytoplasm is activated, but cell division occurs less readily (**Lorch** and **Danielli**, 1960). These experiments have shown that the cytoplasm of a cell cannot survive alone and that its activities are in some manner initiated and regulated by the nucleus.

B. Nucleocytoplasmic relationships in *Acetabularia*. Nuclear transfers similar to amoeba have been made between species of *Acetabularia*, which is a sizable single-celled marine alga which has a foot, a stalk and a cap. The only nucleus in this giant (6 cm long) cell, is located in the basal or rhizoid end. The basal or rhizoid portion can be easily amputated, and in this enucleate condition, survival of the organism may be prolonged for months. During part of this time the enucleate cell can carry on synthetic and morphogenetic activities; indicating that either the cytoplasm is autonomous or that it stores a large reserve of nuclear products. Protein synthesis in enucleate cells remains normal only during the first week. However, photosynthesis and respiration are not affected for several months. The synthesis of individual enzymes (*e.g.,* phosphorylase and phosphatase diminishes at various times; this suggests that the nuclear products may be specific for each protein. From these facts, it has been concluded that in the cytoplasm there would be smaller or larger pools of different mRNAs which have come from nucleus, depending on the amount of protein desired (**Hammerling**, 1963; **Keck**, 1963).

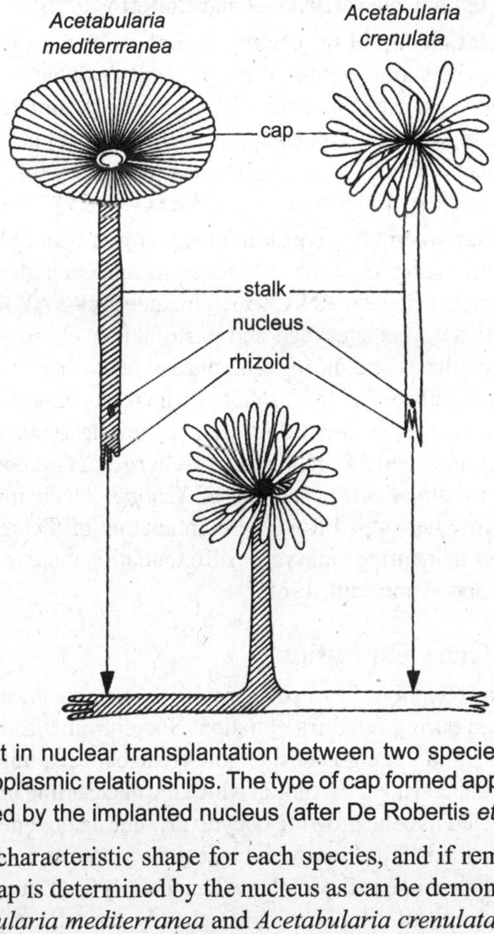

Fig. 25.6. Experiment in nuclear transplantation between two species of *Acetabularia* to show the nucleocytoplasmic relationships. The type of cap formed appears to depend on substances synthesized by the implanted nucleus (after De Robertis *et al* 1975).

The cap has a characteristic shape for each species, and if removed it is easily regenerated. The morphology of cap is determined by the nucleus as can be demonstrated by nuclear transplants. For example, *Acetabularia mediterranea* and *Acetabularia crenulata* have very different caps. If a nucleus from *A. mediterranea* is implanted in an enucleate *A. crenulata*, during the second cycle after the nuclear transplant and intermediary type of cap appears, and in the third cycle the cap will be the *A, mediterranea* type. This experiment and its reciprocal, in which a nucleus of *A. crenulata* (donor) is transplanted into *A. mediterranea* (recipient), demonstrate that a diffusible substance has been produced by the nucleus and that after sometime, it has exerted a morphogenetic effect at the apical end or cap. Further, if more than one nucleus is introduced from the donor species, the cap which regenerates has more resemblance to that of the donor then to that of recipient species. The nucleus, therefore, exerts quantitative morphogenetic influence (**Hammerling**, 1963).

Further, if two nucleate cells of different species (*i.e.*, *A crenulata* and *A. mediterranea*) are grafted, together a hybrid having a cap with intermediary shape is formed (Fig. 25.6). Although the nature of the substance inducing cap differentiation is unknown, it is assumed that it may be a kind of stable messenger RNA that controls the production of specific proteins. In the presence of ribonuclease, the enucleate portion of alga does not regenerate the cap.

Furthermore, the nucleus of *Acetabularia* does not divide until just before gamete formation, at the end of its life cycle. Division of a nucleus from a "young" cell can be induced, however, much before its time, if the nucleus of such a cell is introduced into an enucleated "old" cell of the same species which is about to form gametes. Apparently, in the chain of reactions the cytoplasm gradually develops substances which induce nuclear division. A two-way influence seems to exist—nucleus upon cytoplasm and cytoplasm upon nucleus (**Brachet** and **Bonotto**, 1970).

C. Nucleocytoplasmic relationship in sea urchin. An unfertilized sea urchin egg, enucleated by being cut or centrifuged, may be stimulated to divide, without fertilization, by brief immersion in hypertonic solution. In the total absence of a nucleus it undergoes division to form a multicellular embryonic form which later on regenerates. Apparently, division of cytoplasm, for a limited time, can continue without the presence of a nucleus, but a nucleus is necessary for continued and normal functioning and differentiation of the cytoplasm of a cell (**Harvey**, 1936).

D. Nucleocytoplasmic relationship in amphibian eggs. Amphibian eggs are most useful for the study of mechanism of cell differentiation. During oogenesis, there is a high rate of RNA synthesis (*i.e.,* tRNA, and rRNA heterogeneous nuclear RNA, which includes mRNA). RNA synthesis ceases during maturation and is reinitiated after cleavage and gastrulation. Up to gastrulation maternal ribosomes are used in protein synthesis and during gastrulation new ribosomes become available. Likewise, DNA synthesis begins slightly before fertilization and increases enormously during cleavage. Nuclear transplantation into amphibian eggs have been used to demonstrate that the amount of genetic information remains unchanged during cell differentiation. **Fiscberg** and **Gurdon** (1968) transplanted the nucleus of a differentiated intestinal cell of tadpole of *Xenopus laevis* into an enucleated egg and found that a normal adult frog developed from the combination of the egg cytoplasm and the transplanted nucleus. This shows that during embryonic differentiation there is no permanent loss or inactivation of genes (**Gurdon** and **Woodland**, 1968).

Cytoplasmic Control of Gene Expression

The nuclear transplantation technique has also been used to examine the mechanisms by which genes are activated and expressed during cell differentiation. Nuclei from blastula, gastrula, neurula, or even intestinal epithelium or brain undergo considerable changes when implanted into the egg's cytoplasm. The results obtained depend upon the time at which the nuclear implantation was made. For example, if brain nuclei are injected into the growing oocyte (*i.e.,* during oogenesis) they enlarge, and RNA synthesis is activated within them. If the transfer is made in oocytes with condensed chromosomes (*i.e.*, during maturation there is no change in the implanted nucleus. If the transplant is made at a later period (*i.e.,* during cleavage), when DNA duplication has already started, then the nucleus enlarges and starts to synthesize DNA. These experiments demonstrate that the implanted nucleus responds according to the state of the cytoplasm. It is thought that DNA polymerase enzyme penetrates the transplanted nucleus and induces the DNA synthesis. At the same time, there is a **repressor of RNA synthesis** (*viz.*, transcription) which may suppress it in the implanted nucleus. These experiments of **Gurdon** and his associates during the years 1968 and 1973, clearly demonstrated that in the egg cytoplasm there are molecules that can regulate gene expression.

Heterokaryons. The regulatory role of cytoplasm on the nucleus is also demonstrated by **heterokaryons,** which are the hybrids between two cells. **Harris** (1967) produced the heterokaryons by the introduction of mature nuclei of chicken erythrocytes into **HeLa** cells. The primary event is the enlargement of the transplanted nucleus accompanied by loosening of the condensed chromatin. This nucleus, which had lost the capacity for synthesizing RNA and DNA, resumes both functions in the presence of the HeLa cell's cytoplasm.

The first RNA produced is polydispersed and remains, in the nucleus. 'Two to three days after the transplant, when nucleoli have appeared, the RNA is transferred into the cytoplasm. At this time the information carried by the chicken erythrocyte nucleus may be expressed and produces specific surface antigens in HeLa cell.

Cytoplasmic action during mitosis. The regulatory effect of cytoplasm over genome also becomes apparent during a normal mitotic cycle. At metaphase, besides the consideration of the chromosome, there is a loss of DNA polymerase (**Mazia**, 1966) and non-histone proteins (**Himes**, 1967). At telophase, DNA polymerase and other molecules present in the cytoplasm may become associated with expanding chromatic threads. **Gurdon** and **Woodland** (1968) have suggested that the mixing of chromosomes and cytoplasm during mitosis may thus effectively reprogramme the future genetic activity of the cell.

Mechanisms of Gene Expression in Cell Differentiation

This has become a well established fact now that the diversity of cell phenotypes in Metazoa is derived from the fact that each cell expresses only a limited amount of its full genetic potential and that different cell types express different portions of their genome. Since, all specialized cells (*i.e.,* cells of intestine, blood, brain, etc.) contain the same quantity of genetic information as those that are still undifferentiated (*i.e.,* oocyte, egg, blastomere, etc.), so this implies that cell differentiation does not result in the loss or permanent inactivation of genes. From this fact we can conclude that cell differentiation depends on : (1) a differential transcription of the genes: (2) a differential translation of the particular genes, or (3) both mechanisms of control of gene expression.

The differential transcription of the genes during differentiation has been shown by many direct evidences. One of the most obvious is provided by the polytene chromosomes of insects in which certain bands may show RNA synthesis and other signs of differential gene activity. Likewise, during amphibian oogenesis the chromosomes give out lateral loops in the regions of genes of mRNA, tRNA and rRNA and become lampbrush chromosomes. These genes may be transcribed at different times or stages of oogenesis (*i.e.,* gastrulation) and at different rates. However, the cells (*e.g.,* muscle cells, antibody-producing cell, silk glands, hen oviducts and reticulocytes of mammals) which are specialized for the production of certain proteins remain best suited for isolating a particular mRNA. The isolation of mRNA is helped by the phenomenon of polyadenylation of mRNAs in eukaryotes. For example, reticulocytes (young erythrocytes of mammals) may be produced in large quantities in animals subjected to induced haemorrhage or to drugs that destroy red cells (*e.g.,* phenylhydrazine). Reticulocytes are characterized by the presence of a basophilic substance which contains the polysomes and the mRNA involved in haemoglobin synthesis. After haemolysis, the polysomes are separated and may be dissociated by a chelating agent (*e.g.,* EDTA), releasing a 9S RNA which is the mRNA coding for the α and β globin chains of haemoglobin (**Lebleu** *et al* 1971) This mRNA can be used in a cell-free system to produce haemoglobin. However, **Gurdon** *et al* (1971) injected this 9S mRNA of reticulocyte in the frog oocytes and found that oocytes can translate it into specific haemoglobin molecules. The newly formed haemoglobin contains both α and β globin chains and is specific for the message inoculated. Similar results were obtained when 9S mRNA from the reticulocytes of a rabbit, mouse or duck was injected in frog oocytes, it produces the corresponding haemoglobin molecule (**Lane, Marbaix** and **Gurdon**, 1971). These experiments demonstrate that (1) a living cell is capable of translating a message provided by another cell without loss of specificity; (2) the injected mRNA is very stable and (3) the egg has a spare capacity to translate a foreign mRNA.

We can draw the conclusion from these experiments that synthesis of different kinds of proteins in a differentiating cell does not depend on DNA replication (since there is no loss of genes) or on translation (since nay living cell can translate mRNA of any type and from a different cell), but on a differential transcription of certain genes. Later on, we will see that there are certain post-transcriptional control of gene expression.

25.4 GENE REGULATION IN EUKARYOTES

Eukaryotic cells share with prokaryotes a need to adjust constantly the concentration of enzymes in response to changing conditions. In addition, there is a more basic level of control that establishes the differentiated properties of cells in multicellular organisms. Various kinds of experimental evidence have shown that the activities of eukaryotic genes can be regulated at the level of genome, at the level of transcription and at the level of translation.

1. Gene Regulation at the Level of the Genome

The genome of an eukaryote is much larger than that found in a bacterium and it is divided into several chromosomes, which should be in a proper balance to produce normal development. In Chapter 20 it is discussed that the increase of a single chromosome resulting in trisomy, may result in an abnormal development leading to severe alterations of the nervous system (mongolism).

Organisation of the eukaryotic chromosome. With very few exceptions, each protein has only one structural gene present in a haploid set of chromosomes. Nevertheless, the haploid genome size ranges from about 4×10^8 to 8×10^{10} base pairs among vertebrates, even though there is no reason to believe that a comparable 200-fold ratio exists in the number of proteins made by the different species. Nor is there any clear correlation between our estimate of the complexity of the animal (human) and its genome size. There must be some fundamental difference in the organization of eukaryotic and prokaryotic genomes, for in prokaryotes more DNA in the chromosome means more genes and greater metabolic complexity.

In recent years, the following important observations have been made for eukaryotic DNA which causes complex organization of eukaryotic genome (**R. J. Britten**, 1971):

1. Between 50 and 75% of the DNA consists of gene-sized (*i.e.,* 1000 base pairs or so) segments that are present only once in each haploid set of chromosomes. Exceptions to this rule include the genes for ribosomal RNA, which may be tandemly repeated hundreds of times in the nucleolar organizer region of the chromosome, and the genes for tRNAs and histones, (**K.D. Tartof, 1975**) which are also present in multiple copies. (This is called **gene amplification**). The five histone genes, for example, are present side by side in tandemly repeated sequences that are transcribed as single units.

2. The great majority of these "single-copy" genes never make mRNA and hence do not code for existing proteins. They may be transcribed to hnRNA, but their RNA does not leave the nucleus.

3. Most of the rest of DNA consist of small (about 30 base pair) segments. There are a number of different sequences in these short segments, but copies of most sequences are found at many different places in the genome. Much of this **repetitive** (or **redundant**) DNA is transcribed, but again very little of the RNA ever reaches the cytoplasm.

4. Most, if not all, of the single-copy DNA has adjacent repetitive sequences. The repetitive sequences, in other words, are typically interspersed among the single-copy sequences.

5. A small fraction of genome consists of short (*e.g.,* 20 base pair) simple sequences reported many times. Most of this **highly repetitive DNA** is found in the centromere region, where two

chromatids join. This DNA is frequently different enough from the bulk of the DNA in its base composition to be separable on CsCl gradients as **satellite DNA**.

6. Still another small fraction of the DNA is found in 300—1200 nucleotide **palindromes** scattered throughout the chromosome. A palindrome is a sequence of DNA that would be read the same in either direction, for example:

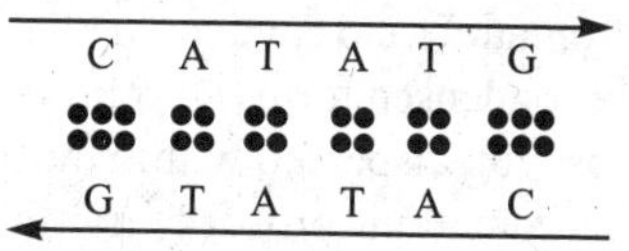

No matter which strand is transcribed (5′ to 3′) the resulting RNA is the same. However, the RNA will be internally complementary and form hydrogen-bonded hairpin loops:

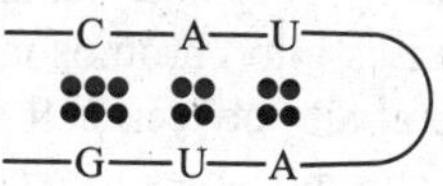

It is still not clear that why most single-copy DNA of gene size does not make mRNA. The function of satellite DNA or palindromes is also not known. However, the logic behind tandemly, repeated segments seems clear, as this pattern provides increased template in those few cases where especially frequent transcription is needed. Some recent findings have suggested a role in gene control for the repetitive sequences interspersed among single-copy genes, such as follows:

Role of repetitive DNA in gene control. The first comprehensive report of repetitive genes was made in 1968 by **R.J. Britten** and **D.E. Kohne**. In 1969, **Britten** and **E.H. Davidson** proposed a theory which provides a satisfying explanation for the existence of repetitive DNA.

Most or all structural genes are assumed to have associated with them multiple control genes. Each cell type in a multicellular organism would produce a set of gene regulators characteristic of that cell type. These regulator molecules would be capable of turning on those genes needed to carry out the differentiated functions of that cell. If a particular structural gene has a control element corresponding to one of the regulators, it will be turned on; otherwise it will be silent perhaps due to associated histones.

In a hypothetical case, a structural gene might has adjacent controlling genes recognized by issue specific activators A, B, E and F, but not by C and D:

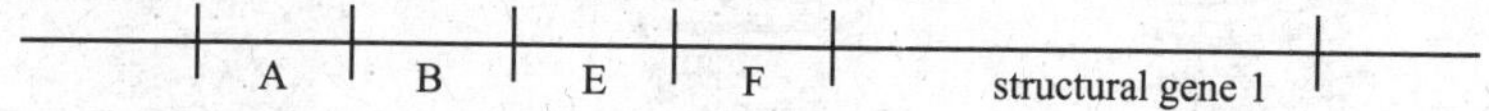

The four control elements in this model permit the gene to be turned on in those tissues having any of the four activators. A second structural gene might have control elements A, C and D:

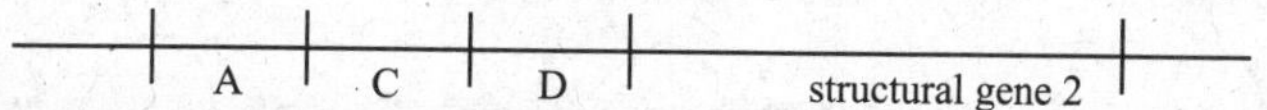

Gene 2 would thus be in those cell types producing one of these three activators. Thus, the two structural genes are recognized by an overlapping but non-directional set of activators. In this way, any combination of structural genes could be selected by a much smaller number of different control genes and their products, which are likely to be non-histone chromosomal proteins.

This theory, though speculative, yet does satisfy most of the observations. It is also consistent with data that have been provide by **Davidson** and **W.H. Klein** (1975). They have demonstrated that only 10-20 percent of the 5000 or so families of repetitive gene sequences in sea urchin are adjacent to structural genes actually expressed at one particular stage in early development. It appears that particular repetitive sequences are associated with specific structural genes, and may well be involved in their control.

2. Gene Regulation at the Level of Transcription

At the level of DNA dependent-RNA synthesis (transcription) the activities of different genes of eukaryotes may be regulated by the following methods:

(1) Transcriptional gene control by heterochromatization and euchromatization of chromatin. During the life span of the cell, most chromatin of eukaryotes is found to undergo the transition between dispersed ("euchromatic") and condensed ("heterochromatic") configurations. Prior to cell division, most chromatin is in condensed form (*i.e.,* chromosomes). Between cell divisions, the bulk of the chromatin in most cells is well dispersed within the nucleus. It has long been felt that the more compact (supercoiled) heterochromatin is probably transcriptionally silent, and that loosening of chromatin structure (*i.e.,* euchromatization) may permit transcription and perhaps even regulate it. Following evidences support this idea:

***(i)* Gene expression and Barr body.** A typical eukaryotic cell ceases to make most RNA at about the time when chromatic condenses into chromosome—*i.e.*, just prior to cell division. The chromatin that does not get dispersed at all between cell divisions may never be transcribed into RNA. For example, one of the two X chromosomes in female mammals is known to fall into that category. It forms a noticeable clump of heterochromatin, called a **Barr body**, in the nucleus between cell divisions. Genes on this heterochromatic X chromosome are not expressed, although their alleles on the euchromatic C chromosome are expressed normally (**M.F. Lyon**, 1970, 1972).

***(ii)* Gene expression and lampbrush chromosomes.** Another example where chromatic unfolding accompanies transcription is found in the lampbrush chromosomes. In the oocytes of some species, especially Amphibia, chromosomes temporarily develop lateral loops extending from a central axis of two DNA helices (see Chapter 19 and Fig. 25.7). It has been demonstrated that transcription is taking place only in the loops and that each homologous pair of chromosomes has its own highly specific pattern of looping, reflecting the activation of genes. After meiosis these chromosomes return to a normal configuration.

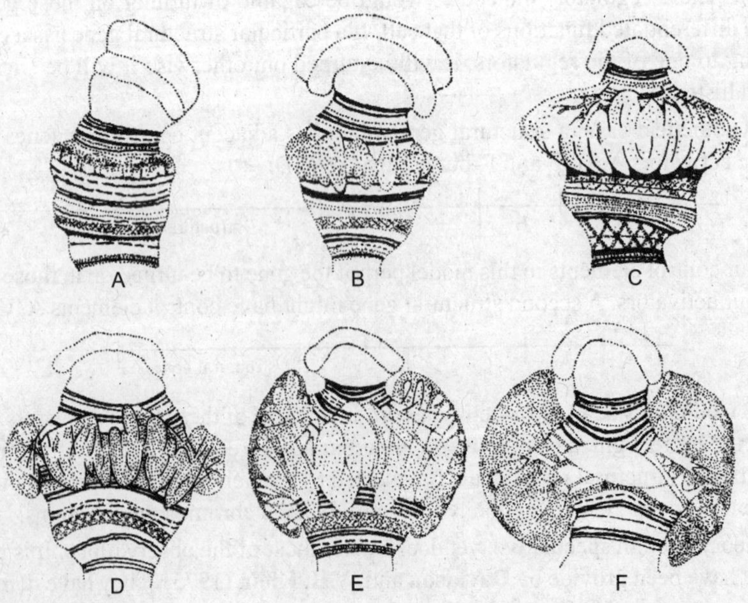

Fig. 25.7. The development of a chromosomal puff in a larval salivary gland cell nucleus of *Chironomous tentans* (after King, 1965).

***(iii)* Gene expression and polytene chromosomes.** One of the earliest correlation between unfolding and transcription was noted in the polytene chromosomes of salivary gland of *Drosophila* and other insects (see Chapter 19). In polytene chromosomes of insect larvae, the expression of gene activity is observed in the so called **puffs** and **Balbiani rings**. Because, puffing is a cyclic and reversible phenomenon; at definite times and in different tissues of the larvae, puffs may appear grow and disappear, therefore, **Beerman** (1952) has interpreted the puffing of polytene chromosomes as an expression of gene activity. At the puffs there is uncoiling of the chromosome bands, followed by the synthesis of RNA (transcription) and accumulation of proteins. Puff formation is stimulated by the steroid hormone **ecdysone**, which become bound to the sites of puffing (**Clever** and **Karlson**, 1960. Experimenters such as **Berendes** (1968) who have used temperature shock to induce certain puffs have observed following successive events in the formation of a complete puff: accumulation of acidic protein, despiralization of DNA, synthesis of RNA, and storage of the newly synthesized RNA. **Berendes** have assumed that cells contain a pool of these acidic proteins which mobilize upon stimulation and which are able to recognize specific regions of the genome.

These examples, all suggest that tightly coiled heterochromatic might be inaccessible to RNA polymerase. The question is what causes the transition back and forth between heterochromatin and euchromatin. Specific role of histone and non-histone proteins have been investigated in this mechanism of gene control (**G. Stein** *et al* 1975, 1976).

(2) Transcriptional gene regulation by histones. As histone proteins form the most abundant material of the chromatin and since they are associated with the phosphate groups of DNA in eukaryotic chromatin, therefore, it has been proposed that they might somehow alter the transcriptional properties of the polynucleotides with which they associate. By the early 1960s biochemical techniques has been artificially developed to study the synthesis of RNA in a cell-free or *in vitro* system. That is, into a test tube were placed a solution of DNA, RNA polymerase and necessary nucleotides for mRNA synthesis **Ru-Chih Huang** and **James Bonner** showed that transcription of DNA into mRNA occurred readily in the absence of histone. Adding histones decreased RNA production. The maximum inhibition was achieved when histones and DNA were present in the same amount (*i.e.,* at a 1 : 1 ratio). This is the same ratio in which DNA and histones are found.

Additional support for the hypothesis that histones inhibit genes was provided by many experiment: **Vincent Allfrey** and **Alfred Mirsky** were able to remove histones from isolated nuclei and they noted an increase in RNA synthesis. **Weissman** and **Hirschhorn** (1969, 1971) have shown that a portion of chromosome becomes active and start transcription of RNA due to the digestion of the histone coat of DNA by a lysosomal enzyme called histonase.

Recently, histone H1 is found to be the major factor in determining higher orders of chromatic structure (**M. Sluyer**, 1977). It is absent or much reduced in chromatin that is uncoiled and actively being transcribed, whereas the other histones seem to be present in the usual concentration. Conversely, untranscribed heterochromatin has much H1. A special case is found in chicken erythrocyte nuclei, where most of the H1 is replaced by a unique histone, H5, that is in many ways similar to H1. As H5 accumulates in the maturing erythrocyte, transcription is progressively inhibited.

All the histones are capable of being reversibly modified by the addition and removal of phosphate or acetate groups, or in some cases by oxidation and reduction of sulfhydryl (—SH) groups. These changes may be responsible for altering the interaction between histone and DNA and hence altering transcriptional ability. **Phosphorylation** is of particular interest because several cyclic AMP (CAMP) dependent histone kinases have been identified. Thus, changes in histones—for example, the phosphorylation of H1 associated with chromatin condensation into chromosomes—can be tied to other regulatory processes through CAMP (It is discussed elsewhere in this chapter).

There is good evidence that histone modification is able to turn blocks of genes off and on. However, they do not have the diversity necessary to be regulators of individual genes the way the *lac* repressor controls the *lac* operon in *E. coli*. For that role there is a need of molecules capable of more specificity—such as non-histone chromosomal proteins.

(3) **Transcriptional gene regulation by non-histone chromosomal proteins.** While the ratio of histone to DNA is relatively constant in cells of many types, the amount of non-histone chromosomal protein (**NHC protein**) varies widely. In general, cells with more active genes tend to have more NHC protein, indicating a role in gene activation. Consistent with this view is the observation that NHC protein also differ from histones in being polydisperse—that is, there are a very large number of individual species.

The most compelling evidences supporting the role of non-histones in gene activation has been developed in the last few years:

(*i*) In 1968, **Tung-Yue Wang** and his colleauges reported that non-histone proteins could reverse the DNA inhibition caused by histones. Working with a solution of DNA, RNA polymerase, and nucleotides as raw materials, they found that histones blocked RNA synthesis; however, the addition of non-histones permitted the RNA synthesis, to proceed by activating the regions of the genome previously suppressed.

(*ii*) In 1970, **R. S. Gilmour** and **J. Paul** provided even more direct evidence of non-histone's activating role. They isolated chromatins from the thymus gland and bone marrow of rabbits and separated the materials into DNA, histones, and non-histone proteins. They were able to reassemble the components back into a functioning chromatin units; in the presence of RNA polymerase each chromatin would synthesize the RNA characteristic of the cell from which it has been originally isolated. That is, the chromatins from thymus manufactured different RNA from bon marrow. Then **Gilmour** and **Paul** put the DNA and the histones from both the thymus and bone marrow together. To some of these solutions they added non-histone proteins from the thymus; to others, they added non-histone proteins from bone marrow. The type of RNA synthesized depended entirely upon the non-histones used : non-histones from thymus promoted thymus—specific RNA; non-histones from bone marrow promoted bone marrow-specific RNA.

(*iii*) In 1973, **Paul, Gilmour** and their colleagues have been able to study the effect of non-histone proteins on the transcription of a single gene. First, chromatin from brain and foetal liver cells of mice were isolated. With appropriate treatment each type of chromatin was tested: the chromatin from liver produced a specific mRNA which coded for the protein globin (the protein of haemoglobin) normally made by liver cells; the chromatin from the brain did not produce mRNA for globin, as the latter is not synthesized by brain cells (though the DNA in both cells was identical). The investigators then showed that the cause of this difference in cell specialization was due to non-histone. They took brain chromatin and mixed it with the non-histones of brain and produced no globin RNA; but when they mixed brain chromatin with the non-histones of foetal liver, mRNA for globin was synthesized.

Further, non-histones activity appears responsible for differences in transcription activity during the cell cycle. Non-histones isolated from different phases of the cell cycle activate RNA synthesis at very different rates. It appears that non-histones have the capacity to bind to regulator sites of specific genes and thus make the genes available for transcription—perhaps by displacing and/or chemically altering histone H1, which would otherwise mask the gene in question.

(4) Transcriptional gene regulation by RNA. Some workers such as **Bekhor** *et al* (1969) and **Huang** and Huang (1969) have proposed that an RNA fraction present in chromatin may regulate gene activity at the level of transcription. Some workers suspected for hnRNA that did not leave the nucleus, a role as **intranuclear activator** to produce the activation of the genes.

(5) Transcriptional gene regulation by hormones. Hormones are molecules that transfer information from one group of cells to another (*i.e.,* target cells). They have been investigated to regulate gene activity at the level of transcription either through cyclic AMP or by directly binding to non-histone chromosomal proteins. Water soluble hormones generally act on their target cells via membrane receptors and cytoplasmic mediators such as cAMP. Lipid-soluble hormones, on the other hand, typically penetrate cells to bind to specific receptors found within the cytoplasm. Hormones having known cytoplasmic receptors include indoleacetic acid (an **auxin**) of plants (**Biswas, Ganguly, Das** and **Roy**, 1975), the sex steroids, cortisol and activated vitamin D of mammals and ecdysone (the molting-hormone of insects)

Hormonal control and cyclic AMP. The molecular bases of hormonal action were very poorly understood until 1956, when the late **E. W. Sutherland** discovered cyclic **adenosine monophosphate** (cAMP) a cyclic nucleotide, that has been found to regulate a large number of metabolic processes. This cyclic nucleotide is synthesized by **adenylate cyclase**, an enzyme that is tightly bound to the cell membrane. Many hormones modify the activity of adenylate cyclase and, therefore produce a change in the intracellular level of cyclic AMP. In Sutherland's model of hormonal action (Fig. 25.8) the hormone is regarded as a **first messenger** hat interacts with specific receptor sites located in the outer surface of cell membrane. This hormone-receptor interaction results in change in adenylate cyclase activity whose active site is on the inner surface and which using ATP as substrate, produces cyclic AMP. This nucleotide is considered as **second messenger** that carries the information to the metabolic machinery of the cell and it activates pre-existing enzymes of cell. The effect of cAMP dependes ont he target organ; for example, an increase in cAMP will produce glycogen degradation in the liver and steroid production in the adrenal cortex.

Role of lipid-soluble hormones in gene control. One of the clearest examples of the mode of action of lipid hormones is seen with the effect of ecdysone on polytene chromosomes of *Drosophila*. Within 5–10 minutes after ecdysone addition, six major new "puffs" are seen in these chromosomes, indicating the transcription of previously silent genes. Some of these early puffs, however, apparently produce not enzymes but regulator molecules that are capable of turning on an additional 100 or so "late puffs" to produce an amplified secondary response to the hormone. In addition, one or more of protein produced by early puffs acts to terminate RNA synthesis in the early puffs. As a result, the original effect of the hormone is transient.

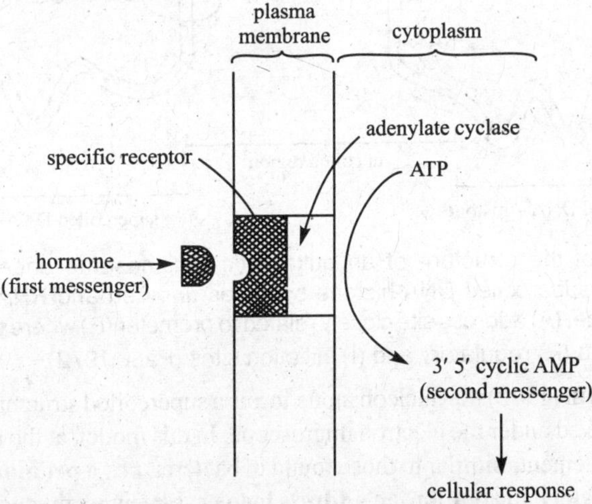

Fig. 25.8. Diagram showing the effect of a hormone (first messenger) upon a specific receptor of the cell membrane and its effect on the enzyme adenylate cyclase (after De Robertis *et al* 1975).

The original early puffs of the ecdysone – stimulated polytene chromosome presumably result from a direct effect of the hormone and its receptor protein on nuclear genes. The actual steps involved have been more clearly define for stimulation of mammalian cells by sex steroids: the steroid penetrates the cell membrane and binds, specifically to a protein receptor in the cytoplasm. This receptor, which is absent in hormone-unresponsive cells (*i.e.,* in other than target cells), is thus activated and becomes capable of penetrating the nucleus to interact with specific acceptor sites on chromatin. Through mechanisms not yet understood, the genes associated with these acceptor sites then become available for transcription (**L. chan** and **B.W.O' Malley, 1976**).

Receptors for estrogens (female hormones), progesterone, androgens (male hormones) and cortisol have been isolated. The estrogen receptor, for example, is a protein of about 80,000 daltons that binds estrogens but not molecules having similar structures but no estrogenic activity. It is activated by binding estrogen in the presence of a second protein, with which it forms a complex (**R. Leake**, 1976).

Various mutations have provided direct evidence for the importance of receptor proteins to steroid function. For example, there is a X-linked recessive condition in humans in which the cytoplasmic receptor for the male hormone dihydrotestosterone is defective. The defective receptor leads to a condition known as **"testicular feminization"** in which the genotype is normal male (46, XY) but the external phenotype is normal female (see **Dyson**, 1978).

(6) Operon-like models of eukaryotic chromosomes. Crick (1972) and **Paul** (1972) have postulated certain molecular models for eukaryotic chromosomes. In these models it is recognized that DNA is a continuous molecule throughout the chromatid and has regions with different degrees of condensation, as in the polytene chromosomes. **Crick** (1971) proposed that the compact regions are involved in control and regulation, whereas the loose regions (*i.e.,* fibrous DNA) are involved in coding.

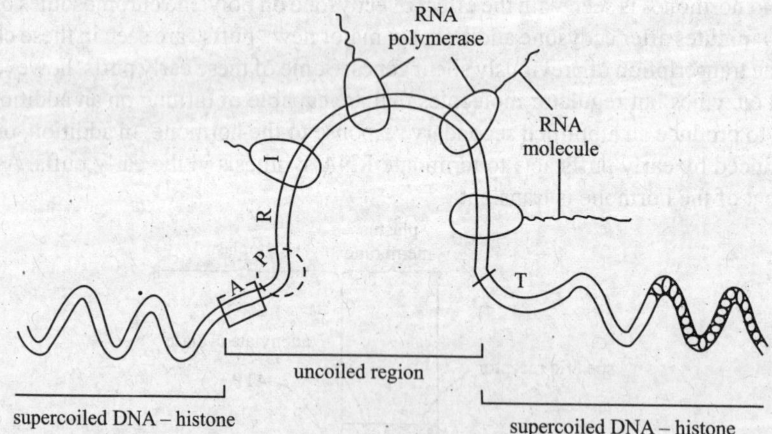

Fig. 25.9. Diagram of the structure of an eukaryotic chromosome undergoing transcription. A region of supercoiled DNA-histone becomes uncoiled and RNA is transcribed by RNA polymerase. (A) address site closely related to promoter (P) where the RNA polymerase first attaches to (R) regulatory and (I) initiation sites (Paul, 1972).

According to **Paul** (1972) the nucleohistone forms a supercoiled structure of about 120 Å, which may actually be observed under the electron microscope. In this model, at the region to be transcribed, there are controlling elements similar to those found in bacteria, *i.e.,* a **promoter, regulator sites,** and an **initiator site** (operator). In addition, an **address locus** has been postulated in which a polyanionic molecule-probably a non-histone protein—binds and produces uncoiling of the DNA. This uncoiling permits the approach of the RNA polymerase to the promotor and the start of transcription. Once the RNA polymerase reaches the initiation site; it could cause further unwinding of the DNA by accumulation of nascent RNA (also a polyanion) and of RNA binding protein.

3. Gene Regulation at the Level of Translation and Protein Turnover

Since many reactions are required to transform the information encoded in DNA to the ultimate polypeptide-gene product, many post-transcriptional gene regulating mechanisms may be considered to exist. According to **Tomkins** *et al* (1970) post-transcriptional gene regulation may be exerted: (1) on nascent mRNA by protecting it or by enhancing degradation; (2) on the transport of mRNA from the nucleus to the cytoplasm; (3) in the association of mRNA to the polyribosomes; (4) in the activation or inactivation of ribosomes; (5) in the process of initiation, elongation and termination of the polypeptide chain; or (6) in alterations in the folding of nascent polypeptide chains either by association with other proteins or with small molecules.

The advantage of translational control is the speed with which protein synthesis can be turned on and off. Its disadvantage lies in the waste involved in making mRNA that is not used before it is degraded. The longer a mRNA can survive intact, the more important it becomes to be able to control its rate of translation. And the more rapidly mRNA turns over, the more wasteful it becomes to avoid translating it without a feedback signal to also control its synthesis. The lifetimes of mRNA in both eukaryotes and prokaryotes are highly variable but usually in a logical way. That is, enzymes whose quantity must be increased or decreased in response to external signals (*e.g.,* diet) have shorter mRNA lifetimes than do enzymes whose synthesis is constitutive. The range of half-lives of most mRNAs in eukaryotes is from roughly an hour to several days. The extreme case of mRNA stability is found in unfertilized eggs, for their mRNA may remain untranslated for very long periods, even years, until fertilization occurs. The analogous situation in plants is the formation of seeds and spores, both of which also contain stable mRNA.

Thus, one way of controlling of the amount of translation of a given message is to regulate the lifetime of the mRNA. Unfortunately, it is not at all clear what makes some mRNAs most stable than others. One possibility is that lifetime is determined by secondary structure. Complementary sequences within the same mRNA molecule result in a specific folding; consisting of loops and hairpins. While these local regions of hydrogen bonding must come apart as the ribosomes pass over them, they probably make an mRNA less attractive to the ribonuclease enzyme that eventually degrade it. An alternative scheme suggests that some mRNAs are transulated a predetermined number of times. A possibly relevant observation in this regard is that the poly A tail on the 3′ end often seems to shorten with life. The early speculation that stable mRNA has an coating of chromosomal protein has been found less attractive to the cytologists.

The level of an enzyme depends not only on the rate of synthesis and translation but on the lifetime of the enzyme. The life times of animal proteins range from a few minutes (about 5 for an enzyme called ornithine decarboxylase) to a few days. These lifetimes not only differ from one protein to another, but seem to be variable for a given protein under different conditions. For example **R.T. Schimke** demonstrated in 1966 that when rats are starved, the amount of the enzyme arginase in their liver doubles in about six days. The change is due entirely to a decreased rate of degradation. In contract, most liver proteins are degraded more rapidly than normal under these same conditions. The increased stability of arginase and decreased stability of other enzymes in the starving rat may be related to the availability of substrates, for it is known that the *in vitro* digestion of enzymes by proteases is hindered by the presence of substrate.

Lastly, certain simple eukaryotes contain a gene regulating mechanism similar to prokaryotes, which can be discussed as follows:

Short-term Genetic Regulation in Simple Eukaryotes

In most simple eukaryotes as fungi, algae and Protozoa several cases of short-term genetic regulations which correspond to bacteria have been reported. For example, the fungi are most like bacteria in their ability to "turn on" and "turn off" particular enzymes in response to the presence or absence of their substrates in the growth medium. Enzymes associated with galactose utilization and with leucine and pyrimidine biosynthesis, for example, have been shown to be variously induced or repressed in several species of fungus. Inducible enzyme systems have been studied in eukaryotic algae, yeast, *Neurospora* and *Aspergillus*. Typically in most fungi, a group of regulated enzymes responds to more than one "effector molecule". For example, **J. Pateman** and **D. Gove** (1969) have found that the *de novo* synthesis of the nitrate reductase enzyme in *Aspergillus nidulans* is induced by nitrate (the substrate) and repressed by ammonium (the end product). Further, in most fungi gene regulation at transcription level by operon-mechanism of Jacob-Monod, has not been reported, however, some kind of post-transcriptional control of gene activity in fungi have been recognized in certain fungi (see **Goodenough** and **Levine**, 1974).

REVISION QUESTIONS

1. Define transcriptional control, transcriptional termination control, and post-translation control.
2. Distinguish between positive and negative transcriptional control.
3. Distinguish between inducible and repressible operons.
4. Give the essential features of the operon theory.
5. Differentiate between end-product repression and end-product inhibition.
6. Why do you suppose tRNAs are important in regulation of amino acid biosynthetic operons rather than carbohydrate utilization operons ?
7. Distinguish between determination and differentiation.
8. Describe an experiment that suggests that the genes are the same in different tissues of a differentiated multicellular eukaryote, although gene expression is quite different in different tissues.
9. List the lines of evidence that indicate condensation of chromatin is an important regulatory process.
10. List evidence in favour of regulation of gene expression (*a*) at the RNA processing level, and (*b*) at the transcription level.
11. Describe the mode of action of steroid hormones.
12. Compare and contrast prokaryotic and eukaryotic gene regulatory systems.
13. What experiments suggest that the pattern of gene expression in a highly differentiated cell is reversible, and that most such cell still contain a complete gene set characteristic of the species ?
14. What experiments, in animals and plants, indicate that nuclear activity is under the control of cytoplasmic factors ?

26 Chapter BIOSYNTHESIS OF LIPIDS AND POLYSACCHARIDES

In certain previous chapters we have discussed the biosynthesis of DNA (*viz.*, DNA replication), biosynthesis of RNA (*viz.*, transcription) and biosynthesis of proteins, all of which are macromolecules and are required by all cells for growth, metabolism and reproduction. But besides these macromolecules, there are many micromolecules (*e.g.*, nucleotides, monosaccharides, amino acids, fatty acids, etc.) and macromolecules (*e.g.*, lipids, polysaccharides, etc.) which are required by all cells as building blocks, energy source substances, etc. Therefore, a brief discussion of biosynthesis of lipids and polysaccharides by cells is earnestly required.

26.1 NUTRITIONAL PATTERNS

Of all the processes in nature, **photosynthesis** is the most fundamental. Transferring the free energy of sunlight, the green plant cells combine carbon dioxide and water, both of which are the end products of metabolism in all organisms, and from them builds carbohydrates, which directly or indirectly serve as the source of free energy of all living beings. However, photosynthesis represents only one aspect of the synthetic activity of a chlorophyll-containing plant cell. The cell can use the products of photosynthesis to synthesize the complex spectrum of small molecules (monosaccharides, oligosaccharides, fatty acids, amino acids, vitamins) and macromolecules (lipids, polysaccharides, proteins, nucleic acids) which it needs for life and reproduction. Colourless plant cells, animal cells, bacteria and viruses ultimately depend upon the products of the green plant cell for their organic supplies—organic carbon, nitrogen and some vitamins. With these and inorganic salts, they too can synthesize the small molecules and macromolecules which are required for maintaining life, and for growth and cell division.

In other words, green plant cells (**photoautotrophic cells**) represent the pattern of nutrition with **maximal synthetic activity**, inasmuch as they synthesize all their organic requirement from the low energy compounds (carbon dioxide, water and salts) at the expense of light energy, all other types of cells (**heterotrophic cells**) may be considered cells in which the capacity for synthetic activities unique to the photoautotrophic cells has been progressively lost, the loss being greatest in heterotrophic cells requiring the most complex media for growth.

There are different degrees of dependence of heterotrophic cells upon supply of organic nutrients. Some organisms (*e.g.,* wild-type *Escherichia coli*), required only organic carbon (usually glucose) and various salts to synthesize all their other organic requirements for life. Others show progressive loss of capacity to synthesize various common molecules needed for functioning or growth and must obtain these directly from their nutrients. In this respect, animal cells generally are much more dependent upon their nutrients than other cels. It does not mean that animal cells are incapable of synthetic activity, as witnesses the genome of such cells which codes for a tremendous number of proteins, but rather that here synthesis start from the level of complex organic molecules which the cells obtain in their nutrients, and from these they synthesize their characteristic complex structures.

26.2 BIOSYNTHESIS OF LIPIDS

The animal and plant cells synthesize the lipids from the fatty acids, glycerol and other accessory substances. These substances are already present in the hyaloplasm of the cell. For the biosynthesis of the lipids, these chemical compounds are first activated by the ATP and CTP and then assembled to form the lipid molecules. For example, the biosynthesis of phosphatidyl choline or lecithin involes following chemical reactions (**Lehninger,** 1965):

1. Activation of Fatty Acids

RCOOH + ATP + CoASH ⟶ RCOSCoA + AMP + Pyrophosphate
Fatty acid Coenzyme A

R′COOH + ATP + CoASH ⟶ R′COSCoA + AMP + Pyrophosphate

2AMP + 2ATP ⟶ 4ADP

2Pyrophosphate + $2H_2O$ ⟶ 4 Phosphate

2. Activation of Glycerol

Clycerol + ATP ⟶ 3 Phosphoglycerol + ADP

3. Activation of Choline

Choline + ATP ⟶ Phosphorylcholine + ADP

Phosphoryl Choline + CTP ⟶ CDP – Choline + Pyrophosphate

Pyrophosphate + H_2O ⟶ 2 Phosphate

4. Assembly Reactions

3-Phosphoglycerol + RCOSCoA ⟶ 1-acyl 3-phosphoglycerol + CoASH

1-acyl 3-phosphoglycerol + R′COSCoA ⟶ α-phosphatidic acid + CoASH

α-phosphotidic acid + H_2O ⟶ 1, 2-diglyceride + phosphate

1, 2-diglyceride + CDP-choline ⟶ phosphatidyl choline + CMP

CMP + ATP ⟶ CDP + ADP

CDP + ATP ⟶ CTP + ADP

These reactions can be summarised as follows:

2 Fatty acids + Glycerol + Choline + 8 ATP ⟶ Phosphatidyl choline (lecithin) + 8 ADP + 8 phosphate

Like the lecithin various other types of lipid molecules are synthesized by various complicated structures.

26.3 BIOSYNTHESIS OF POLYSACCHARIDES

As we have already seen that the molecules of DNA, RNA and proteins can be considered as "informational" molecules, because there is a distinct ordering of units forming the information carrying sequences that form the polymer. In polysaccharides, which are also polymers, however, the molecules are generally not ordered into information carrying sequences, nor are they of a definite chain length. This is perhaps understandable since polysaccharides serve either as storage molecules or as structural components. Polysaccharides, as the name implies, are composed of many subunits. The synthesis of polysaccharides requires that individual subunits be in an activated state. For example, synthesis of sucrose from fructose and glucose in organisms is a result of three enzymatic reactions, the source of energy being the ATP, UTP, etc. The sucrose synthetic reactions can be represented as follows:

$$\text{Glucose + ATP} \xrightarrow[\text{transferring enzyme}]{\text{Phosphate}} \text{Glucose—1—P + ADP}$$

$$\text{Glucose—1—P + UTP} \xrightarrow{\text{Enzyme}} \text{UDP – Glucose + 2P Pyrophosphate}$$

$$\text{UDP – Glucose + Fructose} \xrightarrow{\text{Enzyme}} \text{Sucrose + UDP}$$

$$\text{UDP + ATP} \longrightarrow \text{UTP + ADP}$$

Synthesis of Glycogen

The glycogen is stored food product of animal cells. It comprises may monomer units of glucose molecules. For the synthesis of glycogen, the glucose molecules are phosphorylated by ATP and an enzyme to form glucose–1–phosphate.

$$\text{Glucose + ATP} \xrightarrow{\text{Enzyme}} \text{Glucose–1–phosphate + ADP}$$

The glucose-1-phosphate is activated by UTP and an enzyme:

$$\text{Glucose–1–phosphate + UTP} \xrightarrow{\text{Enzyme}} \text{UDP – Glucose + Pyrophosphate}$$

The enzyme **glycogen synthetase** serves to catalyze the transfer of glucose residues in an activated state from UDP–glucose to the non-reducing ends of a glycogen primer. As a result the chain of glycogen molecule lengthoned and UDP molecules are released. Because glycogen molecule consists of a branching system of linearly arranged glucose units. For the formation of branch points, there occurs the enzyme, **liver-branching enzyme**. Thus, the synthesis of glycogen includes many complex reactions, many enzymes and energy rich chemical compound (ATP, UTP, etc.)

Synthesis of Starch and Cellulose

The starch which is a stored food product of plant cells is a polysaccharide whose main constituent is the unbranched polysaccharide whose main constituent is the unbranched polysaccharide, amylose. Synthesis of starch also requires activated glucose units, ATP and UTP serving as energy sources.

The cellulose which forms the cell wall of plant cell is a polysaccharide in which the glucose units are linked by B–D (1, 4) glucosidic bonds. Its molecules contain the chains of indefinite length. Synthesis of cellulose requires the presence of GTP (guanosine triphosphate) and the synthetic mechanism is still under investigation.

REVISION QUESTIONS

1. Describe, how are lipids synthesized in the cell ?
2. What is glycogen ? Discuss the biosynthesis of some polysaccharides in the cell.

27
Chapter
CELL DIVISION

One of the most important characteristics of the living cells is their power to grow and divide. When a cell reaches the limit of its size peculiar to its species, it divides into two parts. These parts grow to their full size and they divide again. Thus, new cells always arise by the division of the pre-existing cell.

The **cell division** is a process by which the cell duplicates itself for growth and reproduction of organism. In cell division chromosomes occupy a central position. As the vehicles of heredity they determine the characteristics of the cell and its progeny, and it is essential that they should be correctly distributed between the daughter cells. Two basic types of cell divisions are recognized according to the behaviour of the chromosomes. In the first of these, the daughter cells finish up containing exactly the same number of chromosomes as the parent cell. This is called **mitotic cell division** (or **mitosis**) and is the type of cell division which takes place during an organisms growth. In the other type of the cell division, known as **meiotic cell division** (or **meiosis**) the daughter cells finish up with half the total number of chromosomes present in the parent cell. This kind of division generally takes place in the formation of gametes or spores which are required for sexual reproduction.

27.1 HISTORICAL

The first account of mitosis was provided by **A. Schneider** in 1873. **Walter Flemming** observed cell division in the salamander *Titurus maculosus* and in 1879, showed that nuclear division involves a longitudinal splitting of the chromosomes and a migration of the daughter halves to the daughter nuclei. In 1882, he coined the term **mitosis. E. Van Benden** studied cell division in the round worm *Parascaris* in 1883 and showed that the gametes of round worm contain half as many chromosomes as the body cell. In 1892, **T. Boveri** described synapsis and meiosis in *Ascaris*. Further detailed information about cell division came from following cytologists: **Darlington**; **La Cour**; **Revell**; **Comandon** and **Jolly** (1913); **Belar** (1920; **Lewis** and **Lewis**; **Huges**; **A. Bajer** and **J. Bajer** (1950, 1969); and **Abercrombie**, **Ambrose** and **Easty** (1959). In recent years, electron microscopy, polarizing microscopy and other molecular biological studies of the following cytologists have provided modern understanding of cell division: **Swann** and **Mitchison**; **D. Mazia** (1961, 1974); **S. Inoue**; **A. Forer** (1965); **R.S. Brinkley** and **S. Stubblefield** (1970); **J.R. McIntosh** (1971, 1975); **R. Rappaport** (1971); **R. Wettstein** and **J. Sotelo** (1971); **P.B. Moens** (1973); **J. Rattner** and **S.G. Phillips** (1973, 1976); **H. Mohri** (1976) and many others.

27.2 TYPES OF CELL DIVISION

In prokaryotes and eukaryotes the following three types of cell divisions have been distinguished:

1. Direct cell division or amitosis.
2. Indirect cell division or mitosis.
3. Reduction division or meiosis.

However, in protozoans five kinds of cell divisions have been recognized (Table 27.1).

Table 27.1. Types of nuclear division in Protozoa (Meglitsch, 1972).

1.	**Amitosis**	Nuclear divisions with no evidence of chromosomes.
2.	**Cryptomitosis**	Nuclear divisions with a simple or complex spindle but no lining up of chromosomes or chromomeres on an equatorial plate.
3.	**Paramitosis**	Nuclear divisions with definite chromosome-like bodies on the spindle, if it is present, but with no shortening of the chromosomes during prophase.
4.	**Promitosis**	Nuclear divisions with a spindle and chromosomes, differing from mitosis in the persistence of the nuclear membrane throughout division.
5.	**Eumitosis**	Nuclear divisions with a spindle and chromosomes which shorten during prophase, and in which the nuclear membrane disintegrates during division.

Amitosis

The amitosis or direct cell division is the means of asexual reproduction in unicellular organisms like as bacteria and protozoans and also a method of multiplication or growth in foetal membranes of some vertebrates. In amitosis type of cell division the splitting of nucleus is followed by cytoplasmic constriction.

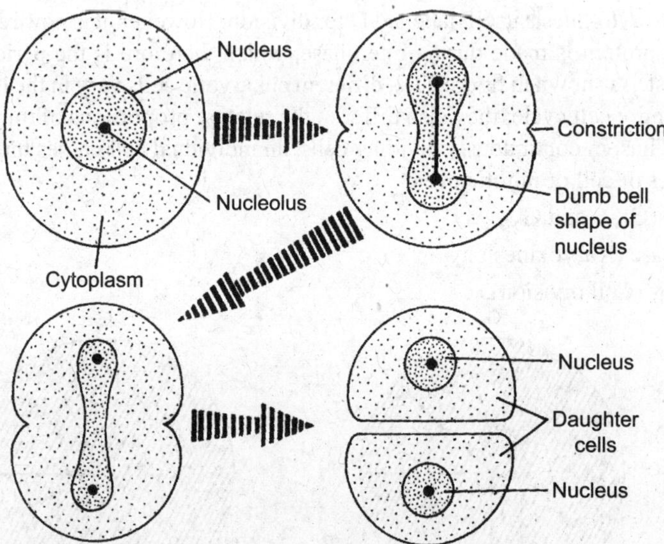

Fig. 27.1. Diagrammatic representation of amitosis.

During amitosis the nucleus elongates first and then assumes dumb-bell-shaped appearance. The depression or constriction increases in size and ultimately divides the nucleus into two nuclei. The division of nucleus is followed by the constriction of cytoplasm which divides the cell into two equal or approximately similar halves. Therefore, without the occurrence of any nuclear event two daughter cells are formed.

In bacteria, the distribution of replicated DNA to daughter cells is quite simple. The molecules are attached to the cell membrane and can be separated and distributed to daughter cells by growth of the membrane between them.

27.3 MITOSIS AND CELL CYCLE

The mitosis (Gr., *mitos*-thread) occurs in the somatic cells and it is meant for the multiplication of cell number during embryogenesis and blastogenesis of plants and animals. Fundamentally, it remains related with the growth of an individual from zygote to adult stage or with the replacement of damaged or destroyed body cells.

One of the basic characteristic of mitotic cell division which is meant for growth due to multiplication is that it gives rise to two daughter cells, which resembles each other and also the parent cell qualitatively and quantitatively (*i.e.*, the chromosome number of mitotic product cells remains the same like the parent cell). The mitosis composed of two apparatuses, *viz.*, **chromatic apparatus** which includes the chromosomes and the nucleolus and the **achromatic apparatus** which in its turn includes the centrioles and spindle. The basic outline of mitosis remains the same in all living organisms. Mitosis is part of the overall **cell cycle** that includes replication of DNA, division of the nucleus (**karyokinesis**), and division of the cell itself (**cytokinesis**).

27.4 THE CELL CYCLE

A complete cell cycle usually consists of five stages, labelled **G_1, S, G_2, M** and **D**. The first-three of these together were originally believed to be a single **interphase**, or period of rest between cell divisions. This concept arose because visible activity is confined to mitosis (M), during which daughter nuclei form and to cytokinesis itself, labelled D for division. However, it is now recognized that most DNA, RNA and protein is made during interphase, which therefore is the period when metabolic activity is greatest. As shown in figure 27.2, different eukaryotic cells vary in the length of time taken to complete an entire cell cycle; they also differ in the relative proportions of time alloted to each of the four stages. Thus, in continuously dividing cells, an individual cell passes through the following three main phases of cell or mitotic cycle.

A. Interphase (G_1, S and G_2),

B. Mitotic phase (Karyokinesis),

C. Cytokinesis (Cell division).

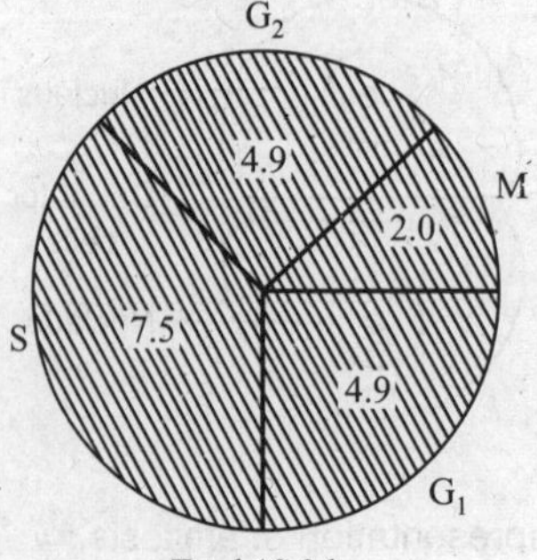

A. Vicia faba root cells

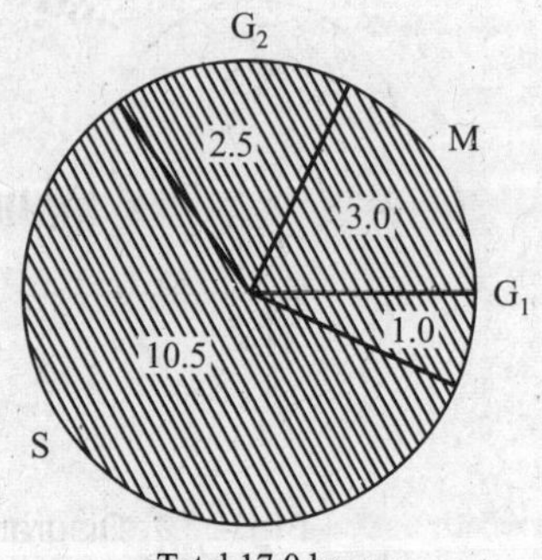

B. Tradescantia paludosa root cells

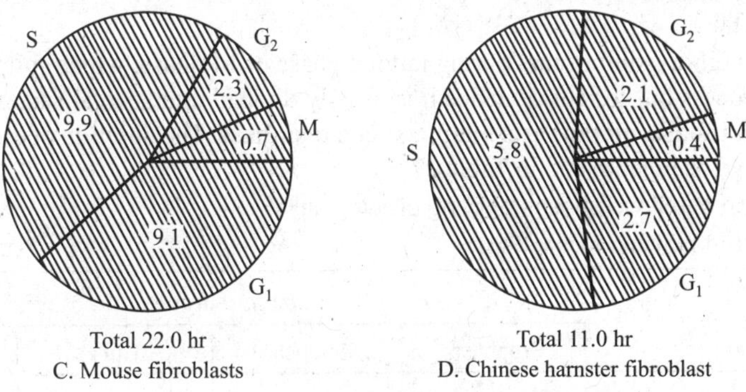

Fig. 27.2. The cell cycle of various cell types

A. Interphase

The resting phase or stage between the two mitotic divisions is called **intermitotic phase** or **interphase** (*L.*, *inter*-between, Gr., *phasis*-appearance). In interphase no division of chromosomes or cytoplasm occurs, but the nucleus and cytoplasm remain metabolically active and due to that an increase in volume of nuclear as well as cytoplasmic substances take place. The interphase is the longest phase of the mitotic cycle, taking one or two days in its completion and including following three sub-phases: 1. G_1 phase; 2. S phase and 3. G_2 phase. **G_1 phase** (G standing for gap) includes the synthesis and organization of the substrate and enzyme necessary for DNA synthesis. Therefore, G_1 is marked by the transcription of rRNA, tRNA, mRNA and synthesis of different types of proteins. During **S phase** (S standing for synthesis) synthesis (replication or duplication) of chromosomal DNA molecules takes place. Since histones are also synthesized during this time, the S phase can be considered a time of chromosomal as well as DNA replication. In contrast, in rapidly growing bacteria DNA synthesis occurs from the time a cell originates at division to the time it gives rise to daughter cells by division. Likewise, in simple eukaryotes such as yeast, DNA synthesis takes place throughout the interphase and ceases only during the brief period of nuclear and cell division (*i.e.*, M phase). **G_2 phase** is the post-DNA synthesis phase during which all the metabolic activities concerning the growth of cytoplasm and of its constituent organelles and macromolecules are performed. Thus, during interphase following events occur: The nuclear envelope remains intact. The chromosomes occur in the form of diffused, long, coiled and indistinctly visible chromatin fibres. The DNA amount becomes double. Due to accumulation of ribosomal RNA (rRNA) and ribosomal proteins in the nucleolus, the size of the latter is greatly increased. During the G_1 stage, prior to mitosis, the two members of the centriole pair separate slightly. Near the beginning of the S stage a smaller procentriole appears adjacent to each mature centriole, with the two at right angles to each other (**Fulton,** 1971; **Rattner and Phillips,** 1973).

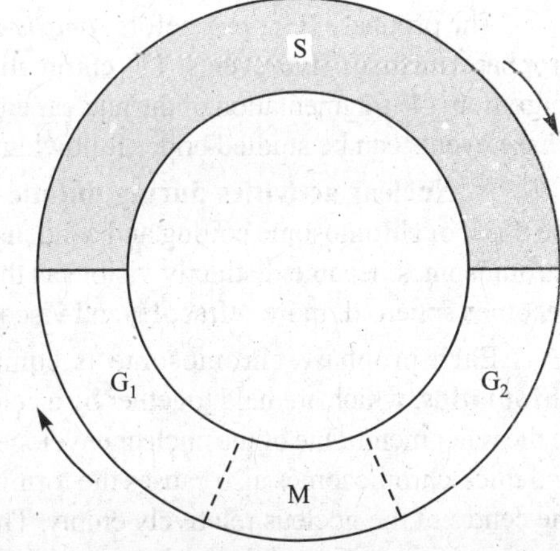

Fig. 27.3. The cell cycle or mitotic cycle, showing relative duration of phases (*e.g.*, interphase and mitotic phase) in a growing cell. S, synthesis of DNA; G_1, the pre-DNA-synthesis phase; G_2, post DNA-synthesis phase; and M, the period occupied by mitotic phase.

B. Mitotic Phase

The main mitotic cell division occurs during mitotic phase or M phase, which follows G_2 phase. It is a continuous process but for convenience it is usually divided into several stages or phases, *viz.*, **prophase, prometaphase, metaphase, anaphase** and **telophase**. The duration of each mitotic phase of certain cells have been tabulated in Table 27.2.

Table 27.2. Duration of mitotic phases of living dividing cells

(Adapted from Maiza, 1961).

Cell		Time in minutes			
		Prophase	Metaphase	Anaphase	Telophase
1.	*Triton* liver fibro-blasts (26%)	18 or more	17-38	14-26	28
2.	Mouse spleen in culture	20-35	6.15	8.14	9.26
3.	*Chortophasge* (grass-hopper neuroblast)	102	13	9	57
4.	Onion roots	71	65	2.4	3.8
5.	Pea endosperm	40	20	12	110
6.	Iris endoplasm	40-65	10-30	12-22	40-75

Mitosis in higher eukaryotes consists of fragmentation of the nucleus and chromatin condensation into visible chromosomes during prophase; alignment of chromosomes at the equatorial plane of the spindle during metaphase; separation of chromosomes into individual chromatids by centromere division at anaphase; and assembly of daughter nuclei during telophase.

Prophase

The prophase (Gr., *pro*-before; *phasis*-appearance) is the actual first phase of the mitosis. The prophase includes five events: (1) chromatin condensation; (2) nucleolar dispersal; (3) centriole migration; (4) fragmentation of the nuclear envelope; and (5) initiation of spindle apparatus assembly. These events can be studied under following heads:

A. Nuclear activities during mitotic prophase. The beginning of prophase is indicated by the onset of chromosome coiling and condensation. As coiling or folding and condensation progress, chromosomes become distinctly visible as thin threads inside the nucleus. At the same time the cell becomes spheroid, more refractile, and viscous.

Each prophase chromosome is composed of two coiled identical filaments, the **sister chromatids**, which are held together by a centromere or kinetochore. Because chromatin is attached to the inner membrane of the nuclear envelope, the progressive coiling and folding that produces short and thick chromosomes also causes the forming chromosomes to move toward the envelope, leaving the centre of the nucleus relatively empty. The centrifugal movement of the chromosomes indicates that the disintegration of the nuclear envelope is approaching, and with it, the end of prophase. During this time, the fibres of the nucleolus usually disperse, so that discrete nucleoli disappear from view.

The nuclear envelope begins to break up during early prophase, starting at the poles. Remnants of the nuclear envelope remain more or less in place throughout prophase. By the end of prophase, fragmentation of the nuclear envelope is complete and in most cells, the fragments are incorporated into the endoplasmic reticulum (ER).

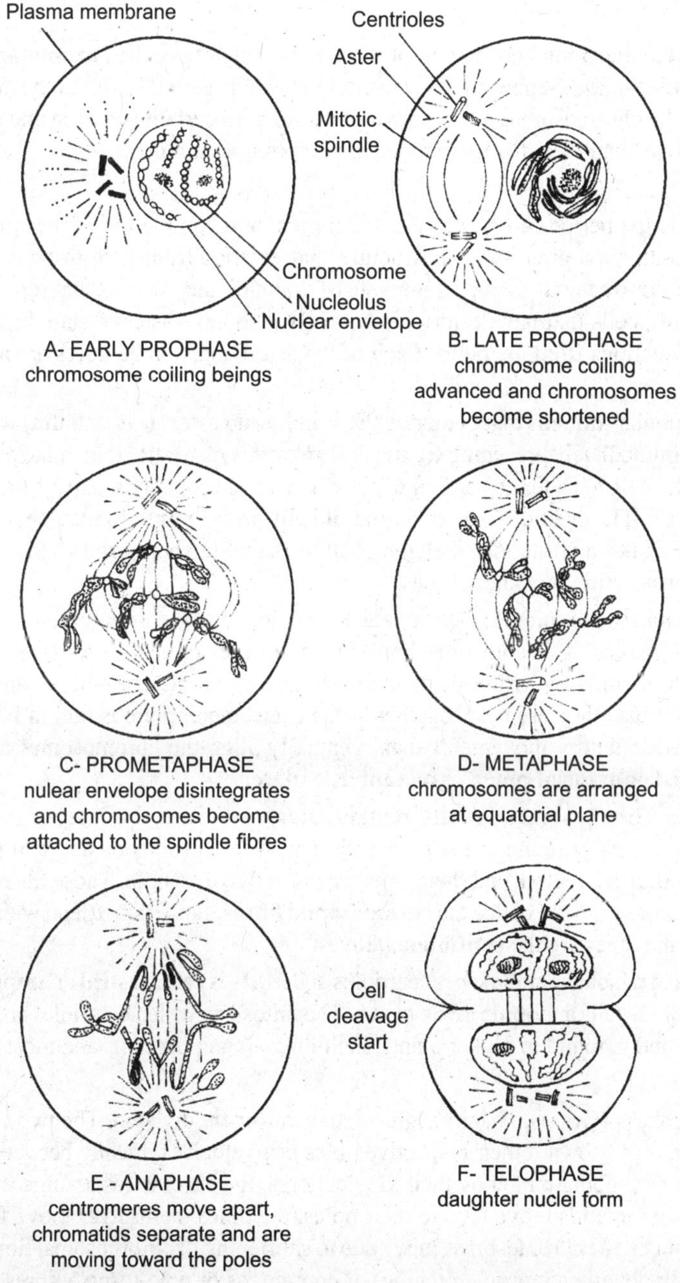

Fig. 27.4. General diagrams of mitosis (after De Robertis *et al.* 1975).

B. Cytoplasmic activities during mitotic prophase. During prophase, procentrioles elongate and the two pairs of centrioles separate and migrate to occupy positions on opposite sides of the nucleus. By the end of prophase there is a pair of full-length centrioles on each side of the nucleus, defining the poles of the cell. Spindle formation begins during prophase, although the spindle is not fully functional until metaphase.

Prometaphase

Sometimes the transition between prophase and metaphase is called **prometaphase** (Gr., *pro*-before; *meta*-between; *phasis*-appearance). This is a very short period in which the nuclear envelope disintegrates and the chromosomes are in apparent disorder. In certain Protozoa and fungi, however, the nuclear envelope characteristically remains intact throughout mitosis.

Metaphase

Metaphase is the period of chromosome alignment and completion of the spindle apparatus. The spindle apparatus is a microtubular structure that extends from pole to pole. It is organized either by centrioles or by the ill-defined aggregate of granules and vesicles that replace centrioles in higher plants. Those cells that have centrioles typically also have asters ("stars"), which are fibres radiating out in directions from the poles. Each of the astral and spindle fibres are actually bundles of microtubules.

The microtubular proteins that comprise the spindle and asters (*i.e.,* tubulin) were synthesized in part during the immediately preceding G_2 stage. However, a major fraction of the proteins involved were present in the cell for a longer period of time and were probably a part of the spindle during the previous mitosis. The characteristic rounding of cells prior to mitosis may be a consequence of depolymerization of the microtubule skeleton used to maintain shape, and to the utilization of its subunits in the construction of spindle fibres.

During metaphase the spindle fibres invade the nucleus and their microtubules extend between the poles. The chromosomes become attached to some of the spindle fibres by their kinetochores. The two sister chromatids by virtue of their kinetochores and attached fibres are pulled toward opposite poles. Because they are held together at the centromere, there is pull in both directions at once, resulting in oscillatory movements that eventually align the chromosomes all in one plane. This plane is called **equatorial plane** or **metaphasic plate.**

The smaller chromosomes usually remain situated toward the interior, while the larger chromosomes are normally found at the periphery. The sister chromatids are held together only at their common centromere region, and their arms are often free to dangle. Those fibres of spindle that connect to the chromosomes are called the **chromosomal fibres;** those that extend without interruption from one pole to the other are the **continuous fibres.**

The mitosis in which the spindle has centrioles and asters is called **astral** or **amphiastral mitosis** and is found in animal cells and some lower plants. The mitosis in which centrioles are absent is called **anastral mitosis** and is found in higher plants, including all angiosperms and most gymnosperms.

Anaphase

Mitotic anaphase (Gr., *ana,* back) begins with centromere division. The two chromatids, now free of each other, move toward their respective poles at a velocity typically between 0.2 and 4 µm/min. Because they are being pulled by their kinetochores, the chromatids assume a V-shape. At the same time as the chromatids move toward their poles, the poles themselves move further apart. As will be explained later, the chromosomes move due to shortening of chromosomal fibres and the poles are pushed apart by lengthening (or stretching) of continuous or pole-to-pole fibres.

Telophase

Telophase finds the two diploid sets of daughter chromosomes gathered at opposite poles. The chromosomes start to uncoil and become less and less condensed (*i.e.,* euchromatic) and ultimately become anastomose mass of chromatin. The nucleoli condense and reappear. The spindle fibres disperse and reappear from view. The nuclear envelope is assembled from elements of the endoplasmic reticulum – in part, from fragments added to the ER during prophase. As the sacs of ER align about the still-condensed chromosomes, ribosomes are lost from the inner (nuclear) surface and at the same time, pores begin to appear. The stimulus for these two changes in the membranes perhaps is associated with reattachment of chromatin to their inner surfaces. When new nuclei are completed by fusion of adjacent ER membranes, mitosis is complete.

Condensation Cycle of Chromosomes During Karyokinesis

Under light optical microscope during metaphase and anaphase chromosomes generally appear as compact structures. During prophase and late telophase chromosomes become less condensed and coiled filaments may be visible (Fig. 27.4). **Wolfe** (1972) has suggested that there may occur built-in information in the unit fibre for the condensation cycle of chromosomes due to coiling. He postulated the existence of special "folders" along the unit fibre of chromosome which are progressively activated as condensation progresses. These folders could be initially attractive regions spaced along the unit fibre.

C. Cytokinesis

Cytokinesis accompanies telophase in most cells and produces two daughter cells. The mechanism of cytokinesis will be discussed in detail elsewhere in this chapter.

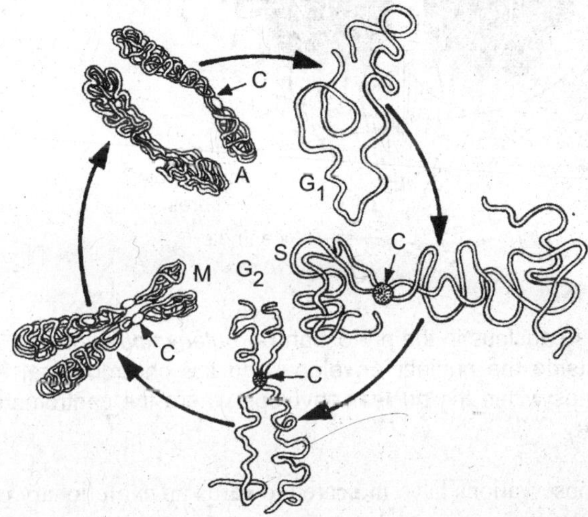

Fig. 27.5. The condensation–decondensation cycle of the chromosomes. G_1, chromosomes are completely dispersed; S, duplication of chromosomes occurs due to synthesis of DNA and histones; and G_2, condensation of chromosomes due to coiling and folding of unit fibre and centromeres (C) become apparent. At metaphase (M) and anaphase (A), the condensation is maximal and two centromeres are clearly visible. – (After De Robertis, *et al* 1975).

The Evolution of Mitosis

As noted earlier, bacterial chromosomes are attached to membranes and are separated by growth of the membrane (the nuclear envelope) and even mitotic mechanism of some lower eukaryotes is very much like that of prokaryotes.

For example, in the dinoflagellates chromosomes are anchored permanently to the nuclear envelope, which remains intact through mitosis. As in bacteria, chromosomes become separated as the envelope elongates and is pinched into two. This pinching-off process seems to be due to growth of microtubules outside the envelope, a feature that has been retained through envolution to shape the nucleus of forming spermatozoa. These external microtubules in the dinoflagellates may also help separate daughter nuclei (Fig. 27.6).

The macronucleus of ciliate protozoa (*e.g., Paramecium, Tetrahymena*) divides by mitotic mechanism just described for dinoflagellates. In the micronucleus of these same cells, however, both chromosomal and pole-to-pole spindles are seen. This latter pattern is found also in the slime mold *Polysphondylium*. In this case, pole-to-pole fibres seem to push the poles apart as the fibres grow, causing elongation of the nucleus in preparation for its division into two daughter nuclei.

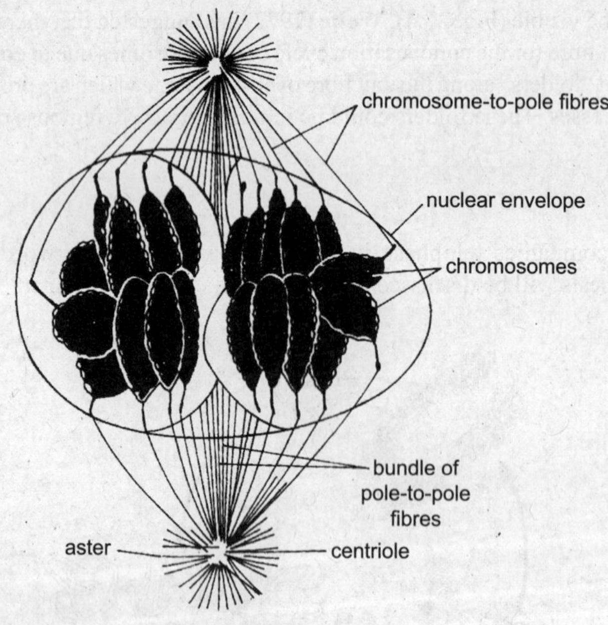

Fig. 27.6. An anaphase nucleus in the protozoan *Barbulanympha* showing the pole-to-pole fibres located outside the nuclear envelope and the chromosomal fibres attached to the chromosomes within the nuclear envelope where the centromeres are attached (after Avers, 1976).

These and other observations have indicated towards an evolutionary progression in mitosis. In the most primitive eukaryotic mitosis, the nuclear envelope remains intact and chromosomes are separated by growth of the nuclear envelope. As one proceeds up the evolutionary ladder, microtubules appear within the nucleus. A first they seem to be relatively unoriented, but in other cells clear attachments to chromosomes are found. The pattern seems to be one of decreasing importance of membrane attachment and increasing importance of the spindle as a mechanism of chromosome separation.

Further, as the need for a nuclear envelope (as a means of separating chromosomes) during mitosis diminishes with evolutionary progression, so does its integrity. For example, cells at intermediate stages in the evolutionary progression have an envelope that develops tears but remains largely intact. Almost all higher eukaryotes, however, have a completely open mitosis, where the envelope breaks down into small fragments at prophase, allowing mixing of nucleoplasm and cytoplasm. Such a nuclear fragmentation also occur during meiosis and fertilization, where there is complete mixing of two nuclei. One possible advantage of nuclear fragmentation is that assembly of the spindle from cytoplasmic proteins is facilitated by absence of a barrier between cytoplasm and nucleoplasm.

Significance of Mitosis

The mitosis has the following significance for living organisms:

1. The mitosis helps the cell in maintaining proper size.
2. It helps in the maintenance of an equilibrium in the amount of DNA and RNA in the cell.
3. The mitosis provides the opportunity for the growth and development to organs and the body of the organisms.
4. The old decaying and dead cells of body are replaced by the help of mitosis.
5. In certain organisms, the mitosis is involved in asexual reproduction.
6. The gonads and the sex cells depend on the mitosis for the increase in their number.
7. The cleavage of egg during embryogenesis and division of blastema during blastogenesis, both involve mitosis.

27.5 MEIOSIS AND REPRODUCTIVE CYCLE

The term meiosis (Gr., *meioum*—to reduce or to diminish) was coined by **J.B. Farmer** in 1905. Meiosis produces a total of four haploid cells from each original diploid cell. These haploid cells either become or give rise to gametes, which through union (fertilization) support sexual reproduction and a new generation of diploid organisms. Thus, meiosis is required to run the **reproductive cycle** of eukaryotes such as microorganisms *Chlamydomonas, Neurospora*); bryophytes; plants and animals. For example, the reproductive cycle of *Chlamydomonas* includes a long haploid generation and a short diploid generation which involves the zygote formation. The zygote undergoes reduction division (*i.e.,* meiosis) resulting in the formation of haploid spores. In higher plants, however, the reproductive cycle includes a long dominant diploid and multicellular generation (called **sporophyte**) and a short, multicellular haploid generation, called **gametophyte** generation. The tiny gametophyte is nurtured in specialized tissues of sporophyte. Male and female haploid cells called **spores,** are produced by meiosis in the diploid (sporophyte) organism. Spores grow into multicellular male and female haploid (gametophyte) structures, which through meiosis produce haploid cells corresponding to the actual gamete.

In both animals and plants, male and female gametes unite during fertilization to produce a **zygote** in which the diploid chromosome number is restored. In animals and simpler plants, the zygote matures to a new diploid organism. In the seed-producing plants, development is arrested at an early multicellular stage as a seed, which may remain stable for long-time before germination permits a continuation of growth. Thus, reproductive cycle includes alternation of two generations: haploid and diploid and involves meiosis.

Kinds of Meiosis

Meiosis occurs in the germ cells of sexually reproducing organisms. In both plants and animals, germ cells are localized in the gonads. The time at which meiosis takes place varies among different organisms, and on this basis the process can be classified into: **terminal, intermediate** or **initial.**

1. Terminal meiosis. It is also called **gametic meiosis** and is found in animals and a few lower plants. In terminal meiosis, the meiotic division occurs immediately before the formation of gametes or **gametogenesis** and will be discussed in detail in Chapter 29.

2. Intermediary or **sporic meiosis**. It is the characteristic of flowering plants. This meiosis takes place at some intermediate time between fertilization and the formation of gametes. It is also involved in the production of microspores in anthers) and megaspores (in ovary or pistil) or in **microsporogenesis** and **megasporogenesis,** respectively.

3. Initial or **zygotic meiosis**. It occurs in some algae, fungi and diatoms. Meiotic division occurs immediately after fertilization; in this case, only the egg is diploid.

Meiocytes. The cells in which meiosis takes place are known as **meiocytes**. The meiocytes of gonads are called **gonocytes** which may be **spermatocytes** in male and **oocytes** in female. The meiocytes of the plant sporangium are called **sporocytes** (*i.e.,* **microsporocytes** and **megasporocytes**).

Process of Meiosis

Meiosis superficially resembles two mitotic divisions without an intervening period of DNA replication. The first meiotic division includes a long prophase in which the homologous chromosomes become closely associated to each other and interchange of hereditary material takes place between them. Further, in the first meiotic division the reduction of chromosome number takes place and thus two haploid cells are resulted by this division. The first meiotic division is also known as the **heterotypic division.** In the second meiotic division, the haploid cell divides mitotically and results into four haploid cells. The second meiotic division is also known as the **homotypic division**. In the homotypic division pairing of chromosomes, exchange of the genetic material and reduction of the chromosome number do not occur.

Both the meiotic divisions occur continuously and each includes the usual stages of the meiosis, *viz*., prophase, metaphase, anaphase and telophase. The prophase of first meiotic division is very significant phase because the most cytogenetical events such as synapsis, crossing over, etc., occur during this phase. The prophase is the longest meiotic phase, therefore, for the sake of convenience it is divided into six substages, *viz*., proleptonema (proleptotene), leptonema (leptotene), zygonema (zygotene), pachynema (pachytene), diplonema (diplotene) and diakinesis. The successive meiotic substages can be represented as follows:

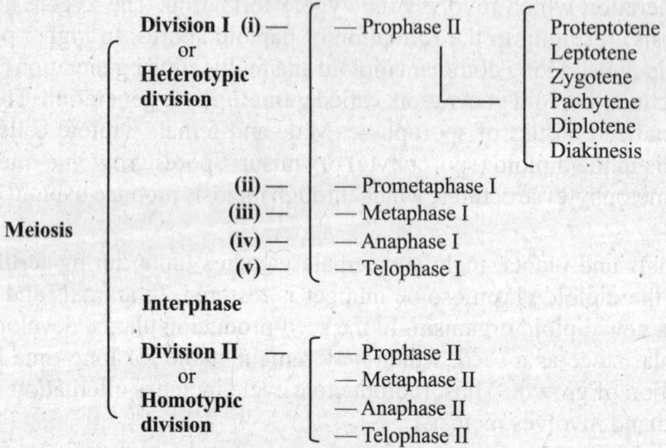

Heterotypic Division or First Meiotic Division

Meiosis starts after an **interphase** which is not very different from that of an intermitotic interphase. During the premeiotic interphase DNA duplication has occurred at the S phase. In the G_2 phase of interphase apparently there is a decisive change that direct the cell toward meiosis, instead of toward mitosis (**Stern** and **Hotta**, 1969). Further, in the beginning of the first meiotic division the nucleus of the meiocyte starts to swell up by absorbing the water from the cytoplasm and the nuclear volume increases about three folds. After these changes the cell passes to the first stage of first meiotic division which is known as prophase.

First Prophase

The first prophase is the longest stage of the meiotic division. It includes following substages:

1. Proleptotene or **Proleptonema.** (Gr., *pro'*,before; *leptas*, thin; *nema,* thread). The proleptotene stage closely resembles with the early mitotic prophase. In this stage the chromosomes are extremely thin, long uncoiled, longitudinally single and slender thread-like structures.

2. Leptotene or **Leptonema**. In this leptotene stage the chromosomes become more uncoiled and assume a long thread-like shape. The chromosomes at this stage take up a specific orientation inside the nucleus; the ends of the chromosomes converge toward one side of the nucleus, that side where the centrosome lies (the **bouquet stage**). The centriole duplicates and each daughter centriole migrates towards the opposite poles of the cell. On reaching at the poles, each centriole duplicates and thus, each pole of cell possesses two centrioles or a single diplosome.

3. Zygotene or **Zygonema**. (Gr., *zygon*, adjoining). In the zygotene stage, the pairing of homologous chromosomes takes place. The homologous chromosomes which come from the mother (by ova) and father (by sperm) are attracted towards each other and their pairing takes place. The pairing of the homologous chromosomes is known as **synapsis** (Gr., *synapsis*-union). The synapsis begins at one or more points along the length of the homologous chromosomes. Three types of synapsis have been recognised.

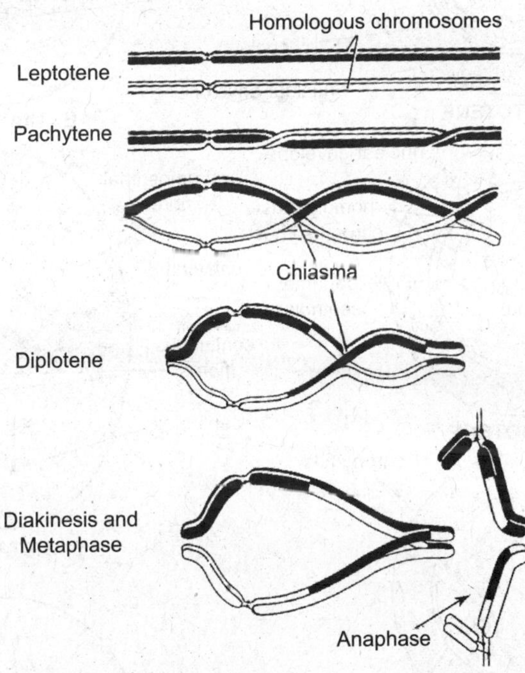

Fig. 27.7. Diagram of chromosomal exchange in the four-strand stage and of terminalization during first meiotic division.

(*i*) **Proterminal synapsis.** In proterminal type of synapsis the pairing in homologous chromosomes starts from the end and continues towards their centromeres.

(*ii*) **Procentric synapsis.** In procentric synapsis the homologous chromosomes start pairing from their centromeres and the pairing progresses towards the ends of the homologues.

(*iii*) **Localized pairing** or **Random synapsis**. The random type of synapsis occurs at various points of the homologous chromosomes.

The pairing of the homologous chromosomes is very exact and specific (*i.e.,* alignment of chromosomes is gene-for-gene exactly). The paired homologous chromosomes are joined by a roughly 0.2 μm thick, protein-containing framework called a **synaptonemal complex**. This complex extends along the whole length of the paired chromosomes and is usually anchored at either end to the nuclear envelope. Synaptonemal pairing produces and opportunity for crossing over that occurs during zygonema and synaptonemal complex facilitates that genetic activity.

4. Pachytene or **Pachynema**. (Gr., *pachus,* thick). In the pachynema stage the pair of chromosomes become twisted spirally around each other and cannot be distinguished separately. In the middle of the pachynema stage each homologous chromosome splits lengthwise to form two chromatids. Actually, the doubling of the DNA molecule strands which is necessary for the subsequent duplication of chromosomes occurs earlier, before the beginning of meiotic prophase. Through the earlier part of the meiotic prophase, however, the DNA molecule in each chromosomes behave as a

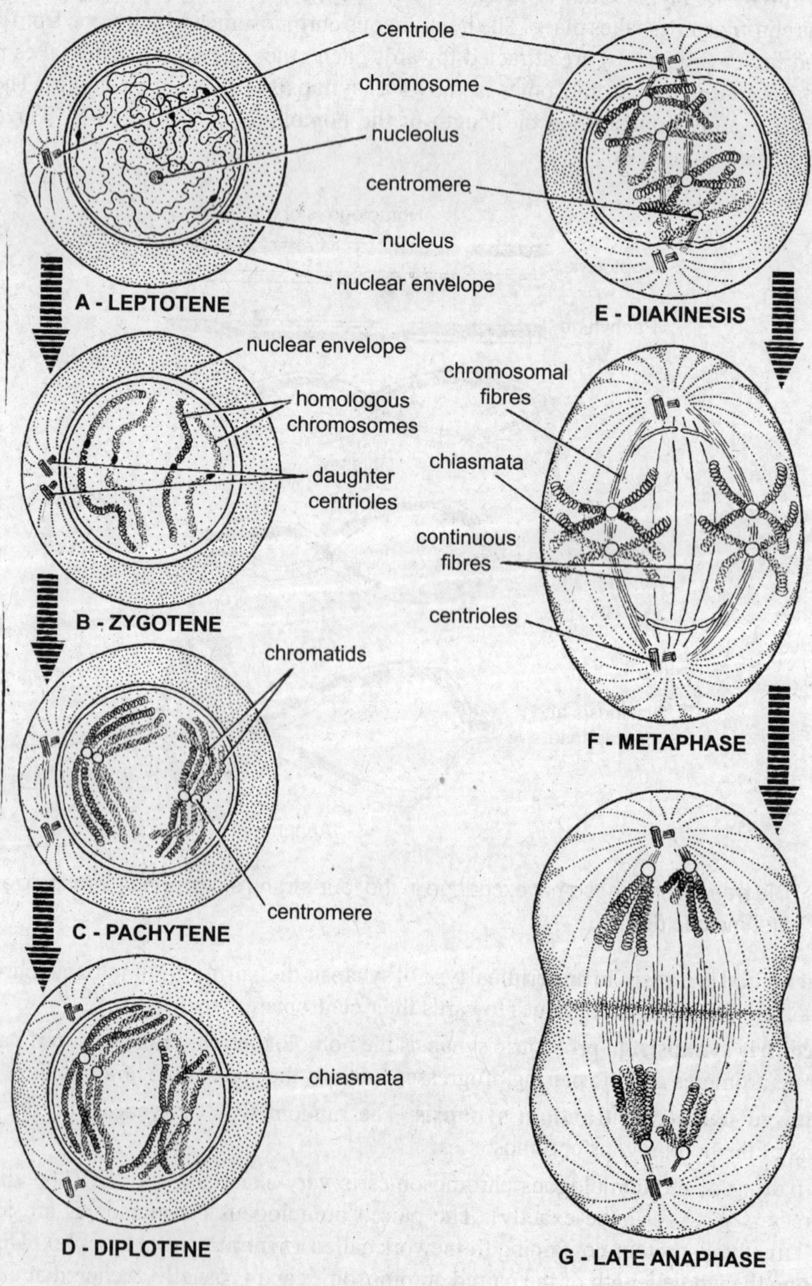

Fig. 27.8. Different stages of first meiotic division (after King, 1965).

single body. In the pachynema stage, this is now changed, the two chromatids of each chromosome containing half of the DNA present in the chromosome at start, become partially independent of one another, although they still continue to be linked together by their common centromere. Each synaptonemal pair at this point is commonly referred to as a **bivalent** because it consists of two visible chromosomes, or as a **tetrad** because of the four visible chromatids.

During pachynema stage an important genetic phenomenon called "crossing over" takes place. The crossing over involves reshuffling, redistribution and mutual exchange of hereditary material of two parents between two homologous chromosomes. According to recent views, one chromatid of each homologous chromosome of a bivalent may divide transversely by the help of an enzyme the **endonuclease** which is reported to increase in the nucleus during this stage by **Stern** and **Hotta** (1969). After the division of chromatids, the interchange of chromatid segments takes place between the non-sister chromatids of the homologous chromosomes. The broken chromatid segments are united with the chromatids due to the presence of an enzyme, **ligase** (**Stern** and **Hotta**, 1969). This process of interchange of chromatin material between one non-sister chromatid of each homologous chromosome is known as the **crossing over** which is accompanied by the **chiasmata formation**.

Stern and **Hotta** (1969) have reported that during the pachytene and zygotene stages, synthesis of small amount of DNA takes place. This DNA amount is utilized in the repairing of broken DNA molecule of the chromatids during the chiasmata formation and crossing over.

The nucleolus remains prominent up to this stage and it is found to be associated with the nucleolar organizer region of the chromosome.

5. Diplotene or **Diplonema**. In diplonema the chromatids of each tetrad are usually clearly visible, but the synaptonemal complex appears to have dissolved, leaving participating chromatids of the paired homologous chromosomes physically joined at one or more discrete points called **chiasmata**. These points are where crossing over took place. Often there is some unfolding of the chromatids at this stage, allowing for RNA synthesis and cellular growth.

6. Diakinesis. In the diakinesis stage the bivalent chromosomes become more condensed and evenly distributed in the nucleus. The nucleolus detaches from the nucleolar organizer and ultimately disappears. The nuclear envelope breaks down. During diakinesis the chaisma moves from the centromere towards the ends of the chromosomes and the intermediate chaismatas diminish. This type of movement of the chiasmata is known as **terminalization.** The chromatids still remain connected by the terminal chiasma and these exist up to the metaphase.

Prometaphase

In the prometaphase the nuclear envelope disintegrates and the microtubules get arranged in the form of spindle in between the two centrioles which occupy the position of two opposite poles of the cell. The chromosomes become greatly coiled in the spiral manner and get arranged on the equator of the spindle.

Metaphase I

Metaphase I consists of spindle fibre attachment to chromosomes and chromosomal alignment at the equator. During metaphase I, the microtubules of the spindle are attached with the centromeres of the homologous chromosomes of each tetrad. The centromere of each chromosome is directed towards the opposite poles. The repulsive forces between the homologous chromosomes increase greatly and the chromosomes become ready to separate.

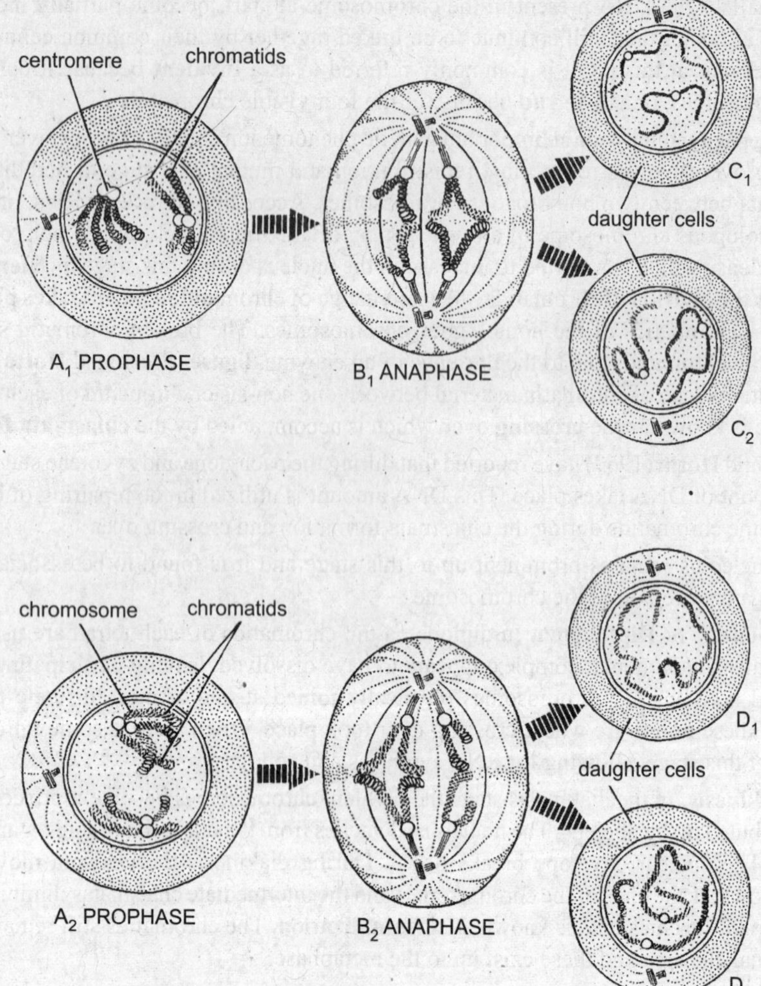

Fig. 27.9. Different stages of second meiotic division (after King, 1965).

Anaphase I

At Anaphase I homologues are free from each other and due to the shortening of chromosomal fibres or microtubules each homologous chromosome with its two chromatids and undivided centromere moves towards the opposite poles of the cell. The chromosomes with single or few terminal chiasma usually separate more frequently than the longer chromosomes containing many chiasma.

The actual reduction occurs at this stage. Here it should be carefully noted that the homologous chromosomes which move towards the opposite poles are the chromosomes of either paternal of maternal origin. Moreover, because during the chiasma formation out of two chromatids of a chromosome, one has changed its counterpart, therefore, the two chromatids of a chromosome do not resemble with each other in the genetical terms.

Telophase I

The arrival of a haploid set of chromosomes at each pole defines the onset of telophase I, during which nuclei are reassembled. The endoplasmic reticulum forms the nuclear envelope around the chromosomes and the chromosomes become uncoil. The nucleolus reappears and thus two daughter chromosomes are formed. After the karyokinesis, cytokinesis occurs and two haploid cells are formed.

Both cells pass through a short resting phase or interphase. During interphase, no DNA replication occurs, so that chromosomes at the second prophase are the same double-stranded structures that disappeared at the first telophase. In case of *Trillium* telophase I and interphase I do not occur and the anaphase I is followed by prophase II directly.

Homotypic or Second Meiotic Division

The homotypic or second meiotic division is actually the mitotic division which divides each haploid meiotic cell into two haploid cells. The second meiotic division includes following four stages:

Prophase II

In the prophase second, each centriole divides into two and thus, two pairs of centrioles are formed. Each pair of centrioles migrates to the opposite pole. The microtubules get arranged in the form of spindle at the right angle of the spindle of first meiosis. The nuclear membrane and the nucleolus disappear. The chromosomes with two chromatids become short and thick.

Metaphase II

During metaphase II, the chromosomes get arranged on the equator of the spindle. The centromere divides into two and thus each chromosome produces two monads or daughter chromosomes. The microtubules of the spindle are attached with the centromere of the chromosomes.

Anaphase II

The daughter chromosomes move towards the opposite poles due to the shortening of chromosomal microtubules and stretching of interzonal microtubules of the spindle.

Telophase II

The chromatids migrate to the opposite poles and now known as chromosomes. The endoplasmic reticulum forms the nuclear envelope around the chromosomes and the nucleolus reappears due to synthesis of ribosomal RNA (rRNA) by rDNA and also due to accumulation of ribosomal proteins.

After the karyokinesis, in each haploid meiotic cell, the cytokinesis occurs and thus, four haploid cells are resulted. These cells have different types of chromosomes due to the crossing over in the prophase I.

Significance of Meiosis

The meiosis have the greatest significance for the biological world because of its following uses:

1. The meiosis maintains a definite and constant number of the chromosomes in the organisms.
2. By crossing over, the meiosis provides an opportunity for the exchange of the genes and thus causes the genetical variations among the species. The variations are the raw materials of the evolutionary process.

27.6 SPINDLE DYNAMICS

The spindle is responsible both for chromosome separation during mitosis and meiosis, and increasing pole-to-pole distance, the latter so that two daughter nuclei have room to form. As noted earlier, spindle fibres are actually bundles of microtubules. These bundles may contain microtubules as few as one (in certain fungi) or 16 in yeast cell and as many as 5000 in higher plant cells. The chromosomal fibres extend from pole to kinetochore, while pole-to-pole fibres span poles without branching (*i.e.,* they extend from a pole past the chromosomes and into the opposite the half spindle).

In recent years, the following facts have been investigated about the behaviour of these microtubular bundles and the way they generate force to separate poles or move chromosomes:

1. The spindle forms from a pool of pre-existing subunits. Assembly is catalyzed by microtubular organizing centres consisting of spindle pole (or centrioles) and kinetochores.

2. Kinetochores, possibly because they participate in microtubule organization, fall under the influence of whichever pole they face and experience a pill toward that pole transmitted by the spindle fibres.

3. Each chromosome has two oppositely facing kinetochores, hence is pulled into a midplane position to form the metaphasic plate in mitosis. However, in the meiosis I, each of the two chromosomes falls completely under the influence of one pole. During this period of alignment, tubulin is constantly being added to the microtubules at the kinetochores and removed at the poles (Fig. 27.10).

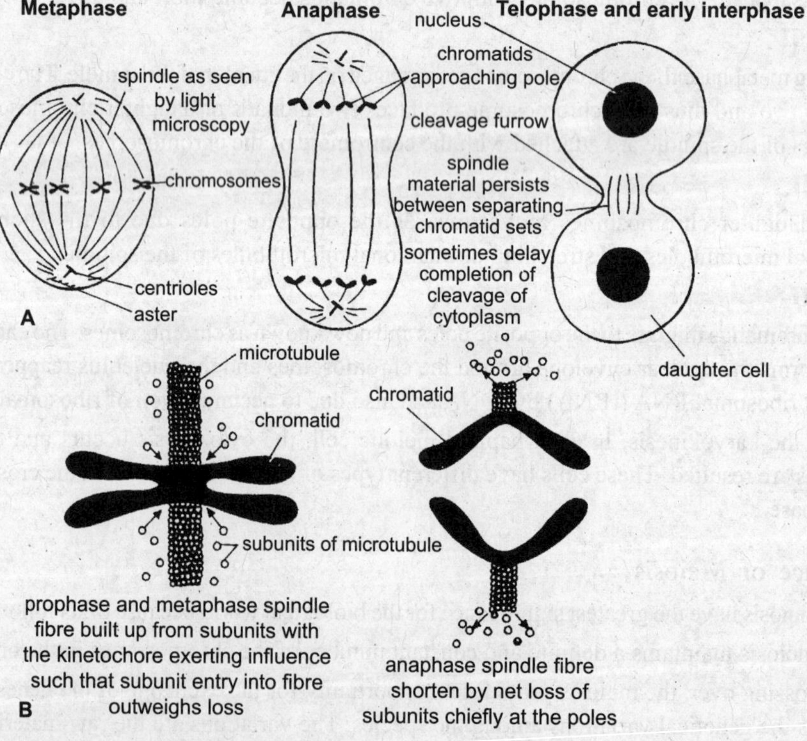

Fig. 27.10. A—Diagram illustrating the functions of microtubules of mitotic spindle in poleward migration of chromosomes during mitosis; B—Mode of functioning of microtubules by adding and deleting of their subunits.

4. At centromere division in mitosis or separation of bivalents in meiosis, tubulin addition at the kinetochores stops. Kinetochores, their chromatids trailing behind them, are pulled toward the poles as their spindle fibres dissolve by continued polar disassembly.

5. In most cells, chromosome movement is accompanied by lengthening of the pole-to-pole distance—as much as a fivefold or sixfold increase in the total span of the mitotic apparatus. It is as if tubulin that is removed from chromosomal spindle fibres is added instead to the pole-to-pole fibres. Thus, one set of fibres shrinks as the other grows, permitting the chromosomes togather at two widely separated points in the cell.

The whole mitotic process and meiosis, therefore, depends on the dynamic nature of spindle microtubules—that is to say, they depend on a shifting equilibrium between assembled microtubules and their pool of subunits.

The amount of force needed to move chromosomes is very small. **Forer** (1969) has calculated that to move a chromosome a force less than 10^{-8} dynes is needed and that the entire displacement from the equator to the pole of a chromosome may require the use of about 30 ATP molecules.

The following three force-generating mechanisms that are required for the poleward movement of chromosomes, have been proposed by different cytologists: **contraction, assembly-disassembly** and **sliding**. Contraction as a mechanism has been discarded since the microtubules do not become thicker with the polar movement of the chromosomes. And over two remaining mechanisms, there exists a lot of controversy.

1. Microtubule disassembly and chromosome movement. S. Inoue and his associates (1967, 1975) have suggested that the rate of mircotubule disassembly may determine the rate of chromosome movement. In fact, disassembly may even be responsible for chromosome movement, as the following reasoning of **R.D. Dyson** (1978) makes clear:

Picture a microtubule anchored at one end to a kinetochore and at the other to a spindle pole. Then remove a tubulin subunit from a region near the pole. If the microtubule is a dynamic structure, as cytologists have supposed, there will be a rearrangement of those subunits left behind, thus filling in the hole. In the process of rearrangement, however, the microtubule is shortend by a distance equivalent to the lost subunit. Conversely, of course, adding a subunit to the pole-to-pole fibre would drive the poles apart.

Further, the amount of force on a chromosome that could be generated by removing a microtubular subunit depends on how much attraction the other subunits have for each other, since it is this attraction that will cause remodelling and hence shortening. According to Inoue's estimates, the attraction is sufficient to cause chromosomal movement.

Lastly, it can also be analysed that if disassembly causes movement and movement takes energy, then disassembly must take energy. Where that energy comes from is not clear. However, it might well be supplied by an ATP-driven phoshporylation of the subunits, causing a conformational change favouring disassembly.

Some support to the idea that disassembly of chromosomal microtubules causes chromosomal movement comes from observations made on developing oocytes of the marine annelid worm, *Chaetopterus*. In this organism, the spindle poles are anchored through asters to the cell cortex, or perhaps to the cell membrane itself. If astral and spindle microtubules are slowly depolymerized or disassembled with any agent (*i.e.,* drug colchicine, low temperature, or high pressure), the poles and attached chromosomes are transported away from each other and toward the cell membrane. Removing the depolymerizing agent allows regrowth of spindle and asters and subsequent return of the chromosomes to their original position.

2. Sliding microtubules and chromosome movement. This idea was first advocated by **J.R. McIntosh** (1970, 1975) and it was conceived by analogy with that of muscle contraction. According to this theory the movement of chromosomes can be explained by having kinetochore microtubules slide along pole-to-pole fibres, the way microtubules in a cilium slide past each other. A similar sliding of pole-to-pole against pole-to-pole microtubules could widen the spindle (as has been observed in dividing human cell by **J. McIntosh**, 1975 and in the diatom *Pinnularia* at telophase by **J. Pickett-Heaps**, 1976). Intermicrotubular bridges that might be dynein-like (or myosin-like) arms have been noted in the spindle by **P. Hepler, J. McIntosh** and **S. Cleland** (1970). These arms may be responsible for the proposed sliding of microtubules. According to a possibility, however, these arms may work not against other microtubules but against actin filaments which are also known to be present in the spindle, localized to kinetochore-attached fibres (**J.W. Sanger**, 1975). In fact, microtubules may even be structural rather than motile components of the spindle, with force generation arising from myosin-actin interactions rather than tubulin-tubulin or tubulin interactions (see **Dyson** 1978).

27.7 CYTOKINESIS

Cytokinesis is generally, but not always, synchronized with anaphase and telophase in both mitosis and meiosis. A notable exception occurs after fertilization of *Drosophila* eggs, for some 4000 nuclei are produced by mitosis without any cell division at all. Then each nucleus is partitioned into a separate cell by multiple cytokinesis. On the other hand, many fungi and some green algae regularly undergo nuclear division without cytokinesis to form a multinucleated cell called a **coenocyte**. Animal cells with more than one nucleus are also seen especially in the liver. Though skeletal muscle cells have multiple nuclei, but they got that way by cell fusion rather than by nuclear proliferation. These multinucleated cells are the exceptions rather than the rule. Most eukaryotic cells couple cytokinesis to karyokinesis.

Cytokinesis occurs differently in animal and plant cells and, therefore, can be studied separately as follows:

1. Cytokinesis in Animal Cells

In those animal cells in which karyokinesis and cytokinesis are normally synchronized the point where the cells actually divide is clearly influenced by position of the centre of the spindle. For example in 1919 **E. G. Conklin** found that when the spindle apparatus of an oocyte was displaced by centrifugation so was the site of division, altering the relative size of the polar body and ovum. In fact, the mitotic apparatus can be experimentally shifted to and fro causing new **division furrows** (indentations) to form in the cell membrane and old ones to regress. The mitotic apparatus is clearly responsible in some way for inducing the formation of these furrows; it determines both their location and it establishes the synchrony between karyokinesis and cytokinesis.

The spindle apparatus itself, however, is not responsible for cytokinesis, only for initiating it. Once the chain of events leading to cytokinesis has been established, the spindle can be surgically removed or dissolved without substantially altering the subsequent division. **Y. Hiramoto** (1965) has dissolved the spindle apparatus of the sea urchin (*Clypeaster*) egg by injecting less than a microliter of sucrose solution in the latter, and found that cytokinesis occurred on schedule and in the position that it would have taken had the spindle been left intact.

The current view is that asters are responsible for establishing the division furrow. (Higher plants do not have asters but neither do they have division furrows, as they divide by cell plate formation). Cytokinesis seems to start at a point on the cell membrane midway between the two asters, and therefore, at a point affected equally by them. In certain experiments, the spindle was surgically removed while leaving asters intact, and then cells were distorted to bring two astersinto close proximity without an intervening spindle. Division furrows in these cases formed midway between the asters.

Fibres radiate out in all directions from asters, often reaching the plasma membrane. It may be this connection between aster and membrane that is responsible for the aster's influence. In cells with very small asters and large spindle, however, spindle fibre themselves may be responsible for initiating division.

Mechanism of cytokinesis. For explaining the method of division furrow formation during cytokinesis, the following theories have been proposed by different cytologists:

***(i)* Contractile ring theory** (or cortical gel contraction theory). This theory holds that cell cortex contains certain contractile proteins. A dividing cell before cytokinesis elongates and the cortical proteins which form a ring-like structure at equator contract and resulted into furrow at the equator (**Marsland** and **Landau**, 1954). The contractile proteins of cortex of sea urchin eggs have been found to contain ATPase activity like the actomyosin proteins of muscle cells (**Oknishi**, 1962). In the contraction of cortical gel the involvement of ATP is also suggested.

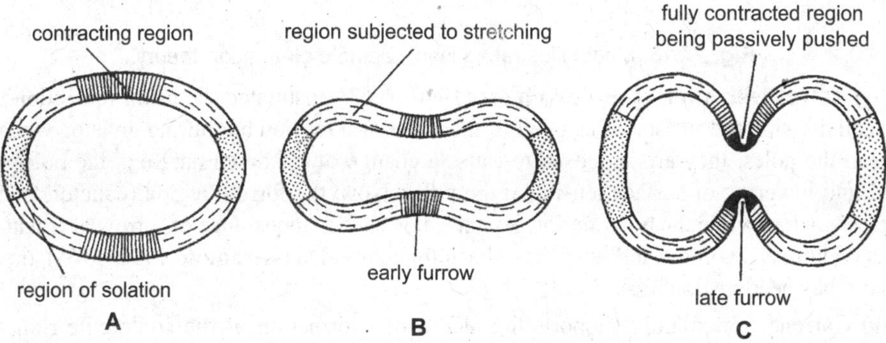

Fig. 27.11. Diagram of the cortical gel contraction theory of Marsland and Landau. A—Early telophase; B—Early furrow; C—Late furrow.

***(ii)* Expanding surface theory.** This theory was postulated by **Mitchison** in 1952 and it holds that a nuclear substance is liberated probably from the chromosomes which cause expansion of the cellular membrane at the poles. As the polar area expands, the equator contracts, leading to division. This theory has been supported by **Dan** and **Dan**, 1947 and **Mitchison,** 1952 by certain experimental evidences. However, there exists controversy about the nuclear origin of excitant substance because the cells without nuclei or chromosomes have been found divided (**Harvey**, 1936; **Hiramoto,** 1956, 1965, and **Nachtwey** 1965). Further, **Selman** and **Waddington** (1955) have postulated that expansion of surface area of cell may occur due to growth.

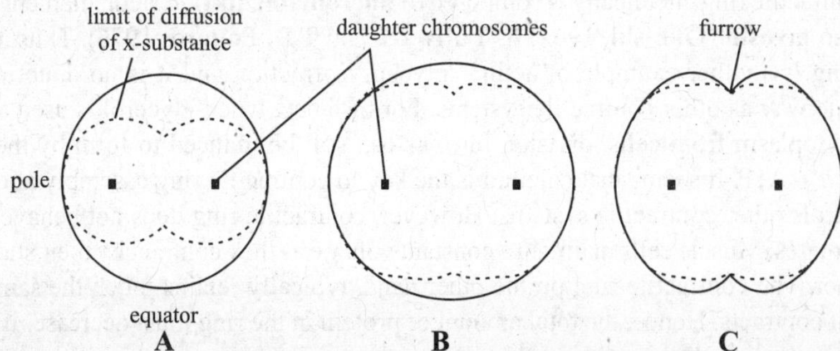

Fig.27.12. Diagram illustrating the expanding membrane theory of cleavage of Mitchison and Swann.

***(iii)* Spindle elongation theory.** This theory is postulated by **Dan** and **Dan**, 1947; **Dan,** 1958 and suggested active participation of spindle and asters in cytokinesis. The microtubules of the spindle elongate and push the centres apart due to that the astral rays which occur at the equator come close together and cause pull at the furrow region. Due to the pull, the furrow appears at the equator of the dividing cell.

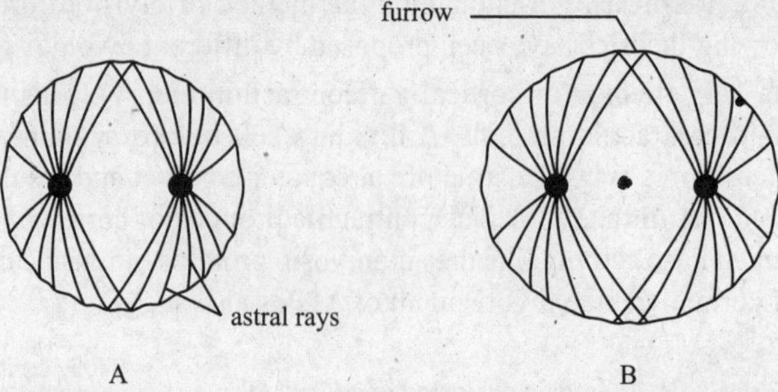

Fig. 27.13. Model illustrating Dan's spindle elongation theory.

***(iv)* Astral relaxation theory. Wolpert** (1960, 1963) postulated the astral relaxation theory. Before cell division the surface of egg cell is under uniform tension but during division when astral rays reach the poles, they are supposed to cause a change of unknown nature at the poles, which resulted into lowering of surface tension at the poles. Now, the furrow region (equator) maintains its surface tension, while the polar region expands, this causes appearance of furrow at equator. But, the cells without any spindle and asters have been found divided (**Hiramoto** 1956, 1965), therefore, this theory has become doubtful.

(*v*) Current view mainly supports the idea of the formation of the contractile ring for the formation of division furrow. The cytoplasm directly beneath a division furrow contains a dense ring of microfilaments arranged circumferentially around the cell like a purse string (**D.G. Scott** and **C.W. Daniel**, 1970). This collection of filaments is referred to as the **contractile ring**.

The contractile ring is assembled when a division furrow forms and it disappears again when the cells are divided. The contractile ring grows ever smaller, dragging the cell membrane with it until division is complete. Where the cell membrane is drawn into the division furrow, it is puckered as has been supported by scanning electron micrography on cleaving frog egg by **H.W. Beams** and **R.G. Kessel** (1976).

As already noted, the assembly of the contractile ring is usually initiated by the presence of a nearby mitotic or spindle apparatus. Once assembly has begun, however, it seems to be self-propagating.

The contractile ring chemically is composed of **microfilaments** (*i.e.,* actin filaments) (**Brinkley,** 1971) and also **myosin** (**Oknishi**, 1962; **K. Fujiwara** and **T.D. Pollard**, 1976). Thus, probably the contractile ring is another example of actin – myosin interaction and it is no doubt controlled in much the same way as other contractile systems. For instance, when glycerol is used to extract the bulk of the cytoplasm from cells, division furrows can still be induced to form by the addition of Ca^{2+} and Mg^{2+} – ATP. It seems that calcium is the key to contractile ring assembly and movement, just as it controls other contractile systems. However, contractile ring does not behave exactly like muscle sarcomeres. Muscle cells maintain a constant volume as they contract by their sliding filament past each other. The contractile ring on the other hand, typically retains much the same width and thickness as it contracts. Hence, the total amount of protein in the ring must decrease. It appears that the filaments in the ring disassemble as the ring contracts.

During the end of cytokinesis, in many cells, remnants of the spindle apparatus called the **midbody** (**Brinkley** and **Cartwright**, 1971) persist in the region below the ring and get compressed into a long lasting, "telophase neck". During this time the contractile ring becomes less and less prominent. The purpose of this persistent midbody is uncertain. However, as it contains an overlap of microtubules from the two poles of the former spindle (**McIntosch** *et al* 1975), the midbody may elongate and serve to help separate the new cells and thus prevent their accidental fusion.

Membrane changes during cytokinesis. Recently it has been calculated that when a spherical cell divides its cytoplasm among two spherical daughter cells, the total surface area of the daughter cells will be 26 per cent larger than the original area of the parent cell. This means that either new membrane must rapidly be made and inserted during division, or the existing membrane must stretch, or our assumption of spherical cell is not quite accurate. Recent findings have supported heavily in the favour of latter.

Some cells remain roughly spherical throughout their cycle, while others round up prior to division. Even the very round cells have numerous surface projections consisting of microvilli, filopodia, lamellipodia and so on. These projections significantly increase the total surface area of the cell. As a consequence there is typically more than enough surface membrane in the parent cell to accommodate the two daughters. From this model, one would expect newly formed daughter cells to be relatively smooth and the amount of surface projections (especially microvilli) to be at a maximum just before division. **S. Knutton, M. Summer** and **C. Pasternak** (1975) have supported this prediction by their studies on dividing cultured mouse mastocytoma cells (tumor cells).

New cell membrane seems to be made and inserted throughout interphase. In non-growing cells, destruction balances synthesis; growing cells, however, accumulate most of their new membrane as microvilli that are unfolded to support cell division.

Due to cytokinesis the cytoplasmic organelles become randomly distributed to daughter cells and might lead to slight variations, such as 120 mitochondria in one cell and 80 mitochondria to other. But because many cytoplasmic organelles such as kappa particles of *Paramecium*, mitochondria, centrioles, chloroplast, etc., have their independent DNA and protein synthetic mechanism, so, have the capacity of self replication. Soon after cytokinesis due to self-replication of these organelles the usual number of organelles is restored.

2. Cytokinesis in Plant Cells

Most cells of higher plants are surrounded by a dense cell wall that establishes shape. The cell membrane is attached to this wall at numerous points. Hence, the division furrow used by animal cells would not be an appropriate mechanism of cytokinesis in plants.

In plants cytokinesis occurs by formation of a **cell plate, usually** at the equatorial plane of the spindle. A collection of vesicles called the **phragmoplast** accumulates around microtubules at the mid-plane of the spindle after chromosomes have been pulled away. These vesicles are derived from Golgi saccules and are brought into position by the microtubules. These vesicles fuse to form a **disc** which then grows outward by fusion of more vesicles at its edges until the cell membrane is reached. Finally, the growing disc fuses with the cell membrane. When this process is completed, the vesicle membranes have become inward extensions of the plasma membrane and two daughter cells have been created. The vesicle contents which are trapped between the two daughter cells, represent the beginning of new cell wall.

The cell wall grows and matures with the cells. It does so by addition of components carried to it in Golgi-derived vesicles and by local polysaccharide synthesis using enzymes and raw materials transported to it from the Golgi apparatus. The new cell wall is rarely completely solid. Rather, as the vesicles coalesce during cell plate formation, they leave channels of cytoplasm. These channels continue to extend between and thus connect daughter cells after cell wall formation. They are the **plasmodesmata** that transfer substances and signals from cell to cell presumably to coordinate growth and function.

27.8 REGULATION OF CELL CYCLE

The rate at which prokaryotic and eukaryotic cells traverse the cell cycle is highly variable. For example, yeast cells can make it in three hours. Cells lining the small intestine of mammals take 17 or 18 hours to traverse the cell cycle, but some mammalian cells never divide (*e.g.*, skeletal muscle cells and neurons). However, even these most stable cells are capable of some degree of progress through the cell cycle when properly stimulated, indicating the presence of some kind of regulatory process that normally holds the cells in check. In recent years, the following facts have been known about the regulatory processes of cell division:

1. Cell Growth and Cell Division

The cell grows to a certain stage and then divides. The rate at which a critical size needed for division is reached depends on the rate of metabolism. That, in turn, will be influenced by such factors as the surface-to-volume ratio, which limits the capacity to bring in food and get rid of wastes. The ratio becomes less favourable as the cell gets larger. Metabolic rate is also dependent on temperature and other environmental factors, including the supply of oxygen and nutrients. The actual rate of growth itself will be a function both of metabolic activity and of kinds of organic molecules the cell must make, as opposed to those that are supplied by the growth medium. Thus, all these things influence the generation time.

However, even under constant conditions, the generation time for a given cell may vary widely in response to external controls. Most of the variation occurs in the length of time the cell spends in the G_1 stage. Very rapidly growing cells may have no noticeable G_1 stage at all. At the other extreme, some cells such as liver cells, skeletal muscle cells, neurons, etc., seem to be more or less permanently arrested in G_1 stage. These observations have led to the concept of a **G_1 checkpoint** at which a cell may be temporarily or permanently halted, thus regulating the time of cell cycle.

2. Cell Cycle Checkpoints

It has been already mentioned that the cell cycle, either prokaryotic or eukaryotic, is an ordered sequence of events (*i.e.,* five events G_1, S, G_2, M and D), where the occurrence of one leads naturally to the next. A **checkpoint** is a critical event in this sequence that represents a barrier to further progress through the cycle.

In the bacterial cell cycle the checkpoint is the initiation of DNA synthesis because once a replication fork has been initiated DNA synthesis will continue until the chromosome has been duplicated, and that event in normal cells invariably leads to cytokinesis. In *E. coli*, replication of DNA takes a constant 40 minutes and cytokinesis follows about 20 minutes after its completion. Hence, the rate of cell division depends on the rate of initiation, which in *E. coli* can be as often as every 20 minutes.

In the eukaryotic cells, the following three kinds of checkpoints have been found:

***(i)* G_1 checkpoint.** In most eukaryotic cells, the major check point is in the G_1 stage. Once it has been passed, the S, G_2, M and D stages usually take place without hesitation and in a length of time that is often relatively fixed for cells of a given species. For example, mouse epithelial cells from various locations in the animal had generation times ranging from 41 to 8000 hours, with the variation almost exclusively attributed to variation in length of the G_1 stage (**W.K. Blenkinsopp**, 1969).

The length of time a cell stays at the G_1 checkpoint and hence remains in the G_1 stage, is speculated to depend on the energy of activation needed to get through it. Controlling the rate of replication, thus, becomes a matter of varying this energy of activation.

It is still not known that what is the G_1 checkpoint, however, it has been reported that passing the G_1 checkpoint, results in accumulation in the cytoplasm of a substance that makes possible entry into the **S** stage. The presence of this substance has been demonstrated by cell fusion and nuclear transplantation experiments: (1) when a nucleus was transplanted from a cell in the G_2 stage to a cell in the S stage, the transplanted nucleus began to replicate its DNA again; (2) when a G_1 and S stage cell were fused, the G_1 nucleus enters the S stage at once; and (3) when mouse and hamster cells were fused, both nuclei entered S stage at the time expected for the hamster cells, which had a much shorter G_1 stage than mouse cells. In fact, in multinucleate cells all nuclei enter the S stage simultaneously, apparently in response to the appearance of some cytoplasmic factor.

***(ii)* G_2 checkpoint.** A second checkpoint exists in the G_2 stage. Cells that are arrested at the G_2 transition will be tetraploid – that is, having passed the S stage they will have twice the usual amount of DNA. Tetraploid nuclei are occasionally found in various tissues; they are common in the liver cells, and they are present as a rule in heart muscle cells of adult humans. In heart muscle, the conversion from diploid to tetraploid occurs during childhood, presumably to support the metabolism of the enlarging cells, which do not divide. This reasoning has been supported by the observation that when adult human beings experience congestive heart failure from abnormal enlargement of heart cells (for example, in response to long-standing high blood pressure), many of the nuclei pass through still another S stage to become octoploid and a few become 16 or 32 ploid (see **Dyson,** 1978).

The critical event at the G_2 checkpoint is concerned with the condensation of chromatin, which necessarily precedes mitosis. In fact, traversal of the G_2 checkpoint leads to accumulation of a cytoplasmic substance capable of causing chromatin condensation. The existence of a chromatin condensing factor was demonstrated by **R.T. Johnson** and **P.N. Rao** (1970, 1974) by using Sendai virus to fuse HeLa cells at different stages in their cell cycle. When a mitotic cell is fused with a cell in the G_2 stage, chromatin condensation takes place at once in the G_2 nucleus, producing normal looking chromosomes. When a mitotic cell is fused instead with a cell at its G_1 stage, chromatin condenses in that nucleus too, but since DNA replication has not occurred only single-stranded chromatids (or chromosomes without two daughter chromatids in each) are seen. Even S-stage nuclei can undergo chromatin condensation in this way, although multiple fragments of condensed chromatin instead of complete chromatids are seen..

Chromatin condensation is thought to be associated with, and perhaps due to, phosphorylation of histone H1 (**Marks, Paik** and **Borun** 1973; **Ord** *et al.,* 1975; **E.M. Bradbury,** 1975). Histone H1, like the other histones, is synthesized at the same time as the DNA to which it binds (in contrast to non-histone chromosomal proteins, which are synthesized at a regular rate throughout the cell cycle). The enzymes capable of phosphorylating H1 however have a peak of activity late in G_2 stage. The phosphate content of both new and old histone H1 rises sharply just prior to chromatin condensation and decreases again when the chromatin disperses after mitosis. Thus, G_2 checkpoint is somehow associated with interrelationship between H1 phosphorylation and chromatin condensation.

***(iii)* G_0 cells.** The term G_0 refers to cells that have completed mitosis but are not proceeding toward another one. These are **quiescent cells** small lymphocytes, liver cells, skeletal muscle cells, neurons and so on. The transition from G_0 to G_1 by definition requires not just the passage of time but a specific stimulus—*i.e.,* a **mitogenic** stimulus, or one that induce mitosis. Mitogenic stimulation is accompanied by biochemical changes in the cell that include increased transcription of DNA and increased level of non-histone chromosomal proteins.

A good example of a G_0 to G_1 transition has been provided by regenerative capacity of liver of rat. The liver parenchymal cells (hepatocyte) of the rat are highly differentiated cells that rarely divide. However, surgical removal of part of the liver (**"partial hepatectomy"**) is followed by an abrupt change in the biochemical activities of the remaining cells. By 24 hours, mitotic figures are seen. Their number peaks rapidly and then drops to almost nothing by 72 hours. The newly divided cells then enlarge and differentiate so that the original mass is regained in about two weeks. Some other examples of quiescent cells and stimuli that can cause them to replicate have been tabulated in Table 27–3.

Table 27.3. Stimulation of quiescent cells (from Dyson, 1978).

	Cell	Stimulus
1.	Liver parenchymal	partial hepatectomy; albumin depletion
2.	Kidney tubule	removal of other kidney
3.	Uterine smooth muscle and endometrium	estrogens
4.	Mammary gland	estrogens
5.	Prostate gland (castrated rat)	5-α-dihydrotestosterone
6.	Adrenal gland	ACTH
7.	Salivary gland	catecholamines
8.	Growth cartilage (to lengthen long bones)	growth hormone/somatomedins
9.	Fibroblasts	epidermal growth factor; fibroblast growth factor
10.	Lymphocytes	lectins; receptor antibodies; specific antigens

3. Growth Factors

Nearly all cultured animal cells require at least a small amount of blood serum in their culture medium. In an attempt to find out why, many substances have been identified in serum that are not nutrients in the usual sense or most not even gain entry to the cytoplasm, but which nevertheless are needed by the cells. These substances are called **growth factors** or **mitotic stimulators**. The typical growth factor can act as a **mitogen** for specific types of quiescent cells (*i.e.,* it can cause G_0 cells to reenter the cell cycle and divide).

Certain cell culture experiments have shown that when a culture of non-cancerous cell was permitted to grow under favourable conditions, replication usually stopped when the cells had approximately covered the dish to a depth of one cell. This phenomenon was originally called **contact inhibition** but is now more often referred to **as density dependent inhibition of growth**, because it seems to have more to do with the ability to transport nutrients into the cell than with cell-to-cell contact as such (**Martz** and **Steinberg**, 1972). The cells in this condition seem to have reverted to the quiescent Go phase, a situation from which they can often be rescued by the addition of appropriate growth factor or by certain less specific manipulations, such as damage of membrane proteins with trypsin. This ability to rescue G_0 cells is commonly used to identify growth factors.

Types of growth factors. Most growth factors are **peptides** or small **proteins. Insulin** is one of the first known mitogen in mammalian systems. **Growth hormone** was one of the first growth factor other than insulin to be investigated. It was long assumed to be directly responsible for cellular proliferation in growth cartilage and hence for elongation of bones during childhood. In fact, a deficiency of growth hormone during childhood results in dwarfism, while an excess results in a pituitary giant. However, it is now considered that growth hormone is only indirectly responsible in the growth of bones and it causes release from other tissues of a family of proteins called **somatomedins**. These secondary proteins appear to be the true mitogens.

Erythropoietin is often listed as a growth factor or mitogen though its target cell, the proerythroblast (precursor of the erythrocyte), is not absolutely dependent on erythropoietin. Nevertheless this glycoprotein, which appears to be made by the kidneys in response to oxygen deprivation, can cause erythrocyte production to be increased as much as seven fold or more.

Other growth factors having specific tissues as their target include **nerve growth factor,** which is an essential mitogen for embryonic sympathetic nerves and necessary for growth and maintenance of these same cells later in life; **epidermal growth factor,** which causes epithelial cell division at various locations; and **fibroblast growth factor**, which stimulates not only fibroblast, but cells lining small blood vessels. There are many other protein growth factors (see **D. Gospodarowicz** and **J. Moran,** 1976).

Certain **non-protein** growth **factors** or **mitogens** such as **steroid hormones** and **polyamines** have also been identified. A particularly interesting non-protein growth factor is the polyamine **putrescine** which has been found in the growth medium of some cultured human cells and is a putrid-smelling mitogen. It is produced by the enzyme **ornithine decarboxylate (ODC)** from ornithine according to the following reaction:

$$\text{Ornithine} \xrightarrow[\text{ODC}]{} \text{Putrescine} \longrightarrow \text{Spermidine} \longrightarrow \text{Spermine}$$

ODC has very short half-life of 5 minutes and so, its concentration rapidly fluctuates in the cell. A rise in ODC activity is one of the first events to be measurable in a mitogenically stimulated cell. In addition, it appears that spermidine fluctuates in concentration with the cell cycle and is essential for the G_1 to S transition. These polyamines are found to bind to DNA and somehow act as mitogens.

Putrescine and steroid hormones penetrate cell membrane and so are able to interact with cytoplasmic receptors. The protein growth factors interact with target cells by binding to specific receptors on the cell surface and their mitogenic effect is mediated by some kind of cytoplasmic "second messengers," such as cAMP and Ca^{2+} (**M. J. Berridge**, 1976).

Mode of action of growth factors. Different growth factors stimulate mitosis by the following methods:

***(i)* Cyclic AMP and other "Second messengers".** The level of cAMP in many cells vary inversely with growth rate; that is, rapidly dividing cells have low levels of cAMP while stationary cell cultures have high levels of cAMP. The direct addition of cAMP or agents that raise cAMP levels (*e.g.,* theophylline or caffeine) often slow growth rates, even in some cancer cells. Conversely, agents associated with a fall in cAMP (*e.g.,* insulin) are often promoters of growth and cellular replication. Certainly the known capacity of cAMP to stimulate protein kinases gives itself readily to a regulatory role, for not only enzymes but gene regulators may be controlled in part by phosphorylation and dephosphorylation. It is also possible that gene repressors having direct need of cAMP will be found in eukaryotes as they have been in prokaryotes.

Another candidate for second messenger is **cGMP**, the level of which also fluctuate during the cell cycle and can be increased by external stimuli. Still another is Ca^{2+} ions. In fact, it is hard to separate the role of Ca^{2+} from that of cyclic nucleotides (*i.e.,* cAMP and cGMP), since there is a strong interaction (**M. Willingham**, 1975; **L. Rebhun**, 1977).

***(ii)* Lymphocyte activation.** A B-lymphocyte cell has little cytoplasm and a dense, shrunken nucleus. When B-lymphocytes come in contact with the right antigen, they may be stimulated to leave their G_0 state—they very quickly change into a more active appearing cell with increased amount of cytoplasm and less condensation of their chromatin. This transformation is called **blastogenesis**, as it leads to a lymphocyte capable of dividing and of differentiating into a mature antibody-producing plasma cell (**J.M. Hanifen** and **M.J. Cline,** 1970). This change can also be brought about by specific antigens, by antibodies to surface receptors and by certain lectins, especially phytohemagglutinin. The key to blastogenesis in each case, however, appears to be cross-linking of surface receptors and a subsequent increase in cytoplasmic Ca^{2+}. It appears that Ca^{2+} uptake is the event causing stimulation, most probably by activating protein kinases (**G.L. Nicolson**, 1974, **P.K. Lauf**, 1975; **M. Crumpton** *et al* 1975; **C. Parker**, 1976).

***(iii)* Steroid hormones.** The steroid hormones, as explained in Chapter 25, are able to enter cells directly, complex with cytoplasmic receptors and then move into the nucleus where the expression of target genes is altered. Steroid hormones apparently do not need cyclic nucleotides or Ca^{2+} to mediate their effect.

Of the various steroids, the estrogens in particular are known for their mitogenic effects on target tissues. For example, smooth muscles of the rodent uterus can be induced to proliferate in the presence of estrogen. And the normal rise and fall of estrogen levels in menstruating women causes, in the first-half of the menstruating cycle, rapid proliferation of cells of endometrium lining the uterus. These cells will be caused to differentiate by progesterone in the latter half of the cycle and then sloughed at menstruation. Similarly, estrogens cause proliferation of ductal cells in the mammary glands, which then differentiate in response to progesterone during pregnancy **(J. Loeb**, 1976).

Growth Factors in Plants

There are certain chemical agents which stimulate mitosis in plant cells. Certain wellknown plant mitogens are the plant hormones such as **gibberellins, ethylene, indoleacetic acid** and **kinetin** (**D. Gross,** 175; **H.N. Krishnamoorthy,** 1975; **S. Osborne,** 1977). For example, kinetin (6-furfurylaminopurine) increases the mitotic rate in meristems of *Allium* and at low concentrations, generally reduces the duration of interphase and increases the mitotic rate.

27.9 MITOTIC POISONS (MITOTIC INHIBITORS)

Certain chemical compounds act like inhibitors of the mitotic and meiotic cell divisions and they are generally called **"mitotic poisons"** (**Biesele, 1958**). These active agents can be endogenous (naturally occurring in tissues) or exogeneous (developed or originating outside the organism). A mitotic poison may inhibit different phases of mitosis or all phases of mitosis with different intensity. One or several mitotic mechanisms may be involved, *e.g.,* nuclear membrane cycle, chromosomal condensation, behaviour of the centromere, formation of the spindle and chromosome movement, chromosome duplication, nuclear cycle and metabolism of nuclear DNA, nuclear and cytoplasmic RNA, proteins and the energy-producing processes for mitosis and meiosis. The mitotic poisons and their effect on cell division can be studied under the following headings:

1. Mitotic Poisons that act at Prophase and Interphase

Some chemical agents produce a change at the critical stages during which the chromosomes duplicate. Certain chemicals inhibit oxidation (cyanide, azide) or uncouple oxidative phosphorylation processes (2, 4-dinitrophenol) that provide the energy for mitosis. Therefore, the prevent mitosis, but not chromosomal duplication. Consequently, the mitotic phase does not take place, but the nuclear volume increases.

Other chemical agents affect carbohydrate metabolism (*e.g.,* the adrenal glucocorticoids) or interfere with chromosomal replication by changing the metabolism of DNA and protein. Certain chemicals such as nitrogen mustards produce a chromosomal fragmentation similar to that caused by ionizing radiation. A chromosomal fracture is readily followed by reorganization. Research with chemical agents indicate that some areas of chromosome (*e.g.,* centromere) are more sensitive than other. **Saez** and **Drets** (1958) have suggested that a highly active chemical agent can cause nuclear disintegration. In this process "DNA droplets" are forced out of the nucleus into the cytoplasm and nuclear vocuolation followed by nuclear lysis finally takes place.

2. Chemical Agents that act at Metaphase and the following Phases

This type of action is called **mitosis C** because it is produced principally by colchicine, cytogenetical affects of which were discovered in animals by **Lits** (1934) and in plants (**Dustin, Havas**, and **Lits**, 1937). This alkaloid affects the formation of the spindle, and also acts on the chromosomes. The action on the spindle leads to different degrees of blockage of chromosomal division in metaphase and anaphase. Since chromosomal duplication is not affected, polyploidy may result. Treated with colchicine, chromosomes may continue the spiralization cycle; the two chromatids are contracted and repel one another, but remain united by the centromeres (ski-configuration). Colchicine bind to tubulin (a monomer protein of microtubules) preventing its polymerization and the formation of microtubules and so, block the mitotic spindle formation. (For the action of certain antibiotics, see Chapter 24).

27.10 CHALONE

Attempt to determine why damage of cells in the skin stimulates their division thus permitting wound healing, led **W.S. Bullough** and **E.B. Laurence** to the discovery in 1960 of a substance, called **chalone.** According to **Bullough**, the name comes from a Greek word meaning "*to slack off the main sheet of a sloop to slow the vessel down.*" Chalones are mostly peptides or glycoproteins and share the following characteristics:

1. They inhibit mitosis both *in vivo* and *in vitro*.
2. They are tissue-specific, but they are remarkably the same from one species to another.
3. The tissue affected by a particular chalone is also a tissue that makes the same chalone.
4. Mitotic suppression by chalones is reversible, apparently without harm to the cell.

Substances fitting this description have now been isolated from a number of animal tissues. Cells are stimulated to divide when chalone production by nearby cells is compromised, as when tissue is damaged. Inhibition is reestablished when an adequate concentration of healthy, chalone-producing cells is again present (**A. Thornley** and **E. Laurence**, 1975; **J. Houck**, 1976) (For more details see Chapter 32).

The subject of mitotic inhibitors is receiving much attention from medically oriented scientists because of its obvious application to the treatment of allergies and tumours. For example, the adrenal glucocorticoids such as cortisol or cortisone are used to treat severe allergies and inflammations, prevent rejection of transplanted organs and treat lymphocytic leukemia, since, lymphocytes are especially sensitive to these mitotic inhibitors. Malignant cells tend to be much less sensitive to mitotic inhibition by chalones and other natural inhibitors, but more sensitive to drugs that tend to have greater effects on rapidly dividing cells.

Comparison Between Mitosis and Meiosis

Mitosis	Meiosis
1. Mitosis occurs continuously in the body or somatic cells.	1. Meiosis occurs in the germ cells (the cells of the testes or ovaries during the process of gametogenesis.
2. The whole process completes in one sequence or phase	2. The whole process completes in two successive divisions which occur one after the other.
Prophase	
3. The prophase is of short duration and includes no substage.	3. The prophase is of longer duration and it completes in six successive stages, *viz*, proleptotene, leptotene, zygotene, pachytene, diplotene and diakinesis.
4. The homologous chromosomes (paternal and maternal) duplicate into two chromatids. The two chromatids separate and form new chromosomes. Each daughter cell receives the daughter chromosomes or chromatids of each homologous chromosome and thus having the chromosome number like the parental cells.	4. Out of two homologous chromosomes only one type of chromosome either maternal or paternal move to the daughter cells. A daughter cell thus receives only a maternal or paternal chromosome of the homologous pair and the number of chromosomes remain half than the paternal cells.
5. No pairing or synapsis takes place between the homologous chromosomes.	5. Paring or synapsis occurs; between the homologous chromosomes.
6. Duplication of chromosomes takes place in the early prophase.	6. Duplication or spliting of chromosomes takes place in the late prophase (pachytene stage).

7. No chiasma formation or crossing over takes place.	7. Chiasma formation or crossing over takes place.
8. The exchange of the genetic material between the homologous chromosomes does not occur.	8. The exchange of the genetic material takes place between the non-sister chromatids of homologous chromosomes.
Metaphase	
9. The chromatids occur in the form of dyads.	9. The chromatids of two homologous chromosomes occur as the tetrads.
10. The centromeres of the chromosomes remain directed towards the equator and the arms of the chromosomes remain directed towards the poles.	10. The centromeres of the chromosomes remain directed towards the poles and the chromosomal arms remain directed towards the equator.
Anaphase	
11. The chromosomes are the monads, *i.e.*, having single chromatid.	11. The chromosomes are the biads. *i.e.*, having two chromatids and single centomere.
12. The chromosomes are long and thin.	12. The chromosomes are short and thick.
Telophase	
13. The telophase always occurs.	13. The first telophase is sometimes omitted.
Significance	
14. The chromosome number in each daughter cell remains the same like the parent cell.	14. In meiotic division the chromosome number is reduced to half in the daughter cells than the parental cells.
15. A diploid cell produces four diploid cells by a mitotic division.	15. A diploid cell produces four haploid cells by a meiotic division.

REVISION QUESTIONS

1. What is the cell division ? How many types of cell divisions occur in living organisms ? Discuss the use and biological significance of each type of cell division ?
2. Define the terms: cell cycle and mitosis. Name the stages of cell cycle. Which is usually the longest stage ? What are the major features of each mitotic phase ?
3. What basic activities occur during mitosis ? How does mitosis differ in animal and plant cells ?
4. What biochemical events take place in cells before visible cellular division occurs. Compare the cytogenetic view of chromatin in interphase, in mitosis, and in meiosis.
5. Describe the behaviour and presumed role of centrioles during mitosis.
6. What is meiosis ? Describe the major features of each meiotic phase. Also discuss, why is meiosis needed for the production of gametes ?
7. Summarize the events of the first meiotic prophase.
8. Which phases of meiosis are the same as the corresponding mitotic phase and which are different ? In what ways to they differ ?
9. What do you mean by "dynamic equilibrium of the spindle fibres"? What experiments establish that concept ?
10. Describe the role of the microtubules in chromosome movement during mitosis and meiosis.
11. What is cytokinesis ? Describe the process of cytokinesis in animal and plant cells.
12. What is a division furrow and contractile ring ? What influences appear to be instrumental in establishing contractile ring ?

13. If one creates two spheres our of one, additional surface would be needed. In cell division, where does this additional surface come from ?

14. Describe the process of cell plate formation. What are plasmodesmata and how are they formed ?

15. What is a “cell cycle checkpoint.” ? What are the possible cell cycle controls ? What events seem to be most directly dependent on passing the G_1 and G_2 checkpoints ?

16. What is meant by a “G_0 cell” ? Growth factor ? Mitogen ? Describe the events leading to lymphocyte blastogenesis.

17. What are some cellular effects of estrogens and glucocorticoids ?

18. Describe mitotic regulation by negative feedback. How do chalones fit into this scheme ?

28
Chapter

REPRODUCTION

This is the inherent property of the living organisms to continue their race by the mechanism of reproduction. The reproduction is a process by which the living beings propagate or duplicate their own kinds. The reproduction may be of following two types:

1. Asexual reproduction
2. Sexual reproduction.

28.1 ASEXUAL REPRODUCTION

The development of new individuals without the fusion of the male and female gametes is known as **asexual reproduction**. The asexual reproduction usually includes amitotic or mitotic division of the body (somatic) cells, therefore, it is also known as **somatogenic** or **blastogenic reproduction**. The asexual reproduction is common only in lower plants and animals and it may be of following types:

1. Fission; 2. Budding; 3. Gemmule formation; and 4. Regeneration.

1. Asexual reproduction by the fission. The fission is the most widely occurring type of asexual reproduction of the protozoans and various metazoans. In this method of reproduction the nuclear and cytoplasmic contents of the cell divide or split completely into smaller-sized daughter individuals. The fission itself may be of following types:

A. Binary fission. In the binary fission the animal body splits or divides in such a plane that two equal and identical halves are produced, It is most common in protozoans but it also occurs in certain lower metazoans. First of all the nucleus divides by amitotic or mitotic division and the division of the nucleus is followed by the division of the cytoplasm. According to the plane of fission the following types of binary fission have been recognized in the organisms:

(*i*) Simple or orthodox type of binary fission. The simple or orthodox type of binary fission occurs in the irregular-shaped organism, *e.g.*, *Amoeba* in which the plane of division is difficult to observe.

(*ii*) Transverse binary fission. The transverse binary fission occurs in some protozoans, *e.g.*, *Paramecium* (Fig. 28.1) and some metazoans such as certain coelenterates, turbellarians and annelids. In transverse binary fission the plane of the division is always transverse to the longitudinal axis of the body of the organisms.

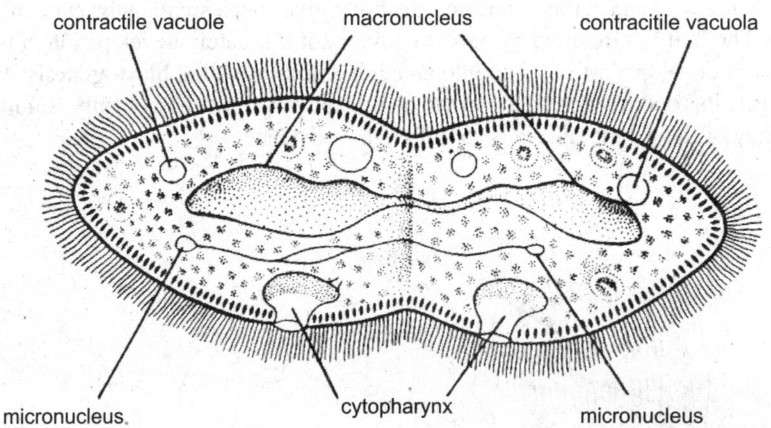

Fig. 28.1. Transverse binary fission in *Paramecium*.

***(iii)* Longitudinal binary fission.** The longitudinal binary fission occurs in certain ciliates and flagellates, *e.g.*, *Vorticella* and *Euglena* (Protozoa; Fig. 28.2) and some corals (Anthozoa). In longitudinal binary fission the nucleus and the cytoplasm divide in the longitudinal plane.

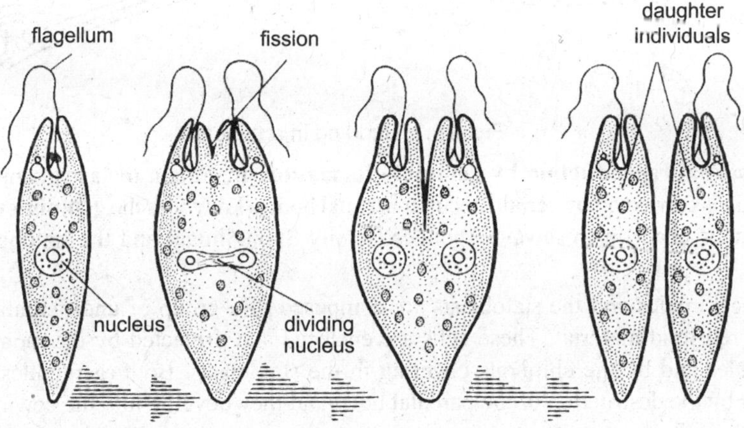

Fig. 28.2. Longitudinal binary fission in *Euglena*.

***(iv)* Oblique binary fission.** The oblique binary fission occurs in most dinoflagellates. In this type of fission the cell or body of the organism divides by the oblique division.

(*v*) Strobilation. In certain metazoan animals a special type of transverse fission known as the strobilation occurs. In the process of the strobilation several transverse fissions occur simultaneously and giving rise to a number of individuals which often do not separate from each other immediately. The strobilation occurs in the scyphozoan (*Aurelia*), certain polychaetes and ascidians. In *Aurelia*, for instance, strobilation occurs during the formation of ephyra larva.

B. Asexual reproduction by multiple fission. In the multiple fission, the nucleus of the cell divides very rapidly into many nuclei. Each daughter nucleus in later stage is surrounded by the little mass of the cytoplasm and forms the asexually reproducing body such as schizogont, gamont, spore, etc. The multiple fission occurs in most algae, fungi and some protozoans, *e.g.*, *Amoeba*, *Plasmodium* and *Monocystis*, etc.

2. Asexual reproduction by budding or gemmation. In certain multicellular animals such as *Hydra* (coelenterates) and certain tunicates, the body gives out a small outgrowth known as the **bud** (Fig. 28.3). The bud is supported by parent body and it ultimately develops into a new individual. The process of development of a bud into an adult animal is called **blastogenesis**. The developing individual gets its food from the body of the parent and when it becomes fully mature it is detached from the body of the parent and leads an individual existence.

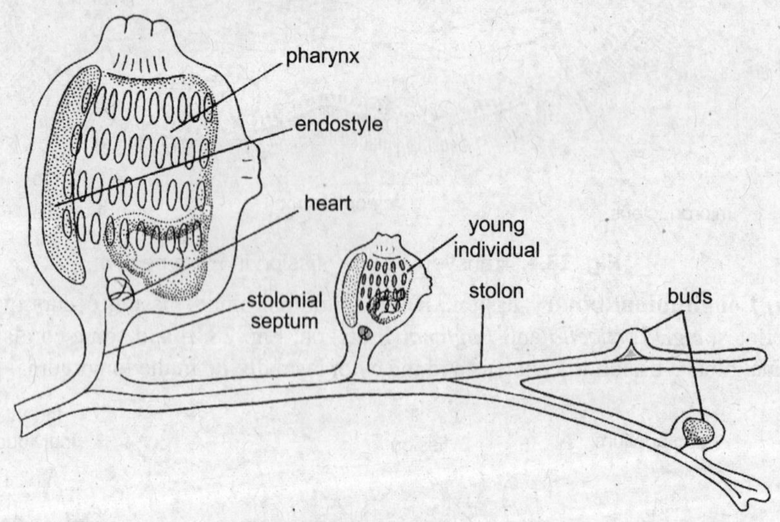

Fig. 28.3. Budding in a tunicate.

3. Asexual reproduction by gemmule formation. In certain metazoan animals the asexual reproduction is carried on by certain peculiar asexual bodies known as the **gemmules** and **statoblasts**. The gemmules occur in freshwater sponges (family Spongilidae) and the statoblasts occur in the bryozoans.

The gemmules and the statoblasts are composed of a group of undifferentiated cells which contain stored food material. These cells are enclosed and protected by the monaxon spicules in the gemmules and by the chitinous covering in the statoblasts. Both (gemmules and statoblasts) are set free by the destruction of the parental body and they develop into the new individuals in the favourable conditions.

4. Asexual reproduction by regeneration. The regeneration is a process by which the organisms develop or regenerate their lost or worn out parts. The regeneration is the best means of asexual reproduction in certain protozoans, sponges, coelenterates, planarians and echinoderms.

28.2 SEXUAL REPRODUCTION

In the sexual reproduction, the development of the new individual takes place by the fusion of the sex cells or male and female gametes. The sexual reproduction is the most common type of reproduction among animals. It may be of following types:

1. Syngamy. The syngamy is the most common type of sexual reproduction in the plants and animals. In syngamy (Gr., *syn* = together; *gam* = marriage) the fusion of two gametes takes place completely and permanently. Following kinds of syngamy is prevalent among the living organisms:

(*i*) **Autogamy.** In autogamy (Gr., *auto* = self; *gam* = marriage) the male and female gametes are produced by the same cell or organisms and both gametes fuse together to form a zygote, *e.g.*, *Actinosphaerium* and *Paramecium*.

(*ii*) **Exogamy.** In exogamy (Gr. *exo* = external; *gam* = marriage) the male and female gametes are produced by different parents and both unite to form a zygote.

(*iii*) **Hologamy.** In the lower organisms, sometimes the entire mature organisms start to act as gametes and the fusion of such mature individuals is known as the **hologamy**.

(*iv*) **Paedogamy.** Paedogamy is the sexual union of young individuals produced immediately after the division of the adult parent cell by mitosis.

(*v*) **Merogamy.** In the merogamy (Gr., *meros* = part; *gam* = marriage), the fusion of smaller-sized and morphologically different gametes (**merogametes**) takes place.

(*vi*) **Isogamy.** In isogamy (Gr., *is* = equal; *gam* = marriage) the fusion of morphologically and physiologically identical gametes (*isogametes*) takes place.

(*vii*) **Anisogamy.** Some organisms produce two types of gametes. Both types of gametes differ from each other in their shape, size and behaviour and are collectively known as the **anisogametes** or **heterogametes**. The male gametes are motile and small in size and known as the **microgametes**. The female gametes are passive and have comparatively large size and known as the **macro-** or **mega-gametes**. The union of micro-and macrogametes is known as the **anisogamy** (Gr. *an* = without; *is* = equal; *gam* = marriage). The anisogamy occurs in higher animals and plants but it is customary to use the term **fertilization** in them instead of the anisogamy or syngamy.

(*viii*) **Macrogamy.** The syngamy or fusion of the macrogametes is known as **macrogamy** (Gr., *macro* = large; *gam* = marriage).

(*ix*) **Microgamy.** The microgamy (Gr., *micro* = small; *gam* = marriage) is common in certain protozoans, *e.g.*, foraminiferns and *Arcella*. In microgamy the fusion of microgametes takes place.

2. Conjugation. The conjugation is the temporary union of the two individuals of the same species. During the union both individuals known as **conjugants** exchange certain amount of nuclear (DNA) material and after which conjugants are separated. The conjugation is most common among the ciliates, *e.g.*, *Paramecium* and bacteria.

3. Automixis. When the gamete nuclei of the same cell unite together to form new individuals this phenomenon is known as the **automixis**.

4. Parthenogenesis. The parthenogenesis (Gr., *parthenos* = virgin, *genesis* = birth) is the special type of sexual reproduction. In parthenogenesis, the eggs of an organism develop into the young individual without the fertilization of the eggs by the sperms. The parthenogenesis occurs in certain insects (wasps and bees, aphids, etc.) and rotifers.

REVISION QUESTIONS

1. What is reproduction ? How many kinds of reproduction occur in the living organisms ?
2. What is asexual reproduction ? Describe various kinds of asexual reproduction.
3. Describe different kinds of sexual reproduction in animals.

29 Chapter GAMETOGENESIS

The gametogenesis (Gr., *gamos*-marriage; *genesis*-origin) is the process of gamete formation in the sextually reproducing animals. The sexually reproducing animals contain two types of cells in their body, *e.g.*, **somatic cells** and the **germinal cells**. Both types of cells have diploid number of chromosomes but each type has its different destiny. The somatic cells form various organs of the body and provide a phase for the maturation, development and formation of the germinal cells. The somatic cells always multiply by mitotic division.

The germinal cells form the gonads (testis and ovaries) in the animal body. These cells produce the gamete cells by successive mitotic and meiotic divisions. The male gamete is known is **spermatozoon** or **sperm** and the female gamete is known as **ovum** or **egg**. The process of sperm production is known as the **spermatogenesis** (Gr., *sperma*-sperm or seed; *genesis*-origin) and the process of production of ovum is known as **oogenesis** (Gr., *oon*-egg; *genesis*-origin). Both the process can be studied in detail under separate headings.

29.1 SPERMATOGENESIS

The process of spermatogenesis occurs in the male gonads of testis. The testis of the vertebrates are composed of many seminiferous tubules which are line by the cells of germinal epithelium. The cells of the germinal epithelium form sperms by the process of spermatogenesis. But in certain animals, *e.g.*, vertebrates including mammals and Mollusca, etc., there are somatic cells lying in between germinal cells. These somatic cells are known as **Sertoli cells**. The Sertoli cells anchor the differentiating cells and provide nourishment to the developing sperms. The insects do not possess Sertoli cells. The spermatogenesis is a continuous process and for the sake of convenience this process can be studied in two different stages:

1. Formation of spermatids,
2. Spermiogenesis.

1. Formation of spermatids

The male germinal cells which produce the sperms are known as the **primary germinal cells** or **primordial cells**. The primordial cells pass through the following three phases for the formation of spermatids:

(*i*) Multiplication phase. The undifferentiated germ cells on primordial cells contain large-sized and chromatin-rich nuclei. These cells multiply by repeated mitotic divisions and produce the cells which are known as the **spermatogonia** (Gr., *sperma*-sperm or seed; *gone*-offspring). Each spermatogonium is diploid and contains 2X number of chromosomes.

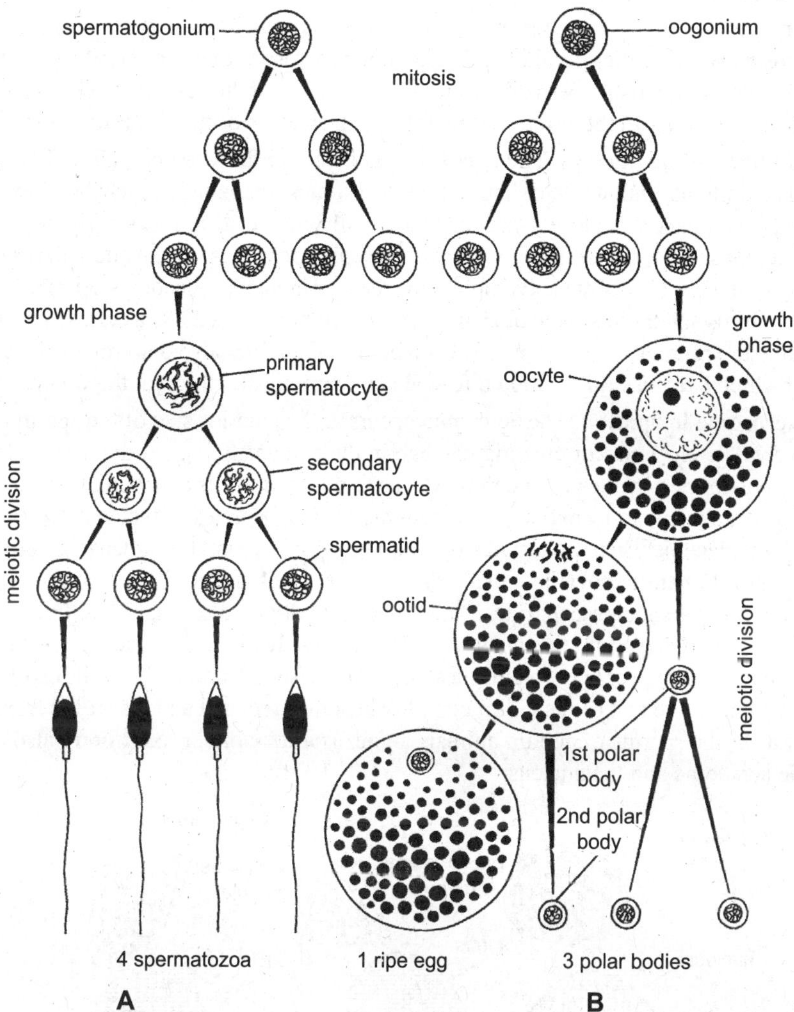

Fig. 29.1. Spermatogenesis and oogenesis. A — Spermatogenesis; B — Oogenesis (after Balinsky, 1970).

***(ii)* The growth phase.** In the growth phase, the spermatogonial cells accumulate large amount of nutrition and chromatin material. Now each spermatogonial cell is known as the **primary spermatocyte**.

***(iii)* The maturation phase.** The primary spermatocytes are ready for first meiotic or maturation division. The homologous chromosomes start pairing (synapsis), each homologous chromosome splits longitudinally and by the chiasma formation the exchange of genetic material or crossing over takes place between the chromatids of the homologous chromosomes. The DNA amount is duplicated in the beginning of the division. By first meiotic division or homotypic division two **secondary spermatocytes** are formed. Each secondary spermatocyte is haploid and contains X number of chromosomes. Each secondary spermatocyte passes through the second maturation or second meiotic or heterotypic division and produces two **spermatids**. Thus by a meiotic or maturation division a diploid spermatogonium produces four haploid spermatids. These spermatids cannot act directly as the gametes so they have to pass through the next phase, the **spermiogenesis.**

2. Spermiogenesis

The metamorphosis or differentiation of the spermatids into the sperms is known as **spermiogenesis.** Because the sperm or spermatozoon is a very active and mobile cell so to provide great amount of mobility to the sperm, the superfluous material of the developing sperms is discarded. For the reduction of the weight of the sperms following changes occur in the spermatids:

(*i*) Changes in the nucleus. The nucleus loses its entire fluid content, all its RNA, nucleolus and most of its proteins. Only DNA of haploid set of chromosomes exist as such, however, chromatin becomes more compact and closely packed into small volume. Due to its shrinkage the nucleus assumes different shapes in the different animals. The sperm nucleus in man and bull becomes ovoid and laterally flattened. In rodents and amphibians the sperm nucleus becomes scimitar-shaped with pointed tip. In birds and molluscs the nucleus becomes spirally twisted like a cork screw. The bivalve molluscs have the round sperm nucleus. The shape of the nucleus also determines the shape of the sperm head which becomes fully adopted for the active propulsion through the water.

(*ii*) Acrosome formation. The acrosome occurs at the anterior side of the sperm nucleus and contains hydrolytic enzymes for creating passage in the contents of egg at the time of fertilization. The acrosome is formed by the Golgi complex. The Golgi complex is concentrated near the anterior end of the sperm nucleus to form the acrosome. One or two vacuoles of the complex become large and occupy the place between the tubules of Golgi complex. Soon after a dense granule known as the **proacrosomal granule** develops inside the vacuole. **Leblond** (1955) found the proacrosomal granule rich in the mucopolysaccharides. The proacrosomal granule attaches with the anterior end of the nucleus and enlarges into the **acrosome**. The membranes of Golgi vacuoles form the double membrane (unit membrane of lipoprotein) sheath around the acrosome and forms the cap-like structure of the spermatozoa. The rest of the Golgi complex becomes reduced and discarded from the sperm as **Golgi rest**. In the sperms of certain animals an **acrosomal cone** or **axial body** also develops in between the acrosome and the nucleus.

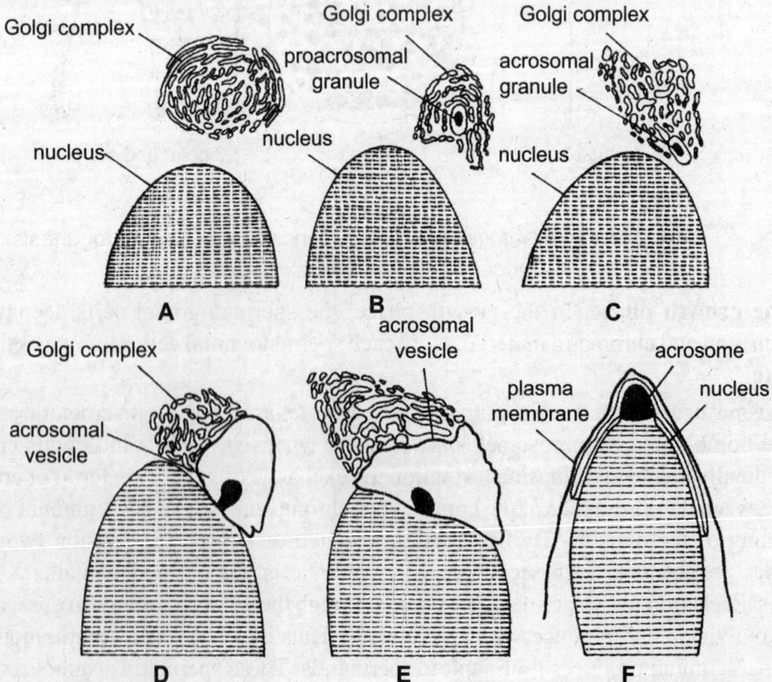

Fig. 29.2. Formation of acrosome of sperm (after Balinsky, 1970).

***(iii)* The centrioles.** The centriole divides into two and the two centrioles of the spermatids become arranged one after the other behind the nucleus. The anterior one is known as the **proximal centriole** and the posterior one is known as the **distal centriole**. The distal centriole changes into the basal body and gives rise to the **axial filament** of the sperm. The axial filament or the flagellum is composed of a pair of central longitudinal fibres and nine peripheral fibres. The distal centriole and the basal part of the axial filament occur in the middle piece of the spermatozoa. The mitochondria of the spermatids fuse together and twist spirally around the base of the axial filament.

Thus, most of the cytoplasmic portion of the spermatid except the nucleus, acrosome, centriole, mitochondria and axial filament is discarded during the spermiogenesis.

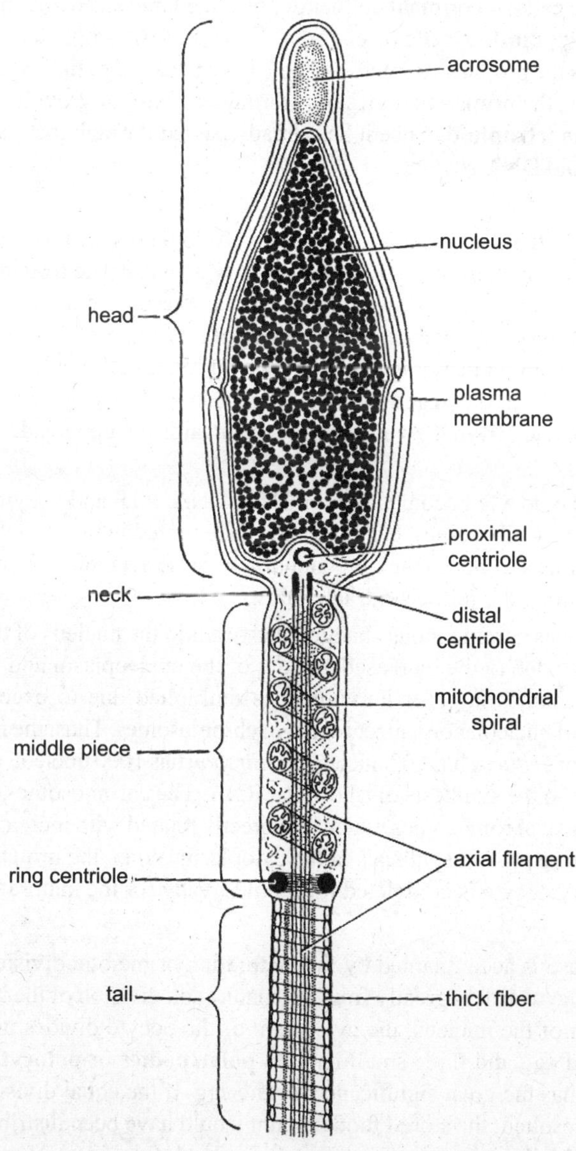

Fig. 29.3. Electron microscopic view of a flagellate spermatozoon (after Balinsky, 1970).

29.2 OOGENESIS

The process of oogenesis occurs in the cells of the germinal epithelium of the ovary, such cells are known as **primordial germinal cells**. The oogenesis is completed in the following three successive stages:

1. Multiplication phase,
2. Growth phase,
3. Maturation phase.

1. Multiplication phase

For oogenesis, some cells of germinal epithelium become large sized and multiply mitotically to form a population of **egg mother cells** or **oogonia**. When mitosis stops, the oogonia are called **oocytes**. The oocyte enters the prophase of meiosis I and now are called **primary oocytes**. Before the completion of first meiosis, the primary oocytes pass through a phase of growth and differentiation. Note that oocyte nucleus is **tetraploid**, since it has already passed through the S stage of interphase to double the normal diploid DNA content.

2. Growth phase

The growth phase of the oogenesis is comparatively longer than the growth phase of the spermatogenesis. In the growth phase, the size of the primary oocyte of the frog in the beginning has the diameter about 50 μm but after the growth phase the diameter of the mature egg reaches about 1000 μm to 2000 μm. In the primary oocyte, large amount of fats and proteins become accumulated in the form of **yolk** and due to its heavy weight (or gravity) it is usually concentrated towards the lower portion of the egg forming the **vegetal pole**. The portion of the cytoplasm containing the egg nucleus remains often separated from the yolk and occurs towards the upper side of the egg forming the **animal pole**.

The cytoplasm of the oocyte becomes rich in RNA, DNA, ATP and enzymes. Moreover, the mitochondria, Golgi complex, ribosomes, etc., become concentrated in the cytoplasm of the oocyte. In certain oocytes (Amphibia and birds) the mitochondria become accumulated at some place in the oocyte cytoplasm and forming the mitochondrial clouds.

During the growth phase, tremendous changes also occur in the nucleus of the primary oocyte. The nucleus becomes large due to the increased amount of the nucleoplasm and is called **germinal vesicle**. The nucleolus becomes large or its number is multiplied due to excessive synthesis of ribosomal RNA by rDNA of nucleolar organizer region of chromosomes. Thus, the nucleus or germinal vesicle of primary oocyte of *Triturus* has 600 nucleoli, of *Siredon* has 1000 nucleoli and of *Xenopus* has 600 to 12000 nucleoli due to the synthesis of ribosomal RNA. The chromosomes change their shape and become giant lampbrush chromosomes which are directly related with increased transcription of mRNA molecules and active protein synthesis in the cytoplasm. When the growth of the cytoplasm and nucleus of the primary oocyte is completed it becomes ready for the maturation phase.

3. Maturation phase

The maturation phase is accompanied by the maturation or meiotic division. The maturation division of the primary oocyte differs greatly from the maturation division of the spermatocyte. Here after the meiotic division of the nucleus, the cytoplasm of the oocyte divides unequally to form a single large-sized haploid egg and three small haploid **polar bodies** or **polocytes** at the end. This type of unequal division has the great significance for the egg. If the equal divisions of the primary oocyte might have been resulted, the stored food amount would have been distributed equally to the four daughter cells and which might prove insufficient for the developing embryo. Therefore, these unequal divisions allow one cell out of the four daughter cells to contain most of the cytoplasm and reserve food material which is sufficient for the developing embryo.

***(i)* First maturation division.** During the first maturation division or first meiosis, the homologous chromosomes of the primary oocyte nucleus pass through the pairing or synapsis, duplication, chiasma formation and crossing over. Soon after the nuclear membrane breaks and the bivalent chromosomes move towards the opposite poles due to contraction of chromosomal fibres. A new nuclear envelope is developed around the daughter chromosomes by the endoplasmic reticulum.

After the karyokinesis the unequal cytokinesis occurs and a small haploid polar body or polocyte and a large haploid **secondary oocyte** or **ootid** are formed.

***(ii)* Second meiotic division.** The haploid secondary oocyte and first polocyte pass through the second meiotic division. Due to the second meiotic division the secondary oocyte forms a mature egg and a second polocyte. By the second meiotic division the first polocyte also divides into two secondary polocytes. These polocytes ooze out from the egg and degenerate, while the haploid egg cell becomes ready for the fertilization.

Structure of Mature Egg

The mature egg has a cell-like structure and composed of the following parts:

1. Plasma membrane. The mature egg is covered by a plasma membrane which is the unit membrane. It is composed of an outer and an inner layer of protein. Both the layers are 50 Å in thickness. Between the proteinous layers there occurs a lipoidous layer of 60° thickness.

2. Primary egg membranes. In addition to the plasma membrane the eggs of most animals except the sponges and certain coelenterates consist of certain other additional egg membranes. These membranes are known as the primary and secondary egg membranes. The primary egg membrane is secreted around the plasma membrane by the oocyte itself. In the insects, molluscs, amphibians and birds the primary egg membrane is known as the **vitelline membrane**, while in tunicates and fishes this membrane is known as the **chorion**. The mammalian eggs contain similar membrane and in them this is known as the **zona pellucida**. The vitelline membrane is composed of mucoproteins and fibrous proteins. The vitelline membrane usually remains closely adhered to the plasma membrane but in later stages a space is known as the **perivitelline space**.

3. Secondary egg membranes. The secondary egg membranes are secreted by the ovarian tissues around the primary egg membranes. They are composed of either jelly-coats in amphibians or chitinous shells in insects, ascidians and cyclostomes.

4. Tertiary egg membranes. The tertiary egg membranes are formed by the oviduct or other accessory parts of female reproductive system. They may be composed of either jelly coats in amphibians, albumen and hard horny capsule in elasmobranch fishes, or albumen, shell membranes and calcareous shell in birds.

5. The ooplasm. The cytoplasm of the egg cell is known as the ooplasm. The ooplasm consists of large amount of reserve food material in the form of **yolk.** It is also composed of a lipoprotein, pigment granules, water, RNA, ribosomes, mitochondria and various other cellular inclusions. The peripheral layer of the ooplasm is known as the **cortex** and it contains many microvilli and cortical granules. The microvilli are formed by the outpushings of the plasma membrane and they help in the transportation of the substances from the follicle cells to the egg during the development of the egg. The cortical granules are spherical bodies of various diameters, *e.g.*, 0.8 μm in the sea urchin eggs and 2.0 μm in the eggs of frog. The cortical granules are surrounded by the unit membranes and are originated from the Golgi complex. They contain homogeneous and granular acid mucopolysaccharides and are present in the eggs of sea urchins, frogs, fishes, bivalve molluscs, some annelids and certain mammals. But they do not occur in the ova of man, rat, guinea pig, gastropod molluscs, urodele amphibians, insects and birds.

Yolk contents of the ooplasm. The amount of the yolk in the ooplasm varies from species to species. According to the amount of the yolk following types of egg cells have been recognised.

1. **Alecithal.** The eggs without the yolk are known as alecithal eggs, *e.g.,* Eutherian mammals.
2. **Microlecithal.** The eggs with very little amount of the yolk are known as the microlecithal eggs, *e.g., Amphioxus*.
3. **Macrolecithal.** The eggs with large amount of the yolk are known as the macrolecithal eggs. The macrolecithal eggs can be grouped into two types on the basis of the distribution of the yolk in the ooplasm.

A. Homolecithal. The eggs with evenly distributed yolk contents in the ooplasm are known as the homolecithal eggs, *e.g.,* eggs of echinoderms.

B. Heterolecithal. The eggs in which the yolk is not evenly distributed in the ooplasm are known as the heterolecithal eggs. The heterolecithal eggs may be of following types.

(*i*) Telolecithal. When the amount of the yolk is concentrated in the one of half of the egg to form the vegetative pole of the egg, then this condition is known as the telolecithal, *e.g.,* eggs of amphibians, etc.

(*ii*) Meiolecithal. In the meiolecithal eggs the amount of the yolk is very large and it occupies the largest portion of the egg except a small disc-shaped portion of the cytoplasm. The cytoplasm contains the zygote nucleus and is known as the germinal disc, *e.g.,* eggs of fishes, reptiles and birds.

(*iii*) Centrolecithal. In the centrolecithal eggs the yolk accumulates in the centre of the ooplasm, *e.g.,* eggs of insects.

Differences Between Spermatogenesis and Oogenesis

Spermatogenesis	Oogenesis
1. This occurs in male gonads, *i.e.,* testes.	1. This occurs in female gonads, *i.e.,* ovaries.
2. Four spermatids are formed from one sperm mother cell.	2. Only one ovum is formed from one primary oocyte.
3. The sperm mother cell divides by meiotic cell division into four equal sized cells and all the four cells transformed into spermatozoa to act as reproductive unit.	3. The oocyte divides unequally and resulted into one large sized ovum and three small sized polar bodies or polocytes which are sexually inert and extruded from the ovum as waste. Only ovum acts as reproductive unit.

REVISION QUESTIONS

1. What is gametogenesis ? Summarize the steps in spermatogenesis and oogenesis.
2. Describe the events of spermiogenesis. Why is it necessary for spermatogenesis ?
3. What are the major features of each step of oogenesis ? Compare the oogenesis with spermatogenesis.
4. Describe different kinds of eggs on the basis of yolk contents.

30
Chapter
FERTILIZATION

The union of the cytoplasm and pronuclei of the male and female gametes is known as the fertilization (L., *fertilis*-to bear). The fertilization is the most commonly used method for the production of the diploid zygotes in the sexually reproducing organisms of Metazoa and Metaphyta.

In the process of the fertilization the haploid male gamete (spermatozoa or pollen), which carries the paternal genetic information, unites with the haploid female gamete (ovum or egg), which carries genetic informations of female parent, to form a diploid zygote. The zygote ultimately, produces a diploid multicellular organism by the several repeated and organized mitotic divisions and cellular differentiation.

30.1 EXTERNAL AND INTERNAL FERTILIZATION

The fertilization always occurs in the aquatic media such as sea water, freshwater or intra-somatic (body) fluid of the maternal individual. If the fertilization occurs outside the body of the organism it is known as **external fertilization** and if it occurs inside the body of the organism then it is termed as **internal fertilization.** The external fertilization is common in various invertebrates and chordates, while the internal fertilization occurs only in those animals which possess specialized sex organs for receiving and transmitting the sperms, *e.g.*, reptiles, birds, mammals and angiosperms, etc.

30.2 FERTILIZIN AND ANTIFERTILIZIN

The process of fertilization is very specific. The sperms of one particular species fertilize the ova of the same species. This type of specificity of male and female gametes is of utmost biological importance and is achieved by the help of certain chemical compounds. It is found that the egg contains a chemical substance known as **fertilizin (Lillie,** 1919). The fertilizin is a glycoprotein which is composed of different types of amino acids and monosaccharides (glucose, fucose, fructose and galactose) according to the species. The molecular weight of the fertilizin is 300,000 and it contains large molecules.

The surface layer of sperm contains another proteinous substance known as **antifertilizin**. The antifertilizin is a protein which is composed of acidic amino acids. It has small molecules and the molecular weight is about 10,0000.

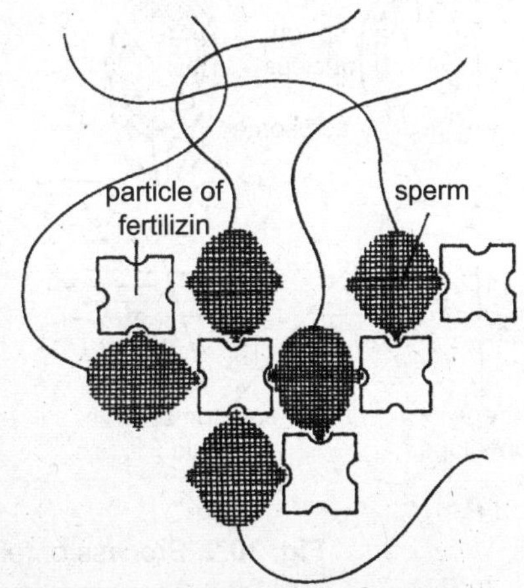

Fig. 30.1. Agglutination of sperms (after Balinsky, 1970).

The fertilizins of the eggs are supposed to attract the sperms which contain a particular type of antifertilizin. It has been found that egg fertilizin of any species reacts efficiently with the sperm antiferilizin of the same species. It has also been reported that the fertilizin in egg-water attracts the sperms of the same species and many sperms adhere together. This type of mutual adhesion of the sperms is known as the **agglutination**.

30.3 PROCESS OF FERTILIZATION

The process of the fertilization includes the following successive steps:

1. Movement of the Sperm Towards the Egg

The sperms which occur in the external or internal fluid media around the egg, swim towards the egg at randomly. The collide with the egg by chance. The chance of colliding of the sperms with the egg occurs regularly in the nature and remains fruitful only due to the large number of the sperms and enormously large size of the ovum. The fertilizins and antifertilizins become active after the chance collision of the sperms with the ova. The egg fertilizin usually occurs in the jelly surrounding the egg. It gradually dissolves in the surrounding water of the egg and forms the so called egg water.

2. Activation of the Sperm

When a sperm with a specific antifertilizin comes in contact with the egg water of its own species then certain significant changes occur in the acrosome of the sperm. The peripheral portion of the acrosome of sperm collapses and its enzymes the **lysins** are extruded and dissolve in the water. The central portion of the acrosome elongates and forms a 1 to 7.5 μm long, thin tube known as the **acrosomal filament** or **tubule**. The acrosomal filament is the rigid tube which protrudes out from the sperm head. When the sperm possesses such as acrosomal filament it is said to be activated for the ready penetration in the unfertilized egg. When the activated sperms reach to the egg the acrosomal filaments penetrate into the egg jelly and vitelline membrane by the help of dissolving action of the sperm lysins. As soon as the tip of the acrosomal filament touches egg plasma membrane, various important morphological and physiological changes are started in the egg.

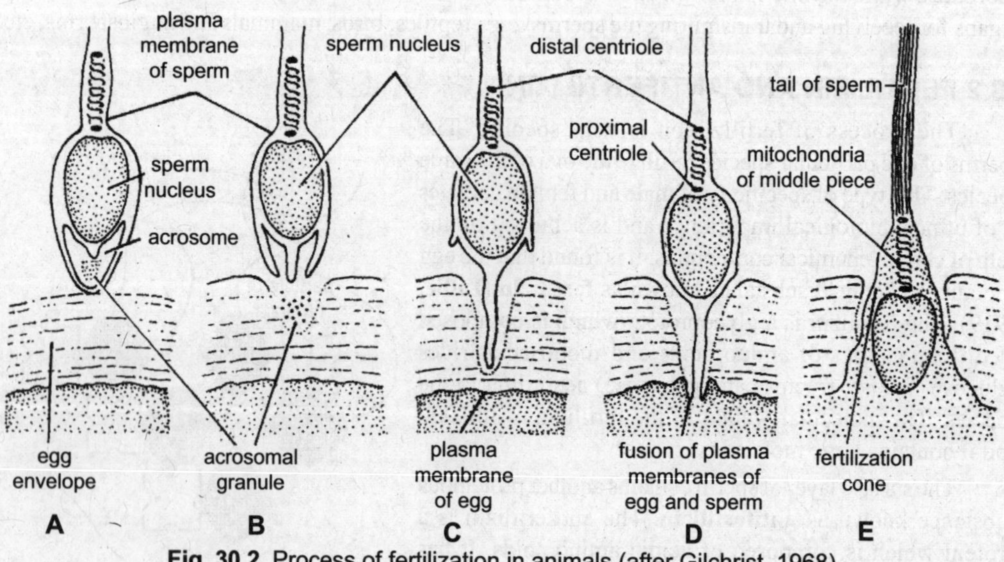

Fig. 30.2. Process of fertilization in animals (after Gilchrist, 1968).

3. Activation of Ovum

Immediately after the apical tip of the acrosomal tubule of a spermatozoon touches the surface of the egg plasma membrane, fusion of both membranes (*i.e.*, plasma membranes of sperm and egg) over this limited area of contact, takes place and a single continuous mosaic membrane is formed. Consequently, the plasma membrane of both gametes become in continuation and forms a single cell, called **zygote**. This event is followed by following activities, are collectively called the **activation of ovum**:

A. Fertilization cone formation. At the place of fusion of plasma membranes of acrosomal tubule and ovum, the cytoplasm of the ovum bulges forward, producing a cone-shaped protrusion called **fertilization cone**. The fertilization cone gradually engulfs the different components of spermatozoon such as periacrosomal granules, sperm nucleus, proximal centriole, mitochondria of mid-piece, etc., and then begins to retract. The plasma membrane of sperm becomes one of the entity of plasma membrane of the egg (see **Berrill**, 1971).

B. Cortical reaction and fertilization membrane formation. The fertilization-cone elevation is followed by a chain of physico-chemical reactions in the cortex of egg cytoplasm, all of which are called **cortical reactions** and which ultimately, culminate into the formation of a membrane, called **fertilization membrane,** outside the egg plasma membrane. For the formation of fertilization membrane, in many animals, the **cortical granules** of egg cortex, which are derived from Golgi-complex during oogenesis and contain mainly mucopolysaccharides, are broken down, their contents are liquefied and extruded on the surface of egg plasma membrane. The fertilization membrane blocks the enterance of late arriving spermatozoa (For details see **Verma, Agarwal** and **Tyagi**, 1980).

C. Metabolic activation. The penetration of spermatozoon's different components in the unfertilized egg, initiates a diverse series of cytoplasmic reactions in egg cytoplasm. Following metabolic changes occur in the egg at fertilization:

(*i*) The permeability of plasma membrane of egg increases for the molecules of water ethylene glycol, phosphate, etc. The enzyme **adenyl cyclase** of egg plasma membrane is activated and the production of cAMP is started. cAMP activates most of the metabolic reactions in a fertilized egg (**Castaneda** and **Tyler,** 1968).

(*ii*) There occur certain intracellular changes in the concentration of cations, especially those of sodium, potassium and calcium. The change in calcium ion concentration in a fertilized egg, has great significance in the metabolic activation of the egg (**Rasmussen**, 1970).

(*iii*) NAD coenzyme of egg is activated (**Epel** and **Iverson,** 1965).

(*iv*) In fertilized egg, the rate of respiration either increase (*e.g.,* sea urchins), or decrease (*e.g., Chaetopterus*, and mollusc, *Cumingia*) or remains static (*e.g., Bufo* and *Fundulus*). The increased oxygen consumption is related with the oxidation of glycogen and other food stuffs of egg and synthesis of numerous ATP molecules.

(*v*) The complete machinery of protein synthesis of unfertilized egg which is repressed or inactivated by certain inhibitor proteins during late oogenesis, is activated by certain proteolytic enzymes during fertilization and start to produce proteins. However, translation of maternal mRNA only occur during this protein synthesis.

(*vi*) DNA replication is started. The pair of centrioles of sperm-origin divides and consequently, two pairs of centrioles are formed. These centrioles form the mitosis spindle of microtubules and thus, initiation of mitosis for cleavage of egg takes place.

(*vii*) **Berrill** (1971) has suggested that the activation of egg is done by periacrosomal material.

4. Migration of Pronuclei and Amphimixis

At the time of penetration of spermatozoon inside the egg cytoplasm, the sperm nucleus remains compact and its mitochondria and centriole remain situated behind it. To perform the act of **amphimixis** or fusion of sperm and egg nuclei, the sperm nucleus has to perform two activities—(*i*) it has to become pronucleus, and (*ii*) it has to migrate from the site of fertilization to the site of amphimixis. Thus, sperm nucleus moves inward from the site of fertilization cone and it soon rotates through the angle of 180°, so that the mitochondria and centriole assume the leading position. During this migration and rotation, the sperm nucleus start swelling by absorbing water from the surrounding ooplasm, and its chromatin, which is very closely packed, becomes finely granular. It ultimately becomes vesicular and has an appearance like the interphase nucleus and is called **male pronucleus**.

Before amphimixis, the haploid nucleus of egg which occurs near the surface of the egg in the form of several vesicles, known as **karyomeres**, undergoes certain changes like the sperm nucleus. Its karyomeres fuse together to form the **female** or **egg pronucleus** which swells, increases in volume and becomes vesicular. It also migrates towards the site of amphimixis which lies either near the centre of microlecithal and mesolecithal eggs or in the centre of the active cytoplasm at the animal pole of macrolecithal or telolecithal eggs.

The amphimixis may differ in detail in different animals. In most animals, the two pronuclei actually fuse together, that is, the nuclear membrane of both pronuclei is broken at the point of their contact and the contents of both pronuclei unite into one mass, which is ultimately bounded by a common nuclear membrane. In other cases (*e.g.*, *Ascaris*, some annelids and molluscs) however, the male and female pronuclei do not fuse as such, but the nuclear membranes in both dissolve and the chromosomes become released. These chromosomes get arranged on the equatorial plane of mitotic spindle and only after the completion of the first mitotic division of first cleavage of the fertilized egg, the paternal and maternal chromosomes of two daughter nuclei of two blastomeres are enclosed by the common nuclear envelope.

30.4 KINDS OF FERTILIZATION

In the organisms following types of fertilization occur:

1. Monospermic fertilization. In most animals usually only one sperm enters in the egg, this type of fertilization is known as **monospermic fertilization.** The monospermic fertilization is common in the coelenterates, annelids, echinoderms, bony fishes, frogs and mammals.

2. Polyspermic fertilization. When many sperms enter in the egg, the fertilization is known as the **polyspermic fertilization**. It may be of two types:

(*i*) **Pathological polyspermy.** Under certain abnormal conditions when in a monospermic type of egg many sperms enter in the egg, the condition is known as the **pathological polyspermy.** This type of egg does not develop further and dies soon.

(*ii*) **Physiological polyspermy.** In the animals with large yolky eggs such as molluscs, selachians, urodels, reptiles and birds the polyspermic fertilization usually occurs. Such polyspermic fertilization is known as the **physiological polyspermy**. In these cases, many sperms enter in the egg but the pronucleus of only one sperm unites with the pronucleus of the egg and rest are degenerated soon. Such eggs are viable and develop further.

3. Polyandry. When two male pronuclei unite with a female pronucleus, the union is known as polyandry, *e.g.,* man and rat.

4. Polygamy. When two egg pronuclei unite with single male pronucleus, the phenomenon is known as polygamy, *e.g.,* sea urchins, polychaete worm, urodels and rabbits.

5. Gynogenesis. When only sperm activates the egg but its pronucleus does not unite with the egg pronucleus, *e.g.,* planarians and nematodes.

30.5 SIGNIFICANCE OF FERTILIZATION

1. The fertilization ensures the usual specific diploidy of the organisms by the fusion of the male and female pronuclei.
2. The fertilization establishes definite polarity in the eggs.
3. The fertilization provides new genetic constitution to the zygote.
4. The fertilization activates the egg for the cleavage.
5. The fertilization increases the metabolic activities and rate of the protein synthesis of the egg.
6. The fertilization initiates the egg to start cleavage and embryogenesis.

REVISION QUESTIONS

1. What is fertilization ? Describe the process of fertilization in animals.

2. What is the function of fertilization ?

3. How many kinds of fertilization occur in the animals ?

31

Chapter

PARTHENOGENESIS

Usually an unfertilized ovum develops into a new individual only after the fertilization but in certain cases the development of the egg takes place without the fertilization. This peculiar mode of sexual reproduction in which egg development occurs without the fertilization is known as the **parthenogenesis** (Gr., *parthenos*-virgin; *genesis*-origin). An organism that has developed parthenogenetically is called a **parthenogenone** or **parthenote**. The phenomenon of the parthenogenesis occurs in different groups of the animals as in certain insects (Hymenoptera, Homoptera, Coleoptera), crustaceans and rotifers.

The parthenogenesis may be of two types:

1. Natural parthenogenesis; 2. Artificial parthenogenesis.

31.1 NATURAL PARTHENOGENESIS

In certain animals the parthenogenesis occurs regularly, constantly and naturally in their life cycles and is known as the **natural parthenogeneris**. The natural parthenogenesis may be of two types, *viz.*, complete or incomplete.

(*i*) Complete parthenogenesis. Certain insects have no sexual phase and no males. They depend exclusively on the parthenogenesis for the self-reproduction. This type of parthenogenesis is known as the **complete parthenogenesis** or **obligatory parthenogenesis.**

(*ii*) Incomplete parthenogenesis. The life cycle of certain insects includes two generations, the sexual generation and parthenogenetic generation, both of which alternate to each other. In such cases, the diploid eggs produce females and the unfertilized egg produce males. This type of parthenogenesis is known as the **partial** or **incomplete** or **cyclic parthenogenesis**.

The complete and incomplete type of natural parthenogenesis may be of following two types:

(*a*) Haploid or arrhenotokous parthenogenesis,

(*b*) Diploid or thelytokous parthenogenesis.

(*a*) Haploid or arrhenotokous parthenogenesis. In the arrhenotokous parthenogenesis, the haploid eggs are not fertilized by the sperms and develop into the haploid individuals. In these cases the haploid individuals are always males and the diploid individuals are the females *e.g.*, 1. Insects: (*i*) Hymenoptera (Bees and Wasps), (*ii*) Homoptera, (*iii*) Coleoptera (*Micromalthus debilis*), (*iv*) Thysanoptera (*Anthothrips verbasi*). 2. Arachnids, *e.g.*, ticks, mites and certain spiders (*Pediculoidas ventricusm*). 3. Rotifers, *e.g.*, *Asplanchne amphora.*

(*b*) Diploid or thelytokous parthenogenesis. In the diploid parthenogenesis, the young individuals develop from the unfertilized diploid eggs.

Following types of the thelytoky have been recognized:

***(i)* Ameiotic parthenogenesis.** Sometimes during the oogenesis, first meiotic or reduction division does not occur but second meiotic division occurs as usual. Such eggs contain **diploid** number of chromosomes and develop into new individuals without the fertilization. This type of parthenogenesis is known as **apomeiotic** or **ameiotic parthenogenesis** and occurs in *Trichoniscus* (Isopoda), *Daphnia pulex* (Crustacea), *Compelona rufum* (Mollusca), weevils and long-horned grasshoppers.

***(ii)* Meiotic parthenogenesis.** Certain eggs develop by the usual process of oogenesis but at certain stages **diplosis** or doubling of chromosome number and production of diploid eggs occur. Such eggs develop into the diploid individuals and this phenomenon is known as the **meiotic parthenogenesis**.

The **diplosis** of the diploid thelytoky may occur by the following methods:

***(a)* By autofertilization.** In certain cases the oocyte divides meiotically upto the formation of ootid and secondary polocyte. But the ootid and the secondary polocyte unite together to form a diploid egg which develops into a new individual, *e.g.*, *Artemia salina* (Crustacea) and various other organisms.

***(b)* By restitution.** Sometimes in primary oocyte karyokinesis forms a nucleus of the secondary oocyte and a nucleus of the first polocyte. But the karyokinesis is not followed by the cytokinesis. The chromosomes of both daughter nuclei are arranged on the equator and undergo second meiotic division to form a diploid ootid and a diploid polocyte. The diploid ootid or ovum develops into a parthenogenetic diploid individual. This type of diplosis is known as the restitution, *e.g.*, insects of order Hymenoptera (*Nemertis conesceus*) and Lepidoptera.

31.2 ARTIFICIAL PARTHENOGENESIS

The eggs which always develop into the young individuals by the fertilization sometimes may develop parthenogenetically under certain artificial conditions. This type of parthenogenesis is known as **artificial parthenogenesis**. The artificial parthenogenesis may be induced by various physical and chemical means.

A. Physical means. The following physical means cause the parthenogenesis:

(i) **Temperature.** The range of temperature may induce parthenogenesis in the eggs. For instance, when the egg is transferred from the 30°C to 0–10°C the parthenogenesis is induced.

(ii) **Electrical shocks can** cause parthenogenesis.

(iii) **Ultraviolet light can** cause parthenogenesis.

(iv) When the eggs are pricked by the fine glass needles the development of young ones takes place parthenogenetically.

B. Chemical means. The following chemicals have been found to cause parthenogenesis in the normal eggs:

1. Chloroform. 2. Strychnine. 3. Hypertonic and Hypotonic sea waters. 4. Chlorides of K^+, Ca^{++}, Na^{++}, Mg^{++}, etc. 5. Acids as butyric acid, lactic acid, oleic acid and other fatty acids. 6. Fat solvents, *e.g.*, toulene, ether, alcohol, benzene and acetone. 7. Urea and sucrose.

The artificial parthenogenesis has been induced by above mentioned physical and chemical means by various workers in the eggs of most echinoderms, molluscs, annelids, amphibians, birds and mammals.

31.3 SIGNIFICANCE OF PARTHENOGENESIS

1. The parthenogenesis serves as the means for the determination of sex in the honey bees, wasps, etc., and it supports the chromosome theory of inheritance.
2. The parthenogenesis is the most simple, stable and easy process of the reproduction, *e.g.*, aphids (insects).
3. The parthenogenesis eliminates the variation from the population, but encourages development of the advantageous mutant characters.
4. The parthenogenesis causes the polyploidy in the organisms.
5. Due to the parthenogenesis, there is no need for the organisms to waste their energy in the process of mating but it allows them to utilize that amount of energy in the feeding and reproduction.

REVISION QUESTIONS

1. What is parthenogenesis ? Describe various kinds of natural parthenogenesis.
2. Describe the artificial parthenogenesis.
3. What is the significance of parthenogenesis ?

32 Chapter CELL GROWTH AND AGING

Because the cells are living, so, they grow like other living beings from within (**intussusception**). However, the growth of the cells depends on the favourable conditions of temperature, oxygen, pH, nutrients, water, light and other conditions. In the absence of water, the cell, may pass into such dormant stages as cysts, spores, etc., and thus remain alive for many years. In the absence of certain nutrients or other environmental factors the growth of cell may stop or become abnormal. Moreover, the poisons, radiations and similar agents which injure the cell or disturb normal cellular functioning may also inhibit the growth of cell.

32.1 GROWTH IN THE CELLS OF UNICELLULAR AND MULTICELLULAR ORGANISMS

Weismann (1913) has postulated that the unicellular organisms are potentially immortal, while in the multicellular organisms the cell of the "germ-plasm", which pass during reproduction from generation to generation, only are potentially immortal. The somatic cells have to die.

Immortality of unicellular organisms. In past, various workers doubted the Weismann's views about the immortality of protozoans and of course they produced certain experimental evidences to show that unicellular organisms age and ultimately die. But culturing experiments of **Lwoff Kidder** and **Dewey, Hall,** 1967, **Brock**, 1946, etc., have supported the view of Weismann and stated that microorganisms are probably potentially immortal and the growth of protoplasm and cell division follows without abatement, if environmental and nutritional conditions are favourable. Under natural conditions, however, the environment does not remain so favourable for the unicellular animals. Limiting factors for a particular unicellular organism may be the light and temperature conditions; there may be a shortage of nitrogen for protein synthesis, or of phosphorus for energy processes, so that cells compete with one another for limited resources and many may die. Motile cells have the advantage of being able to move to new surroundings when there is overcrowding. But because of competition immortality at the molecular level of unicellular organisms is seldom realized in practice. An organism must change with its environment if it is to survive.

32.2 GROWTH IN THE CELLS OF MULTICELLULAR ORGANISMS AND PROCESS OF AGING

In multicellular organisms the situation is very different, because the organisms as a whole is able to outlive the life-span of its individual cells. Apart from the processes of wound healing and repair, which takes place in response to a particular injury, individual cells die and are replaced continually throughout the life of the organism. In mammals and birds, the high body temperature means that there is a high cellular metabolic rate which tends to shorten the life of the individual cells, so that the difference between their life-span and that of the whole animals is more marked than in other organisms (Table 32-1). Exceptions to this are the germ line cells and those of the developing zygote, all of which have high rate of cell division and long life-span. Turnover in the central nervous system and the muscular system is very slow; the cells in the brain and spinal cord are not replaced so that those present in an young animal must last a life-time. This may be connected with the fact that nerve cell replacement would interfere with the maintenance of stable nerve circuits.

Table 32.1. Cellular life spans in the adult mouse (from **Dyson**, 1978).

Cellular life spans
Near or equal to that of the animal itself
Neurons and associated cells
Muscle cells of all types
Brown fat cells
Osteocytes (bone cells)
Kidney medullary tubule cells
Cells of the adrenal medulla
Stomach zymogen cells
Slow renewal (more than 30 days, but less than the mean life span of the animal)
Respiration tract epithelium
Kidney cortical cells
Adrenal cortical cells
Liver hepatocytes
Pancreas acinar and islet cells
Salivary gland cells
Skin connective tissue cells
Stomach parietal cells
Fast renewal (less than 30 days)
Skin (epidermis)
Cornea
Epithelium of the mouth and gastrointestinal tract
Precursors of red and white blood cells

Classification of Cell Populations. Studies of growth and renewal of cell populations of multicellular animals during postnatal life has led to the classification of the different cell types into following three groups (**Leblond**, 1964).

1. Static cell populations. These are homogeneous groups of cells in which no mitotic activity can be detected and in which the total DNA content remains constant. Only the nerve cells were found not to divide after the age of seven days in rat. Some cells of nervous system, such as neuroglial cells and subependymal cells are, however, not static. One of the most important characteristic of static cells is the constant increase in cell volume that runs parallel to the growth of the organism and is proportional to the total volume of the body.

2. Expanding cell populations. These are homogeneous groups of the cells showing scattered mitosis in numbers that account for the increase in the total DNA content. This implies that the life of each cell continues for as long as that of the individual and that new cells are produced by division only to cover the growth of the tissue contrary to early theories, the dividing cells are fully differentiated. Examples of expanding cell populations are found in the pancreas, the thyroid, the kidney, the adrenal, the salivary glands and muscle.

3. Renewing cell populations. These are homogeneous groups of cells in which mitosis is abundant and exceeds that required for the total increase in DNA content. In renewing populations, the high production of cells is balanced by a corresponding cell loss. For example, the white phagocytic cells of the blood exist individually for approximately 1 to 3 weeks, red blood cells live for about 120 days, while bone and cartilage cells are relatively long-lived and their replacement is very slow. Likewise, there occur a rapid renewal of cells of intestine and epidermis. Other renewing cell populations are the testis (which continuously sheds spermatozoa), the lung (which produce "dust cells"), the thymus, the lymph ganglia, the bone marrow and all hematopoietic organs in general.

Thus, in multicellular animals, there is a continuous turnover of certain cell types; even in young animals, the processes of cell death and new cell growth taking place at the same time. With a young organism still in its growth phase the production of new cells must be in excess of the death of the old cells. When the organism reaches maturity, however, a balance is attained between the **birth rate** and **death rate** of the cells in the various tissues. The process of growth and replacement are regulated by various growth controlling mechanisms (such as homeostasis, contact inhibition, growth promoting hormones or **auxins** in plants and thyroid hormone which is released from thyroid by being activated by TSH (thyroid-stimulating hormone) of pituitary gland and which can regulate gene activity at transcription level) which operate to maintain the structure and coordinated function of the various parts of the organism.

Failing disease or injury, a multicellular organism dies from the process of aging or **senescence** (**Ebert** and **Sussex**, 1970), which takes different forms in different types of cell. Aging is still imperfectly understood, but it seems to be connected with the high degree of specialization required for carrying out specific functions, which is known for many cell types to lead to loss of capacity for cell division. There is continued progressive decrease in the production rate with increasing age of the organism, although the life span of individual cells does not appear to alter significantly. This means that not all dying cells are being replaced, and there is a loss of weight and loss of function in tissues and organs; for instance, in animals the heart does not pump so much blood in a given time as it did when the individual was a young adult, the blood is not oxygenated so efficiently as it passes through the lungs, the actual blood volume diminishes, partly because tissues retain less water and partly because the production of red blood cells slows down, and so on. All of this means that a greater burden is thrown on the remaining cells.

Hormonal changes affecting adversely the functioning of various organs, the accumulation of waste material from various metabolic processes inside certain cells, loss of elasticity in elastic fibres, and an increase in the amount of collagen in connective tissues—all play a part in aging, resulting in such well-known changes as stiffening of the joints and hardening of the arteries. Even at subcellular level following changes occur in different cell types due to aging:

32.3 SUBCELLULAR CHANGES DUE TO AGING

Due to the process of aging following changes occur in the different cellular organelles:

1. Mitochondria. Reiner (1947) has reported that due to aging the rate of carbohydrate metabolism (Krebs cycle) is decreased. The aging also affects the glycolysis. Such results have also been reported by **Rafsky** (1952) and **Barrows** (1958). **Dampsey** (1956) has shown that the mitochondria are related with the aging process of the animals and in old tissues the mitochondria become degenerated. **Zeuthen** (1947, 1953) has reported that the rate of respiration in multicellular organisms becomes slow and they become somewhat dehydrated.

2. Endoplasmic reticulum. Due to aging the amount of granular endoplasmic reticulum decreases in the cytoplasm of old cells. In the nerves of older animals and human the decrease of Nissl substance (rRNA) have been reported by various workers.

3. Pigment accumulation and lysosomes. Due to aging various pigmented inclusions such as lipofuscin, yellow pigment, brown degenerations, etc., become accumulated in the cells. The lipofuscin probably is the result of accumulation and autooxidation of lipid components of lysosomes. **Shock** (1962) and **Strehler** (1962, 1963) have reported the accumulation of calcium, various pigments and other inert matter in the aged cell. The inert matter are the accumulated metabolic excretory wastes which might have failed to exit across the plasma membrane.

4. Nucleus. Minot (1970) has suggested that the natural death of the cell is a consequence of cellular differentiation of which a change in nucleocytoplasmic ratio is an important index. **Smallwood** and **Philips** (1916) have shown that fatigue and age do not produce significant changes in the nuclear size. **Falzone** (1959) has studied the effect of the age on the ploidy or DNA contents of the nuclei of rat liver cells and reported that no significant effect of aging on the nuclei. However, various modern cytologists have shown that the age effects the nucleus variously.

5. Nuclear and plasma membrane. Lansing (1942, 1952) has reported that due to aging process the calcium becomes accumulated in the cellular membranes and causes various physiological changes in them.

32.4 CAUSES OF AGING

Over the years, numerous theories have been proposed to explain the causes of aging. The most simplest theory of aging states that it is governed in a major way by an organism's genetic inheritance or by what a sometimes called its **"genetic time table"** or **"genetic clock"** (**B. Pal**, 1975). Heredity helps us in explaining that why fruit flies have a maximum life span of 40 days, golden hamsters 3 years, dogs 20 years, horses 50 years, human 100 years and giant tortoises 180 years. These organisms evidently have coded informations for their respective maximum life-spans in their genomes. There are many investigators, who believe that every organism has **"aging genes"** that control its rate of aging and thus its maximum life-span. Further, to explain that whether the "genetic clock" resides in all cells, or is it present in certain organs which initiate the process of aging to eventually encompass the whole organism, following two kinds of theories have been proposed:

1. Cellular theories of aging,
2. Pacemaker theories of aging.

1. Cellular Theories of Aging. A series of cell-culture experiments begun in 1960's by **L. Hayflick** has invalidated the notion that aging is the property of the whole complex organism and that individual cells, if properly cultured, would be immortal, that is, there would be no limit to the number of times they could divide. **Hayflick** found that cultured human fibroblasts double only a limited number of times before they deteriorate, become senescent (*i.e.,* aged), lose their capacity to divide and finally die. The number of cell divisions of cultured cells is roughly related (*a*) the age of the cell donors and (*b*) the longevity of the species. For example, **Hayflick** found that fibroblasts from the human embryos, when sustained in tissue culture, divide about 50 times before they die. Those taken from persons after birth divide 20 to 30 times.

Transplantation experiments of **Daniel** *et. al.*, (1968), in which they transplanted mouse mammary epithelial cells into the mammary fat pads of female mice, also exhibit that the cells showed a characteristic decline in proliferative capacity with repeated transplantations. From results of tissue culture and cell transplantation studies, **Hayflick** recently has concluded that aging is due to loss of cell functions that occurs before cells reach their maximum division point. As cells malfunction, organs or whole systems suffer adverse effects and eventually the individual dies.

So, at this stage we have to analyse that what causes cells to become senescent and incapable of division. Many theories have been proposed for explaining this question, however, some of the following important theories will throw much light on this problem:

***(a)* Mutation or "error" theories.** Most gerontologists (the biologists of **gerontology,** which is a biological science dealing with the problems of aging or senescence of man and other living beings) believe that as a person grows older, his genetical material (DNA) gradually becomes impaired. This deterioration may in some cases be caused by accumulated errors in the replication of DNA. Thus mutation may cause aging. If the damage to DNA is too subtle for the DNA repair system to detect, or if it accumulates faster than the repair system functions, the cells will gradually be defective in essential control systems or enzymes. Result is the destructive process of aging. Similarly, if mutation in somatic cells are involved in aging, then the efficiency of DNA repair mechanisms may determine susceptibility to aging.

***(b)* "Error catastrophe" theory.** This theory has been proposed by **L.E. Orgel** (1963). According to this theory, an accumulation of errors in the amino acid sequence in proteins, specially errors that affect the specificity of enzymes needed for protein synthesis, will result in further mistakes in protein synthesis and consequently will lead to cell deterioration and death. The mistakes could occur during transcription of mRNA. **Holliday** *et. al.,* (1974) have recently provided certain evidences in favour of this theory. They could shorten the life-span of adult fruit flies by feeding a variety of amino acid analogues (*e.g.,* p-fluorophenylalanine and methionine) to the larvae. These amino acid analogues substitute phenylalanine and methionine respectively in the proteins and interfere with the functions of proteins. **Holliday** has also detected abnormal forms of enzymes in aging fibroblasts, while others have observed reduced specific activities of some enzymes isolated from aged organisms. Certain scientists even have speculated that errors are not the result of blind chance but are purposefully programmed probably by the "aging genes."

***(c)* Free radical reaction theory.** Certain naturally producing free radicals which are extremely unstable molecular fragments and are highly reactive due to the presence of unpaired electrons have been considered significant in causing aging in animals. **Harman** (1956) proposed that certain free radicals generate oxidative reactions which can lead to the deterioration of lipids, collagen, elastin and other body substances and may cause aging. **Chio** *et. al*., (1969) reported the increase in accumulation of **lipofuscin** pigment in aging cells and found that this aging pigment may damage the cells variously. Further, certain free radicals attack specifically on unsaturated lipids in cell membranes and thus, may seriously impede the diffusion of nutrients into the cell and extrusion of waste products out of the cell. This might be associated with cell-death consequent on aging.

2. Pacemaker theories of aging. Evidence is growing that aging is caused, in part, by progressive breakdown in the immunological system. The activities of both **B cells** (bone-marrow derived) and **T cells** (thymus-derived) decrease in aged animals. When properly stimulated, B cells differentiate into plasma cells that secrete antibodies. The T cells form 'killer' lymphocytes that kill foreign cells. T cells also act as B cell 'helpers' that are needed for B cell differentiation. At present, evidences strongly indicate that the age-related decline in the immunological activities of the body is largely due to changes in the environments (activity) of the T cells.

Thymus as the pacemaker. Burnet has recently suggested that the thymus gland is the **biological clock** that determine how fast we age. It is the pacemaker for the whole body and its atrophy would be the programmed event that leads to aging of the animal. It is well known that the thymus begins to atrophy shortly after puberty in humans.

***(a)* Burnet** have also shown that the body can also produce antibodies called **auto-antibodies** that attack not only foreign substances but also substances that occur naturally and desirably in the body. These auto-antibodies are speculated to cause certain age-associated diseases such as rheumatoid arthritis, systemic lupus erythematosus, Hashimoto's thyroiditis, etc. It has been speculated that as a person gets older, his immunological system becomes less able to distinguish "self" from "non-self" and as a result, proceeds to destroy normal and desirable proteins of the body. The consequence is the deterioration of aging.

(*b*) **Brain as the pacemaker. Finch** believed that brain with its role as an overseer for hormone production, may contain the clock that defines the length of life of animals. To support this belief, an evidence is advanced that when the ovary of an old rat is transplanted into an young female it will again produce estrogenic hormones and begin to function normally, even though it had ceased to do so in the older female.

Reconciliation of the Theories of Aging

B. L. Strehler recently reconciled many theories discussed above by postulating aging as a process programmed by the action of "on-off switches" that reside in the genetic machinery. The effect, he suggested, would be to cause first one set of genes, then another to produce special products (enzymes, hormones, antibodies, structural proteins and the like) as the individual matures, ages and dies. The specific off-switch that appears to be central is that which prevents the key body cells found in the thymus, brain, heart and endocrine glands from dividing once maturity has been attained (for more informations on aging see **L.E. Orgel**, 1973; **R.G. Cutler**, 1976; **L. Heyflick**, 1976; **N. Bucher** *et. al.,* 1977; **M. Lamb,** 1977).

Regulation of Form and Size of Cell

In most animals and plants the size of cell is regulated by division, as is most clearly demonstrated with *Amoeba proteus* (**Prescott,** 1956). During growth of an amoeba the mass increases until it just doubles. Then no further increase occurs and after a lapse of time it divides, each daughter cell receiving half the mass of the mother cell. If a part of an amoeba is cut-off during the period of growth, division will not occur at the time it does in control amoebas, but only after the removed mass of protoplasm has been replaced by growth (see **Giese**, 1973).

In multicellular animals the size of particular tissue is regulated **by chalones**, as follows:

Chalones. In normal tissue of a full-grown mammal and equilibrium state is reached in which mitosis is suspended, except in some special tissues, such as the cells of the germinative epithelium of the skin, gametogenic tissues in gonads and blood cell proliferative tissues in the bone marrow. Such **inhibition** of cell **division** is apparently the result of products of the tissues themselves; these are tissue-specific inhibitors of mitosis which have collectively been called **chalones.** Each tissue apparently produces two types of chalones, one of low molecular weight (about 1000 to 3000) and another of high molecular weight (30,000 to 50,000). Chalones are not cytotoxins—their effects are reversible upon removal. When cells in tissue culture are freed of chalones by washing, they resume mitosis and proliferation. Addition of appropriate chalones again stop mitosis. The chalones are produced by different types of tissues and they presumably attach to specific receptor sites on cell membranes and in an unknown manner exert their inhibitory effects (see **Giese**, 1973). **Szent-Gyorgyi** (1967) has suggested that there may be a **growth-promoting substance** (**promine**) and a **growth-inhibiting substance** (**retine**) present in certain tissues of animals. In plant cells growth of cell (*i.e.,* cell size, etc.) is regulated by **auxin** (indole acetic acid) (**Hillman**, 1962).

Lastly heredity plays an important role in the maintenance of size and shape of cells. This is evident since clones of a given species of microorganisms under a given set of evironmental conditions tend to be quite constant in size and form for a long series of generations—a constant nuclear to cytoplasmic ratio is maintained. However, overall size was found to vary with a change in each environmental factor studied (**Adolph,** 1931). Likewise the experimental increase in the number of chromosomes by polyploidy is apparently often attended by an increase in size (**Fankhauser,** 1952)

32.5 PROGRAMMED DEATH

Cell death is not always associated with old age (senescence), but is a normal part of the embryonic shaping of hands, feet and wings. For example, separation of fingers and toes of animals occurs due to the death of tissue between them. Similarly, the chick wing is shaped in part by the death of selected cells. In an elegant set of experiments with this latter system, **J. W. Saunders, Jr.,** (1966), demonstrated that the time of death of these cells is established at a given point during development, in much the same way as other characteristics are determined at given times.

The metamorphosis of insects is another example of programmed death, as is the metamorphosis of amphibians (*e.g.,* the absorption of a tadpole's tail). Thus, it is possible that eventual senescence is programmed into a cell in much the same way as any other function (see **Dyson**, 1978).

REVISION QUESTIONS

1. Define the phenomenon of aging or senescence. Describe the process of aging.
2. Eventual senescence is less common in cells that reproduce themselves as opposed to those that result from the differentiation of a simple stem cell. Give examples that support this statement.
3. Discuss different theories of the possible causes of senescence.
4. What role might programmed death play in normal development ?

33 Chapter
CELLULAR INTERACTION

In a multicellular organism the cells of the different tissues cooperate in a harmonious way and among them there is a high degree of functional interdependence. Cells may interact over long distances by way of diffusion of some chemical substances (*e.g.,* hormones, etc.), but in many cases their interaction depends on a short range action, as by **cell contact**.

During embryonic development there is considerable cell motility and mass movement of cells (*i.e.,* morphogenetic movements during blastulation, gastrulation, neurulation and organogenesis). One of the most interesting example of cell migration is the case of the germinal cells. In avian embryos germinal cells differentiate in the extraembryonic endoderm while the rest of the gonad develops in the embryonic mesodermal ridge. The germinal cells enter the blood stream and are carried through all parts of the embryo, but they selectively adhere and accumulate at the germinal ridges. It may be postulated that there is a **specific recognition** between these cells. This kind of recognition is very important in the development (morphogenesis) of the nervous system, in which millions of neurons must find their specific partners to establish synaptic junctions.

33.1 CELL ADHESION

In order to aggregate, cells must first come in contact (adhere) with one another. **Harris** (1961) has enlisted following three kinds of contacts between the cells which lead to their aggregation in a tissue:

1. The aggregation may form by the inclusion of the cell in a common matrix. In most cases this extra-cellular matrix consists of the **extraneous coat** of the cell. These substances (*e.g.,* cellulose, hyaluronic acid, and so forth) accumulate after the cells have made contact with each other.

2. The aggregation of cells may have little or no demonstrable intracellular material. In many tissue there is a space of 150 A° between adjacent cell membranes that contain mucoproteins. These mucoproteins account for the specificity of cell association.

3. The aggregation may imply the presence of intercellular channels. Cells in a tissue use these channels to interchange more or less freely. For example, in plant cells, cytoplasmic bridges or plasmodesmata provide narrow connections between the cells and across the cellulose walls and permit the free passage of ions and probably macromolecules.

33.2 INTERCELLULAR COMMUNICATIONS

In many animal cells, there are intercellular communications as have been demonstrated by **Loewenstein** and **Kanno** (1964) by introducing intracellular microelectrodes into adjacent cells of a tissue. In such a case the cells are found to be **electrically coupled** and they have regions of low resistance in the membrane through which there is a rather free flow of electrical current carried by ions (**Loewenstein**, 1967). The parts of the cell membrane, which are not coupled, show a much higher resistance. This type of coupling called **junctional communication**, is found extensively in embryonic cells (**Potter** *et. al.*, 1966), but also in certain adult tissues such as epithelia (**Loewenstein**, 1966), cardiac cells and liver cells (**Penn**, 1966). Skeletal muscle and most neurons do not show electrical coupling. The giant-cells of the salivary glands of *Chironomus* are excellent for demonstrating electrical coupling (**Oliveiracastro** and **Loewenstein**, 1971). Between these cells there are **septate junctions** that establish a direct communication between two adjacent cell membranes. While in most other junctional communications, the so-called **gap junctions** are found.

Structure of coupling. The essential compo nents of the coupling between two cells are represented in fig. 33.1. Each passageway unit consists of a pair of membrane regions of high permeability (**junction membranes**) circumscribed by a kind of seal (**junction seal**) that insulates the junctional region from the extracellular space.

It has been found that the junctional communications depend on the energy provided by oxidative phosphorylation (*i.e.*, ATP). Treatments which inhibit cell metabolism, such as cooling at 8°C, dinitrophenol, cyanide, and olgiomicin, produce uncoupling between the cells and this may be reversed by injection of ATP. **Politoff** *et. al.*, (1969) have suggested that during the action of inhibitors, the uncoupling of cells occur due to the influx of Ca^{2+} either from the medium or from mitochondria.

Loewenstein (1973) have shown that besides ions molecules as large as 10,000 daltons *e.g.*, peroxidase enzyme go through the junctional communications of *Chironomus*.

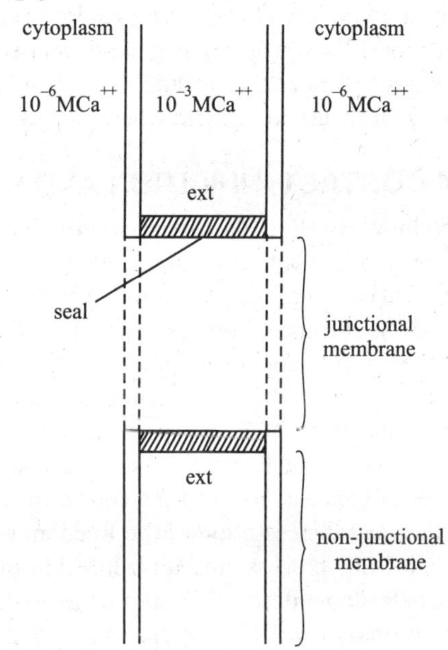

Fig. 33.1. Diagram showing different components of the coupling between cells (after De Robertis *et. al.*, 1975).

Functions of Intercellular Communications

Intercellular junctional communications perform many important functions. In cardiac muscle, and in electrical synapses between certain neurons they are related to communication of electrical signals between these cells. Junctional interconnections are particularly widespread during embryonic development at stages in which cell differentiation takes place. Because diffusion of molecules can readily take place through them, these junctions are well suited for the dissemination of signals (*i.e.*, embryonic inductions) controlling growth and differentiation at close range (**Loewenstein**, 1973).

33.3 CELL DISSOCIATION AND REASSOCIATION

In a classical experiment **Wilson** (1908) forced living sponges through a fine silk mesh and found that they disaggregated into isolated motile cells which upon standing reaggregated to form fresh sponges. Similarly, **Moscona** (1957) found that embryonic tissues treated with trypsin dissociate into individual cells and then reaggregate to form the specific patterns of the original tissue. Later on, in 1962 he reported that if the cells of a chick embryo are dissociated with trypsin and allowed to stand, they will reaggregate. When similar cells attach to each other, they form aggregates that are characteristic for a given cell population, *e.g.*, retinal cell, kidney or bone.

The process of reassociation or reaggregation is not species specific. For instance, if cells of chick and mouse embryos are mixed, they reaggregate according to the cell population rather than the species. Reassociation of cells does not occur in the absence of calcium ions, or in the presence of blocked carbohydrates or glycoproteins. The mechanism by which a cell remains able to 'recognize' and aggregate with another cell of similar kind, takes place at the cell surface, but its intimate nature is unknown. **Steinberg** (1962) has suggested that the surface of the cell is highly ordered in the tangential direction and that this is reflected in the spatial organization of ionized acid groups that bind Ca^{2+} and Mg^{2+}. The surface material of the adjacent cells may have a molecular fit of reactive groupings. However, **Burnet** (1961) has postulated that glycoproteins and glycolipids present in the cell coat are involved in the **'molecular' recognition** of cells of similar type by immunochemical interactions. This property is gene-dependent and is phenotypically expressed at the cell surface. According to **Singer** and **Rothfield** (1973) molecular recognition is highly developed between neurons of the central nervous system where specific neuronal circuits of immense complexity are formed.

33.4 CONTACT INHIBITION AND CONTACT GUIDANCE

Several investigators like **Abercrombie, Heaysmann, Ambrose** and **Easty** in 1960's have studied the movement of both fibroblasts and epithelial cells in culture and in each case, they found that the movement of a single cell is controlled by the movement of other like cells with which it makes contact (Fig. 33.2). The upper fibroblast is at first moving downwards, the process being characterized by the formation of pseudopodia on the leading edge. When the upper fibroblast touches the lower one, an adhesion is formed between the membranes. The two cells may try to move in different directions, resulting in considerable tension in the contact, and sometimes in breakage, resulting again in freedom of movement of the two cells. As mitosis occurs in culture, and the density increases, an increasing number of contacts between the cells will be formed. This leads to stabilization of the culture by contacts, and the cessation of the freedom of movement of individual cells. **Abercrombie** (1966) has called this process **contact inhibition** of movement. The contact inhibition is now referred to as **density dependent inhibition of growth**, because it seems to be more related to transport of nutrients into the cell than with cell-to-cell contact as such (**Dyson**, 1978). A similar type of control occurs in epithelial cells.

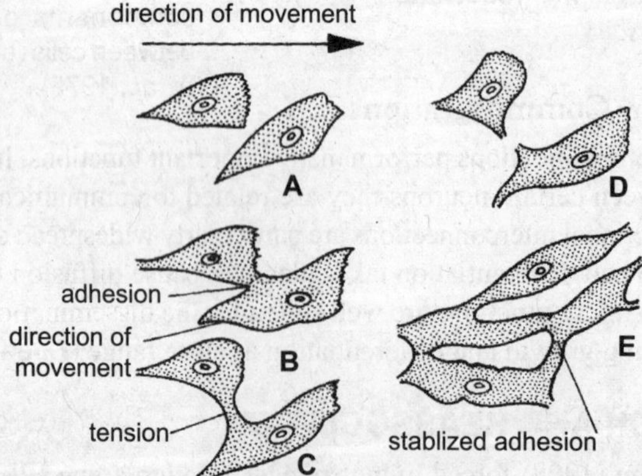

Fig. 33.2. Successive stages in the making and breaking of a contact between fibroblasts (after Ambrose and Easty, 1970).

Thus, the phenomenon of contact inhibition refers to the inhibition of cell mortality and also of mitotic activity in normal cells grown in tissue culture at the time they come into contact. The inhibition depends on some unknown signals between cells in contact, and not on a diffusible substance acting at a distance.

Certain workers reported a correlation between adhesion between cells and substrate on which they are moving. The direction of movement of cells is found to be regulated by the substrate. **Weiss** (1926) found that when fibroblasts are cultured on glass, which has fine surface grooves (or on fish scales) the cells tend to elongate and move along the grooves. This control of direction is known as **contact guidance**.

REVISION QUESTIONS

1. Define the following terms: cell adhesion, contact inhibition and cell dissociation.
2. Describe the phenomena of cell adhesion and intercellular communications.
3. Write brief notes on the (*i*) cell dissociation; and (*ii*) contact inhibition and contact guidance.

34 Chapter

CANCER

Usually the cells and animals have controlled growth but in certain special circumstances, the cells begin to grow and multiply continuously, forming a **tumour**, or a **cancerous growth** (**Congdon** and **Mari-chavez**, 1963; **Gaus**, 1966; **Tadaro** *et. al.*, 1966). A **tumour** is a **neoplasm**,or abnormal growth of new tissue. Such growths can arise anywhere in the body and may be quite **benign**, or harmless (*e.g.,* the common wart). On the other hand, a tumour may become malignant, in which case it invades and destroys the supporting tissue on which it grows, eventually causing the death of the host. In addition, a malignant tumour or **cancer**, may slough cells that are carried to other parts of the body by way of the lymph or blood where they establish new colonies of malignant cells. This process, called **metastasis,** spreads the tumour and hastens the time when a vital function will be interrupted by one of the growths.

Cancers are named according to the tissues from which they arise, usually with the suffix "**—oma,**" added. Most common are the **carcinomas**, which are derived from epithelial cells; the **sarcomas,** which originate in connective tissue; the **lymphomas**, which are derived from lymphatic tissue; and the **lipomas** that are originated from adipose or fatty tissues. However, not all malignancies result in solid tumours. **Leukemia**, for example, is a malignant disease involving the proliferation of white blood cells or leukocytes (**Dyson**, 1978).

Cancer has received much attention from biological and medical scientists not only because the disease is a major medical problem, but because it represents an aberration in some very basic mechanisms involving the regulation of cellular activity, including growth and differentiation.

Most of the cytology of cancer or tumour cells has been worked out by working on 30 years old human cell-line culture called **HeLa** after **Henrietta Lacks,** the unfortunate donor of cells, who died from a very malignant cancer soon after the cells from her tumour were put in culture (see **Bodmer** and **Cavallisforza**, 1976).

34.1 CHARACTERISTICS OF CANCER CELLS

A tumour or cancerous growth consists of undifferentiated cells which grow and disorganize the tissue in which it occurs. Electron microscopy of cancer tissues and cancer cells has visualized many fine structural variations or abnormalities of cellular organelles, but none of the hitherto observed changes can be considered as constant and specifically linked with the malignant (cancerous) process. Following changes have been observed to occur in different cellular organelles of the cancer cells.

1. Nucleus

The nucleus of the cancer cell has a more irregular outline and is usually enlarged. The irregularities in the distribution of chromatin have been observed frequently. In between the chromatin and around the chromatin there occur some particles or granules which usually contain RNA and proteins and known as **interchromatin** and **perichromatin granules** respectively. Such granules though occur in the nucleus of normal cells but are specially abundant and unchangeable in the nucleus of cancer cell. The nucleus of tumour cells sometimes possesses some **nuclear bodies** having the diameter 0.2 - 2 μm and characterized by concentric fibrillar or granular or lamellar structures which may have dense granules in their centres (discovered by **De The** *et. al.*, and frequently observed by **Bouteille** *et. al.*, 1967 in tumour cells). The nuclear membrane is characterized by deep infolding or by bleb formations and contain cytoplasmic material (mitochondria, fat droplets, Golgi material, myelin figures, etc). Other nuclear inclusions of cancer cell nucleus may contain proteins, glycogen, lipids or in rare cases viruses.

The nucleolus of cancer cell nucleus display hypertrophy. The increased size of this organelle together with the enlarged and irregularly shaped nucleus are considered as characteristics of cancerous growth. The shape of nucleolus is more irregular than in normal cells and quite frequently there are several nucleoli present within ones nucleus. Its fine structure may be either unchanged or show any type of abnormality (**Bernhard** and **Granboulan**, 1963 and 1968). Vacuoles or granular inclusions may be found in it. No fine structural changes have so far been observed in cancer chromosomes or in the achromatic apparatus (**W. Bernhard**, 1969).

2. Cytoplasm

In the cytoplasm of a cancer cell following alterations have been frequently observed:

1. Mitochondria. Among all fine structural changes in tumour cells, mitochondrial alterations are the most frequent and striking ones. More often the cancer cell mitochondria have been found to be swollen and lacking in its various structures. For example, the cancer cell mitochondria have fewer irregular or parallel tubular cristae (**Leduc** and **Wilson**), concentric cristae (**Seljelid** and **Ericsson**, 1965), unhomogeneous matrix, myelin figures and irregular (*e.g.*, cup-like) shape. Their number may be increased or on the contrary decreased.

2. Ergastoplasm and ribosomes. Because cancer cells grow rapidly and therefore have to produce an increased amount of proteins comparable to embryonic cells. In the cytoplasm the formation of polyribosomes or polysomes by the union of various ribosomes is very frequent. Usually the cytoplasm of cancer cells is filled with ergastroplasm and ribosomes.

3. Golgi apparatus. The Golgi apparatus of a cancer cell of a exocrine gland (*e.g.*, pancreas, thyroid, etc.), have been found considerably developed. But as a rule the cancer cells have a poorly developed Golgi complex.

4. Other cytoplasmic organelles. Annulate lamellae and paired cisternae are more frequently found in cancer cells.

5. Pathological cytoplasmic inclusions. The cytoplasm of cancer cells have many types of inclusions. For example, milk droplet in mammary tumours, mucus in gastric cancer, colloidal substance in thyroid tumours, secretion granules in intestinal carcinoids (cancer) (**Luse** and **Lacy**, 1960; **Schumacher** and **Schulz**, 1963) and bronchial carcinoids (**Bouteille** *et. al.*, 1964; **Verley**, 1965), in insulinomas (**Lazarus** and **Volk**, 1962; **Bencosme** *et. al.*, 1963; **Greider** and **Elliott**, 1964). Melanin pigment is found in melanomas (**Rappaport** *et. al.*, 1963); mast cell granules in mastocytomas ((**Mengel** and **Trier**, 1961; **Christensen** *et al.*, 1963); eosinophilic granules in certain human leukemias (**De Harven** *et. al.*, 1967); lipids and glycogen in hypernephromas (**Oberling** *et. al.*, 1959), mucopolysaccharides in myxosarcomas, large protein droplets in hepatomas (**Hruban** *et. al.*, 1966) or protein crystals in ancocytomas (**Tendlear** and **Shipkey**,1966). Bundles or tiny cytoplasmic fibrils may be seen in leukemia cells, in reticulosarcomas, gliomas, or in ascites tumours. Myofilaments may persist in myoepithelial cells from mammary tumours or in rhabdomyosarcomas.

Many cancer cells have phagocytic activity. Cell debris of all kinds may be found in the cytoplasm in various stages of disintegration and digestion. Certain cancer cells have many lysosomes.

3. Cell or Plasma Membrane

The cell or plasma membrane of the cancer cells usually remain unaltered except a few cases in which mucopolysaccharide production is increased at cell surface. Intercellular connections may be normal or desmosomes may be more numerous in keratinizing epitheliomas (a cancer). In certain cases, there are fewer tight junctions than usual and therefore these cancer cells show no intercellular coupling and they fail to communicate with normal cells (**Azarnia** and **Loewenstein**, 1971). It is assumed that these cancer cells have a genetic defect which has interrupted the passage of growth-controlling molecules between them. Recently, **Harris** (1971) has produced heterokaryons between a cancer cell and normal cell by **cell-fusion technique** and obtained non-cancerous hybrid. In this hybrid the intercellular communications, which were established between the hybrid cells (**Azarnia** and **Loewenstein**, 1973). The cancerous cells also lack the phenomenon of **contact inhibition** (**De Robertis** *et. al.*, 1975).

4. Anaplasia

In the rapidly growing tumours, a very low degree of differentiation of cancer cells occurs. This is known as **anaplasia**. Malignant tissues gradually lose the architecture of the normal homologous tissue. On cellular level the fine structure of cytoplasm is much less organised. The polarization of cells may be inverted or is gradually lost. The number of mitochondria varies, but has the tendency to decrease. Ergastoplasmic lamellae are rare or disappear completely, as well as the Golgi complex. The cytoplasm may have a hydropic appearance. The nucleus has very irregular outline. Anaplasia is possibly caused due to rapid division of cancer cells which may have not enough time to build up the complete cellular architecture which would enable the cancer cells to function normally. The different functioning of genes responsible for cellular metabolism have also been held responsible for the phenomenon of anaplasia.

5. In cancer cells, the mitotic rate is not inhibited and in cultures the cells tend to pile up, forming irregular masses several layers deep. These cells show less adhesion to the solid support or among themselves and motility is more pronounced.

Further, in cancerous or malignant tissue less chalone is produced and that is released into the blood rather than attached to receptor sites, so that, paradoxically, the blood draining their normal counterparts (**Paukovits**, 1969; **Bullough** and **Laurence**, 1970; **Maugh**, 1972).

34.2 POSSIBLE CAUSES OF CANCEROUS GROWTH OR CARCINOGENESIS

The cancerous growth, tumorigenesis, or carcinogenesis has around great problems before the cytologists, physiologists and doctors. The search for the causes of above discussed changes in malignant cells has been complicated by what appears to be a multiplicity of unrelated mechanisms. In the first decade of this century, **V. Ellermann** and **O. Bang** succeeded in transferring leukemia from one bird to the next with a cell-free filterate. At about the same time, **P.F. Rous** demonstrated that cell-free filterates can also transmit some solid tumours (sarcomas) between birds. The causative agent in both cases is a virus. Within a year of these discoveries, **Erwin F. Smith** and **C.O. Townsend** showed that a specific bacterium, not a virus, is responsible for the initiation of a plant tumour called **crown gall disease**. And now, we recognize that cancer can arise not only from certain infectious agents, but also from a wide variety of radiations, chemicals, and physical irritants. Some plastics, silicon, stainless steel films, etc., also have been shown to elicit tumours in laboratory animals when implanted in their tissues. Therefore, various theories have been put forward for the carcinogenesis. We are giving few important theories of carcinogenesis which are as follows:

1. Mutation theory,
2. Virus theory,
3. Metabolic theory,
4. Hormonal disturbance theory,
5. Irritation theory.

1. Mutation Theory of Carcinogenesis

Jacobson (1958) has suggested that mutation may cause genetic disorders in a normal cell which may become incapable to control the hormones and enzymes necessary for the repression of multiplication in normal cells. For example, in between the bone marrow cells of a normal individual and bone marrow cells of a leukemic individual (an individual with the disease leukema, caused due to mutation) occur various genetical and physiological differences.

A number of chemical substances, which are also **mutagens** (a substance which cause mutation), have been found to cause cancer and so known as **carcinogenic agents**. The carcinogenic chemical compounds are as follows:

1. Polycyclic hydrocarbons which occur in tars, such as benzpyrene, certain dye stuffs such as "butter yellow" and other azo dyes.
2. Mustard gas [S $(CH_2.CH_2.Cl)_2$] and analogous compounds such as nitogen "mustard", *e.g.*, $CH_3N\ (CH_2.CH_2Cl_2)$.
3. β-napthylamine and aminophenol. The aminophenol is formed naturally in the human bladder in some abnormal conditions and gives rise to bladder cancer.
4. Plastic films of various materials, ionizing radiations from X-ray sets or certain other radioactive substances may also cause cancerous growth in normal cells.

2. Virus Theory of Carcinogenesis

According to some workers viruses have been claimed as the possible sources of carcinogenesis. **Murphey** and **Peyton Rous** in 1910 have seen the possibilities of transmission of certain avian tumours by injecting cell free extracts of the tumour cells into healthy birds. Viruses that produce leukemia and other tumours in mice and birds belong to the so called **myxoviruses** which have a single-strand chain of RNA to their genome.

Certain oncogenic viruses (*i.e.*, viruses capable of inducing cancer) such as polyoma or SV40 (*i.e.*, semian virus 40) are commonly used to transform normal culture cells into cancer cells. Polyoma virus has a circular double-stranded DNA genome of only 1.6 µm in length and a capsid with 72 capsomeres. When a polyoma virus is infected a normal cell in culture, its DNA becomes integrated into the genome of the cell in regions in which there is some genetic homology. The viral genome contains only 5000 nucleotides to codify a few viral proteins such as genes to code for DNA replication, for the protein of the capsid, for an internal protein and for two antigens occurring in viral DNA.

With cell transformation, the host cell (cancer cell) shows a lack of control of cell division and of cell motility, and changes in cell contact and cell surface. Further, two viral-specific antigens make cell their appearance in host cell or cancer cell. One viral antigen remains in host nucleus and other in the membrane of host (see **De Robertis** *et. al.*, 1975). Thus, the viruses disturb the cellular functions so that the cell losts its balance over the rate of multiplication and other functions and become cancerous in nature (for details see **Ablashi** *et. al.*, 1976; **A. M. Campbell**, 1976; **R. Dulbecco**, 1976; and **G. Fareed**, 1977).

Cells may also be transformed by certain RNA viruses such as the leukemia viruses or Rous sarcoma virus (RSV). This observation immediately raises the question of how a RNA virus might function from a provirus state since there is no reason to believe that RNA can incorporate directly into cellular DNA. The answer was suggested in 1964 by **Howard Temin**, who shared the 1975 Noble Prize with fellow cancer virologists **Renato Dulbecco** and **David Baltimore. Temin** proposed, and with others later proved, that certain virus-specific enzymes exist that can polymerize DNA complementary to an RNA template. With these RNA-dependent DNA polymerases, or **reverse transcriptases**, one can postulate that all oncogenic viruses insert new genetic information into the chromosome of the host. The added gene may result in altered cellular properties (such as loss of contact inhibition), either directly or by interfering with the normal scheme of gene expression in the host.

For example, in the case of RSV, a single gene (the *src*-for sarcoma-gene) seems to be the key to malignant transformation. The product of this gene is thought to be a protein essential for the malignant change (**E. Vang** and **A. Goldberg**, 1976). Without the *src* gene, RSV can multiply but cannot transform its host. Malignancy, therefore, may result from loss of the associated repressor (for further information consult **Aaronson** and **Stephenson**, 1976; **D. Baltimore**, 1976; **R. Hehlmann**, 1976; **H. Temin**, 1976, 1977; and **I.M. Verma**, 1977).

3. Metabolic Theory of Carcinogenesis

Warburg (1956) has suggested that the cancer is caused due to the injury of the cellular respiratory equipment. The poisons and other carcinogenic agents are supposed to effect the respiratory mechanism of cell. Due to injured aerobic respiratory mechanism (Krebs cycle) the rate of anaerobic metabolism (glycolysis) increases. The glycolysis is a energy liberating mechanism of lower grade and it is incapable to maintain the structural integrity and organisation of the cells of multicellular organisms. **Oppenheimer** found that if plastic film is embedded in the skin of an animal a cancerous growth may be found. But, when the plastic film is made porous no cancerous growth occur because in that condition cells get ample amount of oxygen for their aerobic respiration.

But certain experiments of culturing have suggested that the injury of aerobic respiratory mechanism do not cause cancerous growth but the cancerous growth itself disturb the aerobic respiratory mechanism. Because it has been found that the tumour cells synthesize protoplasm so actively that soon they exhaust the supplies of high energy phosphate which may be required for normal pathways of aerobic respiration.

4. Hormonal Disturbance Theory of Carcinogenesis

In aged persons, the hormonal balance become upset and that may cause cancerous growth in normal body cells. Mammary cancers are very common in certain strain of mice but removal of their ovaries reduces the incidence of the mammary tumours. Therefore, the ovaries produced some hormone which stimulate cancerous growth in mammary glands. Likewise, the cancer of uterus and prostrate glands may be caused by sex hormones.

5. Irritation Theory of Carcinogenesis

According to some cytologists the cancer may also be formed by continual irritation of a tissue or if a wound is prevented from healing. It is possible that lip cancer caused by contact with pipe stems, or hooka stems with this. The chemical action of tobacco may be another possibility of lip cancer. Recently, the betels have been found to be possible cause of tongue and throat cancer in Indians who take betels regularly.

Differentiation of Tumour Cells

The nuclei of tumour cells may have a full set of normal genes in addition to whatever viral genes they harbour, if any. This condition has been demonstrated by transplanting nuclei and by causing the tumour cells themselves to differentiate. For example, in a nuclei transplanting experiment, hydrostatic pressure was used to produce a diploid egg which after fertilization, became a triploid frog (Fig. 34.1). Nuclear transplantation from a cancer cell of this triploid frog with kidney tumour to an enucleated but otherwise normal egg produced a triploid tadpole, thus demonstrating the development potential of the tumour nucleus (**McKinnel** *et. al.*, 1969).

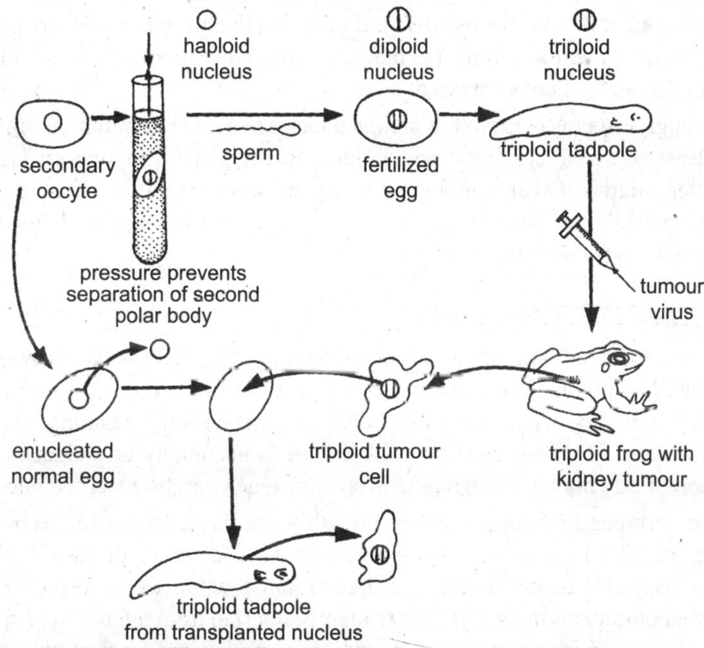

Fig. 34.1. Diagram showing the prototype of experiment which was conducted to demonstrate the development potential of a tumour nucleus (after Dyson, 1978).

In another experiment, **A.C. Braun** succeeded in causing complete new plants to develop from single cell taken from a portion of a crown gall tumour. He proceeded by forming a clone of the malignant tissue and then grafting a small amount to the cut stem of a tobacco plant tip. Under the influence of the host plant, the grafted tissue regained a portion of its ability to organize mature structures. When some of this still-abnormal growth was grafted to a second tobacco plant even more normal function was regained, culminating in the production of seeds from which perfectly normal, healthy plants were grown.

The genetic potential of the cancerous cell has also been demonstrated with amphibian regeneration. When a fragment of the Lucke adenocarcinoma (an adenocarcinoma is a cancer of gland tissue) is transplanted from the leopard frog, ***Rana pipiens***, to the regeneration blastema of an adult newt amputee, the tumour cell differentiate into muscle, cartilage and connective tissue as the new limb forms. Further, to establish that tumour cells themselves are involved in the differentiation. **M. Mizell** in 1965 amputated a newt tail by cutting through a transplanted tumour already growing in the region. The tumour cells had been heavily labelled with tritium isotope before transplantation, so autoradiographs of the regenerating tissue could be used to determine the fate of tumour nuclei. By this experiment he proved that tumour cells had been influenced to differentiate into a variety of normal tissues.

The genetic potential of malignant cells in mammals cannot be easily demonstrated because of their relative lack of regenerative power. However, differentiated (and therefore non-cancerous) cell types are often associated with and derived from, certain kinds of malignancies. For example, teratocarcinoma, which is a cancer derived from embryonic tissue, commonly has associated with it differentiated cells of many types (muscle, teeth, hair, fat, etc.). Clones derived from single teratocarcinoma cells show this same pleuropotential capacity when transplanted to susceptible hosts.

In many other tumours such a spontaneous reversion of malignant cells to mature cell types has also been observed. For example, when grown in culture, cells of neuroblastema (a cancer of neuroblasts and most common in small children) can be caused to revert to cells having many characteristics of mature neurons, including the production of neurotransmitters and formation of cell-cell contacts (**J. Morgan** and **N.W. Seeds**, 1975). It indicates that the genes conferring differentiated properties are always on in neuroblastoma, but that some step subsequent to RNA synthesis is blocked when the differentiated state is not expressed.

Further, although it seems certain that malignancies can be due to mutation of genes, it is thus probable that at least some cancers represent failures in the genetic regulatory mechanisms that govern normal differentiation and are not the result of gene loss or mutation. Thus, there seems to be a possibility of curing cancers not by killing the malignant cells, but by causing them to differentiated to mature, benign cell types (**Dyson**, 1978).

34.3 IS CANCER CONTAGIOUS ?

Cancer is a much-feared human disease of modern age. Its victims typically feel frightened, depressed and alone. Just at this time in their lives when contact with other humans is so important, they are too often shunned by friends and relatives who worry about "catching" the disease. This tragedy might be averted if people understand that there is absolutely no evidence for person-to-person transmission of any human malignancy in spite of much careful research into the question.

Although some types of human cancers probably are caused by viruses, making them an infectious disease, an infectious disease is not necessarily a contagious disease. Even with known tumour viruses, **horizontal transmission** (*i.e.,* animal to animal within the same generation) of cancer is very rare among laboratory animals. **Vertical transmission** (*i.e,* from mother to offspring) however is very common *e.g.,* transmission of mouse mammary tumour virus from mother to offspring by breast milk (**Moore** and **Charrey**, 1975).

REVISION QUESTIONS

1. Define the terms–tumour and cancer. How is naming of the cancer types done ? Describe the peculiar features of the cancer cells.
2. Describe various theories of the possible causes of carcinogenesis.
3. Is cancer contagious ?
4. Of what significance of our understanding of cancer are studies of the differentiation ?
5. Why is it believed that at least some malignant cells still carry a full complement of normal genes ?

35 Chapter

EFFECT OF RADIATION ON THE CELL

This is an evident fact that all life of earth is ultimately dependent upon the sun's radiant energy that is stored by green plant cells during photosynthesis. In addition to this primary role of light in the living economy, a persistent environment of various radiations produces other effects, reactions and adaptations, which may influence the life activities of the organisms living within this environment.

Muller (1927, 1928), **Stadler** (1928) and **Altenburg** (1928) independently discovered the mutagenic effect of radiation. Experimenting with X-rays on *Drosophila melanogaster*, barley and maize, they found a considerable increase in the frequency of mutation. Radiation—X-rays, γ-rays, β rays, fast neutrons, slow neutrons and ultraviolet rays can induce point mutations at the DNA level or chromosomal aberrations and thus, has a cytogenetical effect.

35.1 SOURCES OF RADIATIONS

In nature there are many sources of radiant energy. The natural radiations include the radiation of the sun's spectrum, radiowaves from the sun and the stars, ionizing radiations from the breakdown of the radioactive elements in the earth's crust and the cosmic rays coming from the sun and from depth of the space. Solar flares and about 120 celestial bodies are the sources of X-rays which on absorption produce ionization 60 miles high in the earth's atmosphere (**Frier** and **Webber**, 1963; **Schnopper** and **Delvaille** 1972).

1. Radiations of sunlight. Sunlight is the major source of radiations on earth. Its spectrum includes ultraviolet radiation,visible light, infrared rays and radiowaves. The sun is also the major source of earth heat without which life as we know would be impossible on earth.

Here we have great concern with ultraviolet radiations only because that have great amount of effect on the biological world.

2. Ultraviolet radiations. The sun radiates three types of ultraviolet radiations, *e.g.*, very short, short and long, from it. The ultraviolet rays with very short wavelengths are absorbed in earth's atmosphere before they reach the surface of the earth. High in the atmosphere the oxygen absorbs ultraviolet radiations and forming a layer of ozone. The ozone in turn absorbs somewhat longer ultraviolet rays and reforming oxygen. The layer of ozone forming the so called **ozone umbrella** at the height of 25 to 30 miles in the atmosphere. The ozone umbrella is the agent which removes the ultraviolet radiations of very short wavelength (**Cadle** and **Allen,** 1971). The ultraviolet radiations of long wavelengths, however, reach the earth surface and effect biological world variously. The ultraviolet rays transmit their energy almost entirely by excitation and not by ionization.

Effect of ultraviolet radiations on the cells. The ultraviolet radiations cause the most commonly known abnormality such as **sun burn** in the human beings. In such a case ultraviolet radiations kill the epidermal cells of skin and the injured cells (prickle cell layer) of a sunburned epidermis liberate chemicals which diffuse out and cause a relaxation of the wall of blood vessels in the dermis, resulting in the reddening of the skin (erythema). If the injury is slight, the red or pink colour soon disappears and in most individuals after a few hour's delay a small amount of pigment (melanin) develops (**tanning**). If the injury is very severe, the prickle cells may die, where upon the layer is invaded by white cells and serum accumulates, causing a blister which later dries and the skin "peels" off and a thicker new epidermis takes the place of the old (**Johnson** *et. al.*, 1968). **Johnson** and his associates have also reported that UV radiation affect lysosomes of cell epidermis which lyse and release their hydrolytic enzymes and so digesting the internal contents.

Sometimes, UV radiation of sunlight induces changes in the dermis which appear later as premature aging of the skin-wrinkling, moulting, change in suppleness of the skin, dryness and alterations in the blood vessels (**Klingman**, 1969).

Another injurious effect of UV radiation is the **eye-burn** or snow **blindness**. UV radiation directly striking the eye, reinforced by similar radiation reflected from snow (or the surface of water), may kill the superficial layers of cells covering the cornea. These cells become opaque, blinding the individual until the layer of dead cells is shed after few days.

Prolong exposure of UV radiation is found to induce superficial skin cancer (**carcinomas**) in rats, mice and man. The relative frequency of carcinomas in man is statistically correlated with the latitude, the frequency for people with the same heredity increasing with proximity to the equator. The fair individuals who are burned by sun but do not tan are most susceptible. Such individuals are most frequently Irish, Scotch, Welsh and Swedes. Conversely, people with rich skin pigment, yellow or black, are essentially immune to such tumours (**Epstein**, 1970).

The effect of ultraviolet radiations of sunlight on cell and unicellular organisms is much more drastic. **Downes** and **Blunt** (1877) discovered that ultraviolet radiations kill bacteria, all types of cells, such as microbes, protozoans, eggs of marine animals, algae, fungi and cells in tissue culture. **Giese** (1968) has suggested that all drastic effects of UV radiation on cell such as retardation of cell division, induction of mutation, killing of bacteria, etc., are caused by the effects of this radiation on nucleic acids in cells. Experiments have shown that inhibition of DNA synthesis by ultraviolet radiations stops cell division. They also inhibit the synthesis of RNA, proteins and other chemical molecules (**Giese**, 1964).

3. Ionizing radiations. The radiant energy which is released due to breakdown of radioactive elements such as polonium, uranium, radium, etc., are known as **ionizing radiations**. For better understanding of the ionizing radiation one should be clear about the structure of atom.

All the matter (solid, liquid and gases) is composed of different elemental, substances and identical atoms comprise these elements. The atom is composed of a positively charged nucleus and one or more negatively charged electrons orbiting in an elliptical or circular pathway around the nucleus. Although at least 32 elementary particles and antiparticles have been described in the nucleus, it may be viewed as essentially composed of uncharged neutrons and protons each of which contains a single positive charge. The number of protons in an atomic nucleus equals the number of orbital electrons which usually move in definite orbits around the nucleus. But, the electrons may be moved from one orbit to another unoccupied orbit. To jump to a higher energy level an electron must absorb energy. When an electron moves to a lower energy level, there is a release of energy equal to the difference in energy between the two levels. Thc energy from the atom (atomic energy) is released in the form of electromagnetic radiations.

The atomic radiations are usually known as **ionizing radiations**. An atom can radiate out the ionising radiations in the following two forms:

(*i*) Particulate radiations. The ionizing radiations which are caused by subatomic particles such as alpha particles, beta particles, fast and slow neutrons, protons and heavy nuclei of the atoms are known as **particulate radiations**.

(*ii*) **Electromagnetic radiations.** The radiations which beside having particulate composition have electromagnetic vibrations or waves are known as **electromagnetic radiations**. They include gamma rays, hard or soft X-rays, ultraviolet light, visible light, infrared rays and radiowaves.

4. Characteristics of ionizing radiations. Alpha particles. The alpha particles are positively charged helium particles or helium nucleus produced by radioactive disintegration of natural or artificial radioactive elements. Since alpha particles are heavy and have a double charge, so they travel slowly and loss high amount of energy. A positively charged alpha particle loses energy by exciting and ionizing atoms of the substance through which it passes. The alpha particles has a strong attraction for a negatively charged orbiting electron. The electron may be excited, *i.e.*, pulled into a higher energy orbit, or pulled completely away to ionize the atoms. An alpha particle can penetrate the cell upto 100 μm deep. Alpha particles travelling slowly through the cell, excite and ionize atoms in a cell. The alpha particles cause breaks in the chromosomes and when their energy is completely lost, they capture two electrons in their outer orbit and become helium atoms.

Beta particles. The beta particles are the electrons emitted with high velocity from the nucleus of a radioactive atom. They have negative charge and known as beta-minus particles. The beta-positive particles (positrons) have a similar mass to electrons, but a different charge (positive). Both electrons and positrons transmit energy to matter in a similar way. They vary in speed and energy depending on the voltage by which they are accelerated. They can ionize the matter and are generally absorbed by superficial tissues.

Fast neutrons. They are uncharged, highly energetic particles produced by bombarding low molecular weight substances with protons and deutrons. They may give rise to gamma rays on an inelastic collision with some matter, but in tissue of organisms which consists of nuclei of atoms of low atomic weight, collision give rise to protons. The protons are positively charged particles which may pass through tissue and cause ionization.

Slow neutrons. They are also called **thermal neutrons** and are much less energetic. Consequently they do not cause ionization or dislodge atomic nuclei but react atomic nuclei to form **a new isotope which may disintegrate to give rise to ionizing particles.**

X-rays and gamma rays. The gamma rays and X-rays produce both excitation and ionization of the substance through which they pass. Both types of rays are photons and have wave lengths from 10^{-3} to 10 A°. Gamma rays are electromagnetic radiations emitted by atomic nuclei during certain nuclear transformations. They are produced when an unstable nucleus gains stability by releasing energy. X-rays are produced when any substance, like tungsten is irradiated by high energy electrons. The electrons in the target substance are deflected from their path by the approaching high energy electrons in the form of electromagnetic radiations. X-rays energy, therefore, depends on the kinetic energy of the impinging electrons which produce X-rays of various energies. The X-rays and gamma radiations behave as if they were small bundles of energy travelling close to the speed of light. A bundle of this energy is called a **quantum** or **photon**. The amount of energy carried by the proton is directly proportional to the frequency of the wave form.

Ionizing radiations caused by X-rays and gamma rays transfer their energy to the media primarily by excitation and formation of ion pairs. When a gamma rays photon passes close to a nucleus it suddenly disappears and an electron and positron appears in its place. Energy (e) and mass (m) are related to each other according to the **Einstein formula** $E = mc^2$, where c is the velocity of light. Some energy is used in pair production, the rest is transferred to the medium by excitation and ionization.

35.2 THEORIES OF ACTION

The biological effects produced in cells by all types of ionizing radiations are qualitatively the same. The physical events causing these biological effects do so by exciting and ionizing atoms. Thus, excitation and ionization are the two major mechanisms whereby energy is transferred in radiation. In excitation, an electron in an atom is raised to a higher energy level. In ionization, an orbital electron is ejected from an atom. An atom can receive energy directly from the incident radiation or an atom may, however, receive energy indirectly by transfer from another atom. It is indirect transfer effect which is important in aqueous solutions in that free radical formation in water occurs. A free radical is extremely reactive. It is an atom or group of atoms containing an unpaired electrons. Usually free radicals are formed in radiation as intermediates between final chemical products and ion pairs. During an ionizing radiation an electron is ejected from a water molecule as follows:

$$H_2O \longrightarrow H_2O^+ + e^-$$

This high energy electron may be picked up by another water molecule as shown in the following reaction.

$$e^- + H_2O \longrightarrow H_2O^-$$

In this way an ion pair, H_2O^+ and H_2O^-, are formed. Each ion thus may, in the presence of another water molecule, form a hydrogen ion and a free radical as shown in the following reaction.

$$H_2O^+ \xrightarrow{C-H_2O} H^+ + OH^\circ$$

or as

$$H_2O^- \xrightarrow{C-H_2O} HH^\circ + OH^-$$

The H^+ and OH^- will combine to form water. The H° and OH^c free radicals are very reactive. In fact many of them can react to form H_2O_2. In cells containing catalase and peroxidases (enzymes) the hydrogen peroxide formation may not be significant but in other cells without these nuclei the H_2O_2 may have biological importance.

Effect of Ionizing Radiations on Cells

Brief exposure of the cells of the skin to ionizing radiation leads to a reddening or erythema which is followed by slight tanning. However, the effect of ionizing radiation is not confined to the surface (except in the action of alpha rays or very soft X-rays), and cells deep in the body may be injured. Certain kinds of cells such as lymphocytes, synthetically active cells and proliferating cells (*e.g.*, gametogenic cells, cells of germinative layer in the skin, blood forming cells, etc.) are specifically sensitive to ionizing radiation; they are destroyed and killed by it (**Haber** and **Rothstein**, 1969).

The radiosensitivity of cells in an organism depends on various biological and chemical factors. The biological factors are age, sex, genetic constitution, body weight, health, diurnal variation, stress, and diet. Generally, radiosensitivity decreases as an organism gets older. When old age, however, is attained the organism again becomes more radiosensitive. The females are slightly less sensitive to radiation than males. The organism of lesser body weight seems more susceptible to radiation than an organism of greater body weight. Unhealthy animals are less resistant to radiation' than healthy ones.

Recently, the effect of radiation on cellular organelles have been extensively studied. The ionizing radiation have following types of effects on different cellular organelles:

1. Cytoplasm. The ionizing radiations have small effect on cytoplasm. However, the endoplasmic reticulum vesicles, cellular membranes and mitochondria are affected by the radiations. The endoplasmic reticulum are dilated due to radiations. Membranes of lysosomes and plasma membrane are found much sensitive for ionizing radiations. Lysosome membrane are probably damaged by irradiation induced oxidation of the sulphydral groups of amino acid residues in proteins; very large doses induce peroxidation of membrane lipids. Consequently lysosomes are broken down and hydrolytic enzymes are set free, causing cellular damage (**Harris**, 1970).

The ionizing radiation injures the mitochondrial membranes. However, the oxidative phosphorylating system in mitochondria does not appear to be involved in primary radiation damage. Due to radiation the mitochondria swell and their cristae rupture.

2. Nucleus. The nucleus is more sensitive to ionising radiations than the cellular cytoplasm. The effect of ionizing radiations on chromosomes and DNA is drastic. The ionizing radiations cause mutation and chromosomal aberration in the chromosomes. The DNA is greatly effected by ionizing radiations. They change the genetic codes of DNA by affecting the nitrogen bases. The purines of DNA are less sensitive to radiation than the pyrimidines. Of these, thymine is the most sensitive pyrimidine. In fact, large doses of ionizing radiation destroy thymine, cytosine and uracil in aqueous solutions.

Ionizing radiations cause depolymerization of DNA. In doing so, it may prevent DNA replication and halt genetic transcription. Mutagenesis or death or both, may be the biological consequence of such damage to DNA. Depending on the nature and amount of DNA damage, complete reconstruction of the genome can occur. In some cells there exist a multienzyme mechanism which repairs DNA lesions caused not only by ionizing radiation, but also by ultraviolet irradiation, chemical mutagens and carcinogens.

The radiations destroy DNA either directly or indirectly. There are various types of direct destruction by radiation to DNA molecules. Hydrogen bonds break between chains. A base may be deleted, or changed in some way as in deamination. Single or double chain fracture may occur. And crosslinking may occur within the DNA double helix, or with protein molecules. Indirect damage can be done from peroxides, or free radicals, formed from water or organic compounds by ionizing radiation to act on nucleic acids or other precursors. Inhibition of DNA synthesis results from a direct effect. If the cell is irradiated in the 'S' phase (DNA synthesis phase of interphase) there is an inhibition of DNA replication which prevents mitosis and results in cell death.

3. Mitotic apparatus. The radiations may delay mitosis by inhibiting spindle formation and DNA synthesis during cell divisions.

4. Other influencing factors. No living cell is completely resistant to radiation. But several factors seem to be related to radiation effects in a cell. A clear correlation is apparent between lethal exposure and chromosome volume. Because the cells with the largest chromosome volumes are the most radiosensitive. Further, the haploid cells are more radiosensitive than diploid cells and polyploid cells are most radioresistant. There are fewer chromosomal aberrations in those cells having extra nucleoli. It appears that the nuclear cytoplasmic volume is an influencing factor. These cells with a large cytoplasmic volume as compared to their nuclear volume are more radioresistant than those with a small cytoplasmic volume. The cells with large number of mitochondria are also more radioresistant. Younger cells of particular tissue are more radioresistant than mature cells. The cells with a rapid mitotic rate are less radioresistant than those cells having a low rate of mitosis. The less differentiated cells seem more radiosensitive than highly specialized cells, but many exceptions occur.

35.3 GROSS EFFECTS OF RADIATIONS

The effects of radiations on the various organisms are as follows:

1. Viruses. The ultraviolet radiations inactivate viruses and destroy their infectivity and immunizing capacity. Both ultraviolet and ionizing radiations produce mutations in viruses. Viruses with DNA are more radiosensitive than viruses having RNA.

2. Microorganisms. Nearly all microorganisms are radioresistant. However, the radiations may cause inactivation and death in the microorganisms.

3. Plants. Generally plants are more radioresistant than animals. They remain more radioresistant in dormant stage, but gradually become more radiosensitive in the early development and growth stages. When growing plants are irradiated, they may be killed, their growth inhibited or mutations may result. Modifications of roots, stems, leaves and flowers in regard to both gross morphology and histology have been seen to occur in irradiated plants. Ionizing radiations also increases the incidence of tumour formation in plants.

4. Animals. In animals the effect of radiation is not only mutagenic and chemogenic but is also carcinogenic. A quantitative relation exists between the amount of radiation tolerated by different groups of organisms and their nucleic acid contents. A decreasing order of sensitivity has been reported for viruses, with single stranded DNA and RNA, double stranded DNA viruses, haploid cells of bacteria and yeast, diploid yeast cells and avian and mammalian cells. In fact, mammals are more sensitive to radiations than birds, reptiles, amphibians and fishes.

Effect of Radiations on Mammals

Among mammals, the tissue of bone marrow, lymphoid organs and the lining of intestine are most radiosensitive. The radiations cause radiation syndromes which may be haemopoietic, gastrointestinal, central nervous system and cardiovascular. They may cause lymphopenia and leukemia diseases in man. Due to radiations, the rate of mitosis decreases in the epithelial cells lining the mucosa of small intestine of mammals and results the denude mucosa which ulcerates, haemorrhages and becomes an inflamed gangrenous tissue. Death can ensue.

The ionizing radiations affect the skin by injuring the basal layer, *i.e.*, the stratum germinativum of the stratum malpighii to inhibit mitosis. As a result erythema may occur. Cells forming hair are also radiosensitive. When damaged, a loss of hair occurs. Although spermatozoa are somewhat radioresistant, spermatogonia are not and are very radiosensitive. Oocytes are relatively radiosensitive. Large doses of radiation injure the brain and nervous system as well the heart and blood vessels.

Ionizing Radiation and Human Cancer

In human, heavy medical irradiation, atomic accidents or radioactive substances may produce chromosomal aberrations. An interesting example of this is provided by a study of radium-dial painters, who put luminescent paint on watch dials. They retain small amounts of radioactive radium, which accumulate in their bones. The resulting radiation doubles the frequency of chromosomes breaks observed in their lymphocytes and these individuals have a high risk of developing bone cancer (see **Bodmer** and **Cavallisforza**, 1976).

Further, the survivors of the atom bombs dropped on Hiroshima and Nagasaki at the end of World War II are another group of people who have been studied intensively in order to find out more about the genetic and other effects of radiation.

Biological Effects of Atom Bombs

An atomic bomb explosion lasts about 10^{-6} seconds and develops in its centre a temperature of about 1,000,000°C. Its destructive effects are the result of its extreme heat, the ultraviolet flash, shock waves and ionizing radiation. The temperature of the surface of an object such as human skin at about 400 yards from the bomb may be raised to about 50°C. The ultraviolet flash burn may be severe and surface cells of the organisms are most rapidly damaged. The shock waves rip the capillaries of the sense organs and lungs and cause haemorrhages throughout the entire digestive system. The ionizing radiations consists of about 15 per cent neutrons, about 15 per cent alpha and beta particles and the remainder consists of short gamma rays.

A characteristic set of symptoms in a person injured by ionizing radiations is nausea accompanied by vomiting, prostration, after a latent period, fever, bloody diarrhoea, loss of hair and appearance of purple haemorrhagic spots in the skin. Should the individual survive, various skin lesions appear in areas where the germinative epithelium has been killed by the radiations. Ionizing radiation of atomic bomb also caused chromosomal abnormalities and cancer (*e.g.*, leukemia) in Hiroshima survivors.

Economic Uses of Radiations

Besides, their deleterious biological effects, the radiations have economic value. They are employed in medicine, dentistry and radiotherapy. Various types of diseases and cancer have been treated adequately by the radiations.

In the production of new antibiotics and plants, irradiation is being used to economic advantage.

REVISION QUESTIONS

1. What is a radiation? Describe different sources of radiation.
2. How do various radiations effect the cells?
3. Discuss the gross effects of radiation on living organisms.
4. What are the effects of ultraviolet rays on cells?

Glossary

Acentric A part of the whole chromosome which is without the centromere.

Acetyl CoA A metabolic intermediate produced through catabolism of compounds, including fatty acids, and used as the initial substrate for the central respiratory pathway, the TCA (Krebs cycle).

Acrocentric A chromosome with centromere near one end, so that one arm is very short.

Actin A globular cytoskeletal protein that polymerizes to form a flexible, helical filament capabl of interacting with myosin. Actin filaments provide mechanical support for eukaryoti cells, determine's the cell's shape, and enable cell movements.

Actin-binding proteins Any of nearly 100 different proteins belonging to numerous families that affect th assembly of actin filament, their physical properties, and their interactions with on another and with other cellular organelles.

Action potential The collective changes in membrane potential, beginning with depolarization to threshol and ending with return to resting potential, that occur with stimulation of an excitabl cell and act as the basis for neural communication.

Activation energy The minimal kinetic energy needed for a reactant to undergo a chemical reaction.

Active site The part of an enzyme molecule that is directly involved in binding the substrate.

Active transport It is a energy-requiring process in which a substance binds to a specific transmembran protein, changing its conformation to allow passage of the substance through th membrane against the electrochemical gradient for that substance.

Adenine A nitrogen having purine base which occur in DNA, and RNA. Pairs normally wit thymine in DNA.

Adenosine triphosphate (ATP) It is a nucleotide consisting of adenosine binding to three phosphate groups; it is th principal immediate-energy source for prokaryotic and eukaryotic cells.

Adherens junctions (Zonulae adherens) Adherens junctions are a type of specialized adhesive junctions particularly common i epithelia. The plasma membranes in this region are separated by 20 to 35 nm and a sites where cadherin molecules are concentrated. The cells are held together by linkag between the extra cellular domains of cadherin molecules that bridge the gap betwee neighbouring cells.

Aerobes Organisms dependent on the presence of oxygen to metabolize energy-rich compound

Allele (also allelomorph; adj. allelic or allelomorphic). One member of a pair or a series of genes that can occur at a particular locus o homologous chromosomes.

Allopolyploid A polyploid having whole chromosome sets from different species.

Allosteric modulation Modification of the activity of an enzyme through interaction with a compound that bin to a site (*i.e.*, allosteric site) other than the active site.

Alpha (α) helix One possible secondary structure of polypeptides, in which the backbone of the cha forms a spiral (*i.e.*, helical) conformation.

Alternative splicing Widespread mechanism by which a single gene can encode two or more related protein

Amide bond The chemical bond that forms between carboxylic acids and amines (or acidic and amino functional groups) while producing a molecule of water.

Amino acids The monomeric units of proteins; each is composed of three functional groups attached to a central, α carbon: an amino group, a defining side chain, and a carboxyl group.

Aminoacyl-tRNA synthetase (AARS) An enzyme that covalently links amino acids to the 3′ ends of their cognate tRNAS. Each amino acid is recognized by a specific aminoacyl-tRNA synthetase.

Amitosis Direct nuclear division, without the separation of daughter chromosomes.

Amphidiploid A tetraploid individual having two sets of chromosomes from each of two known ancestral species.

Amphimixis To bring together the elements from two gametes in fertilization.

Amphipathic Molecules having spatially separated hydrophilic and hydrophobic regions.

Amphoteric Structural property allowing the same molecule to act as an acid or as a base.

Anabolic pathway A metabolic pathway resulting in the synthesis of relatively complex products.

Anaerobes Organisms that utilize energy-rich compounds through oxygen-independent metabolic pathways such as glycolysis and fermentation.

Anaphase The stage of mitosis during which sister chromatids separate from one another.

Anaphase A The movement of chromosomes toward the poles during mitosis.

Anaphase B Elongation of the mitotic spindle, which causes the two spindle poles to move farther apart.

Androgenesis The phenomenon of parthenogenesis by male.

Aneuploidy A karyotypic abnormality or variation in chromosome number by whole chromosomes, but less than an entire set, *e.g.*, 2n+l (trisomy), 2n–1 (monosomy).

Angiogenesis The formation of new blood vessels.

Angstrom (A°) 0.1 nanometer (nm) or 0.0000001 millimeter.

Animal models Laboratory animals that exhibit characteristics of a particular human disease.

Animal pole That portion of egg which has active cytoplasm and zygote nucleus.

Anion An ionised atom or molecule with a negative charge.

Anisogamy The fusion of unequal sized gametes.

Annulate lamellae The pores and lamellae (*i.e.*, the pore complex of nuclear envelope of most eukaryotes and endoplasmic reticulum of invertebrate and oocytes and spermatocytes of vertebrates).

Antibody An immunoglobulin protein produced by plasma cells derived from B lymphocytes that interacts with the surface of a pathogen or foreign substance to facilitate its destruction.

Anticodon A triplet of nucleotides specific to each tRNA corresponding to a particular amino acid and complimentary to the codon of mRNA.

Antigen Any substance recognised by an immune system as foreign to the organism.

Antiserum Fluid containing desired antibodies that remains after the removal of the cells and clotting factors from whole blood that has been exposed to given antigen.

Apoenzyme The protein component of a holoenzyme which also contains a nonprotein coenzyme or prosthetic group.

Apomixis The occurrence of the external form of sexual reproduction without the occurrence of meiosis and fertilization.

Apoptosis A type of orderly or programmed cell death in which the cell responds to certain signals by initiating a normal response that leads to the death of the cell. Death by apoptosis is characterised by overall compaction of the cell and its nucleus, the orderly dissection of the chromatin into pieces at the hands of a special DNA-splitting endonuclease, and the rapid engulfment of the dying cell by phagocytosis.

Artifact	A structure seen in a microscopic image that results from the coagulation or precipitaion of materials that had no existence in the living cell.
Asexual reproduction	The process of reproduction that does not involve fusion of cells.
Assay	Some identifiable feature of a specific protein such as the catalytic activity of an enzyme, used to determine the relative amount of that protein in a sample.
Aster	"Sunburst" arrangement of microtubules around each centrosome during mitosis.
ATP synthase	The ATP-synthesizing enzyme of the inner mitochondrial membrane, which is composed of two chief components: The F_1 of headpiece and the F_0 basal piece, the latter of which is embedded in the membrane itself.
Auto-antibodies	Antibodies against components of the body's own tissues.
Autoimmune diseases	Diseases characterized by an attack of the immune system against the body's own tissues. Includes multiple sclerosis, insulin-dependent diabetes.
Autophagy	The destruction of organelles and their replacement during which an organelle is surrounded by a double membrane. The membrane surrounding the organelle then fuses with a lysosome.
Autopolyploidy	A polyploidy all of whose sets of chromosomes are those of the same species.
Autoradiography	A method for localizing radioactive atoms in microscope preparations of biological materials by exposing of a photographic film emulsion to radioactive atoms incorporated in the biological specimen including cell.
Autosome	A chromosome not associated with the sex of the individual and therefore possessed in matching pairs by diploid members of both sexes.
Auxotroph	An individual unable to carry on some particular synthesis hence requiring supplementing of minimal medium by some growth factor.
Axon	A single, prominent extension that emerges from the cell body and conducts outgoing impulses away from the cell body and towards the target cell(s).
Axonal transport	Process by which vesicles, cytoskeletal polymers, and macromolecules are moved along microtubules within the axon of a neuron. Anterograde transport moves materials from the cell body toward the synaptic terminals, whereas retrograde transport moves materials in the opposite direction.
Axoneme	The central, microtubule-containing core of a cilium or flagellum. Most axonemes consist of nine peripheral doublets, two central microtubules and numerous accessory structures.
Bacillus	Rod-shaped bacterium.
Bacteriophage	The viruses attacking the bacterial cells.
Barr body (sex chromatin)	A mass of chromatin in the nucleus of resting cells, resulting from inactivation of an X chromosome.
Basal body	A structure that resides at the base of the cilium or flagellum and which generates their outer microtubules. Basal bodies are identical in structure to centrioles. Both can give rise to one another.
Base excision repair (BER)	A cut and patch mechanism for the removal from the DNA of altered nucleotides, *e.g.* uracil (formed from cytosine) and 8-oxoguanine.
Basement membrane (basal lamina)	Thickened layer of approximately 50 to 200 nm of extra-cellular matrix that surrounds muscle and fat cells and underlies the basal surface of epithelial tissues such as the skin the inner lining of the digestive and respiratory tracts, and the inner lining of blood vessels
Beta (β) clamps	One of the non-catalytic components of the replisome that encircles DNA and keeps the polymerase associated with DNA template.
Beta-oxidation	Splitting of fatty acids into two carbon units.

Bioenergetics The study of the various types of energy transformations that occur in living organisms.

Biogenesis The production or orgin of livings from living things.

Bivalent A pair of synapsed homologous chromosomes, whether or not these have yet replicated to form chromatids.

Budding A mode of asexual reproduction in which new organisms develops from the parent body in the form of an outgrowth.

C_3 pathway The metabolic pathway by which carbon dioxide is assimilated into the organic molecules of the cell during photosynthesis. RuBP (= ribulose 1,5 biphosphate) is used by Rubisco as the initial CO_2 acceptor. The product then fragments into two three-carbon PGA molecules.

C_4 pathway Alternate pathway for carbon fixation utilizing phosphoenolypyruvate as the CO_2 acceptor to produce four carbon compounds (predominantly malate and oxaloacetate).

Cadherins A family of related glycoproteins that mediate Ca^{2+}-depends cell-cell adhesion.

Calmodulin A small calcium-binding protein that is widely distributed. Each molecule of calmodulin contains four binding sites for calcium.

Calvin cycle (or Calvin-Benson cycle) The pathway for conversion of CO_2 into carbohydrates, the cycle occurs in cyanobacteria and all eukaryotic photosynthetic cells.

Carbohydrates (Glycans) Organic molecules including simple sugars (monosaccharides, *e.g.*, glucose) and multisaccharide polymers, which largely serve as energy-storage (*e.g.*, starch, glycogen) and structural compounds (*e.g.*, cellulose) in cells.

Carcinogen A chemical substance or physical agent (Such as radiation) that causes cancer.

Carotenoid Any of a group of yellow, orange or red pigments associated with chlorophylls in plants and in animal fat.

Carrier A transport protein within the membrane that binds temporarily with a molecule to be transported across the membrane.

Caspases A family of cysteine proteases that are activated at an early stage of apoptosis and are responsible for the degradative events observed during cell death.

Catabolism Breakdown of organic molecules within the cell with the release of energy.

Catalyst A substance that affects the rate of chemical reaction but is not effected itself in the process.

Cation An ionized atom or molecule with an extra positive charge.

Cell A structural and physiological unit of living organisms (Bacteria, plants and animals) which have protoplasm.

Cell concept A generalization of the cell theory, stating that the cell is the ultimate structural unit of the organism.

Cell culture The technique used to grow cells outside the organisms.

Cell cycle The sequence of events in dividing cells in which an interphase consisting of G_1, S and G_2 periods separates one mitosis from the mitosis of successive cell cycle.

Cell division A method by which new cells are originated from preexisting cells.

Cell fractionation Bulk separation of the various cell organelles by differential centrifugation.

Cell-free system An experimental system to study cellular activities that do not require whole cell. Such systems typically contain a preparation of purified proteins and/or subcellular fractions and are amenable to experimental manipulation.

Cell fusion Technique whereby two different types of cells (from one organism or from different species) are joined to produce one cell with one, continuous plasma membrane.

Cell-mediated immunity Carried out by T lymphocytes, that when activated, can specifically recognize and kill an infected (or foreign) cell.

Cell line Cells that are commonly used in tissue culture studies that have undergone genetic modifications that allow them to be grown indefinitely.

Cell plate Structure between the cytoplasm of two newly formed daughter cells that gives rise to a new cell wall in plant cells.

Cell signaling Communication in which information is relayed across the plasma membrane to the cell interior and often to the cell nucleus by means a series of molecular interactions.

Cell theory Theory of biological organization, which has three tenets: all organisms are made up of one or more cells; the cell is the structural unit of life, cells only arise from the division of preexisting cells.

Cell wall A rigid, nonliving (Karp 2010) or dynamic (Buchanan *et al.*, 2000) structure that provides support and protection for the cell it surrounds.

Cellulose Unbranched glucose polymer with $\beta(1 \rightarrow 4)$ linkages that assembles into cables and serves as a principal structural element of plant cell walls.

Centrioles Cylindrical structures, about 0.2 μm across and typically about twice as long, that contain nine evenly spaced fibrils, each of which appears in cross section as a band of three microtubules. Centrioles are nearly always found in pairs, with each of the members situated at right angles to one another.

Centromere Marked identation on a mitotic chromosome that serves as the site of kinetochore formation.

Centrosome A complex structure that contains two barrel-shaped centrioles surrounded by amorphous electron-dense pericentriolar material (or PCM) where microtubules are nucleated.

Chaperones Proteins that bind to other polypeptides, preventing their aggregation and promoting their folding and/or assembly into multimeric proteins.

Chaperonins Members of the Hsp60 class of chaperones, *e.g.*, GroEl, that form a cylindrical complex of 14 subunits within which the polypeptide folding reaction takes place.

Check point Mechanism that halt the progress of the cell cycle if (1) any of the chromosomal DNA is damaged, or (2) certain critical processes, such as DNA replication or chromosome alignment during mitosis have not been properly completed.

Chemiosmotic mechanism The mechanism for ATP synthesis whereby the movement of electrons through the electron-transport chain results in establishment of a proton gradient across the bacterial, thylakoid, or inner mitochondrial membrane, with the gradient acting as a high-energy intermediate, linking oxidation of substrates to the phosphorylation of ADP.

Chiasma (pl. chiasmata) The point of contact and interchange between the chromatids of two homologous chromosomes during prophases of meiosis.

Chloroplasts Cytoplasmic organelles containing several pigments, particularly the light absorbing chlorophylls.

Chromatid One of the two identical, longitudinal halves of a chromosome which share a common centromere with a sister chromatid,; results from the replication of chromosomes during a nuclear division.

Chromatin Nuclear material (DNA, RNA, histone and non-histone proteins) composing the chromosomes.

Chromatography A term used for a wide variety of techniques in which a mixture of dissolved components is fractionated as it moved through some type of immobile matrix.

Chromocentre Irregular mass of heterochromatin.

Chromomere Small, stainable thickenings arranged linearly along a chromosome.

Chromonema (pl. chromonemata) One of the delicate, helically coiled, thread-like filaments composing a chromosome.

Chromosome Nucleoprotein structures, generally more or less rod-like during nuclear division, the physical sites of nuclear genes which are arranged in linear order. Each species has a characteristic number of chromosomes although individuals with fewer or more than this characteristic number occur, specially in plants.

Cilia Hair like motile organelles that project from the surface of a variety of eukaryotic cells. Cilia tend to occur in large numbers on a cell's surface.

Ciliary or axonemal dynein A huge protein (MW about 2 million daltons) responsible for conversion of the chemical energy of ATP into the mechanical energy of ciliary locomotion.

***Cis* cisternae** The cisternae of the Golgi complex closer to the endoplasmic reticulum.

Cistron A segment of DNA specifying one polypeptide chain in protein synthesis. Under the concept of triplet code, one cistron must contain three times as many nucleotide pair as amino acids in the chain it specifies.

Clonal selection theory Well supported theory that B and T lymphocytes develop their ability to produce specific antibodies or T cell receptors prior to exposure to antigen.

Clone A line of cells derived from a single cell and presumed to contain same genetic information. The multicellular organisms that are propagated by vegetative (non-sexual) reproduction are also called clones.

Coated vesicles Vesicle that bud from a membrane compartment typically possess a multi-subunit protein coat that promotes the budding process. COPI–, COPII– and clathrin-coated vehicles.

Codon Sequences of three nucleotides (nucleotide triplets) in mRNAs that specify amino acids.

Coenocyte Mass of cytoplasm, containing nuclei, formed as a result of repeated divisions of the cytoplasm.

Coenzyme An organic nonprotein component of an enzyme.

Cofactor The nonprotein component of an enzyme, it can be either inorganic or organic.

Cohesin A multiprotein complex that keeps replicated chromatids associated with one another until they are separated during cell division.

Co-linearity The spatial correlation between codons in DNA and amino acids in the polypeptide translated from the DNA blueprint.

Collagens A family of fibrous glycoproteins known for their high tensile strength that function exclusively as part of the extracellular matrix.

Colloid A chemical substance having particles which range from 1 mm to 100 mm in size.

Complementary base pairing Specific hydrogen bond interactions between a particular purine and a particular pyrimidine component in nucleic acids; for example, guanine and cytosine or adenine and thymine or uracil.

Compound A chemical substance formed by the chemical combination of two or more simple substances.

Conductance The movement of small ions across membranes.

Conformation The three dimensional arrangement of the atoms within a molecule, often important in understanding the biological activity of proteins and other molecules in a living cell.

Congression The movement of duplicated chromosomes to the metaphase plate during prometaphase of mitosis.

Conjugation Side by side temporary association of two bodies, as of synapsed chromosomes in meiosis, or of two organisms during sexual reproduction.

Connexon Multisubunit complex of a gap junction formed from the clustering within the plasma membrane of an integral membrane protein called connexin. Each connexon is composed of six connexin subunits arranged around a central opening (or annulus) about 1.5 nm in diameter.

Consensus sequence The most common version of a conserved sequence. The TTGACA sequence of a bacterial promoter (known as the—35 element) is an example of a consensus sequence.

Conserved sequences Refers to the amino acid sequences of particular polypeptides or the nucleotide sequences of particular nucleic acids. If two sequences are similar to one another, *i.e.*, homologous, they are said to be conserved, which indicates that they have not diverged very much from a common an ancestral sequence over long periods of evolutionary time.

Constitutive heterochromatin Chromatin that remains in the compacted state in all cells at all times and, thus, represents DNA that is permanently silenced. It consists primarily of highly repeated sequences.

Constitutive Constant or unchanging; for example, a constitutive enzyme which is synthesized at a constant rate and not subject to regulation.

Conventional (or type II) myosins A family of myosins, first identified in muscle tissue, that are the primary motors for muscle contraction but are also found in a variety of non-muscle cells. Type II myosins are needed for spitting a cell in two during cell division and generating tension at focal adhesions.

Cotransport A process that couples the movement of two solutes across a membrane, termed symport if the two solutes are moved in the same direction and antiport if the two move in the opposite directions.

Covalent bonds Strong chemical bonds between atoms created when they share pairs of electrons (*e.g.*, bond between carbon and hydrogen, C—H).

Cristae The many deep folds that are characteristic of the inner mitochondrial membrane, which contain the molecular machinery of oxidative phosphorylation.

Crossing over (genetic recombination)
1. Reshuffling of the genes on chromosomes (thereby disrupting linkage groups) that occurs during meiosis as a result of breakage and reunion of segments of homologous chromosomes.
2. A process in which genes are exchanged between non-sister chromatids of homologous chromosomes. Chiasmatas are visible evidences of crossing over.

Cyclic AMP (cAMP) Adenosine monophosphate molecule arranged in cyclic form; its formation within cells is triggered by the action of hormones; cAMP functions to control cellular biochemistry.

Cyclin-dependent kinases (Cdks) Enzymes that control progression of cells through the cell cycle.

Cytochrome system Group of iron-bearing enzymes located in mitocbondria through which electrons pass; in the process energy is trapped into ATP molecules.

Cytochromes A type of electron carrier consisting of a protein bound to a heme group.

Cytogenetics Study of the cellular structures and mechanisms associated with genetics.

Cytokines Proteins secreted by cells of the immune system that alter the behaviour of other immune cells.

Cytokinesis The division of cytoplasm during cell division.

Cytology The study of structure and function of cell.

Cytoplasm The portion of cellular protoplasm which occurs between the plasma membrane and nuclear membrane.

Cytosine A pyrimidine base occurring in DNA and RNA. Pairs with guanine in DNA.

Dalton A measure of molecular mass, with one dalton equivalent to one unit of atomic mass (*e.g.*, the mass of a H atom).

Dehydrogenase An enzyme that catalyzes a redox reaction by removing a hydrogen atom from one reactant.

Deletion At the molecular level, the removal of one or more bases from a DNA sequence. At the cytological level, the absence of segment of a chromosome (also known as deficiency).

Denaturation 1. Separation of DNA double helix into its two component strands. 2. The unfolding or disorganization of a protein from its native or fully folded state.

Dendrites Fine extensions from the cell bodies of most neurons; dendrites receive incoming information from external sources, typically other neurons.

Deoxyribonucleic acid (DNA) A usually double-stranded, helically coiled, nucleic acid molecule, composed of phosphate-deoxyribose "back bones" which are connected by paired nitrogen bases (purines and pyrimidines) attached to the deoxyribose sugar, the genetic material of all living organisms and many viruses.

Depolarization A decrease in the electrical potential difference across a membrane.

Desmosome (maculae adherens) Disc-shaped adhesive junction containing cadherins found in a variety of tissues, but most notably epithelia, where they are located basal to the adherens junction. Dense cytoplasmic plaques on the inner surface of the plasma membranes in this region serve as sites of anchorage for looping intermediate filaments that extend into the cytoplasm.

Diakinesis A stage of prophase-I of meiosis in which paired chromosomes are much shortened and thickened.

Dictyosome The Golgi complex of plant cells which has no secretory function.

Differentiation Specialization of cells to perform specific functions in the organism.

Diffusion Migration or molecules or ions as a result of their own random movements from a region of higher concentration to a region of lower concentration. It requires no energy (also called free diffusion).

Dioecious Individuals producing either sperm or egg, but not both. In dioecious species, the sexes are separate.

Diploid An individual or cell having two complete sets of chromosomes.

Diplotene A stage of prophase–1 of meiosis in which each of the synaptic chromosomes gets doubled by splitting.

Disjunction The separation of homologous chromosomes during anaphase–1 of meiosis.

DNA gyrase A type II topoisomerase that is able to change the state of supercoiling in a DNA molecule by relieving the tension that builds up during replication. It does this by traveling along the DNA and acting like a "swivel", changing the positively supercoiled DNA into negatively supercoiled DNA.

DNA methylation An epigenetic process in which methyl groups are added to cytosine residue in DNA by DNA methyltransferases. In vertebrates, DNA methylation occurs on certain CpG residues in the promoter regions of genes and is associated with inactivation of gene expression.

DNA polymerases The enzymes responsible for constructing new DNA strands during replication or DNA repair.

DNA tumor viruses Viruses capable of infecting vertebrate cells, transforming them into cancer cells.

DNA-dependent RNA polymerases (RNA) The enzymes responsible for transcription in both prokaryotic and eukaryotic cells.

Domain A region within a protein (or RNA) that folds and functions in a semi-independent manner.

Double-strand breaks (DSBs) DNA damage often resulting from ionizing radiation involving a fracture of both strands of the double helix.

Duplication The occurrence of the segment twice in the same chromosome or in the same complement.

Dyad A pair of homologous chromosomes before their duplication in the meiosis.

Dynein An exceptionally large, cargo-carrying multisubunit motor protein that moves along microtubules toward their minus end. This family of proteins occurs as cytoplasmic dyneins and ciliary or axonemal dyneins.

Effector	A substance that brings about a cellular response to a signal.
Egg (egg cell)	The female gamete.
Electrophoresis	A technique for separating molecules, particularly proteins, according to over all electric charge of the molecules.
Embryonic stem (ES) cells	A type of cell that has virtually unlimited powers of differentiation, found in the mammalian blastocyst, which is an early stage of embryonic development comparable to the blastula of other animals.
Endergonic reactions	Reactions that are thermodynamically unfavorable and cannot occur spontaneously, possessing a $+\Delta G$ value.
Endocytosis	Mechanism for the uptake of fluid and solutes into a cell. Can be divided into two types: bulk-phase endocytosis, which is non-specific, and receptor-mediated endocytosis, which requires the binding of solute molecules such as LDL or transferrin to a specific cell-surface receptor.
Endomembrane system	Functionally and structurally interrelated group of membranous cytoplasmic organelles including the endoplasmic reticulum, Golgi complex, endosomes, lysosomes and vacuoles.
Endoplasmic reticulum (ER)	A tubular double membrane system in the cytoplasm, continuous with the nuclear membrane and bearing many ribosomes. Contain many enzymes and have skeletal, transporting and biosynthetic functions of the cytoplasm.
Endosomes	Organelles of the endocytic pathway. Materials taken up by endocytosis are transported to early endosomes where they are sorted, and then on to late endosomes and ultimately to lysosomes. Late endosomes also function as destination sites of lysosomal enzymes transported from the Golgi complex.
Endosymbiont theory	Proposal, which is based on considerable evidence, that mitochondria and chloroplasts arose from symbiotic prokaryotes that took up residence within a primitive host cell.
End-product inhibition	A sequence of chemical reactions wherein the last product formed inhibits one of the early steps; a form of negative feedback which limits the rate of chemical reactions.
Energy	Capacity for doing work. It exists in two forms: potential and kinetic.
Enhancer	A regulatory site in the DNA that may be located at considerable distance either upstream or downstream from the promoter that it regulates. Binding of one or more transcriptional factors to the enhancer can dramatically increase the rate of transcription of the gene.
Entropy (S)	A measure of the relative disorder of the system or universe associated with random movements of matter; because all movements cease at absolute zero (OK), entropy is zero only at that temperature.
Enzyme inhibitor	Any molecule that can bind to an enzyme and decrease its activity. It is of two types: noncompetitive or competitive.
Enzyme	Any substance, protein in whole or in part that regulate the rate of a specific biochemical reaction in living organisms.
Epigenetic inheritance	Heritable changes, *i.e.*, changes that can be transmitted from one cell to its progeny, that do not involve changes in DNA sequence. Epigenetic changes can result from DNA methylation, covalent modification of histones, and likely other types of chromatin modifications.
Equatorial plate	The figure formed at the spindle equator in nuclear division.
Euchromatin	Chromatin that returns to its dispersed state during interphase.
Eukaryotes	Organisms (*e.g.*, plants, animals, protists and fungi) with a well-defined nucleus enclosed in a nuclear membrane and usually having one or more other membranous subcellular compartments.

Euploidy Variation in chromosome number by whole sets or exact multiple of the monoploid (haploid) number, *e.g.*, diploid, triploid. Euploids above the diploid level may be referred to collectively as polyploids.

Exocytosis A mode of transport of substances out of the cell by enclosure in a portion of the plasma membrane and subsequent expulsion to the outside.

Exons Those parts of a split gene that contribute to a mature RNA product.

Exonuclease A DNA or RNA-digesting enzyme that attaches to either the 5′ or 3′ end of the nucleic acid strand and removes one nucleotide at a time from that shrinking end.

Extracellular matrix (ECM) An organised network of extracellular materials that is present beyond the immediate vicinity of the plasma membrane. It may play an integral role in determining the shape and activities of the cell.

Facilitated diffusion Assisted passage (transport) of molecules across the membrane towards their lower concentration along a gradient.

Feedback inhibition A mechanism to control metabolic pathways where the end product interacts with an enzyme in the pathway, resulting in inactivation of the enzyme.

Fermentation Anaerobic decomposition of an organic substance in the body of a living organism.

Fertilization The fusion of cytoplasm and male and female pronuclei of male gamete (sperm or pollen) and a female gamete (ovum) to form a zygote in sexually reproducing organisms.

Feulgen reaction Chemical staining process which reacts specifically with genetic material (DNA) in cells.

Fission A mode of asexual reproduction in which the body of the organism divides transversely or longitudinally into two or more equal parts.

Flagella Hairlike motile organelles that project from the surface of a variety of eukaryotic cells.

Fluid-mosaic model Model presenting membranes as dynamic structures in which both lipids and associated proteins are mobile and capable of moving within the membrane to engage in interactions with other membrane molecules.

Fractionated Disassembly of a preparation into its component ingredients so that the properties of individual species of molecules can be examined.

Free radical Highly reactive atom or molecule that contains a single unpaired electron.

Gamete A protoplast (sex cell) which in the process of sexual reproduction, fuses with another protoplast. One of them may be termed as male and another female.

Gametogenesis The origin, maturation and differentiation of gametes from the generative cells.

Gel Jelly-like state of protoplasm.

Gene amplification Differential replication of some genes, producing many copies of these genes.

Gene The particulate determiner of a hereditary trait; a particular segment of DNA molecule, generally located in the chromosome.

Genetic code The code that relates nucleotide sequences in nucleic acids to amino acid sequences. Each triplet of nucleotide designates a particular amino acid; thus, the genetic code allows the translation of information stored in DNA and the use of that information in protein synthesis.

Genome A complete set of chromosomes or of chromosomal genes, inherited as an unit from one parent.

Gluconeogenesis Synthesis of carbohydrates from noncarbohydrate precursors such as fats or proteins.

Glycolysis The oxidation of sugar (glucose) or glycogen to pyruvic acid without the use of oxygen; also known as the Embden-Meyerhof pathway.

Golgi apparatus (complex) A cytoplasmic organelle which have a complex system of tubules and vesicles and which is related with the production of cellular secretions, also called Golgi apparatus complex.

Guanine A purine base occurring in DNA and RNA. Pairs normally with cytosine in DNA.

Haemoglobin An iron protein pigment of blood functioning in oxygen-carbon dioxide exchange of living cells.

Haploid An organism or cell that has one copy of each chromosome.

Hard keratin A keratin used for production of structures such as hair, nails and horns.

Heat-shock proteins A highly conserved group of chaperone proteins expressed in cells exposed to elevated temperatures or other forms of environmental stress.

Hedgehog A secreted signaling molecule that stimulates a pathway regulating cell fate during embryonic development.

Helicase An enzyme that catalyzes the unwinding of DNA.

Helix-loop-helix A transcription factor DNA-binding domain formed by the dimerization of two polypeptide chains. The dimerization domains of these proteins consists of two helical regions separated by a loop.

Helix-turn-helix A transcription factor DNA-binding domain in which three or four helical regions contact DNA.

Hemicellulose A polysaccharide that cross links cellulose microfibrils in plant cell wall.

Hemidesmosome A region of contact between cells and the extra cellular matrix at which keratin filaments are attached to integrin.

Hepatitis B viruses A family of DNA viruses that infect liver cells and can lead to the development of liver cancer.

Hepatitis C viruses A family of RNA viruses that infect liver cells and can lead to the development of liver cancer.

Heterochromatin Darkly stained part of chromatin in interphase nucleus the condensed transcriptionally inactive chromatin.

Hetero-chromosomes Chromosomes with exceptional form or behaviour especially at meiosis, such as a sex chromosomes fragments.

Heterogamy Union of two unlike gametes.

Heterokaryon A cell having two different types of nuclei, as a result of fusion of two cell types without nuclear fusion.

Heterozygote An individual whose chromosomes bear unlike genes of a given allelic pair. Heterozygote produces more than one kind of gametes with respect to a particular locus (gene).

Histone acetylation The modification of histones by the addition of acetyl groups to specific lysine residues.

Histone Any of several proteins that can combine with DNA to form chromosomes, having a high content of the basic amino acids arginine and lysine.

Holliday junction The central intermediate in recombination, consisting of a crossed-strand structure formed by homologous base pairing between strands of two DNA molecule.

Holliday model A molecular model of genetic recombination involving the formation of heteroduplex regions.

Homeobox Conserved DNA sequences of 180 base pairs that encode homeodomains.

Homeodomain A type of DNA binding domain found in transcription factors that regulate gene expression during embryonic development.

Homologous chromosomes Chromosomes occurring in pairs, one derived from each of two parents, normally (except in case of chromosomes associated with sex such as X and Y chromosomes) morphologically alike and bearing the same gene loci. Each member of such a pair is the homolog of the other.

Homozygote An individual whose chromosomes bear identical genes of a given allelic pair or series. Homozygotes produce only one kind of gamete with respect to a particular locus and therefore "breed true".

Hormones Signaling molecules produced by endocrine glands that act on cells at distant body sites.

Hyaloplasm The ground substance of cytoplasm which is colloidal and contain enzymes for glycolysis and structural material, such as sugars-amino acids, water, vitamins, nucleotides, etc., commonly known as cytoplasmic matrix, nutrient soup or cell sap.

Hybridization molecular Formation of a double-stranded structure, DNA-DNA, RNA-DNA, or RNA-RNA, by hydrogen bonding of complementary single stranded molecules or parts of molecules.

Hydrolysis The process by which one molecule is processed into two smaller molecules by the addition of water, usually resulting in the release of energy.

Hydrophilic Soluble in water.

Hydrophobic Not soluble in water.

Idiogram A diagrammatic representation of the complete chromosome set of an individual, arranged according to (decreasing) size and/or accepted numbering system. Idiograms may be drawn from suitable microscope preparations, or these may be photographed and various chromosomes arranged in order (and in homologous pairs in diploid organisms).

Immune system Physiological system consisting of organs, scattered tissues, and independent cells that protect the body from invading pathogens and foreign materials.

Immunity State in which the body is not susceptible to infection by a particular pathogen.

Immunoblotting A method that uses antibodies to detect proteins separated by SDS-polyacrylamide gel electrophoresis.

Importin A karyopherin that recognizes nuclear localization signals and directs nuclear import.

In utero (Latin) in the womb.

In vitro (Latin in glass), pertaining to experiments done on cells grown outside of the organisms.

In vivo (Latin, in the living) pertaining to experiments on a whole living organism.

Induced fit A model of enzyme action in which the configurations of both the enzyme and the substrate are altered by substrate binding.

Inducer (Effector) A substance inactivating a repressor.

Inducer A compound that binds to a protein repressor and activates transcription of a bacterial operon.

Inducible operon An operon in which the presence of the key metabolic substance induces transcription of the structural genes.

Initiation codon The triplet AUG, the site to which the ribosome attaches to the mRNA to assure that the ribosome is in the proper reading frame to correctly read the entire message.

Initiation factors Soluble proteins (IFs in bacteria and eIFs in eukaryotes) that make initiation of translation possible.

Inositol, 1, 4, 5-triphosphate (IP3) A second messenger, formed from the hydrolysis of PIP2, that signals the release of calcium ions from the endoplasmic reticulum.

Insulator A sequence that divides chromatin into independent domains and prevents an enhancer from acting on a promoter in a separate domain.

Integral protein A membrane-associated protein that penetrates or spans the lipid bilayer.

Integrin A transmembrane protein that mediates the adhesion of cells to the extracellular matrix.

Interchange An exchange of non-homologous terminal segments of chromosomes.

Interference The reduction in likelihood of a second crossover closely adjacent to another. Interference ordinarily increases with decreased distance.

Interkinesis See interphase, resting stage.

Intermediate filaments (IFs) Strong, ropelike cytoskeletal fibers about 10 nm in diameter that provide mechanical strength to cells in tissues.

Interphase 1. The stage of cell life during which that cell is not dividing.
2. A period of the cell cycle between cell division that include G_1, S and G_2 phases.

Introns Non-coding sequences of split gene that interrupt exons.

Inversion A chromosomal aberration that results after a chromosome is broken in two places and the resulting center segment is reincorporated into the chromosome in reverse order.

Ion channel A transmembranous structure (*e.g.*, an integral protein with an aqueous pore) permeable to a specific ion or ions.

Ion pump A protein that couples ATP hydrolysis to the transport of ions across a membrane.

Ion A atom or molecule with a net positive or negative charge because it has lost or gained one or more electrons during a chemical reaction.

Ionic bond A noncovalent bond occurring between oppositely charged ions, also called a salt bridge.

Isochromosome A chromosome with two morphologically identical chromosomes.

Isoforms Different versions of a protein. Isoforms may be encoded by separate, closely related genes, or formed as splice variants by alternative splicing from a single gene.

Isogametes Gametes not differentiated as to sex. Fusing isogametes are physically similar but, in some species are chemically differentiated.

Isotonic Property of one compartment having the same solute concentration compared with that in a given compartment.

Isozymes Multiple forms of an enzyme with varying activity.

Junctional complex A region of cell-cell contact containing a tight junction, an adherens junction and a desmosome.

Karyokinesis The division of the nucleus during cell division.

Karyology The biology of the nucleus.

Karyolymph A clear fluid material within the nuclear membrane; nuclear sap.

Karyopherin A nuclear transport receptor.

Karyotype A distribution of photographed metaphase chromosomes from a cell or individual showing chromosomes in pairs and in order of decreasing size, the size shape and appearance of metaphase chromosomes.

Keratin A type of intermediate filament protein of epithelial cells.

Kilobase (kb) One thousand nucleotides or nucleotide base pairs.

Kinesin A motor protein that moves along microtubules toward plus end. It moves membranous vesicles and other organelles along microtubules through the cytoplasm.

Kinetic energy Energy released from a substance through atomic or molecular movements.

Kinetochore microtubules Microtubules of the mitotic spindle that attach to condensed chromosones at their centromeres.

Kinetochore A button-like structure situated at the outer surface of the centromere to which the microtubules of the spindle attach.

Knockout Inactivation of a chromosomal gene by homologous recombination with a cloned mutant allele.

Krebs cycle Continuation of glycolysis; oxidative metabolism of pyruvic acid which is an end product of glucose fermentation (glycolysis), occurring within mitocbondria, requiring O_2 and yielding large quantities of energy that eventually trapped in the bounds of ATP; also called tricarboxylic acid cycle or citric add cycle.

Lagging strand The newly synthesized daughter DNA strand that is synthesized discontinuously, so called because the initiation of each fragment must wait for the parent strands to separate and expose additional template.

Lamellipodium The leading actin-base edge of a moving fibroblast, which is extended out from the cell as a broad, flattened, veil-like projection that glides over the substratum.

Laminin The principal adhesion protein of basal laminae.

Lamins Intermediate filament proteins that form the nuclear lamina.

Lampbrush chromosomes Giant bivalents with extensively looped-out regions of chromatin fibres, especially prominent in amphibian oocyte nuclei during the diplotene stage of meiosis I propase.

Lateral gene transfer Transfer of genes from one species to another.

Leading strand The newly synthesized daughter DNA strand that is synthesized continuously in the direction of movement of the replication fork.

Leptotene The first stage of the extended prophase of meiosis I during which homologous chromosomes pair before condensation.

Leucoplast A plastid that stores energy sources in non-photosynthetic plant tissues.

Ligand Any molecule that can bind to a receptor because it has a complementary structure

Ligand-gated channels Ion channels that open in response to the binding of signaling molecules.

Ligase Enzyme that joins together the parts of single strands of DNA between the 5′ end of one strand and the 3′ end of another.

Locus (pl., loci) The position or place on a chromosome occupied by a particular gene or one of its alleles.

Lysis (n.) v.i. or vt. lyse Disintegration or dissolution; usually the destruction of a bacterial host cell by infecting phase particles.

Lysogenic bacteria Living bacterial cells harbouring temperate phages (viruses).

Lysosomes Cytoplasmic organelles of animal cells which contain digestive enzymes for intracellular digestion of bacteria and other foreign bodies which enter the cells by the process of phagocytosis or pinocytosis. They may cause cell destruction if ruptured.

M phase The part of the cell cycle that includes two events: the process of mitosis, during which duplicated chromosones are separated into two nuclei, and cytokinesis, during which the entire cell is physically divided into two daughter cells.

Macromolecules Large, highly organised molecules crucial to the structure and function of cells; divided into polysaccharides, certain lipids, proteins and nucleic acids.

Major histocompatibility complex (MHC) A region of genome that encode MHC proteins. The genes that encode these proteins tend to be highly polymorphic, being represented by a large number of different alleles. These genetic differences between humans account for the tendency of a person to reject a transplant from another person other than an identical twin.

Mass spectrometry Methodology to identify molecules (including proteins). A proteins or mixture of proteins is fragmented, converted into gaseous ions, and propelled through a tubular component of a mass spectrometer, causing the ions to separate according to their mass/charge (m/z) ratio. Identification of the protein(s) is made by comparison with a computer database of the sequence of proteins encoded by a particular genome.

Matrix One of two aqueous compartments of a mitochondrion; the matrix is located within the interior of the organelle; the second compartment is called the intermembrane space and is located between the outer and inner mitochondrial membrane.

Meiocyte Any cell that undergoes meiosis.

Meiosis Nuclear division in which the diploid or somatic chromosome number is reduced by half. In the first of the two meiotic divisions homologous chromosomes first replicate, then pair (synapse), and finally separate to different daughter nuclei, which thus have half as many chromosomes as the parent nucleus, and one of each kind instead of two. A second division, in which chromosome replicates separate into daughter nuclei, follows so that meiosis produces four monoploid daughter nuclei from one diploid nucleus.

Meiospore In plants, one of the asexual reproductive cells produced by meiosis from a meiocyte.

Membrane fluidity A property of the physical state of the lipid bilayer of a membrane that allows diffusion of membrane lipids and proteins within the plane of the membrane. Inversely related to membrane viscosity. Membrane fluidity increases as the temperature rises and in bilayers with more unsaturated lipids.

Membrane potential The electrical potential difference across a membrane.

Meristem A cellular region in plants characterized by repeated cell division and wherein therefore, growth in size originates.

Mesosome An extensively infolded portion of the prokaryotic plasma membrane which has been implicated in respiratory and cell division functions.

Messenger RNA (mRNA) 1. Ribonucleic acid transcribed by DNA and conferring amino acid specificity on a ribosome.

2. The intermediate molecule between a gene and the polypeptide for which it codes. Messenger RNA is assemblage as a complementary copy of one of the two DNA strands that encodes the gene.

Metabolism The total of the chemical reactions occuring within a cell.

Metaphase The stage of nuclear division in which the chromosomes are located in the equatorial plane of the spindle prior to centromere division.

Metastasis Spread of cancer cells from a primary tumor to distant sites in the body where the formation of secondary tumors may arise.

Micro RNAs (mi RNAs) Small RNAs (20–23 nucleotide long) that are synthesized from many sites in the genome and involved in inhibiting translation or increasing degradation of complementary mRNAs.

Microfibrils Bundles of cellulose molecules that confer rigidity to the cell wall and provide resistance to pulling forces.

Microfilaments Solid 8-nm thick, cytoskeletal structures composed of a double-helical polymer of the protein actin. They play a key role in virtually all types of contractility and motility within cells.

Microscope An instrument that provides a magnified image of a tiny object.

Microsome A heterogenous collection of vesicles formed from the endomembrane system (primarily the endoplastic reticulum and golgi complex) after homogenization.

Microtubule An unbranched proteinous hollow cylindrical assembly of protofilaments which is involved in cell movement phenomena; spindle fibres, ciliary subfibres and centriole-subfibres are microtubules.

Microtubule-associated proteins (MAPs) Proteins other than tubulin contained in microtubules obtained from cells. MAPs may interconnect microtubules to form bundles and can be seen as cross-bridges connecting microtubules to each other. Other MAPs may increase the stability of microtubules, alter their rigidity and influence the rate of their assembly.

Microtubule-organizing centers (MTOCs) A variety of specialized structures that exert a role in initiating microtubule formation.

Microvilli Finger-like projections of plasma membranes of animal ethithelial cells, particularly of the gut.

Mitochondrion (Pl. mitochondria) The small cytoplasmic organelles in which aerobic cellular respiration occur and which are related with the production of energy by Krebs cycle, electron transport chain, beta oxidation of fatty acids, etc.

Mitosis Nuclear division in which replication of chromosomes is followed by separation of the products of replication and their incorporation into two daughter nuclei. Daughter nuclei are normally identical with each other and with the original parent nucleus in both kind and number of chromosomes. Mitosis may or may not involve cytoplasmic division.

Model organism Organisms that have been widely used for research so that a great deal is known about their biology. These organisms have properties that have made them excellent research subjects. Such organisms include the bacterium, *E.coli*; the budding yeast, *S. cerevisiae*; the nematode, *C. elegans*; the fruit fly, *D. melanogaster*; the mustard plant, *A. thaliana* and the mouse, *M. musculus*.

Molecular chaperons Various families of proteins whose role is to assist the folding the assembly of proteins by preventing undesirable interactions.

Monoecious Individual producing both sperms and eggs.

Monoploid An individual having a single complete set of chromosomes. Synonym, haploid.

Monosomic An individual lacking one chromosome of a set ($2n - 1$).

Motor proteins Proteins that utilise the energy of ATP hydrolysis to generate mechanical forces that propel the protein, as well as attached cargo, along one of the components of the cytoskeleton. Three families of motor proteins are known kinesins and dyneins move along microtubules and myosins move along microfilaments.

Mutation A sudden change in genotype having no relation to the individual's ancestry. Used for changes in single gene itself ("point mutation") and for chromosomal aberrations.

Muton A smallest segment of DNA or subunit of a cistron that can be changed and thereby bring about a mutation; probably as small as one nucleotide pair.

Myeloma A tumour consisting of a clone of antibody-forming cells.

Myosin 1. The muscle protein making up the thick filaments of striated muscle and of a few other cell systems; has ATPase activity.

2. A large family of motor proteins that moves along actin-containing microfilaments. Most myosins are plus-end directed motors. **Conventional myosin (myosin II)** is the protein that mediates muscle contractility as well as certain types of nonmuscle motility, such as cytokinesis. **Unconventional myosins** (myosin I and III–XVIII) have many diverse roles including organelle transport.

Nanometer Measure of length equaling 10^{-9} meters.

Nascent protein A protein in the process of being synthesized, *i.e.*, not yet complete.

Negative staining Procedures in which heavy-metal deposits are collected everywhere on the specimen grid except in the locations of very small particulate materials, including high-molecular-weight aggregates such as viruses, ribosomes, multisubunit enzymes, cytoskeletal elements and protein complexes.

Non-disjunction The failure of homologous chromosomes to separate at anaphase-1 of meiosis.

Nucleosomes Repeating subunits of chromatin. Each nucleosome of 146 base pairs of supercoiled DNA wrapped almost twice around a disc-shaped complex of eight histone molecules. The nucleosome core particles are connected to one another by a stretch of linker DNA.

Nuclear lamina A thin meshwork composed of intermediate filaments that lines the inner surface of the nuclear envelope.

Nuclear localization signal (NLS) Sequence of amino acids in a protein that is recognised by a transport receptor leading to translocation of the protein from the cytoplasm to the nucleus.

Nucleic acid Polymers composed nucleotides, which in living organisms are based on one of two sugars, ribose or deoxyribose, yielding the terms ribonucleic acid (RNA) and deoxyribonucleic acid (DNA).

Nucleoid The poorly defined region of a prokaryotic cell that contains its genetic material.

Nucleolar organising region (NOR) The specific part of the nucleolar organizing chromosome where ribosomal RNA genes are situated and where the nucleolus is produced.

Nucleolus Deeply staining nuclear body which is involved in rRNA synthesis; it is usually associated with secondary constrictions or nucleolar organizers of certain chromosomes and has important role in the biogenesis of ribosomes.

Nucleoplasm The unstructured matrix portion of the nucleus in which the chromosomes and nucleoli are bathed.

Nucleoside Portion of DNA or RNA molecule composed of one deoxyribose molecule (in DNA) or ribose (in RNA) plus a purine or a pyrimidine.

Nucleotide Portion of DNA or RNA molecule composed of one deoxyribose phosphate unit (in DNA) or one ribose phosphate unit (in RNA) plus a purine or a pyrimidine.

Nucleus A membrane-bounded cellular organelle having chromatin, nucleolus and nucleoplasm and regulating growth and reproduction of the cell.

Nullisomy The absence of a particular chromosome.

Okazaki fragments Small segments of DNA that are rapidly linked to longer pieces that have been synthesized previously, to form the lagging strand.

Oncogenes Genes that encode proteins that promote the loss of growth control and the conversion of the cell to a malignant state. These genes have the ability to transform cells.

Oncogenic Having a tendency to "cause" cancer.

Ontogeny The complete development of the individual from zygote, spore, etc., to adult form.

Oocyte The egg mother cell.

Oogenesis The process of development and differentiation of the ovum from the oogonium.

Operator site A segment of DNA in one operon that affects activity or non-activity of associated cistrons; it may be combined with a repressor and thereby 'turn off' the associated cistrons.

Operon A system of cistrons operator and promoter sites by which a given genetically controlled metabolic activity is regulated.

Organelle A structural differentiation of the cell (*e.g.*, mitochondria, chloroplasts, ribosomes, etc.) containing particular enzymes and performing particular functions for the whole cell or individual.

Orientation The movement of chromosomes so that their centromere lie axially with respect to the spindle.

Ovary The female gonad in animals or the ovule containing portion of the pistil of a flower.

Ovule Structure within the ovary of pistil of a flower, which becomes a seed.

Oxidation Reactions involving loss of electrons or hydrogens or gain of oxygen.

Oxidative phosphorylation In cellular respiration, oxidation in the cytochrome system accompanied by the addition of phosphate molecules to ADP forming ATP.

Pachytene A stage of prophase-I of meiosis in which the chromosomes are visible as long paired threads.

Parthenogenesis Development of a new individual from an unfertilized egg.

Pectins A heterogeneous class of negatively charged polysaccharides that make up the matrix of the plant cell wall. Pectins hold water and form a gel that fills in the spaces between the fibrous elements.

Peptide bond A chemical bond (CONH) linking amino acid residues together in a protein.

Peptide A string of a few amino acids joined by peptide bonds.

Peptidyl transferase That portion of the large ribosomal subunit that is responsible for catalyzing peptide bond formation; peptidyl transferase activity resides in the large ribosomal RNA molecule.

Perosixomes (microbodies) Simple, membrane-bound, multifunctional organelles of the cytoplam that carry out a diverse array of metabolic reactions, including substrate oxidation leading to formation of hydrogen peroxide. For example, peroxisomes are the site of oxidation of uric acid, and the synthesis of plasmalogens. Plant glyoxysomes, which carry out the glyoxylate cycle are a type of peroxisome.

pH Expression of the relative abundance of H^+ in solution (*i.e.*, negative logarithm of H^+ concentration); relative acidity of a solution. Neutral pH is 7; lower levels are acidic, higher are basic.

Phagocytosis Process by which particulate materials are taken into cells. Materials are enclosed within a fold of the plasma membrane, which buds into cytoplasm to form a vesicle called a phagosome.

Photon Energy quantum or packet of light energy

Photorespiration A series of reactions in which O_2 is attached to RuBP and eventually resulting in the release of recently fixed CO_2 from the plant.

Photosynthesis Manufacture of sugar from CO_2 and H_2O in the light and in the presence of chlorophyll in eukaryotic chloroplasts or within prokaryotic photosynthetic membranes.

Phragmoplast Dense material roughly aligned in the equatorial plane of the previous metaphase plate in plant cells, consisting of clusters of interdigitating microtubules oriented perpendicular to the future cell plate, together with vesicles and associated electrondense material.

Phylogeny The evolutionary development of a species or other taxonomic group.

Pinocytosis A process by which the cell engulf droplets of liquids.

Plasma membrane The differentially permeable and limiting membrane of the cell through which extracellular substances may be selectively sampled and cell products may be liberated.

Plasmodesmata Cytoplasmic channels between plant cells.

Plastids Structures for storage of starch, pigment and other cellular products in plant cell.

Ploidy Variation in number of whole chromosomes.

Polar bodies The expelled products of the division of the oocyte nucleus in animals during oogenesis.

Polymer A chemical compound composed of two or more units of the same compound.

Polymerase An enzyme that catalyzes polymerization. In particular, DNA and RNA polymerases catalyze the formation of the nucleic acids from the nucleotide constituents on the basis of a single-stranded DNA template.

Polypeptide A compound containing amino acid residues jointed by peptide bonds. A protein may consists of one or more specific polypeptide chains.

Polyploid An individual having more than two complete sets of chromosomes, *e.g.*, triploid (3n), tetraploid (4n).

Polysome Polyribosome, an aggregation of ribosomes, connected by a strand of messenger RNA, which is active in protein synthesis.

Polytene chromosomes A multistranded endoreplicated chromosomes

Porins Integral proteins found in bacterial, mitochondrial and chloroplast outer membranes that act as large, relatively nonselective channels.

Primary structure The sequence of amino acids in a polypeptide chain.

Primase Type of RNA polymerase that assembles the short RNA primers that begin the synthesis of each Okazaki fragment of the lagging strand.

Prion An infectious agent associated with certain mammalian neurodegenerative disease that is composed solely of protein.

Procentriole An immature centriole.

Processive A term applied to proteins (*e.g.*, kinesin of RNA polymerase) that are capable of moving considerable distances along their track or template (*e.g.*, a microtubule or a DNA molecule) without dissociating from it.

Prokaryotes Organisms of the bacteria and blue-green algae groups lacking a nucleus separated from the cytoplasm by a membrane.

Promoter site Site on DNA at which mRNA synthesis initiated in an operon. May be combined with a repressor to inhibit mRNA synthesis by associated cistrons.

Prophase The first stage of nuclear division, including all events upto arrival of chromosomes at the equator of the spindle.

Proteasome Barrel-shaped, multiprotein complex in which cytoplasmic proteins are degraded. Proteins selected for destruction are linked to ubiquitin molecules and threaded into the central chamber of the proteasome.

Proteome The entire inventory of proteins in a particular organism, cell type, or organelle.

Protoplasm The living material of the cell.

Protoplast A structural unit of protoplasm; all the living (protoplasmic) material of the cell. Its two principal parts are nucleus and cytoplasm.

Puff A region of expanded chromosome undergoing active transcription, usually observed in giant polyene chromosomes.

Pumps, ion Systems that underwrite active transport of molecules across membrane by expelling one substance out of the cell and thereby helping to drive many kinds of molecules into the cell along an energy gradient.

Purine Nitrogen base occurring in DNA and RNA; these are adenine and guanine.

Pyrimidline Nitrogenous base occurring in DNA (thymine and cytosine) or RNA (uracil and cytosine).

Quality control Cells contains various mechanisms that ensure that the proteins and nucleic acids they synthesize have the appropriate structure. For example, misfolded proteins are translocated out of the ER and destroyed by proteasomes in the cytosol; mRNAs that contain premature termination codons are recognised and repaired.

Quantum The energy of a photon, its amount being, inversely proportional to the wavelength of emitted radiation.

Quaternary structure Specific assemblages of different polypeptide chains which, when combined in the protein, do not have the same structural or chemical properties as in the individual chains.

Rabs A family of small G proteins involved in vesicle transfecting. (For example, in humans more than 60 Rabs (rab proteins) have been isolated, each of which become associated with different membrane compartment to give each of them a unique surface identity).

Ran A GTP binding protein that exists in an active GTP-bound form or an inactive GDP-bound form. RAN ragulates nucleocytoplasmic transport of proteins, and works in association with importin proteins.

Ras Ras protein is a part of a superfamily of more than 150 small G proteins including Rabs, Sar 1 and Ran. These proteins are involved in the regulation of numerous processes including cell division, differentiation, gene expression, cytoskeletal organization, vesicle trafficking and nucleocytoplasmic transport.

Ras is a small GTPase (protein) that is anchored at the inner side of the plasma membrane by a lipid group. It acts similar to G proteins but also acts both as a switch and a molecular timer. Mutations in human *RAS* gene that lead to tumor formation prevent the Ras protein from hydrolyzing the bound GTP back to GDP form. As a result, the mutant version of Ras protein remained in the "on" position, sending a continuous message downstream along the signaling pathway, keeping the cell in proliferative mode.

Ras-MAP kinase cascade A cascade that is turned on in response to a wide variety of extracellular signals and plays a key role in regulating vital activities such as cell proliferation and differentiation.

Receptor Any substance that can bind to a specific molecule (ligand), often leading to uptake or signal transduction.

Recombination The new association in one individual of phenotype traits from both parents (*i.e.*, a non-parental individual). Also random combinations of genes from different linkage groups resulting from meiosis.

Recon The smallest segment of DNA or unit of a cistron that is capable of recombination; probably as one nucleotide pair.

Reduction division See meiosis.

Regulated secretion Discharge of materials synthesized in the cell that have been stored in membrane-bound secretory granules in the peripheral regions of the cytoplasm, occuring in response to an appropriate stimulus.

Regulatory gene A gene responsible for "switching on or off" other genes, usually through production of a repressor that regulates the activity of the other gene.

Replicate To form replicas; applies to synthesis of new DNA from preexisting DNA as part of nuclear division.

Replication fork A site within a replicating duplex DNA molecule at which synthesis of complementary strands is proceeding at that moment.

Repressible enzyme Type of enzyme that is synthesized in the absence of its substrate which represses synthesis of enzyme.

Repressor A protein produced by a regulatory gene that can combine with and repress action of an associated operator gene.

Resolution The ability to see two neighboring points in the visual field as distinct entities.

Restriction endonuclease (restriction enzyme) Nuclease occuring in bacteria that recognize short nucleotide sequences within duplex DNA and cleave the backbone at highly specific sites on both strands of the duplex.

Reverse transcriptase An RNA-dependent DNA polyerase. An enzyme that uses RNA as a template to synthesize a complementary strand of DNA. (An enzyme that is found in RNA-containing viruses and used in the laboratory to synthesize cDNAs).

Ribonucleic acid (RNA) A single-stranded nucleic acid molecule, synthesized principally in the nucleus from deoxyribonucleic acid, composed of a phosphate-ribose backbone with purines (adenine and guanine) and pyrimidines (uracil and cytosine) attached to the sugar ribose. RNA is of several kinds and functions to carry the "genetic message" from nuclear DNA to the ribosomes.

Ribonucleotide	Portion of RNA molecule composed of one ribose-phosphate unit plus a purine or a pyrimidine.
Ribosomal RNAs (or rRNAs)	The RNAs of a ribosome. rRNAs recognise and bind other molecules, provide structural support and catalyse the chemical reaction in which amino acids are covalently linked to one another
Ribosome	A complex structure composed of RNA and protein which is the site of protein synthesis in the cytoplasm, mitochondria and chloroplasts.
Ribozyme	A RNA molecule that functions as a catalyst in cellular reactions.
RNA polymerase-I	The transcribing enzyme found in eukaryotic cells that synthesizes the large (28S, 18S and 5.8S) ribosomal RNAs.
RNA polymerase-II	The transcribing enzymes in the eukaroytic cells that synthesizes messenger RNAs and most small nuclear RNAs.
RNA polymerase-III	The transcribing enzyme found in eukaryotic cells that synthesis the various transfer RNAs and the 5S ribosomal RNA.
RNA splicing	The process of removing the intervening DNA sequences (*i.e.*, introns) from a primary transcript.
RNA World	A proposed stage in the early evolution of life before the appearance of DNA and proteins in which RNA molecules served both as genetic material and catalysts.
Rough endoplasmic reticulum (RER)	That part of endoplasmic reticulum that has ribosomes attached. The RER appears as an extensive membranous organelle composed primarily of flattened sacs (cisternae) separated by a cytosolic space. RER functions include synthesis of secretory proteins, lysosomal proteins, integral membrane proteins and membrane lipids.
Satellite region	A region of DNA that contains highly repetitive base sequences.
Second messenger	A substance that is formed in the cell as the result of the binding of a first messenger—a hormone or other ligand-to a receptor at the surface of the cell.
Secondary structure	The local structure of the polypeptide chain, over a distance of only a few amino acid residues; may exist either as an irregular chains or as a regular and repeating shape such as the α-helix.
Secreted	Discharge outside the cell.
Secretory granule	Large, densely packed, membrane-bound structure containing highly concentrated secretory materials that are discharged into the extracellular space (secreted) following a stimulatory signal.
Sedimentation coefficient (s)	A quantitative measure of the rate of sedimentation of a given substance in a centrifugal field, expressed in Svedberg unit.
Self-assembly	The property of proteins (or other structures) to assume the correct (native) conformation based on the chemical behaviour dictated by the amino acid sequence.
Self-fertilization	Functioning of a single individual as both male and female parent. Plants are "selfed" if sperm and egg supplied by the same individual.
Semiconservative replication	The usual mode of duplex DNA synthesis resulting in daughter duplex molecules which contain one parental strand and one newly formed strand.
Sex chromosomes	Chromosomes not occurring in individual pairs in both sexes in diploid organism; in human beings and fruit fly these are designated as X and Y chromosomes.
Sexual reproduction	Mode of reproduction which is accomplished by the union of male and female gametes.
Sliding filament mechanism	A proposal applied to explanation of cellular movement phenomena, particularly to muscle contraction and to ciliary bending.
Signal transduction	The overall process in which information carried by extracellular messenger molecules is translated into changes that occur inside a cell.

Smooth endoplasmic reticulum (SER)	That part of endoplasmic reticulum that is without attached ribosomes. The membraneous elements of the SER are typically tubular and form an interconnecting system of pipelines curving through the cytoplasm in which they occur. The SER functions vary form cell to cell and include the synthesis of steroid hormones, detoxification of a wide variety of organic compounds, mobilization of glucose from glucose 6-phosphate, and separation of calcium ions.
Sodium-potassium pump (Na^+/K^+-ATPase)	Transport protein that uses ATP as the energy source for transporting sodium and potassium ions, with the result that each conformational change transports three sodium ions out of the cell and two potassium ions into the cell.
Sol	Colloidal solution.
Soma (adj. Somatic)	The body, cells of which in mammals and flowering plants normally have two sets of chromosomes, one derived from each parent.
Spermatocyte	The cell that undergoes meiosis to produce four spermatids.
Spermigenesis	Differentiation of the spermatozoa.
Spermatogenesis	Development of sperms.
Spindle	The axially differentiated part of the cytoplasm within which the centromere of the chromosomes are held during metaphase.
Spliceosome	A macromolecular complex containing a variety of proteins and a number of distinct ribonucleoprotein particles that functions in removal of introns from a primary transcript.
Split genes	Genes with intervening sequences.
Spore	An asexual reproductive protoplast capable of developing into a new individual.
Stem cells	Cells situated in various tissues of the body that constitute a reserve population capable of giving rise to the various cells of that tissue. Stem cells can be defined as undifferentiated cells that are capable of both 1. self-renewal, that is, production of cells like themselves, and 2. differentiation into two mature cell types.
Stereoisomers	Two molecules that structurally are mirror images of each other and may have vastly different biological activity.
Stroma	Space outside the thylakoid but within the relatively impermeable inner membrane of the chloroplast envelope.
Structural gene	A cistron.
Subcellular fractionation	An approach that allows different organelles (*e.g.*, nucleus, mitochondria, plasma membrane, endoplasmic reticulum) having different properties, to be separated from one another.
Substrate	The reactant bound by an enzyme.
Synapse	The specialized junction of a neuron with its target cell.
Synapsis	The pairing of homologous chromosomes occurring in prophase I of meiosis.
Synaptonemal complex (SC)	A ladder-like structure composed of three parallel bars with many cross fibers. The SC holds each pair of homologous chromosomes in the proper position to allow the continuation of genetic recombination between strands of DNA.
Syngamy	The union of sex cells (gametes) in reproduction.
tDNA	The DNA encoding tRNAs.
Telocentric	A chromosome with the centromere located at one end.
Telomerase	A rare enzyme that can add new repeat units of DNA to the 3′ end of the over hanging strand of a telomere. Telomerase is a reverse transcriptase that synthesizes DNA using an RNA template.
Telophase	The concluding stage of nuclear division characterized by the reorganization or interphase nuclei.

Template	1. A model, mold, or pattern; DNA act as a template for RNA synthesis. 2. A single strand of DNA (or RNA) that contains the information (encoded as a nucleotide sequence) for construction of a complementary strand.
Terminalization	Expansion of the association of two pairs of chromatids on one side of the chiasma at the expense of that on the other side.
Tertiary structure	The three-dimensional folding of the polypeptide chain into a complex structural form brought about by interactions among side chains of amino acids at some distance from one another in the primary structure.
Tetrad	The four monoploid (haploid) cells arising from meiosis of a megaspore or microsporocyte in plants; also group of four associated chromatids during synapsis.
Thermodynamics	Study of the changes in energy accompanying events in the physical universe.
Thylakoids	Flattened, membraneous sacs formed by the chloroplast's internal membrane, which contain the energy-transducing machinery for photosynthesis.
Thymine	A pyrimidine base occurring in DNA, pairs normally with adenine.
Tonoplast	The membrane that bounds the vacuole of a plant cell. Plant vacuoles store a large variety of molecules including inorganic ions, organic ions, organic acids, sugars, enzymes (some like the lysosomes), storage proteins and many types of secondary metabolites. Proteins in the tonoplast transport all of these molecules except for storage proteins—into the vacuole.
Transcription	The formation of a complementary RNA from a DNA template.
Transcriptosome	The entire inventory of RNA's transcribed by a particular cell, tissue, or organism.
Transduction	The incorporation of a gene into a cellular genome by means of a virus.
Transfer RNA (tRNA)	Amino acid-specific RNA which transfers activated amino acids to mRNA where protein synthesis takes place.
Transfer RNAs (tRNAs)	A family of small RNAs that translate the information encoded in nucleotide "alphabet" of an mRNA into the amino acid "alphabet" of a polypeptide.
Translation	The process by which the sequence of amino acids is assembled into a polypeptide at the ribosome, under the direction of the coded base sequence copied from DNA into messenger RNA.
Translocation	The shift of a portion of a chromosome to another part of the same chromosome or to an entirely different chromosome.
Translocation	The step in the translation elongation cycle that involves (1) ejection of the uncharged tRNA from the P site and (2) the movement of the ribosome three nucleotides (one codon) along the mRNA in the 3′ direction.
Translocon	A protein-lined channel embedded in the ER membrane; the nascent polypeptide is able to move through the translocon in its passage from the cytosol to the ER lumen.
Transport vesicles	The shuttles, formed by budding from a membrane compartment, that carry materials between organelles.
Transposons	DNA segments capable of moving from one place in the genome to another.
Transverse (T) tubules	Membranous folds along which the impulse generated in a skeletal muscle cell is propagated into the interior of the cell.
Tricarboxylic acid cycle (TCA cycle)	The circular metabolic pathway that oxidizes acetyl CoA, conserving its energy; the cycle is also known as the Krebs cycle or the citric acid cycle.
Trisomy	A chromosome complement that has one extra chromosome, *i.e.*, a third homologous chromosome.
Tritium (^3H)	The radioactive isotope of hydrogen.
Tubulin	The protein that forms the walls of microtubules. Isoforms include α, β and γ tubulin.

Tumor-suppressor genes Genes that encode proteins that restrain cell growth and prevent cells from becoming malignant.

Turnover The regulated destruction of cellular materials and their replacement.

Ubiquitin A small, highly conserved protein that is linked to proteins targeted for internalization by endocytosis or degradation in proteasomes.

Unfolded protein response (UPR) Comprehensive response that occurs in cells whose ER cisternae contain an excessively high concentration of unfolded or misfolded proteins. Sensors that detect this situation trigger a pathway that leads to the synthesis of proteins (*e.g.*, molecular chaperones such as BiP), that can alleviate the stress.

Unineme Concept of chromosome structure having only one chromatin fibre in the unreplicated chromosome or in each chromatid of a replicated chromosome.

Unit membrane A membrane formed of two layers of lipid molecules sandwiched between the two layers or protein molecules. It forms the outer boundary of cell and almost all cellular organelles.

Untranslated regions (UTRs) Non-coding segments contained at both 5′ and 3′ ends of mRNA.

Unwinding protein Structural protein that binds to single-stranded regions of duplex DNA during replication and recombination.

Uracil A pyrimidine base occurring in RNA.

Vacuole A single membrane-bound, fluid filled cytoplasmic structure that comprises as much as 90% of the volume of many plant cells

Vesicle A small, spherical membranous element filled with protein in a watery medium.

Viruses Small, obligatory intracellular pathogens that are not considered to be alive because they cannot divide directly, which is required by the cell theory of life.

Vitamin Organic compounds found in small amounts in all living organisms and which are essentially required by body for its normal working.

Wobble hypothesis Crick's proposal that the steric requirement between the anticodon of the tRNA and the codon of the mRNA is flexible at the third position, which allows two codons that differ only at the third position to share the same tRNA during protein synthesis.

Zygote The protoplast resulting from the fusion of two gametes in sexual reproduction; a fertilized egg.

Zygotene A stage of prophase I of meiosis which is characterized by the synapsis or paring of the homologous chromosomes.

Selected Reading

Ambrose E.J. and Dorothy MEasty, 1970, *Cell Biology,* The English Language Book Society & Nelson, London.

Avers, C.J., 1976, *Cell Biology,* D. Van Nostrand Company, New York.

Balinsky, B.I., 1970, *An Introduction to Embryology*, W.B. Saunders Company, Philadelphia and London.

Barry, J.M. and E.M. Barry, 1973, *Molecular Biology: An Introduction to Chemical Genetics.* Prentice-Hall of India Private Limited. New Delhi.

Berrill, N.J., 1971. *Developmental Biology*, McGraw-Hill Book Company, New York.

Bodmer, W.F., and L.L. Cavalli-Sforza 1976, *Genetics, Evolution, and Man,* W. H. Freeman and Company, Sanfrancisco, London.

Bostok., C.J. and A.T. Sumner, 1978. *The Eukaryotic Chromosomes,* North Holland Publishing Company, Amsterdam.

Bowen, W.R., 1969, *Experimental Cell Biology,* The Macmillian Company, New York.

Brachet, J. and A.E. Mirsky 1959-64. *The Cell (I—V Volumes),* Academic Press, New York.

Bradbury, E.M. N. Maclean and H.R. Mattews, 1981, *DNA, Chromatin and Chromosomes,* Blackwell Scientific Publications, Oxford.

Branton, D. and D. Deamer 1972, *Membrane Structure,* Springer-Verlag, New York.

Branton, D. and R. Park 1968, *Papers on Biological Membrane Structure,* Little Brown & CO. Boston.

Burns, G. W., 1980, *The Science of Genetics* (4th ed). The Macmillan Company, New York.

Butler, J.A.V., 1959, *Inside the Living Cell,* George Allen and Unwin Ltd., London.

1964, *The Life of the Cell,* George Allen and Unwin Ltd., London.

1968, *Gene Control in the Living Cell,* George Allen and Unwin Ltd., London.

Cockrum, E. L., and W.J. McCauely, 1965, *Zoology,* W.B. Saunders Company, Philadelphia.

Cohn, N.S., 1969, *Element of Cytology*, Harcourt, Brace and World, Inc., New York.

DeRobertis, E.D.P., W.Nowinski and F.A. Saez., 1970, *Cell Biology*, W.B. Saunders Company, Philadelphia.

DeRobertis, E.D.P., F.A. Saez and E.M.F 1975, *Cell Biology,* W.B. Saunders Company, Philadelphia.

DeRobertis

De Witt, William, 1977, *Biology of the Cell,* W.B. Saunders Company, Philadelphia.

Dowben, R.M., 1971, *Cell Biology,* Harper & Row, Publishers, New York.

Dupraw, E.J., 1969, *Cell and Molecular Biology,* Academic Press, New York.

Dyson, R.D., 1978, *Cell Biology,* Allyn and Bacon, Inc., Boston.

Fairley, J.L., 1966, *Essentials of Biological Chemistry,* Reinhold Publishing Corporation,

Fairley, New York.

Fawcett, D.W., 1966, *The cell: Its organelles and Inclusions,* W.B. Saunders Philadelphia.

Fraser, Dean, 1967, *Viruses and Molecular Biology,* The Macmillan Company, New York.

Freeman, J.A., 1964, *Cellular Fine Structure,* McGraw-Hill Book Company, New York.

Garber, E.D., 1972. *Cytogenetics,* McGraw-Hill Book Company. New York.

Gerking, S.D. 1969 *Biological Systems,* W.B. Sauders Company Philadelphia.

Giese, A.C., 1973, *Cell Physiology,* W.B. Saunders Company Philadelphia.

Goodenough V. and R.P. Levine, 1974, *Genetics,* Holt Reinhard and Winston, Inc., New York.

Gunning, B. and M.W. Steer, 1975, *Plant Cell Biology,* Crane, Russak, New York.

Harris, H., 1970, *Nucleus and Cytoplasm,* Clarendon Press, Oxford.

Harrison, R. and G. Lunt 1976, *Biological Membranes: Their Structure and Function,* Halsted Press, New York.

Haggis, C.H., 1964, *Introduction to Molecular Biology,* Longmans London.

Hanawalt, P.C. and Robert H. Haynes, 1970, *The Chemical Basis of Life,* W.H. Freeman and Company, San Francisco.

Herreid II, C.F., 1977, *Biology,* Macmillan Publishing Co; Inc., New York.

Khorana H.G. 1978, *Synthetic Nucleic Acids and the Genetic Code.* J Am. Med. Assoc., 206, Lasker Award, 1968.

Kimball, J.W., 1970, *Cell Biology,* Addison-Wesley Publishing Company, California.

Kornberg. A., 1974, *DNA Synthesis* W.H. Freeman & Co., San Franscisco.

Kornberg, R.D. and A. Clug, 1981, *The Nucleosome,* Scientific American, Feb. 1981 48-60.

Lima-de-Faria A., 1969, *Handbook of Molecular Cytology,* North Holland Publishing Company, Amsterdam.

Mays, Laura Livingston, 1981, *Genetics,* Macmillan Publishing Co., Inc., New York.

Lehman, I, and D. Uyemura 1976, *DNA Polymerase I : Essential Replication Enzymes,* Science, 193 : 1963.

Meglitsch, P.A. 1972, *Invertebrate Zoology,* Oxford University Press Oxford.

Mercer, E.H., 1965, *Cell and Cells Structure,* Hutchinson. Educational, London.

Nass, Gisela, 1970, *The Molecules of Life,* Weiden Feld and Nicolson London.

Nomura, M., A. Tissieres, and P. Lengyel, 1974, *Ribosomes.* Cold Spring Harbour Laboratory, New York.

Perry, R., 1976, *Processing of RNA,* Ann. Rev Biochem ; 45 : 605.

Quinn, P.J., 1976, *The Molecular Biology of Cell Membranes,* Macmillan Press, London.

Rabinowitch, E. I. and Govindjee, 1965, *The Role of Chlorophyll in Photosynthesis,* Scientific American, July, 1965.

Reinert. J. and H. Ursprung 1971, *Origin and Continuity of Cell Organelles,* Springer Verlag, Berlin.

Rosenberg, E., 1971, *Cell and Molecular Biology,* Holt, Rinehart and Winston, Inc. New York.

Sager, Ruth, 1972, *Cytoplasmic Genes and Organelles,* Academic Press, New York.

Smith, C.U.M., 1968, *Molecular Biology,* Faber and Faber, London.

Spencer, J.H., 1972, *The Physics and Chemistry of DNA or RNA,* W.B. Saunders Company, Philadelphia.

Spirin, A.S. and L.P. Gavrilova 1969, *The Ribosomes,* Springer-Verlag Inc., New York.

Stern, H. and D.L. Nanney, 1965, *The Biology of Cells,* Wiley Estern Private Ltd., New Delhi.

Sybenga, J., 1972, *General Cytogenetics,* North-Holland Publishing Company, Amsterdam.

Taylor, J.H., 1974, *Units of DNA Replication in Chromosomes of Eukaryotes,* Int. Rev. Cytol., 37 : 1.

Tedeschi, H., 1974, *Cell Physiology,* Academic Press, New York.

Toner, P.G. and K.E. Carr 1971, *Cell Structure,* Churchill Livingston, Edinburg and London.

Verma P.S., V.K. Agarwal and B.S. Tyagi 1980, *Chordate Embryology,* S. Chand & Co. Pvt. Ltd., New Delhi.

Watson, J.D., 1976, *Molecular Biology of the Gene,* (3rd ed.) W.A. Benjamin, Inc., New York.

Weisz, P.B. 1971, *The Science of Biology,* Tata McGraw-Hill Publishing Company Ltd., Bombay.

Werner, D.D., 1977, *The Molecular Biology of Plant Cells,* Blackwell Scientific, Oxford.

Literary Sources in Cytology

A. Journals

1. Journal of Cell Biology.
2. Experimental Cell Research.
3. Journal of Molecular Biology.
4. Journal of Ultrastructure Research.
5. Journal of Cell Science.
6. Journal of Cellular and Comparative Physiology.
7. Journal of General Physiology.
8. Chromosomes.
9. Cytogenetics.
10. Heredity and Hereditary.
11. Nature.
12. Science.
13. Proceedings of the Royal Society.
14. Proceedings of National Academy of Science (Washington).
15. Biochemical et. Biophysica.
16. Biochemical Journal or Journal of Biological Chemistry.
17. Life Sciences.
18. American Scientist.
19. Bioscience.
20. Hospital Practice.
21. New Scientist.
22. The Sciences.
23. Science News.

B. Reviews

24. International Review of Biology.
25. Quarterly Review of Biology.
26. Physiological Review.
27. Biological Review (Cambridge).
28. Advances in Genetics.
29. Plant Physiology.
30. Science Progress (Oxford)
31. Bacteriological Reviews.
32. Biomedicine.

33. Biomembrane.
34. Cell.
35. Life Sciences.
36. New England Journal of Medicine.
37. Reviews of Physiology, Biochemistry and Pharmacology.
38. Sub-cellular Biochemistry.

C. Abstracts.

39. Biological Abstracts.
40. Index Medicus.
41. Excerpta Medica.
42. Chemical Abstracts.

D. Monographs

43. The cell (5 volumes) By Brachet and Mirsky.
44. Handbook of Molecular Cytology By A. Lima-de-Faria (1969).
45. Ciba Foundation symposia (Each volume a separate topic).

INDEX

A

D

E

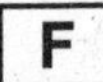

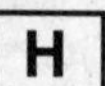

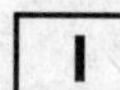

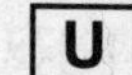

V

W

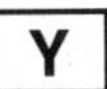

NOTES

NOTES

NOTES

NOTES